Microfluidic Devices for Biomedical Applications

Woodhead Publishing Series in Biomaterials

Microfluidic Devices for Biomedical Applications

Second Edition

Edited by

XiuJun (James) Li
Department of Chemistry and Biochemistry, University of Texas at El Paso, El Paso, TX, United States

Yu Zhou
R&D, Siemens, Tarrytown, NY, United States

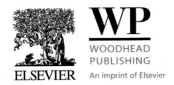

Woodhead Publishing is an imprint of Elsevier
The Officers' Mess Business Centre, Royston Road, Duxford, CB22 4QH, United Kingdom
50 Hampshire Street, 5th Floor, Cambridge, MA 02139, United States
The Boulevard, Langford Lane, Kidlington, OX5 1GB, United Kingdom

Copyright © 2021 Elsevier Ltd. All rights reserved.

No part of this publication may be reproduced or transmitted in any form or by any means, electronic or mechanical, including photocopying, recording, or any information storage and retrieval system, without permission in writing from the publisher. Details on how to seek permission, further information about the Publisher's permissions policies and our arrangements with organizations such as the Copyright Clearance Center and the Copyright Licensing Agency, can be found at our website: www.elsevier.com/permissions.

This book and the individual contributions contained in it are protected under copyright by the Publisher (other than as may be noted herein).

Notices
Knowledge and best practice in this field are constantly changing. As new research and experience broaden our understanding, changes in research methods, professional practices, or medical treatment may become necessary.

Practitioners and researchers must always rely on their own experience and knowledge in evaluating and using any information, methods, compounds, or experiments described herein. In using such information or methods they should be mindful of their own safety and the safety of others, including parties for whom they have a professional responsibility.

To the fullest extent of the law, neither the Publisher nor the authors, contributors, or editors, assume any liability for any injury and/or damage to persons or property as a matter of products liability, negligence or otherwise, or from any use or operation of any methods, products, instructions, or ideas contained in the material herein.

Library of Congress Cataloging-in-Publication Data
A catalog record for this book is available from the Library of Congress

British Library Cataloguing-in-Publication Data
A catalogue record for this book is available from the British Library

ISBN: 978-0-12-819971-8

For information on all Woodhead Publishing publications visit our website at https://www.elsevier.com/books-and-journals

Publisher: Matthew Deans
Acquisitions Editor: Sabrina Webber
Editorial Project Manager: Emily Thomson
Production Project Manager: Surya Narayanan Jayachandran
Cover Designer: Mark Rogers

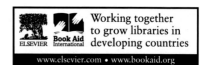

Typeset by TNQ Technologies

Contents

Contributors		xi
Editor Biographies		xv
Preface to the first edition		xvii
Preface to the second edition		xxi

1 Materials and methods for microfabrication of microfluidic devices — 1
Sreekant Damodara, Shadi Shahriari, Wen-I Wu, Pouya Rezai, Huan-Hsuan Hsu and Ravi Selvaganapathy
- 1.1 Introduction — 1
- 1.2 Microfabrication methods — 2
- 1.3 Materials — 8
- 1.4 Conclusion and future trends — 46
- 1.5 Acronyms — 48
- References — 49

2 Surface coatings for microfluidic biomedical devices — 79
M. Sonker, B.G. Abdallah and A. Ros
- 2.1 Introduction — 79
- 2.2 Covalent immobilization strategies: polymer devices — 81
- 2.3 Covalent immobilization strategies: glass devices — 92
- 2.4 Adsorption strategies — 96
- 2.5 Other strategies utilizing surface treatments — 102
- 2.6 Examples of applications — 104
- 2.7 Conclusions and future trends — 108
- 2.8 Sources of further information and advice — 110
- References — 111

3 Actuation mechanisms for microfluidic biomedical devices — 125
A. Rezk, J. Friend, L. Yeo and Yu Zhou
- 3.1 Introduction — 125
- 3.2 Electrokinetics — 126
- 3.3 Acoustics — 143
- 3.4 Limitations and future trends — 152
- References — 153

4	**Droplet microfluidics for biomedical devices**	**163**
	Marie Hébert and Carolyn L. Ren	
	4.1 Introduction—droplets in the wider context of microfluidics	163
	4.2 Fundamental principles of droplet microfluidics	165
	4.3 Droplet microfluidic approaches	171
	4.4 Biomedical applications	175
	4.5 Conclusion—perspective on the future of biomedical applications using droplet microfluidics	188
	References	190
5	**Controlled drug delivery using microdevices**	**205**
	Ning Gao and XiuJun (James) Li	
	5.1 Introduction	205
	5.2 Microreservoir-based drug delivery systems	207
	5.3 Micro/nanofluidics-based drug delivery systems	212
	5.4 Future trends and challenges	220
	References	221
6	**Microneedles for drug delivery and monitoring**	**225**
	Emma McAlister, Melissa Kirkby and Ryan F. Donnelly	
	6.1 Introduction	225
	6.2 Microneedle design parameters and structure	226
	6.3 Drug delivery strategies using microneedle arrays	230
	6.4 Other microneedle array applications	237
	6.5 Microneedle-mediated patient monitoring and diagnosis	239
	6.6 Clinical translation and commercialisation of microneedle products	247
	6.7 Conclusion	250
	References	250
7	**Microfluidic systems for drug discovery, pharmaceutical analysis, and diagnostic applications**	**261**
	Dawei Ding, Sol Park, Jaspreet Singh Kochhar, Sui Yung Chan, Pei Shi Ong, Won Gu Lee and Lifeng Kang	
	7.1 Introduction	261
	7.2 Microfluidics for drug discovery	263
	7.3 Microfluidics for pharmaceutical analysis and diagnostic applications	289
	7.4 Examples of commercial microfluidic devices	310
	7.5 Future trends	311
	References	312
8	**Microfluidic devices for cell manipulation**	**329**
	H.O. Fatoyinbo and XiuJun (James) Li	
	8.1 Introduction	329

	8.2	Microenvironment on cell integrity	330
	8.3	Microscale fluid dynamics	332
	8.4	Manipulation technologies	338
	8.5	Manipulation of cancer cells in microfluidic systems	368
	8.6	Conclusion and future trends	374
	8.7	Sources of further information and advice	374
		References	375
9	**Microfluidic devices for immobilization and micromanipulation of single cells and small organisms**		391
	Peng Pan, Pengfei Song, Xianke Dong, Weize Zhang, Yu Sun and Xinyu Liu	
	9.1	Introduction	391
	9.2	Glass microfluidic device for rapid single cell immobilization and microinjection	393
	9.3	Microfluidic device for automated, high-speed microinjection of *C. elegans*	397
	9.4	Microfabricated device for immobilization and mechanical stimulation of *Drosophila* larvae	401
	9.5	Conclusions and outlook	406
		References	407
10	**Microfluidic devices for developing tissue scaffolds**	413
	L.T. Chau, J.E. Frith, R.J. Mills, D.J. Menzies, D.M. Titmarsh, J.J. Cooper-White and Yu Zhou	
	10.1	Introduction	413
	10.2	Key issues and technical challenges for successful tissue engineering	414
	10.3	Microfluidic device platforms	419
	10.4	Conclusion and future trends	428
		References	429
11	**Microfluidic devices for stem cell analysis**	437
	D.-K. Kang, J. Lu, W. Zhang, E. Chang, M.A. Eckert, M.M. Ali, W. Zhao and XiuJun (James) Li	
	11.1	Introduction	437
	11.2	Technologies used in stem cell analysis	440
	11.3	Examples of microfluidic platform for stem cell analysis: stem cell culture platform—mimicking in vivo culture conditions in vitro	450
	11.4	Examples of microfluidic platform for stem cell analysis: single stem cell analysis	458
	11.5	Microdevices for label-free and noninvasive monitoring of stem cell differentiation	461
	11.6	Microfluidics stem cell separation technology	467

	11.7	Conclusion and future trends	475
	11.8	Sources of further information and advice	478
		References	478
12	**Development of the immunoassay of antibodies and cytokines on nanobioarray chips**		489
	Samar Haroun, Jonathan Lee and Paul C.H. Li		
	12.1	Introduction to immunoassays	489
	12.2	Technologies	491
	12.3	Immobilization chemistry	494
	12.4	Detection methods	497
	12.5	Applications	499
	12.6	Conclusion and future trends	507
		References	507
13	**Integrated microfluidic systems for genetic analysis**		511
	Siwat Jakaratanopas, Bin Zhuang, Wupeng Gan and Peng Liu		
	13.1	Introduction	511
	13.2	Integrated microfluidic systems	513
	13.3	Development of integrated microdevices	513
	13.4	Applications of fully integrated systems in genetic analysis	518
	13.5	Future of integrated microfluidic systems	535
		References	536
14	**Paper-based microfluidic devices for low-cost assays**		551
	Merwan Benhabib and XiuJun (James) Li		
	14.1	Introduction	551
	14.2	Fabrication techniques for paper-based microfluidic devices	552
	14.3	Detection and read-out technologies	563
	14.4	Application of paper-based microfluidic devices	573
	14.5	Current limitations and future perspectives in paper-based microfluidics	579
		References	581
15	**Microfluidic devices for viral detection**		587
	Wenfu Zheng, Jiashu Sun and Xingyu Jiang		
	15.1	Introduction	587
	15.2	Microfluidic technologies used for viral detection	588
	15.3	Examples of applications	603
	15.4	Conclusion and future trends	609
		Acknowledgments	610
		References	610

16 Microfluidic applications on pancreatic islets and β-cells study for human islet transplant — 617
Yuan Xing, Pu Zhang, Yi He, Xiaoyu Yu, Sharon Lu, Farid Ghamsari, Sarah Innis, Joshua E. Mendoza-Elias, Melur K. Ramasubramanian, Yong Wang and José Oberholzer

- 16.1 Introduction — 617
- 16.2 Microfluidic technologies: the emergence of microfluidics applied to islet transplantation — 623
- 16.3 Design and validation of microfluidic devices for islet study and transplantation — 632
- 16.4 Protocol: materials — 639
- 16.5 Protocol: procedures — 643
- 16.6 Conclusion and future trends — 651
- Acknowledgments — 652
- References — 652

17 3D printed microfluidic devices and applications — 659
Sui Ching Phung, Qingfu Zhu, Kimberly Plevniak and Mei He

- 17.1 Introduction — 659
- 17.2 Direct 3D printing of microfluidic devices and applications — 663
- 17.3 3D-printing of molds for fabricating PDMS microfluidic devices and applications — 671
- 17.4 Conclusions and future trends — 677
- References — 678

Index — 681

Contributors

B.G. Abdallah School of Molecular Sciences, Arizona State University, Tempe, AZ, United States

M.M. Ali University of California, Irvine, CA, United States

Merwan Benhabib Telegraph Technologies, llc, San Francisco, CA, United States

Sui Yung Chan Department of Pharmacy, National University of Singapore, Singapore, Republic of Singapore

E. Chang University of California, Irvine, CA, United States

L.T. Chau The University of Queensland, Brisbane, QLD, Australia

J.J. Cooper−White The University of Queensland, Brisbane, QLD, Australia

Sreekant Damodara McMaster University, Hamilton, Ontario, Canada

Dawei Ding College of Pharmaceutical Sciences, Soochow University, Suzhou, Jiangsu, China

Xianke Dong Department of Mechanical and Industrial Engineering, University of Toronto, Toronto, Ontario, Canada; Department of Mechanical Engineering, McGill University, Montreal, Quebec, Canada

Ryan F. Donnelly School of Pharmacy, Queen's University Belfast, Belfast, United Kingdom

M.A. Eckert University of California, Irvine, CA, United States

H.O. Fatoyinbo University of Surrey, Guildford, United Kingdom

J. Friend RMIT University, Melbourne, Australia

J.E. Frith The University of Queensland, Brisbane, QLD, Australia

Wupeng Gan Department of Biomedical Engineering, Tsinghua University, School of Medicine, Haidian District, Beijing, China

Ning Gao RD&E Dispensing Systems Engineering, Sensor Technology, Ecolab, Naperville, IL, United States

Farid Ghamsari Department of Surgery, University of Virginia, Charlottesville, VA, United States

Samar Haroun Department of Chemistry, Simon Fraser University, Burnaby, BC, Canada

Yi He Department of Surgery, University of Virginia, Charlottesville, VA, United States

Mei He Department of Chemical and Petroleum Engineering, Department of Chemistry, University of Kansas, Lawrence, KS, United States

Marie Hébert Mechanical and Mechatronics Engineering, University of Waterloo, Waterloo, Ontario, Canada

Huan-Hsuan Hsu Tufts University, Medford, Massachusetts, United States

Sarah Innis Department of Surgery, University of Virginia, Charlottesville, VA, United States

Siwat Jakaratanopas Department of Biomedical Engineering, Tsinghua University, School of Medicine, Haidian District, Beijing, China

Xingyu Jiang Department of Biomedical Engineering, Southern University of Science and Technology, Shenzhen, Guangdong, P.R. China

D.-K. Kang University of California, Irvine, CA, United States

Lifeng Kang School of Pharmacy, Faculty of Medicine and Health, University of Sydney, Sydney, NSW, Australia

Melissa Kirkby School of Pharmacy, Queen's University Belfast, Belfast, United Kingdom

Jaspreet Singh Kochhar Procter & Gamble, Singapore, Republic of Singapore

Jonathan Lee Department of Chemistry, Simon Fraser University, Burnaby, BC, Canada

Won Gu Lee Department of Mechanical Engineering, College of Engineering, Yongin, Gyeonggi, Republic of Korea

Paul C.H. Li Department of Chemistry, Simon Fraser University, Burnaby, BC, Canada

XiuJun (James) Li Department of Chemistry and Biochemistry, University of Texas at El Paso, El Paso, TX, United States

Peng Liu Department of Biomedical Engineering, Tsinghua University, School of Medicine, Haidian District, Beijing, China

Xinyu Liu Department of Mechanical and Industrial Engineering, University of Toronto, Toronto, Ontario, Canada; Institute of Biomedical Engineering, University of Toronto, Toronto, Ontario, Canada

Contributors

J. Lu University of California, Irvine, CA, United States

Sharon Lu Department of Surgery, University of Virginia, Charlottesville, VA, United States

Emma McAlister School of Pharmacy, Queen's University Belfast, Belfast, United Kingdom

Joshua E. Mendoza-Elias Department of Surgery, San Joaquin General Hospital, French Camp, CA, United States

D.J. Menzies The University of Queensland, Brisbane, QLD, Australia

R.J. Mills The University of Queensland, Brisbane, QLD, Australia

José Oberholzer Department of Surgery, University of Virginia, Charlottesville, VA, United States

Pei Shi Ong Department of Pharmacy, National University of Singapore, Singapore, Republic of Singapore

Peng Pan Department of Mechanical and Industrial Engineering, University of Toronto, Toronto, Ontario, Canada; Department of Mechanical Engineering, McGill University, Montreal, Quebec, Canada

Sol Park School of Pharmacy, Faculty of Medicine and Health, University of Sydney, Sydney, NSW, Australia

Sui Ching Phung Department of Chemical and Petroleum Engineering, Department of Chemistry, University of Kansas, Lawrence, KS, United States

Kimberly Plevniak Department of Chemical and Petroleum Engineering, Department of Chemistry, University of Kansas, Lawrence, KS, United States

Melur K. Ramasubramanian Department of Mechanical and Aerospace Engineering, University of Virginia, Charlottesville, VA, United States

Carolyn L. Ren Mechanical and Mechatronics Engineering, University of Waterloo, Waterloo, Ontario, Canada

Pouya Rezai York University, Toronto, Ontario, Canada

A. Rezk RMIT University, Melbourne, Australia

A. Ros School of Molecular Sciences, Arizona State University, Tempe, AZ, United States; Center for Applied Structural Discovery, The Biodesign Institute, Tempe, AZ, United States

Ravi Selvaganapathy McMaster University, Hamilton, Ontario, Canada

Shadi Shahriari McMaster University, Hamilton, Ontario, Canada

Pengfei Song Department of Mechanical and Industrial Engineering, University of Toronto, Toronto, Ontario, Canada; Department of Electrical and Electronic Engineering, Xi'an Jiaotong-Liverpool University, Suzhou, Jiangsu, China

M. Sonker School of Molecular Sciences, Arizona State University, Tempe, AZ, United States; Center for Applied Structural Discovery, The Biodesign Institute, Tempe, AZ, United States

Jiashu Sun CAS Key Laboratory for Biomedical Effects of Nanomaterials and Nanosafety, CAS Center for Excellence in Nanoscience, National Center for NanoScience and Technology, Beijing, P.R. China

Yu Sun Department of Mechanical and Industrial Engineering, University of Toronto, Toronto, Ontario, Canada; Institute of Biomedical Engineering, University of Toronto, Toronto, Ontario, Canada

D.M. Titmarsh The University of Queensland, Brisbane, QLD, Australia

Yong Wang Department of Surgery, University of Virginia, Charlottesville, VA, United States

Wen-I Wu Bio Rad Laboratories, Mississauga, Ontario, Canada

Yuan Xing Department of Surgery, University of Virginia, Charlottesville, VA, United States

L. Yeo RMIT University, Melbourne, Australia

Xiaoyu Yu Department of Surgery, University of Virginia, Charlottesville, VA, United States

Pu Zhang Department of Mechanical and Aerospace Engineering, University of Virginia, Charlottesville, VA, United States

W. Zhang University of California, Irvine, CA, United States

Weize Zhang Department of Mechanical Engineering, McGill University, Montreal, Quebec, Canada

W. Zhao University of California, Irvine, CA, United States

Wenfu Zheng CAS Key Laboratory for Biomedical Effects of Nanomaterials and Nanosafety, CAS Center for Excellence in Nanoscience, National Center for NanoScience and Technology, Beijing, P.R. China

Yu Zhou R&D, Siemens, Tarrytown, NY, United States

Qingfu Zhu Department of Chemical and Petroleum Engineering, Department of Chemistry, University of Kansas, Lawrence, KS, United States

Bin Zhuang Department of Biomedical Engineering, Tsinghua University, School of Medicine, Haidian District, Beijing, China

Editor Biographies

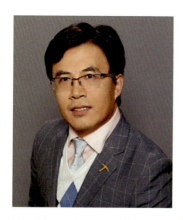

XiuJun (James) Li, Ph.D., is an Associate Professor with early tenure in the Department of Chemistry and Biochemistry, Biomedical Engineering, and Border Biomedical Research Center at the University of Texas at El Paso (UTEP), US. After he obtained his Ph.D. degree in Microfluidic Lab-on-a-Chip Bioanalysis from Simon Fraser University (SFU) in Canada in 2008, he pursued his postdoctoral research with Prof. Richard Mathies at University of California, Berkeley, and Prof. George Whitesides at Harvard University, while holding a Postdoctoral Fellowship from Natural Sciences and Engineering Research Council (NSERC) of Canada. He has gained extensive experience in bioanalysis using microfluidic systems, such as single-cell analysis, genetic analysis, low-cost diagnosis, pathogen detection, 3D cell culture, and so on. Dr. Li's current research interest is centered on the development of innovative microfluidic lab-on-a-chip and nanotechnology for bioanalysis, biomaterial, biomedical engineering, and environmental applications, including but not limited to low-cost diagnosis, nanobiosensing, tissue engineering, and single-cell analysis. He has coauthored about 100 publications in high-impact journals (such as *Advanced Drug Delivery Reviews*, *Applied Catalysis B: Environmental*, *Analytical Chemistry*, *Lab on a Chip*, and *Biosensors and Bioelectronics*) and 22 patents. He is an Advisory Board member of *Lab on a Chip* and *Analyst*, the Founder of microBioChip Diagnostics LLC, and an editor of six journals including *Scientific Reports* from the Nature publishing group, *Micromachines*, etc. He is the recipient of the "Bioanalysis New Investigator Award" in 2014, UT STARS Award in 2012, NSERC Postdoctoral Fellow Award in 2009, and so on. For more information, please visit http://li.utep.edu.

Yu Zhou is a R&D technology leader at Siemens Healthineers and stands at the forefront of the fast-moving in vitro diagnostics (IVD) industry. He has spent the past 4 years developing innovative IVD technologies for immunoassay and clinical chemistry analyzers. Dr. Zhou holds a doctoral degree in mechanical engineering. He is a former R&D professional with Becton Dickson (BD) and has 18+ combined years of experience in BioMEMS, microfluidics, and medical instrument systems. He is a BD Innovation Award winner for Advanced Technology Development in 2017. Also, he holds seven patents and has been recognized for leading the development of microfluidics flow cytometry instrument for the dairy herd genetic application at Genus plc.

Preface to the first edition

Biomedical applications ranging from drug discovery and delivery and disease diagnosis to point of care (POC) devices and tissue engineering have attracted increasing attention since the last few decades. Biomedical engineering, closely related to biomedical applications, has only recently emerged as its own discipline. Conventional biomedical techniques however often face increasing challenges in different biomedical applications, such as high cost, slow diagnosis, expensive instrumentation, low drug delivery efficiency, and high failure rates in drug discovery due to the discrepancy between 2D cell based assays and living tissues. Additionally, many cases of global diseases (e.g. malaria, tuberculosis or TB, meningitis, and hepatitis B) happen in high poverty areas, such as rural areas and developing nations which often cannot afford expensive and high-precision instruments. For instance, according to World Health Organization (WHO) data in 2012, "one million cases of bacterial meningitis are estimated to occur and 200,000 of these die annually." All these pose great challenges to conventional biomedical techniques.

Microfluidic or lab-on-a-chip (LOC) devices emerged in the 1990s and have grown explosively in the last 2 decades due to their inherent advantages associated with miniaturization, integration, parallelization, as well as portability and automation, including low consumption of reagents and samples, rapid analysis, cost-effectiveness, high efficiency, and less human interference during operation. Microfluidics offers great potential in addressing those challenges in biomedical applications. Countless microfluidic systems have been developed for high-throughput genetic analysis, single-cell analysis, proteomics, low-cost diagnosis, pathogen detection, controlled-drug release, and tissue engineering. After a concise introduction of the fundamentals of microfluidic technologies, this book highlights current cutting-edge research of microfluidic devices or LOC platforms in biomedical applications.

Part I mainly aims to introduce the fundamentals of microfluidic technologies. Suitability of device construction materials and methods is highly critical to the success of different biomedical applications. Chapter 1 is dedicated to introduce a variety of widely used materials in microfluidic devices and their corresponding fabrication methods. Because stable and well-characterized surfaces are essential to achieve desired performance in some biomedical applications, Chapter 2 provides an overview of strategies used to accomplish surface coating. Covalent and adsorptive coating strategies are included. Actuators are responsible for sophisticated manipulation of fluids and particles in microfluidic systems and have been proved to be of significant importance in the successful implement of microfluidic operations. Chapter 3 summarizes major actuation principles used in medical devices and concentrates on two mechanisms, namely, electrokinetics and acoustics. Digital microfluidics has recently emerged as a popular approach to transport individual droplets on an array of patterned electrodes. Therefore, Chapter 4 discusses the most recent development of this technology with attention to actuation and sensing scalability.

Part II focuses on applications of microfluidic devices for drug delivery and discovery. The applications of microfluidics technology in drug delivery and discovery have experienced a sustainable growth in the past 2 decades. Microfluidic devices have become an increasingly important tool to improve the efficiency of drug delivery and reduce side effects of treatment. Chapter 5 provides an overview of controlled drug delivery with various microfluidic devices and triggering mechanisms. In particular, Chapter 6 is dedicated to the study of the transdermal delivery of drug molecules and monitoring biological fluids using microfabricated needles and provides an overview of recent progress on the microneedle technology. The last chapter in Part II, Chapter 7, presents the roles of microfluidic chips in current drug discovery and in high-throughput screening, identification of drug targets and preclinical testing. Potential applications of microfluidic devices in chemical analysis as well as analysis of metabolites in blood for studying pathology are also discussed herein.

The cell is the basic organization unit of living organisms, capable of many basic life processes. Part III is dedicated to applications of microfluidic devices related to cellular analysis and tissue engineering. The behaviors of particles or cells in microfluidic channels have been found important to understand the motion of particles or cells of interest. Chapter 8 describes the fundamentals of microscale fluid dynamics and key issues relating to biological cell behaviors within microfluidic chips. Different mechanisms available to manipulate cells and recent development in these areas are presented in detail. Chapter 9 describes an application of a glass-based microfluidic device in trapping and automated injection of single mouse embryos for large scale biomolecule testing. Many efforts have also been dedicated to the study of cells and the surrounding culture microenvironments, which is the key to understand the complex cell biology and tissue genesis. Chapter 10 is more relative to current advances of microfluidic platforms for tissue engineering and regenerative medicine applications. Stem cells, special types of biological cells that can divide and differentiate into diverse specialized cell types, are the basic building blocks of the human body, and the research on stem cells is one of the most fascinating areas. Chapter 11 focuses on the applications of microfluidics technology for molecular and cellular analysis of stem cells.

Part IV focuses on applications of microfluidic devices in diagnostic sensing. Miniaturization helps investigators get rid of the restrictions of low concentration, low volume of samples in protein detection and clinical diagnostics. The focus of Chapter 12 is on the development of immunoassays for antibodies and cytokines analysis on nanobioarray chips. The impact of fully integrated microfluidic systems on high performance genetic analysis is described in Chapter 13. Recent development in DNA sequencing, gene expression analysis, infectious disease detection and forensic short tandem repeat (STR) typing with integrated microfluidic platforms has been reviewed. Many conventional diagnostic methods require bulky and expensive instruments, limiting their applications in resource-poor settings, especially in developing nations. Paper-based analytical devices have been developed for low cost and easy-to-use diagnostic applications. The ability to fabricate microfluidic channels in paper to perform parallel analysis of various biochemical analysts has been demonstrated. Chapter 14 summarizes recent advances in paper-based microfluidic devices. In addition, rapid and multiplexed detection of viral infection is highly desired in many diagnostic applications. Thus, attention has been given to microfluidic POC devices for sensitive viral detection with high specificity based on immunoassays and nucleic acid-based testing in Chapter 15. Furthermore, microfluidic devices have been applied in the field of pancreatic islet transplantation as a clinical therapy for diabetes and radiochemical synthesis for medical imaging in clinical practices, as discussed in Chapters 16 and 17, respectively. In Chapter 16, microfluidic devices are used for the study of pancreatic islet and β-cell physiology and disease pathophysiology. Chapter 17 focuses on the topic of microfluidic devices for radiochemical synthesis in production of radioactively labeled tracers for Positron Emission Tomography and SinglePhoton Emission Computed Tomography, which are commonly used to quantify biochemical processes in live organisms.

Xiujun James Li and Yu Zhou
August, 2013

Preface to the second edition

Microfluidic technology has advanced rapidly in the past decade, particularly in the field of biomedical application. Thus, the second edition of *Microfluidic Devices for Biomedical Applications* aims to provide readers with the latest information about microfluidic advances for biomedical applications. Major changes in this new edition include but are not limited to the following. (1) New microfluidics advances have been updated in every chapter including updated literature, figures, and reference list. (2) Two new chapters pertaining to emerging microfluidic techniques have been added, namely, Chapter 4 and 17. Chapter 4 focuses on droplet-based microfluidic technologies that have wide applications in biomedical applications, including high-throughput single-cell capture and analysis. Chapter 17 introduces three-dimensional printing technologies for microfluidic device and applications, which is a hot research area that has brought increasing attention. (3) We also have added two to three questions at the beginning of each chapter for guided reading. Those questions can also be used for your teaching if you choose this comprehensive book as a textbook. I hope you will find these updates informative and enjoyable.

By XiuJun (James) Li
September 12, 2020

Materials and methods for microfabrication of microfluidic devices

Sreekant Damodara[1], Shadi Shahriari[1], Wen-I Wu[2], Pouya Rezai[3], Huan-Hsuan Hsu[4], Ravi Selvaganapathy[1]
[1]McMaster University, Hamilton, Ontario, Canada; [2]Bio Rad Laboratories, Mississauga, Ontario, Canada; [3]York University, Toronto, Ontario, Canada; [4]Tufts University, Medford, Massachusetts, United States

Guided reading questions:

1. What are the most widely used methods to fabricate microfluidic devices and their advantages?
2. How did the need to integrate new functional materials in microfluidic devices enable fabrication technique to evolve?
3. What are the advantages of new substrates such as paper and threads in the context of microfluidic devices?

1.1 Introduction

Advanced microfluidic and lab-on-a-chip devices have been extensively studied and developed in the last 2 decades due to their inherent advantages such as low consumption of chemicals, rapid analysis, biocompatibility, low cost, and automation in biological, biomedical, and analytical chemistry studies. Since the technology for developing these devices was initially adapted from conventional semiconductor microelectronic industry, initial devices were primarily made in silicon and glass. Many of the commercially available microfluidic devices are made from this technology. However, these materials are expensive and have high fabrication costs. New materials have been investigated, and fabrication processes developed especially in the context of rapid prototyping and disposable applications. Polymers are macromolecules polymerized from smaller molecules called monomers through a series of chemical reactions. They can be categorized based on their structure and behavior (Nicholson, 1997) but mostly classified in accordance to their response to thermal treatment. They have a low cost (suited for disposable devices), can be easily mass-produced by various rapid prototyping techniques, have a wide range of material properties (chemical inertness, low electrical and thermal conductivity, etc.) that can also be tailored (surface modification techniques) in favor of the targeted experimental substance,

Microfluidic Devices for Biomedical Applications. https://doi.org/10.1016/B978-0-12-819971-8.00008-1
Copyright © 2021 Elsevier Ltd. All rights reserved.

and more importantly have been already used in tools and laboratory equipment where conventional biological and chemical assays have been conducted. The devices made of polymers are well amenable to automation and high throughput screening. The impetus to further lower costs associated with microfluidic devices led to the use of paper and threads as alternative materials for microfluidic fabrication. These devices are used primarily for disposable assays and leverage preexisting technologies (inkjet printing, screen printing, etc.) to further reduce fabrication costs. This chapter describes some of the widely used materials in biomicrofluidic and microelectromechanical systems (MEMS), their properties, and fabrication methods.

1.2 Microfabrication methods

The microfabrication techniques used in construction of microfluidic devices can be broadly classified into three types. These are (1) Photolithography-based, (2) Replication-based, and (3) Xurography-based. In photolithographic microfabrication, light is used to define patterns on a photosensitive material, and its resolution is determined by the wavelength of light used, limitations of optical components such as the numerical aperture of the lens and the polarity of photoresist. The photosensitive material itself can be used as a structural feature of the device, or this pattern is transferred onto another structural material. In the replication method, a master mold is made using either the photolithographic process or traditional machining processes. This mold, which could be of any material, can withstand the operating conditions of the process and is used to replicate the pattern or feature onto another softer material through direct physical contact. In Xurography-based method, several layers of pressure sensitive adhesives (PSAs), polymer films, or glass slide are attached to form the microfluidic device. Each layer is individually cut, aligned, and laminated together to create the device. Cutting is done using a cutting plotter. The choice of the fabrication method in any application depends on various factors such as the desired substrate, cost, speed, feature size, and profile. The following sections will briefly describe existing microfabrication technologies and materials used in microfluidic applications along with their advantages and limitations.

1.2.1 Photolithography-based microfabrication

Photolithography is the technique of using light to define features on a photodefinable material. This technique along with established semiconductor manufacturing process of thin film deposition and etching were initially adapted to produce the first microfluidic devices on silicon (Manz, Verpoorte, Fettinger, Ludi, & Widmer, 1991; Terry, Jerman, & Angell, 1979) and glass (Fan, Ludi, & Widmers, 1992; Jacobson, Roland, Koutny, & Ramsey, 1994) substrates. New methods to fabricate high aspect ratio open microchannel structures in silicon or glass substrate using various etching techniques such as reactive-ion etching (RIE), hydrofluoric acid (HF) wet etching, or potassium hydroxide (KOH) wet etching were simultaneously developed. Subsequently, the microchannels were enclosed using bonding techniques such as electromagnetic induction heating (Thompson et al., 2002), hydrophobic silicon bonding (Tong et al., 1994), fusion bonding (Harendt et al., 1992), and anodic bonding (Kutchoukov et al., 2003). Although these processes are well developed, the cost of the substrates and of microfabrication in a cleanroom facility makes them unsuitable for disposable microfluidic devices. These microfabrication techniques have been extensively reviewed in these review articles (Bustillo, Howe, Muller, & Fellow, 1998; Gad-El-Hak, 2002; Hoffmann & Voges, 2002; Judy, 2001, p. 1115; Lang, 1996; Maluf, 2002; Miki, 2005; Petersen, 1982; Rai-Choudhury, 1997; Stokes & Palmer, 2006).

The cost consideration led to the investigation and use of photodefinable polymers such as conventional photoresists that have been used for patterning in microelectronics industry as structural elements in microfluidic devices. For instance, these photoresists were applied to create manifolds for microfluidic devices (Burns et al., 1998) though channel height is limited to <3 µm due to their physical parameters. Even earlier, X-rays have been used to define features in photoresist using a process known as LIGA (Lithographie, Galvanoformung, Abformung) to obtain >350 µm microstructures with an aspect ratio of >100:1 (Becker, Ehrfeld, Hagmann, Maner, & Münchmeyer, 1986). Later, the photoresist SU-8 which requires no complex X-ray facility was developed for high microstructures using standard photolithography process (Lin et al., 2002; Sikanen et al., 2005; Yang et al., 2004). A channel height of 100 and aspect ratio of >10:1 is achievable according to its manufacturer (Microchem, 2012). Moreover, Pinto et al. have fabricated low-cost SU-8 microstructures with aspect ratios >20:1 in the absence of cleanroom facilities. Therefore, obtaining 100 µm width structures up to 2 mm height is possible (Pinto, Sousa, Cardoso, & Minas, 2014).

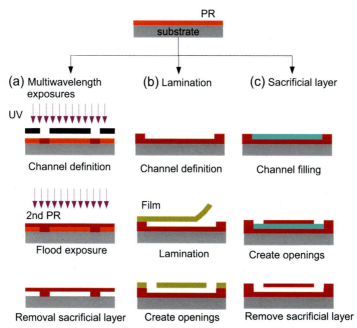

Figure 1.1 Microfabrication processes for (a) Multiwavelength exposures, (b) Lamination, and (c) Sacrificial layer.

Various methods have been adopted for fabrication of photoresist-based microfluidic devices. The first method shown in Fig. 1.1(c) begins with a spin coating of photoresist onto a substrate and patterning with a photomask (Metz, Jiguet, Bertsch, & Renaud, 2004; Tay et al., 2001). Once the open microchannels are created, a sacrificial material is filled into the space of microchannel. Subsequently, a second layer of photoresist is spin-coated and patterned on top to define the access holes for inlet and outlet. Finally, the sacrificial layer is dissolved to create the closed microchannels. The major disadvantage in this process is the slow dissolution; therefore, only short microchannels are applicable. The second method shown in Fig. 1.1(b) laminates a dry SU-8 or Kapton film on top of the open microchannels (Agirregabiria, 2005). Although this process is relative simple, the alignment and the bonding strength of lamination could be challenging. The third method shown in Fig. 1.1(a) uses two exposures at different wavelengths to create the embedded microchannels in SU-8 (Dykes et al., 2007). The first exposure (365 nm) defines the sidewalls of microchannels while the second exposure (254 nm) creates the encapsulation layer for the microchannels due to its shallower absorption depth. The exposure with two wavelengths could be inconvenient in certain circumstances, and similar slow dissolution problem in the first method could happen here.

Alternatively, stereolithography (Morimoto, Tan, & Takeuchi, 2009; Tse et al., 2003) and laser ablation are also used for the microfabrication for microfluidic devices. The former method is an additive manufacturing process which employs liquid resins and high intensity light beams to build 3D microstructures. The photo-induced cross-linking happens upon the exposure of the liquid resin. The process time depends on the complexity of the 3D microstructures; therefore, it is commonly used for prototyping. An extensive review on stereolithography can be found here (Bertsch et al., 2002; Martinez, Basit, & Gaisford, 2018; Melchels, Feijen, & Grijpma, 2010). The latter method is a subtractive manufacturing process which uses a focused high intensity laser beam to evaporate the material from the surface (Jensen et al., 2004; Khan Malek, 2006; Rihakova & Chmelickova, 2015). Laser ablation is mostly used to fabricate microchannels in thermosetting polymers like polyimide (PI) due to its physical properties (Metz et al., 2004; Metz, Holzer, & Renaud, 2001; Yin et al., 2005). Microstructures with nanometer scale have been demonstrated (Kim et al., 2005); however, the surface roughness and properties using laser ablation are difficult to control and highly dependent on the manufacturing parameters. An extensive review on laser micromachining can be found here (Dubey & Yadava, 2008; Gattass & Mazur, 2008; Rihakova & Chmelickova, 2015; Rizvi, 2003; Shiu et al., 2008).

1.2.2 Replication-based methods

One of the major advantages of using polymers in microfabrication is largely owing to the low-cost, high-volume replication methods such as soft lithography, hot embossing, and injection molding. A master (also called as mold) is the most essential tool for all replication methods, and it can be fabricated through conventional photolithography, silicon etching, LIGA, laser ablation, or micro-EDM (electrode discharge machining). The selection of mold fabrication method depends on the available material, resolution, aspect ratio, and processing conditions. In the following sections, brief description of various replication methods and their performance characteristics are given.

1.2.2.1 Soft lithography

Due to its simple process, excellent material properties, low manufacturing cost, high replicating accuracy, soft lithography process has become one of the main rapid prototyping methods (Xia & Whitesides, 1998) used in microfluidics. Commonly used materials, like Sylgard 184 by Dow Corning and RTV 615 by Elastosil, contain two components, base elastomer and curing agent. The mixture is degassed to prevent the formation of air bubbles and then cast on the mold. After curing, the elastomer is peeled from the mold and bonded to a glass slide or other polymer sheets to create closed microchannels. Various methods have been developed to increase the bonding strength for each polymer. For example, a treatment with oxygen or air plasma can lead to a permanent bond between two polydimethylsiloxane (PDMS) layers. A replication accuracy of <10 nm feature has been demonstrated using this method (Hua et al., 2006). In additional to elastomers, other polymers like polyurethane (PU) and polyester can also be used in casting microfluidic structures since they can be cured through temperature or ultraviolet (UV) exposure (Fiorini et al., 2007; Wu et al., 2012). Furthermore, Sticker et al. used a thermoset polymer as an alternative to PDMS to fabricate multilayer structures (Sticker et al., 2015). An extensive review on soft lithography can be found here (Lakshminarayanan, 2018; Qin, Xia, & Whitesides, 2010; Rogers & Nuzzo, 2005).

1.2.2.2 Hot embossing

Hot embossing has been commonly used for the microstructuring of polymers in industry before it is adapted for microfluidic applications due to its relatively simple process, wide selection of materials, and availability of facility. As shown in Figs. 1.2 and 1.3, the microstructures are transferred from the master to the polymer

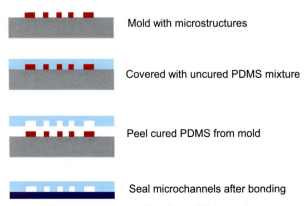

Figure 1.2 Process flow for soft lithography.

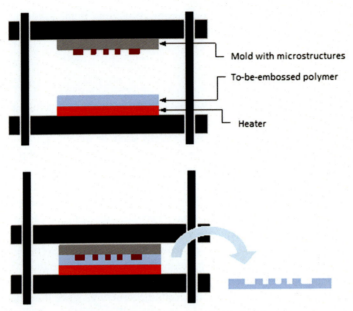

Figure 1.3 Process flow for hot embossing.

by stamping the master into the polymer softened by raising the temperature above its glass transition temperature. This method is limited to thermoplastic polymers, and a variety of polymers have been successfully hot embossed with microstructures, including polycarbonate (PC) (Klintberg et al., 2003), PI (Youn et al., 2008), cyclic olefin copolymers (COC) (Jeon et al., 2011), and Poly(methyl methacrylate) (PMMA) (Becker, 2000). The surface quality, temperature uniformity, and chemical compatibility of the master determine the success of the hot embossing. A replication accuracy of few tens of nanometers has been achieved using this method (Kolew et al., 2010; Roos et al., 2002; Schift et al., 2000; Weerakoon-Ratnayake, O'Neil, Uba, & Soper, 2017). A variation of this method is known as "nanoimprinting" where the feature size is in few tens to hundreds of nanometer. An extensive review on hot embossing and nanoimprint lithography can be found here (Gale et al., 2018; Guo, 2007; Traub, Longsine, & Truskett, 2016; Worgull, 2009; Worgull, Heckele, & Schomburg, 2005).

1.2.2.3 Injection molding

Similar to hot embossing, injection molding is well established as the most suitable fabrication process for polymers in high volume production due to its fast process time and high replication accuracy. As shown in Fig. 1.4, the polymer is fed into a chamber and melted upon heating (200–350°C depending on the melting temperature of polymer). It is then injected into the mold cavity and cooled to form a replica. In the microfluidic application, a good filling without trapping air bubbles is one of the key requirements for successful molding. Although the cycle times for injection molding

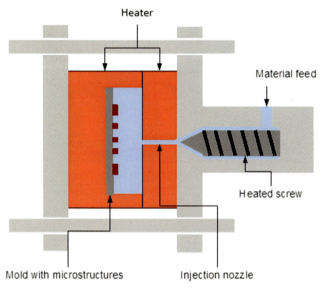

Figure 1.4 Setup for injection molding.

can be fast as several seconds, insufficient cooling time for polymers can lead to thermal stress and defect formation. The process control over various parameters like injection pressure, molding temperatures and their duration, cycle times etc. increases its complexity. Moreover, the relatively high cost for the mold material to ensure it is capable of withstanding high temperature process is also one of its disadvantages. However, the major advantage of injection molding over other replication methods is its ability to form 3D microstructures without geometrical constraints using both thermosetting and thermoplastic polymers. Additional fluidic components such as interconnections and connectors can also be integrated together (Gartner, Klemm, & Becker, 2007; Mair et al., 2006). Number of researches has been done to improve the functionality of this method. For example, Wiedemeier et al. fabricated a superhydrophobic surface during injection molding which is essential in stable generation and movement of liquid droplets in droplet-based microfluidic devices (Wiedemeier et al., 2017).

An extensive review on injection molding can be found here (Attia & Alcock, 2011; Attia, Marson, & Alcock, 2009; Heckele & Schomburg, 2004).

1.2.3 Xurography-based microfabrication

Xurography was first introduced by Bartholomeusz, Boutté, and Andrade (2005) for creating microstructures in films. The technique is used to make devices that consist of multiple cut layers that are bonded together using PSAs. Each layer is individually cut using a cutting plotter. The layers are then aligned and laminated together to create a multilayer stack that constitutes the complete device. Fig. 1.5 shows this process. In this method, as a physical blade is used to cut the material based on a premade design, compared to laser cutting which uses a focused beam for cutting, xurography is less

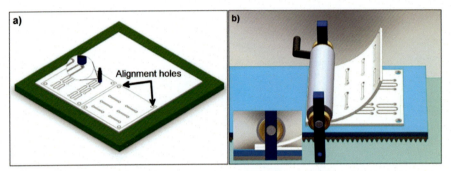

Figure 1.5 (a) Cutting the pattern using a cutting plotter, (b) Assembly of the layers by using lamination (Mohammadzadeh et al., 2018).

expensive and easier to set up. However, it operates at a lower resolution (Gale et al., 2018). Laser cutters have a higher resolution but require a vacuum pump and may leave burn residue (Nath et al., 2010). An extensive review on xurography can be found here (Walsh III, David, Kong, Murthy, & Carr, 2017).

This microfabrication method offers a few advantages over photolithographic fabrication. Some of these are the ability to integrate different materials into a single device, the use of inexpensive materials, rapid fabrication, and simple processing steps (Mohammadzadeh, Fox-Robichaud, & Selvaganapathy, 2018). Additionally, this method enables the integration of electrodes into microfluidic devices. Embedding electrodes in microfluidic devices is essential for numerous applications. However, most methods for electrode fabrication in microfluidic devices are based on expensive photolithography and sputtering processes. Using xurography to cut and integrate metal films into microfluidic devices reduces the cost of fabrication of devices (Mohammadzadeh, Robichaud, & Ravi Selvaganapathy, 2019).

PSAs with different surface energy and properties and polymer films such as polyvinyl chloride (PVC) and polyethylene terephthalate (PET) with different thicknesses are extensively used in this fabrication method and are further detailed in Section 3.6.

The fabrication techniques that are briefly described here represent a few commonly used methods for fabrication of microfluidic devices. In addition, there are a wide range of other methods such as microthermoforming, microelectro discharge machining, LIGA machining, micromilling, and precision machining that have also been used for fabrication of microfluidic devices. These methods are reviewed in works by Ehrfeld et al., 1996, Faustino, Catarino, Lima, and Minas (2016), Gale et al. (2018), Giselbrecht et al., 2004, Hupert et al., 2006, Malek and Saile (2004), Nikumb et al. (2005), Truckenmuller et al. (2002).

1.3 Materials

Numerous materials have been used in the fabrication of microfluidic devices. They have been broadly classified into glass, silicon, polymeric, paper, thread, and PSAs. Glass and silicon are the traditional materials derived from the origin of microfluidic devices from its history in MEMS. The impetus for reducing fabrication and prototyping costs led to the use of materials ranging from commonly used polymers to low cost, mass manufactured products like paper, thread, and PSAs. The physical properties of some of these materials are listed in Table 1.1.

1.3.1 Glass

Glass is an amorphous solid silicon compound that can be also applied in fabricating microfluidic devices. This material has number of favorable features i.e., chemically inert, insulated, transparent, and low fluorescence emission that make it suitable for microfluidic devices used in biological or optical application. The most commonly used glass for microfluidic device manufacturing is Pyrex Corning 7740, due to its compatibility in thermal expansion with silicon (Paoletti, Roth, & De Rooij, 2007, pp. 219–222). Fused silica (quartz) is another attractive material in certain applications which require UV-transparency; however, it is expensive. Also quartz has crystalline structure that make anisotropic etching possible. Apart from these, there are two other kinds of glasses that have been used to fabricate microfluidic devices, Soda lime glass and FOTURAN glass, which would be introduced in following sections.

1.3.1.1 Fabrication

The fabrication techniques of glass-based microfluidic devices have not been extensively investigated and are not as well developed as silicon. Due to the amorphous nature of most glass substrates, the etching using wet chemicals is usually isotropic, and hence, the aspect ratios obtainable are typically lower than silicon. Despite this factor, glass has been used for fabrication of microfluidic devices as many biochemical reactions have been characterized and standardized in these substrates. Various methods including wet chemical etching (Zhang, Tan, Hong, Yang, & Gong, 2001), plasma etching (Li, Abe, & Esashi, 2001), powder machining (Schlautmann, Wensink, Schasfoort, Elwenspoek, & Van Den Berg, 2001), laser micromachining (Ke, Hasselbrink, & Hunt, 2005), and ultrasonic drilling (Egashira, Mizutani, & Nagao, 2002), glass reflow (Lee, Lee, Lee, & Park, 2013; Razi-ul & Wise, 2013) have been used to microstructure glass. An extensive review on microdrilling and microstructuring methods for glass can be found here (Hof & Abou Ziki, 2017).

1.3.1.2 Wet chemical etching

Wet chemical etching is the most common strategy for glass microfabrication. In most cases, the HF is used as the main etchant for any type of silicate glass. Some other components such as HCl, HNO_3, and NH_4F-buffer may also be added to control the etch rate (Spierings, 1993). The chemical reaction for etching is shown below:

$$SiO_2 + 6HF \rightarrow H_2SiF_6 + 2H_2O \tag{1.1}$$

Table 1.1 Physical properties.

	Silicon	Glass	PDMS	Parylene C	PC	PMMA	PI	PU	COC/COP	Paper
T_m (°C)	1414	700 (Soda lime) 1750 (Quartz) 820 (Pyrex) 465 (Foturan)	−40	290	260	250–260	None	Unavailable	190–320	N/A
T_g (°C)	3265	2239 (SiO_2)	−125	90	150	100–122	>400	Unavailable	70–155	N/A
CTE (10^{-6} °C^{-1})	2.49	9.2 (Soda lime) 0.54 (Quartz) 3.3 (Pyrex) 8.6 (Foturan)	310 μm/(m·°C)	35	60–70	70–150	20	150	60–80	111 (cellulose)
Moisture absorption (%)	N/A	N/A	0.03	0.06	0.12–0.34	0.3–0.6	0.32	<0.2	<0.01	75% (porosity)
Solvent resistance	Good	Good	Soluble in toluene, swell in nonpolar organic solvent	Insoluble in all organic solvents up to 150°C, can be dissolved in chloro-naphthalene at 175°C	Good	Good	Good	Good	Excellent	Good
UV transmission	Moderate	Poor below 300 nm (Quartz is excellent) (Foturan absorb UV for curing)	Transparent; UV cutoff 240 nm. Optical detection from 240 to 1100 nm	Transparent, strong absorption below 280 nm	Poor	Good	Good >425 nm	Poor	Excellent	N/A

Hardness	12–13 (Gpa)	585 kg/mm² (Soda lime) 522 kg/mm² (Quartz) 418 kg/mm² (Pyrex) 469 kg/mm² (Foturan)			M70–M75	RM92	E53–99, R129, M95	Shore 85A	130–180 N/mm²	39.1 (N/15 mm)
Thermal conductivity (10^{-4} g cal-cm s^{-1} cm^{-2o}C)	150(W/mK)	1.12 (Soda lime) 1.4 (Quartz) 1.1 (Pyrex) 1.35 (Foturan)	0.15–0.2 W/mK	0.082 W/mK	4.7	0.167–0.25	2.3–4.2	0.209 W/mK	0.12–0.15 W/mK	10^{-4} (W/mK)
Dielectric strength (MV m^{-1})	N/A	10 (Soda lime) 8 (Quartz) 14 (Pyrex) 1.2 (Foturan)	2.3–2.8		15–16	25	16–22	12–20	Unavailable	16
Young's modulus (MPa)	160(Gpa)	70 (Soda lime) 107 (Quartz) 64 (Pyrex) 78 (Foturan)	0.360–0.870	69	2200	1800–3100	2550	55	3000	3600–3800
Tensile or fracture strength(MPa)	2000	20 (Soda lime) 48 (Quartz) 20.7 (Pyrex) 60 (Foturan)	2.24	3200	65	48–76	90	50	60	Wet:0.002 Dry:0.011

Continued

Table 1.1 Continued

	Silicon	Glass	PDMS	Parylene C	PC	PMMA	PI	PU	COC/COP	Paper
References	Kohlmann & Vogel (1979)	Kohlmann & Vogel (1979)	Clarson & Semlyen (1993); McDonald, Metallo, & Whitesides (2001); McDonald & Whitesides (2002); Chuang & Wereley (2009); Armani, Liu, & Aluru (1999); Mata, Fleischman, & Roy (2005)	Tan and Craighead (2010); Noh, Huang, & Hesketh (2004a); Noh, Moon, Cannon, Hesketh, & Wong (2004b); Shin et al. (2003)	Mark (2007); Utracki (2002); Rabek (1995); Minges (1989)	Tsao and DeVoe (2009); Assael, Botsios, Gialou, & Metaxa (2005); Boger, Bisig, Bohner, Heini, & Schneider (2008)	Mark (2007); Utracki (2002); Rabek (1995); Minges (1989)	Wu et al. (2012); Mark (2007); Utracki (2002); Rabek (1995); Minges (1989)	Todo & Kashiwa, 1996; Sastri (2010); Biron (2007); Shin (2005)	Hori & Wada, 2005; Mark (2001); Pelton (2009); Rigden (1996); Schröder & Bensarsa (2002)

The wet chemical etching is isotropic and produces rounded sidewall microchannels. The shape and angel of sidewall may be adjusted by apply titanium as a receding mask during wet etching (Fig. 1.6) (Pekas, Zhang, Nannini, & Juncker, 2010). The depth of channel is controlled by etch rate and etch duration. Furthermore, the width of channel can be estimated by mask opening plus twice of channel depth. Gold (Au) is a suitable masking material for HF etching because of its inert nature. Usually, a patterned Chromium (Cr)/Au thin film is used as a mask for glass wet etching where Cr provides the adhesion between glass and Au polysilicon layer patterned by plasma dry etching, and photolithography is another popular masking method. In the case of some shallow etches, a thick layer of negative photoresists (i.e., SU-8) may be a simple, low cost but suitable masking material. In another research, a positive photoresist (AZ4330) in combination with a Cr/Au mask was used in order to wet etch glass in 49 wt% HF solution (Jin, Yoo, Bae, & Kim, 2013). Anisotropic wet etching of glass is possible if crystalline quartz is used as the substrate material. Z-cut wafers are typically used as the etch rate in this direction and is significantly greater than any other direction. With proper design and tuning of etch conditions (i.e., etchant concentration and temperature) (Rangsten, Hedlund, & Katardjiev, 1998), appropriate shapes required for microfluidic structures can be obtained.

1.3.1.3 Plasma etching

The fundamental principle of RIE and deep reactive-ion etching (DRIE) of glass are similar to that for Silicon. During RIE etching, gas phase etchants such as CHF, CHF_3, CF_4, or their combination are introduced in a plasma to produce fluorine radicals that directionally bombard and etch the glass substrate. The chemical reaction for etching is presented below:

$$SiO_2 + CF_4 \rightarrow CO_2 + SiF_4 \qquad (1.2)$$

The etching rate decreases strongly with increasing proportion of nonvolatile oxides produced during etching resulting in a low etch rate (10 nm/min) (Ronggui, 1991). High speed directional etching of glass was achieved by applying high density inductively coupled plasma (ICP) and strong permanent magnet to stabilize plasma. By doing so, the 0.3 μm/min etching rate of glass and 1 μm/min for quartz can be obtained (Li et al., 2001). Alexandrov et al. reported a combination of glass poling and plasma etching technique to produce submicron relief structures on glass surfaces (Fig. 1.7) (Alexandrov, Lipovskii, Osipov, Reduto, & Tagantsev, 2017).

1.3.1.4 Other methods

A simple method of micromachining glass has been devised through the use of the dicing process. Diamond blades (Blade widths can be very thin (below 100 μm) depending on the diameter of the blade) are used in this process with low depth of cuts to precisely define microchannels. Photoresist coating on the dicing substrate is used to prevent redeposition of debris from the dicing process onto the substrate

14 Microfluidic Devices for Biomedical Applications

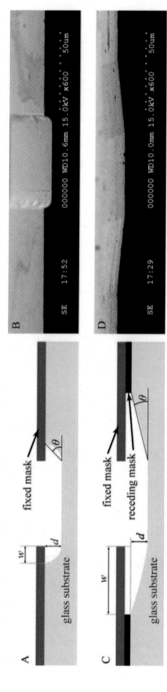

Figure 1.6 (a) Schematic representation of etching of glass using a Si passive etch mask and (b) scanning electron microscope (SEM) image of the cross section of a isotropic glass etching using a fixed a-Si as the etch mask. (c) Schematic representation of etching of glass with a bilayer mask made of a fixed mask and a receding mask. (d) SEM image of the cross section of a channel etched in glass using a 10-nm layer of Ti as a receding mask. Reprint from Pekas et al. (2010) with permission.

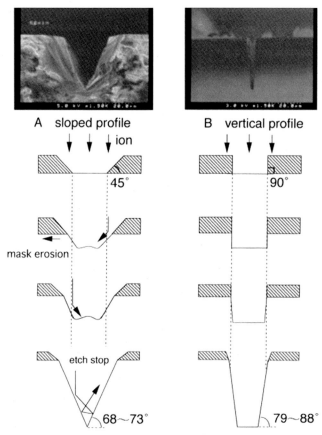

Figure 1.7 Scanning electron microscope (SEM) images and schematic illustrations of the observed etched profiles of ICP-RIE (inductively coupled plasma-reactive ion etching) (pressure 0.2 Pa, self-bias voltage 390 V, etching time 1 h).
Reprint from Li et al. (2001) with permission.

(Ngoi & Sreejith, 2000). However, this method is usually limited to fabricating simple straight microchannel structures. The aspect ratio of structures produced by dicing can be further improved by introducing ultrasonic vibration during cutting since it can reduce cutting force thus preventing the breakage of glass (Egashira et al., 2002).

Powder machining is another technique that is used for making interconnect through-holes in glass. In this process, sharp indenting particle jets are shot at high speeds on to the substrate protected by a thick layer of masking material (Ordyl BF410 resist foil). The impingement of these sharp particles generate microcracks that erode the exposed regions (defined by polymer mask) of glass substrates (Belloy, Thurre, Walckiers, Sayah, & Gijs, 2000). This procedure is able to provide fast etching rate (25 μm/min), but the process requires special facilities and produces features with high surface roughness (Schlautmann et al., 2001).

Laser micromachining has been used for making number of through-holes in glass. In this method, glass is removed by targeted ablation with a pulsed laser. The removed materials usually form debris that redeposit on the substrate which limits its application in fabrication channel shape features (Bu, Melvin, Ensell, Wilkinson, & Evans, 2004). Two approaches have been used to resolve this limitation. One, shown by, Ke et al. performed laser micromachining under fluid where the debris can be carried away from the machining site and avoid redeposition, later called water-assisted femtosecond laser drilling: WAFLD. By this approach, the microchannel features were successfully synthesized in glass without any postprocessing (Ke et al., 2005). Femtosecond laser machining has been applied for nanofabrication of glass with a resolution down to several hundred nanometers (100−500 nm) (Korte et al., 2003). In this process, the debris formed per pulse is small, and they solidify before redeposition. By applying this technique, micro- and nanochannels with high aspect ratios and good wall-surface quality were successfully made (Hwang, Choi, & Grigoropoulos, 2004; Kudryashov, Mourou, Joglekar, Herbstman, & Hunt, 2007). Jedrkiewicz et al. presented single-shot glass modification by means of high-order Bessel beams in the picosecond pulsed regime (Jedrkiewicz, Bonanomi, Selva, & Di Trapani, 2015). One limitation that was observed at this point was a clogging when channels over 1 mm long were fabricated. This was resolved by used porous glass as the substrate (Sugioka et al., 2014). This allowed the removal of the debris through the pores which enabled longer channel lengths to be fabricated. However, the fabricated device had to be annealed after the process to close the pores in the glass device. This has been used to fabricate devices with a resolution of under 50 nm (Liao et al., 2013). Another method is to use selective laser-induced etching (SLE) process which is a combination of laser direct patterning and wet chemical etching. In this process, a femtosecond laser is used to locally irradiate either photosensitive glass (Masuda et al., 2003) or fused silica (Burshtein, Chan, Toda-Peters, Shen, & Haward, 2019). The chemical etch rate of fused silica can be increased up to 1000 times (Burshtein et al., 2019). Kim et al. used this technique to fabricate 3D microfluidic channels. KOH was used as wet etchant on a substrate of fused silica, and the etch rate of 166 μm/h was obtained (Kim et al., 2019). FOTURAN glass is an example of photosensitive glass made by components that contain CeO_2, Ag_2O, and Sb_2O_3 that crystallizes after exposure to UV light, and the etch rates of the crystallized regions are increased significantly. Thus, high aspect ratio (20) glass microfluidic features can be obtained by using this material. More details on FOTURAN microfabrication and mechanism can be obtained here (Dietrich, Ehrfeld, Lacher, Kramer, & Speit, 1996). In comparison to using fused silica, photosensitive glass has a higher scanning rate and requires lower peak intensity but requires thermal treatment prior to use. A detailed review of femtosecond laser micromachining is available here (Sugioka et al., 2014).

1.3.1.5 Bonding

The glass−glass, glass−silicon wafer bondings are usually employed for sealing the fabricated glass microfluidic features. Wafer bonding can also be used to assemble several wafers with different microfeatures on them to construct a complex and tall microfluidic design. Other materials such as GaAs and SiC can also bonded on wafer to create versatile devices i.e., electrodes heaters, sensors, and detectors. Bonding techniques used for glass include fusion bonding, anodic bonding, and adhesive bonding. The details of these wafer bonding approaches can be found in the following review paper (Gösele & Tong, 1998; Schmidt, 1998; Silverio & de Freitas, 2018).

Soda lime glass is a multicomponent mixture consisting of small amounts of Na_2O, CaO, MgO, and Al_2O_3 apart from SiO_2. This material is also employed in glass microfluidic device fabrication for facilitating the glass-to-glass fusion bonding procedures (for enclosing the microfluidic channel) as well as reducing the fabrication cost (Lin, Lee, Lin, & Chang, 2001).

1.3.1.6 Applications and future trends

Since glass is one of the most widely used substrate material in biology, biomedical microfluidic devices such as those used for DNA stretch and capture device (Sidorova, Li, Schwartz, Folch, & Monnat, 2009), DNA mass spectrometry (Erickson & Li, 2004), and micro-DNA amplification (polymerase chain reaction (PCR)) devices (Lagally, Simpson, & Mathies, 2000) have typically been microfabricated in glass. Many components such as monolithic membrane valves/diaphragm pumps for high throughput assays, micropumps microflow, and pressure sensors (Grover, Skelley, Liu, Lagally, & Mathies, 2003) have also been integrated with glass microfluidic devices. Moreover, because glass is transparent under a wide wavelength range (glass: Vis-Near IR transparent; quartz: UV-Near IR transparent), it is widely used in making microoptical bioanalytical devices (Fan & White, 2011).

With its unique properties, glass is the very suitable substrate for microfluidic devices with biological and biomedical application. The surface properties of glass have been well characterized for surface functionalization as well as for electrophoretic and electrokinetic assays. Additionally, by applying the laser microfabrication, glass-based microfluidic device can be made in a single step. However, widespread use of glass is constrained due to the: (1) Complicated bonding steps for glass devices manufactured by planar fabrication methods, (2) Limited length of channels that can be fabricated by femtosecond laser etching, (3) Surface roughness of glass after processing is large and needs to be minimized to reduce disturbance to biological samples, (4) High resolution fabrication techniques can only be used to fabricate small devices (Sugioka et al., 2014). Methods have been developed to resolve individual challenges such as the use of porous glass to increase length of channels that can be fabricated using a femtosecond laser and postannealing to reduce surface roughness. However, the combination of challenges has yet to be resolved.

1.3.2 Silicon

Silicon is the second most abundant element in the Earth's crust after oxygen. Highly pure silicon is usually extracted directly from silica (SiO_2) or other silicon compounds by molten salt electrolysis and refined by the Czochralski process into ultrahigh purity single crystals which are used in semiconductor industry and for manufacture of MEMS (Lang, 1996) and microfluidic devices. The widespread availability of single crystal silicon wafers and the techniques developed for their processing in the semiconductor industry facilitated the development of some of the first microfluidic devices such as inkjet print heads (Kim, Son, Choi, Byun, & Lee, 2008) and gas chromatography (GC) columns (Goldstein et al., 1979, pp. 1880–1886) on this substrate. Subsequently, numerous silicon-based microfluidic devices with applications in chemical and biochemical assays (Lion et al., 2003), disease diagnostics (Lee, Kim, Chung, Demirci, & Ali, 2010), drug delivery (Keohane, Brennan, Galvin, & Griffin, 2014; Zafar Razzacki, Thwar, Yang, Ugaz, & Burns, 2004), and environmental monitoring (Jang, Zou, Lee, Ahn, & Bishop, 2011) have been developed.

1.3.2.1 Fabrication

Microfabrication of silicon-based devices can be broadly classified as bulk micromachining and surface micromachining. In bulk micromachining, single crystal silicon is used as a substrate, and various etching processes (wet and dry etching) are used to etch into the substrate to create the microchannel structure. In surface micromachining, the substrate provides a stable and flat base upon which the microchannel structure is constructed by depositing various materials in the thin film form.

1.3.2.2 Bulk micromachining

In this process (Fig. 1.8(a)), photolithography is used to define patterns on a silicon wafer. Subsequently, the microscale features, thus, patterned such as microfluidic

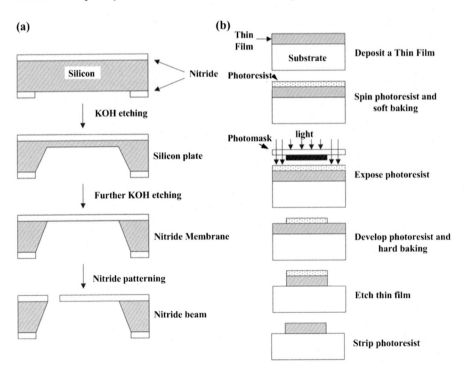

Figure 1.8 (a) Bulk micromachining and (b) Surface micromachining. Reprint from Ziaie (2004) with permission.

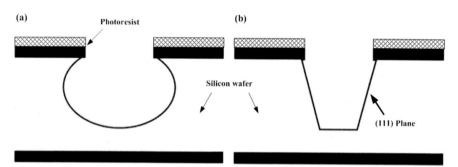

Figure 1.9 (a) Isotropic and (b) anisotropic etching
Reprint from Ziaie (2004) with permission.

channels and chambers are constructed by etching into the exposed regions in the silicon substrates. Finally, another silicon or glass wafer is bonded to the microstructured wafer to form closed microfluidic structures. The etching process used in bulk micromachining can be classified as wet (liquid) and dry (gas) etching based on the phase of the reactants used. Depending on the etchants used, isotropic or anisotropic etching is possible (Fig. 1.9) (Petersen, 1982).

For instance, the combination of HF, nitric acid (HNO$_3$), and acetic acid (CH$_3$COOH) etches silicon without any directional dependence (isotropic). The HNO$_3$ oxidizes the exposed silicon surface into SiO$_2$ which is then subsequently etched by HF and the reaction products dissolve into the etchant solution. The etch rate can be controlled from 0.1 to over 100 μm/min by varying the ratio of acid mixture in HNA (Hydrofluoric, Nitric, Acetic acid mixture) (Maluf, 2002). Alternatively, KOH, Sodium hydroxide (NaOH), Ammonium hydroxide (NH$_4$OH), and Ethylene diamine pyrocatechol (EDP) produce anisotropic etching. The etch rate is related to the surface density of silicon atoms which are different along various crystallographic directions in single crystal silicon. In general, the etching rate in <111> direction is two–three orders of magnitude slower than <110> and <100> direction. The <111> planes serve as etch stop and 3D structures with submicrometer resolution can be obtained using these etches. Microfluidic channels with sloping sidewalls (54.74°) made of (111) planes have been made using <100> wafers while <110> wafers are used for vertical sidewalls (90°). An extensive review on wet chemical etching based silicon bulk micromachining can be found here (Pal & Sato, 2015).

Dry etching of silicon is typically carried out by using reactants (etchants) in the gaseous form to the wafer and using a plasma to energize and direct them toward the wafer. This process is known as RIE. This process can be either isotropic or anisotropic depending on the pressure in the plasma chamber and the electric field that provides directionality to the ionic species in the plasma (Verpoorte & De Rooij, 2003). One of the most popular RIE process is the Bosch process which involves the alternative plasma etching and protection layer deposition step. DRIE using the Bosch process can obtain very high aspect-ratio structures with anisotropies in the order of 30:1 and sidewall angles of 90 ± 2° with the typical etch rates of 2–3 μm/min (Kovacs, Maluf, & Petersen, 1998). Veselove et al. studied DRIE of silicon by using diode plasma etcher system with a low power source and etch rate of 2 μm/min was achieved (Veselov, Bakun, & Voronov, 2016). An extensive review of bulk micromachining processes are detailed here (Fu et al., 2009).

1.3.2.3 Surface micromachining

In this process (Fig. 1.8(b)), silicon-based materials are deposited in the thin film form using chemical vapor deposition processes to produce structural features on a substrate. Two kinds of materials are deposited alternatively till the entire structure is built. Polysilicon (Poly-Si) is generally used as a structural material while Silicon di oxide (SiO_2) and Silicon nitride (Si_3N_4) is used as the sacrificial material. First, the sacrificial material (SiO_2) is deposited and patterned using photolithography to produce the features of the microfluidic channels or networks. Then, Poly-Si is deposited over it and patterned, again using photolithography, to expose the structural material only in the reservoir or interconnect regions. Several layers of microchannels or microscale features could be built by alternatingly depositing and patterning the structural and sacrificial materials. Finally, the fabricated devices is exposed to HF which etches all of the patterned SiO_2 leaving behind the Poly-Si structure which forms the microfluidic network. The process requires highly compatible materials and chemical etchants with high etch selectivity so that the etching of one would not affect the other. An extensive review of various surface micromachining methods and process are detailed here (Bustillo et al., 1998).

1.3.2.4 Applications and future trends

Many essential components of microfluidic devices have been fabricated in silicon such as (Rival et al., 2014) (1) microvalves (Oh & Ahn, 2006); (2) micropumps (Laser & Santiago, 2004); and (3) channels (Verpoorte & De Rooij, 2003) using a combination of the various micromachining methods. Silicon-based microfluidic devices have found applications in inkjet printing (Petersen, 1979), liquid chromatography (LC) (Manz et al., 1990), GC (Terry et al., 1979), mass spectroscopy (MS) (Schultz, Corso, Prosser, & Zhang, 2000), cell detection (Verpoorte et al., 1992), disease diagnostics (Ma et al., 2019; Vo-Dinh & Cullum, 2000), DNA extraction (Tian, Hühmer, & Landers, 2000), drug delivery (Chung, Kim, & Erickson, 2008), quantitative polymerase chain reaction (qPCR) (Rival et al., 2014), miniaturized flow injection analysis (FIA) (Search et al., 1994, p. 246), highly parallelized three-dimensional microfluidics (Yadavali, Lee, & Issadore, 2019), and filter microfluidic chip (Le, Huynh, Hue Phan, Dung Dang, & Dang, 2017, p. 25).

Silicon is one of the first materials used for fabricating microfluidic devices. There are several advantages that make silicon suitable: (1) The micromachining technology for silicon is well-developed; (2) Oxidation of silicon surface produces SiO_2 which is an ideal surface that is suitable for biochemical analysis; (3) Various surface modification chemistries are available for silicon and SiO_2 that make it suitable for functionalization of biomolecules. However, the cost associated with clean room processing and time involved with micromachining along with the cost of the substrate itself makes devices made of silicon expensive. Still, the advantages that silicon possesses makes it an ideal material of choice for microfluidic components and some devices in the commercial domain.

1.3.3 Polymers

Polymers used in fabrication of microfluidic devices can broadly be classified into siloxane elastomers, thermosetting polymers, thermoplastic polymers, paper, and thread devices.

1.3.3.1 Siloxane elastomers

These elastomers are synthetic polymers with a dimethyl siloxane repeating element along the backbone. Of these, PDMS is the most popular polymer used in microfluidic devices (Seethapathy & Górecki, 2012).

Polydimethylsiloxane
PDMS exists in various forms such as fluid, gel, elastomer, resin, and rubber (Brook, 2000) and has been used extensively in microfluidic applications for analytical chemistry (Seethapathy & Górecki, 2012), biology (Kartalov, Anderson & Scherer, 2006; Sia & Whitesides, 2003), biomedical devices, and medicine. PDMS consists of repeating Si−O backbones with two CH_3 organic side arms linked in the polymeric chain. PDMS can be made into its elastomeric form by a process of crosslinking long chain siloxane oligomers containing vinyl terminated end groups (base) with short chain crosslinkers. The reaction mixture also contains platinum-based catalyst, inhibitors, and silica filler (Fu et al., 2003). The process of crosslinking and polymerization is accelerated by heat treatment and increasing the volumetric ratio of crosslinker to base that also increases the rigidity of the final elastomer (Campbell et al., 1999).

Fabrication of microfluidic devices using PDMS
The process used to fabricate microdevices in PDMS material is termed as soft lithography (McDonald et al., 2000; Xia & Whitesides, 1998). In this process, a master mold is created where the microchannel geometry is defined on photoresists photolithographically on a silicon wafer as protruded features (Duffy, Mcdonald, Schueller & Whitesides, 1998; Qin, Xia & Whitesides, 1996; Xia & Whitesides, 1998). Master molds have also been fabricated using silicon bulk micromachining methods (Effenhauser, Bruin, Paulus & Ehrat, 1997). More recently, low cost fabrication of master molds outside cleanroom facilities using techniques like 3D printing (Gale et al., 2018), micro-EDM, micromilling, laser ablation, and xurography has become more common (Faustino et al., 2016). Components of commercially available PDMS base and agent (Sylgard 184 Kit, Dow Corning, USA) are mixed in an appropriate volumetric ratio and cast over the master mold. Crosslinking and polymerization is achieved through the application of heat (65−90°C for 2−4 h) after which the PDMS elastomer formed is peeled off the master mold forming a negative replica. Fluid access ports are punctured, and the microstructured substrate is bonded to a

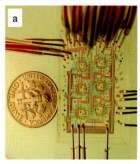 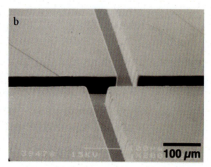

Figure 1.10 (a) A bioreactor fabricated from polydimethylsiloxane (PDMS) with multiple side input/output interconnects. (b) Scanning electron microscopy view of the microchannels of another capillary electrophoresis device made of PDMS.
(a) Reprinted with permission from Balagadde, You, Hansen, Arnold, and Quake (2005), (b) Duffy et al. (1998), Copyright (1998) American Chemical Society.

second PDMS layer for enclosure. Chemical surface treatment (i.e., silanized in 3% v/v dimethyloctadecylchlorosilane in toluene for 2 h) of the master mold before casting can serve as a mold release layer and improve the reliability of the casting process. The process flow is depicted in Fig. 1.2. Fabricated PDMS microchannels are shown in Fig. 1.10.

A replication accuracy of <10 nm has been demonstrated for PDMS casting itself (Hua et al., 2006). Therefore, the feature size that can be obtained largely depends on the resolution and capability of the process creating master molds. Table 1.2 summarizes the minimum feature sizes and maximum aspect ratios achieved in PDMS replication using various processes that are commonly used to make master molds.

PDMS has also been used to fabricate membranes using a spin coater to spin a known quantity of PDMS mix at a high revolutions per minute (rpm) to make sheets

Table 1.2 Minimum feature sizes (MFS) and maximum aspect ratios (AR) fabricated in polydimethylsiloxane (PDMS).

Fabrication method	MFS (μm)	AR	References
Multispinning of SU8 for photolithography and soft lithography	20	17	Natarajan, Chang-Yen, and Gale (2008)
Lithographie, Galvanoformung, Abformung (LIGA) and polydimethylsiloxane (PDMS) casting	20	15	Kim et al. (2002)
Laser and electron discharge micromachining followed by PDMS casting	<20	4	Shiu, Knopf, and Ostojic (2010)
Proton beam writing for Ni masters and PDMS casting	2.5	5.2	van Kan, Wang, Shao, Bettiol, and Watt (2007)

of a thickness dependant on the rpm which are then cured (Jang et al., 2019). The resultant sheets demonstrate enhanced physical properties such as increased elasticity and air porosity. These properties have been leveraged to fabricate capillary channels that deform and aid capillary flow (Anoop & Sen, 2015). The porosity of the membrane is a function of its thickness and has been used to increase oxygenation of blood flowing through a PDMS device (Dabaghi et al., 2019).

Interconnection and bonding

One of the contributing factors toward the popularity of PDMS as a rapid prototyping material is the ease with which strong bonding to various substrates can be obtained as well as the variety of methods for interconnection. Interconnection is used to connect microfluidic networks in chips to macroscale devices, ports, and fittings. Various methods have been developed for interconnection to PDMS devices including manual or machine-based coring and insertion of needles or tubing such as low density polyethylene (LDPE) tube as well as the usage of more standardized world-to-chip interface sockets. These have yielded interconnects that withstand pressure of 100–700 kPa without leakage (Bhagat et al., 2007; Christensen et al., 2005; Fredrickson & Fan, 2004; Quaglio et al., 2008; Westwood, Jaffer & Gray, 2008). The strength of the interconnect has also been enhanced through plasma oxidization prior to interconnection, intermediate adhesive layers, and usage of fastening o-rings (Bhagat, Jothimuthu, Pais, & Papautsky, 2007; Christensen et al., 2005; Frederickson & Fan, 2004; Li & Chen, 2003; Quaglio et al., 2008; Saarela et al., 2006).

Reversible and irreversible bonding of PDMS to itself as well as a variety of other materials has been realized. Some of the widely used methods of bonding PDMS include:

Plasma Treatment: After peeling off the master mold, surface of the PDMS is inertly hydrophobic due to the presence of the surface methyl groups. Exposure to oxygen plasma opens up hydrophilic hydroxyl radicals on the surface which upon conformal contact with another oxidized PDMS surface will form irreversible Si—O—Si bonds (Duffy, Mcdonald, Schueller, & Whitesides, 1998). The plasma exposed surfaces have to be brought into contact immediately to ensure strong bonding. Delay after exposure leads to diffusion of PDMS chains from the bulk onto the surface which reduces the surface density of hydroxyl groups responsible for bonding (Hillborg et al., 2000). In addition to PDMS (Duffy et al., 1998; Eddings, Johnson, & Gale, 2008), bonding to glass, Si (Bhattacharya, Datta, Berg, & Gangopadhyay, 2005) and passivated layers on Si (i.e., phosphosilicate glass (PSG), undoped silicate glass (USG), Si_3N_4, and SiO_2 (Tang et al., 2006) has also been achieved by this method. Plasma treatment with other gases (1:2 argon:oxygen) have also been employed to investigate the bond between polyethylene terephthalate glycol (PETG), COC, and polystyrene (PS) with PDMS and PU layers (Mehta et al., 2009). PDMS and parylene have been bonded using exposure to SF_6: N_2 plasma (Rezai, Selvaganapathy, & Rwohl, 2011). In addition to surface oxidization for making the PDMS surface hydrophilic, methods involving treatment of PDMS surface with sodium silicate (low temperature adhesive for glass bonding applications) (Ito, Soubue, & Ohya, 2002; Wang, Foote,

Jacobson, Schneibel, & Ramsey, 1997), sol—gel techniques (Roman, Hlaus, Bass, Seelhammer, & Culbertson, 2005), silanization (Papra et al., 2001), chemical vapor deposition (Lahann et al., 2003), atom transfer radical polymerization (Xiao, Zhang, & Wirth, 2002), and polyelectrolyte multilayers (Liu et al., 2000) have also been investigated.

Chemical treatment: Eddings et al. (2008) used other chemical-based methods such as partial PDMS curing, varying base: agent mixing ratio, and uncured PDMS adhesive to bond two PDMS layers. Fabrication of multilayer microfluidic 3D networks has been achieved by the "multilayer soft lithography" method (Unger, Chou, Thorsen, Scherer, & Quake, 2000). Each layer containing an excess amount of PDMS base or crosslinker chemical is cast over its mold, peeled off, and bonded to the other layer with an opposite chemical composition. Migration of excess molecules toward the interface forms a bond resulting in a monolithic elastomeric device.

PDMS-PDMS and PDMS-PMMA bonds were realized by immersing or spin-coating the surfaces with a thin layer of diluted silane solution (5% 3-aminopropyltriethoxysilane, APTES, in water), plasma oxidizing, and physically attaching together (Vlachopoulou et al., 2009). An elaboration of this technique was used to bond PDMS to PMMA, PC, PET, U-PET, and PI (Tang & Lee, 2010).

Mechanical: PDMS-PMMA and PDMS-parylene bonding has been achieved by low temperature and applied mechanical pressures on the assembly (Chow, Lei, Shi, Li, & Huang, 2006; Kim & Najafi, 2005; Ko et al., 2003).

A comprehensive view of the various bonding methods used, methodology, and the bond strengths obtained are summarized in Table 1.3.

Applications and future trends

PDMS is considerably cheaper compared to traditional MEMS substrates such as silicon or glass; can be easily replicated and bonded to a diverse range of substrates; has been used to develop various fluidic components (Ng, Gitlin, Stroock, & Whitesides, 2002); has satisfactory optical transparency, mechanical stability (Armani & Liu, 2000), gas permeability, and biocompatibility (Chang et al., 2007). The ease of fabrication combined with increasing prevalence of 3D printed molds combined with these characteristics make PDMS the material of choice for rapid prototyping of microfluidic devices. The evidence of this is its extensive use in prototyping of microfluidic devices for chemistry, biology, and medicine-based applications (Kartalov et al., 2006; Seethapathy & Górecki, 2012; Sia & Whitesides, 2003). The primary drawbacks of PDMS lie in its instability at high temperatures, vulnerability to defects in the master mold, and the lack of scalability to mass production. Despite these drawbacks, PDMS will continue to be used as a popular rapid prototyping material for microfluidic devices in a variety of academic and industrial setting.

1.3.3.2 *Thermosetting polymers*

Thermosetting polymers are polymers that irreversibly harden when crosslinked from an initial viscous liquid or soft solid. This crosslinking is called curing and can be initiated by either heat or exposure to light of specific wavelengths. Depending on the polymer used, and its sensitivity to light or heat, different fabrication methods have

Table 1.3 PDMS bonding to various materials (Rezai et al.,2011).

PDMS bonded to	Bond quality	Bonding method	Parameters	Description	References
Glass	74 psi	Oxygen Plasma	Time: 5–60 s, Power: 5–150 W, Pressure: 20–1000 mTorr	Optimum: Time 20 s, pressure >700 mTorr, power 20 W	Bhattacharya et al. (2005)
PSG USG Si3N4	100% bonded area	Oxygen plasma	Power: 20–140 W, Pressure: 30–500 mTorr, Time: 10–40 s, Temperature ineffective	Optimum: Pressure 30 mTorr, power 60 W for PSG, USG, Si3N4.	Tang et al. (2006)
SiO$_2$	0% bonded area				
LTCC[a]	No leakage	Oxygen plasma	1.5 mL/min flow (1 kPa) into PDMS/LTCC channel		Malecha, Gancarz, and Golonka (2009)
PDMS	300 kPa	Oxygen plasma			Eddings et al. (2008)
	290 kPa	Corona discharge			
	650 kPa	Partial PDMS curing			
	470 kPa	PDMS base:agent ratio	With optimum ratio of 15:1 base: agent		
	670 kPa	Uncured PDMS adhesive			

Continued

Table 1.3 Continued

PDMS bonded to	Bond quality	Bonding method	Parameters	Description	References
PETG[b], COC[c], PS[d]	120 kPa for PETG–PU bonds	Plasma	1:2 argon:oxygen Plasma and overnight 60°C heat and 1 lb pressure	PDMS bonding to these materials was stable over several months	Mehta et al. (2009)
PDMS	400 kpa	Chemical + Plasma	5% APTES[e] in water		Vlachopoulou et al. (2009)
PMMA	1100 kPa				
PC	178 and 579 kPa	Chemical gluing + Plasma	APTES[d] and GPTES[f]	U-PET is PET with a urethane functionality on the surface	Tang and Lee (2010)
PET	579 kPa				
U-PET	607 kPa				
Parylene	1.7 MPa	SF_6 and N_2 plasma		Parts fabricated, then bonded	Rezai et al. (2011)

[a] low-temperature cofired ceramics.
[b] polyethylene terephthalate glycol.
[c] cyclic olefin copolymer.
[d] polystyrene.
[e] 3-aminopropyltriethoxysilane.
[f] 3-glycidoxypropyltriethoxysilane.

been developed for thermosetting polymers. As a result of their irreversible shaping, they are generally stronger than thermoplastic polymers and have higher temperature stability. The most used thermosetting polymers in microfluidic devices are parylene, polyimide, and polyurethane.

Parylene

Parylene has a para-xylylene backbone and is commercially available in the forms of basic N (poly-para-xylylene) or C and D that have one and two chlorine atom replaced in their benzene backbone, respectively. Parylene has been widely used in fabrication of microchannels (Man, Jones, & Mastrangelo, 1997; Webster & Mastrangelo, 1997), microvalves (Carlen & Mastrangelo, 2002; Chen, 2007; Rich & Wise, 1999; Wang, Lin, & Tai, 1999), membrane filters (Yang et al., 1998), peel-off masks for protein and cell micropatterning (Delivopoulos, Murray, Macleod, & Curtis, 2009; Ilic & Craighead, 2000; Jinno et al., 2008; Tan, Cipriany, Lin, & Craighead, 2010; Wright et al., 2008; Wright, Rajalingam, Selvarasah, Dokmeci, & Khademhosseini, 2007, 2008), functionalized coated surfaces for 3D patterning of proteins (Chen & Lahann, 2005), spatially-selective coating of microchannels for surface functionalizing (Chen, Elkasabi, & Lahann, 2006; Chen & Lahann, 2007), microelectronic circuits (Lin & Wong, 1992; Olson, 1989), biological sample encapsulations (Nosal et al., 2009), dielectric interlayers (Selbrede & Zucker, 1997),wire bond enforcement (Flaherty, 1995) in microchip packaging, tunable microlens array and as a flexible microfluidic device as a composite with PDMS (Fallahi, Zhang, Phan, & Nguyen, 2019). Readers are referred to articles by Tan and Craighead (2010), and Fallahi et al. (2019), for more elaborate review of parylene applications.

Fabrication of microfluidic devices using parylene Parylene has a high molecular weight, and its structure is linear and highly crystalline; therefore, it cannot be molded (high T_g) in a process similar to PDMS. As a result, it can only be vapor deposited in the form of thin conformal layers (Gorham, 1966) with an inherent hydrophobic property (surface free energy of 19.6 mN/m). Deposition is done through thermal sublimation of dimers at 140–160°C (in furnace), vapor phase splitting into monomers at 680°C (in pyrolysis chamber), and conformal deposition (Lee et al., 1995) and polymerization on the surfaces under vacuum at room temperature (in deposition chamber).

Complex structures can be microfabricated after parylene deposition using surface (Fig. 1.11(a)) (Webster, Burke, Burns, & Mastrangelo, 1998) and bulk (Tacito & Steinbruchel, 1996) micromachining as well as micromolding (Fig. 1.11(b)) (Noh, Huang, & Hesketh, 2004a) techniques. Since it is resistant against solvents, it can be used in lithographic processes as the main structural layer (using patterned photoresist as sacrificial layers, Fig. 1.11(a)) or can be dry etched in oxygen- and/or fluorine-based plasmas.

Similar to many other materials, various applications require high aspect ratio and microscopic structures fabricated in parylene (few examples listed in Table 1.4).

Interconnection and bonding Interconnection to parylene-based micro and nano-fluidic channels has been achieved using a variety of methods. Peeled off parylene

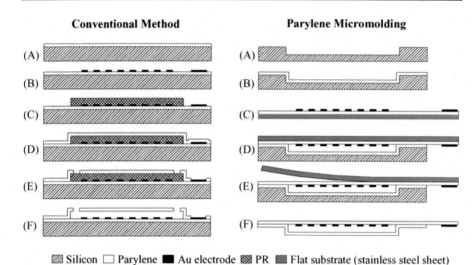

Figure 1.11 Parylene microfabrication, (a) Surface micromachining: parylene deposition, electrode patterning, photolithography, 2nd parylene deposition and photoresist etch away, (b) micromolding: substrate etching, parylene deposition, electrode patterning, 2nd parylene lamination, and base peel off.
Permission Noh et al. (2004a).

Table 1.4 Minimum feature sizes (MFS) and maximum aspect ratios (AR) fabricated in Parylene.

Fabrication method	MFS (μm)	AR	References
O_2 and Ar ICP[a]	6	9	Selvarasah et al. (2008)
DRIE-based Si molds, parylene deposition, and release by Si wet etching	10	10–30	Suzuki and Tai (2003, 2006)
DRIE Si etching, parylene deposition, and back plasma release etching	20	10	Zoumpoulidis, Bartek, Graaf, and Dekker (2009)

[a]ICP: Inductively Coupled Plasma, DRIE: Deep Reactive-Ion Etching

channels were punched by needles and polyimide-coated silica microtube were attached and epoxy glued to them withstanding up to 0.2 SCCM water flows (Noh et al., 2004a). Photocurable adhesives have also been used for interfacing parylene microtubes to microfluidic reservoirs (Ilic, Czaplewski, Zalalutdinov, Schmidt, & Craighead, 2002). In order to interface surface micromachined parylene channels, SU-8 anchors housing multiple PDMS sockets at the end of the parylene channel were used that each received a syringe needle horizontally as the interconnects (Lo & Meng, 2011). Most of these methods tend to fail at high flow or high pressure conditions making interconnection to parylene devices a more difficult task compared with PDMS.

Bonding of parylene to other materials is somewhat more challenging due to the strong chemical backbone structure of this material; however, a number of bonding methods have been introduced (Rezai et al., 2011) that are listed in Table 1.5. Here are the most popular methods used for parylene bonding to other materials:

Silanization: Parylene adhesion to silicon oxide and nitride layers as well as metals such as Au, Cr, and Ti was enhanced by using a surface silanization pretreatment step. However, this method was not as effective in bonding parylene to Silicon and Al.

Plasma treatment: Similar to PDMS-based bonding methods discussed before, surface plasma treatment (using Ar, CH_4, O_2. SF_6, and N_2 gases) of various surfaces (Parylene, PTFE, PP, PE, PMMA, glass, SiO_2, Si_3N_4, PDMS, Au, and Pt as the most widely used materials), followed by an immediate parylene deposition process, has been extensively studied and used for bonding purposes (Ciftlik & Gijs, 2011, 2012; Hassler, Metzen, Ruther, & Stieglitz, 2010; Rezai et al., 2011; Sharma & Yasuda, 1982). Plasma treatment of parylene results in etching a thin layer off the surface and a subsequent exposure of active nucleation sites that can enhance bonding. Hassler et al. (2010) used oxygen plasma treatment to successfully bond parylene to itself, Si_3N_4 and Pt as an encapsulation material for neural prostheses. In this study, oxygen plasma exposure alone was ineffective in bonding parylene to Si_3N_4 and Pt and a pretreatment with silane A-174 before deposition was required. In the study by Sharma and Yasuda (1982), it has been reported that Ar and CH_4 plasma treatments are more effective in bonding parylene to several other materials (Table 1.5) than that of O_2 plasma due to generation of more radical species on the surfaces for covalent bonding to parylene.

Most of the plasma-based methods introduced above are followed immediately by parylene deposition without breaking the vacuum pressure conditions of the chamber. With this, it is not possible to perform post-parylene-deposition processes such as patterning of the surfaces. Rezai et al. (2011) introduced a method to bond already cured PDMS and parylene surfaces together using a plasma enhanced method. With this, fabrication of dual-material PDMS-parylene microchannels in an easy way without a need for sacrificial layers was made possible.

Thermomechanical: Another method that has been widely used for parylene bonding is the application of heat and compressive forces mostly in order to bond already deposit parylene layers to other surfaces such as nitrides and oxides. This is useful when patterning of the parylene layer is required before bonding such as fabrication of microfluidic channels (Ciftlik & Gijs, 2011, 2012). The heat can be generated externally or internally on the chip by using reactive multilayer Ni/Al foils for exothermic reaction−based heat generation (Qiu et al., 2009). This method has been widely applied to bonding silicon wafers to each other by the application of a parylene interfacial layer (Kim & Najafi, 2005).

Applications and future trends Parylene is inherently hydrophobic. The hydrophobicity can be enhanced by buffered hydrofluoric acid (BHF) and HF exposure or changed to hydrophilicity by chromium etchant or oxygen plasma (Hwang et al.,

Table 1.5 Parylene bonding to various materials (Rezai et al., 2011) Permission.

Parylene bonded to	Bond quality	Evaluation method	Bonding method	Parameters	Description	References
PTFE[a], PP[b], PE[c], PMMA, glass	4–5 (ANSI/ASTM D3354-76)	Qualitative 0–5 scale, 5 being best bonding	Argon and methane plasma	Plasma treatment was followed by direct parylene layer deposition	Thin hydrocarbon formed after exposure	Sharma and Yasuda (1982)
Parylene	3.6 MPa	Tensile	Thermocompressive	Heat + 0.1 MPa pressure	For bonding Si wafers	Kim and Najafi (2005)
PDMS	1.7 MPa	Tensile	SF_6 and N_2 plasma		Parts fabricated, then bonded, interface bond stronger than PDMS itself	Rezai et al. (2011)
Au, PI Si_3N_4, Pt	Weak 1000 mN/cm	Peel test: Bond strength (mN/cm) = peel force/ sample width	Oxygen plasma and dispersion in the silane A-174 before deposition	Effect of annealing, deposition pressure and steam sterilization after deposition was studied	Enhanced 3 magnitude orders just by silane	Hassler et al. (2010)
Parylene C	2000 mN/cm				Generally strong, PO distracting bond	
Parylene	Strong	Qualitative	Thermocompressive	545 K heat + 1.1 kPa pressure	Reactive multilayer Ni/Al foils	Qiu et al. (2009)
SiO_2	10 MPa	Tensile	O_2 plasma + Thermocompression	200W, 15 s + 280°C–100 KPa, 40 min	Should start bonding with 1 h after plasma	Ciftlik and Gijs (2011)
Si_3N_4	23 MPa	Tensile	O_2 plasma + Thermocompression	200W, 15 s + 280°C–100 KPa, 40 min	Should start bonding with 1 h after plasma	Ciftlik and Gijs (2012)

[a]Polytetrafluoroethylene.
[b]polypropylene.
[c]polyethylene.

Materials and methods for microfabrication of microfluidic devices

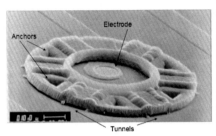 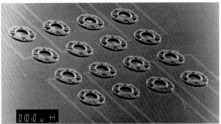

Figure 1.12 Scanning electron microscope (SEM) pictures of (a) a single and (b) an array of microfabricated neurocages made out of 4 μm of parylene integrated with electrodes. Cages were used to study neuronal signaling actuated by electrical stimuli. Scale bars = 10 μm. Permission Erickson et al. (2008).

2004) exposure. Due to vacuum-based fabrication process and lack of initiators and catalysts in parylene polymerization, chemically pure parylene layers can be deposited. Room temperature deposition process leads to formation of mechanical stress-free layers with no pin-holes (useful for PDMS coating for long gas permeability (Lei, Liu, Wang, Wu, & Li, 2011)) and good dielectric breakdown properties especially below 1 μm. As opposed to other porous polymers such as PDMS, parylene has low gas permeability (moisture vapor permeability of 1.7×10^{-16} kg-m/N.s) and a well stability against organic solvents. Parylene is also optically transparent (low optical absorption above 280 nm wavelengths) with a low autofluorescence behavior (Sasaki, Onoe, Osaki, Kawano, & Takeuchi, 2010) as well as chemically and biologically inert (Chang et al., 2007; Tooker, Meng, Erickson, Tai, & Pine, 2005) that makes it an ideal material for biomicrofluidic and biomedical applications. Using these fabrication processes, parylene-based devices have been used for DNA separation (Webster, Burke, Burns, & Mastrangelo, 1998), PCR (Man, Jones, & Mastrangelo, 1997), cochlear implants (Bell, Wise, & Anderson, 1997), biochemical reactions (Brahmasandra et al., 1998), biological materials surfaces protection (Nosal et al., 2009), microvalves for drug delivery (Carlen & Mastrangelo, 2002; Rich & Wise, 1999), electroosmotic pumping (Freire, Yang, Luk, & O'brien, 2011), microneedles, microtubes (Ilic et al., 2002), microchannels (Chen, Shih, & Tai, 2006), 3D microfluidic mixers (Liu et al., 2008), and neurocages (Fig. 1.12) (Erickson, Tooker, Tai, & Pine, 2008). Although the properties of parylene make it suitable for some applications especially that require chemical inertness, minimal adsorption or electrical insulation, the lack of a simple yet strong bonding and interconnection method has prevented its continued widespread use in rapid prototyping of a wide variety of microfluidic devices.

Polyimide
PI is the thermosetting plastic and exhibits very low creep and high tensile strength compared to other thermoplastics. PI also has an excellent thermal stability ($T_g > 400°C$) and chemical resistance, thus it has been used as the insulation film in the flexible printed circuit board (PCB) for the electronics industry, and adhesive and photoresist in the semiconductor industry (Fig. 1.13).

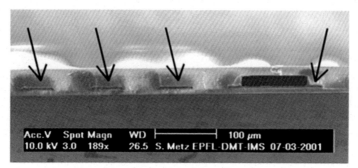

Figure 1.13 Cross section of a polyimide device with three adjacent interconnection lines (left side) and a microchannel (width 100 μm, height 20 μm) with an electrode inside the channel (right side).
Metz et al. (2001) -Reproduced by permission of The Royal Society of Chemistry.

Due to PI's photosensitive property, structural features can be fabricated in them using conventional photolithography processes which is a significant advantage. Open microfluidic channel structures using PI can be micromachined by direct structuring techniques like laser ablation (Khan Malek, 2006; Yin, 2004), hot embossing (Youn et al., 2008), dry etching (Mimoun, Pham, Vincent, & Dekker, 2013; Nguyen & Lee, 2007), or photolithography (Lake, Cambron, Walsh, & McNamara, 2011; Metz, Trautmann et al., 2004; Metz et al., 2001) and subsequently closed by laminating a cover layer. Various lamination techniques have been developed to fabricate PI-based microfluidic devices. For instance, solvent bonding (Glasgow, Beebe, & White, 1999) was used to laminate a PI microstructured layer between two wafers. Similarly, a thin layer of PI precursor as adhesive can be used for PI bonding (Mangriotis et al., 1999; Metz et al., 2001). This was taken further with partially cured PI being studied as a substrate material for etching. Two of these layers could then be bonded together using the unlinked chains to form a stronger bond than was possible through using cured PI (Zulfiqar, Pfreundt, Svendsen, & Dimaki, 2015).

Alternatively, microfluidic channels can be made by applying surface micromachining techniques which use sacrificial resist layers embedded in PI to form microchannels. The sacrificial layer is then removed by solvent dissolution (Man et al., 1997), dry etching (Bagolini et al., 2002), or heating (Metz, Jiguet, Bertsch, & Renaud, 2004; Suh, Bharathi, Beebe, & Moore, 2000) to reveal the microchannel structure. Materials like silicon oxide, metals, and photoresists have been used as sacrificial layers for the construction of PI microchannels although this method usually is a time-consuming process especially when fabricating submicron channels where dissolution is limited by diffusion.

Due to its mechanical flexibility and good adhesion to metal layers, PI has been already widely used in flexible PCBs such as DuPont Kapton. In a similar vein, PI has been used to make flexible microfluidic devices with embedded electronic circuits such as neural electrode (Kato et al., 2012), microfluidic mass spectrometry (Spectrometry et al., 2010, pp. 605–607), bioelectric activity monitoring (Metz et al., 2004), liquid flow sensor (Kuoni et al., 2003), impedance spectroscopy flow cytometer (Gawad, Schild, & Renaud, 2001), and for building implantable microprobes (Phan et al., 2019).

Polyurethane

PU is a polymer composed of a chain of organic units joined by urethane links. Because urethane is available in a broad hardness range, PU can be synthesized to offer the specific elasticity combined with the toughness and durability. Therefore, its mechanical properties are superior, namely higher tensile strength (62 MPa), Young's modulus (55 MPa), and hardness (94 Shore A). It has density (1.15 g/cc) and melting point (215.5°C) similar to PDMS. Its dielectric constant is similar to that of PDMS, and it performs well as an insulator. PU is commercially available either in pellet or sheet as raw materials from various manufacturers (Fig. 1.14).

Traditionally, solvent molding techniques such as vertical dipping, rotating mandrel, and rotating plate are used to fabricate PU parts such as sheets, membranes, and tubing. The rotating plate method is used for fabricating PU films and sheets, while vertical dipping and rotating mandrel are used for fabricating cylindrical parts, like tubing. However, these fabrication techniques are not suitable for replicating the

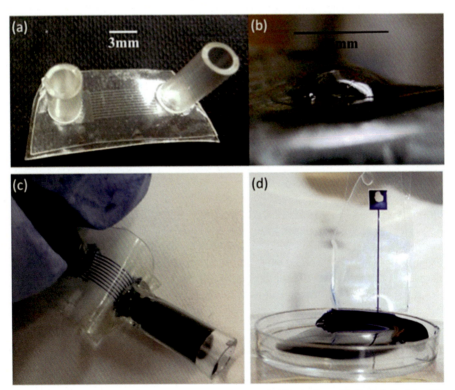

Figure 1.14 Photos of polyurethane (PU)-based microfluidic devices. (a) Sealed device with integrated interconnect, (b) a deflected PU membrane under a pressure of 200 kPa (⌀5 mm and membrane thickness = 25 μm), (c) a flexible and bendable device with colored microchannels for visualization, (d) self-priming microchannel (4 cm × 500 mm × 80 mm) filled with deionized water (dyed with methylene blue) due to its hydrophilicity.
Wu et al. (2012)—Reproduced by permission of The Royal Society of Chemistry.

intricate and detailed microscale features present in microfluidics devices. PU-based microfabrication typically involves injection molding (Folch, Mezzour, & Du, 2000; Kuo et al., 2009), hot embossing (Shen et al., 2006), imprinting (Xu et al., 2000), plasma etching (Rossier et al., 2002), sacrificial material (Haraldsson et al., 2006), and reaction polymerization (Haraldsson et al., 2006; Kim, Lee, & Hammond, 2003; Kuo et al., 2009; Piccin et al., 2007; Thorsen et al., 2001). These methods are not suited for rapid prototyping as they use high-cost intermediate molds and expensive fabrication equipment. Furthermore, the substrates produced are rigid and not transparent. Solvent casting is more suitable since intermediate molds can be fabricated using photolithography and the fabrication equipment is low cost (Wu et al., 2012).

To achieve irreversible bonding, semicured parts of PU have been placed in contact and heated above the glass transition temperature causing fusion of the two parts (Kuo et al., 2009; Piccin et al., 2007). However, this method is not suitable for retaining the fine structural features needed in microchannels. Recently, dry and wet bonding methods using plasma treatment and solvent welding have been developed to overcome this issue. A highest bonding strength of 326.4 kPa using wet bonding was reported (Wu et al., 2012).

PU, since its development in the 1930s (Brash, Fritzinger, & Bruck, 1973; Lyman et al., 1971), has been widely used in various blood-contact applications such as the artificial heart (Lyman et al., 1971), intraaortic balloons (Brash, Fritzinger, & Bruck, 1973), pacemaker leads (Devanathan, Sluetz, & Young, 1980), heart valves (Tsutsui, Imamura, & Kayanagi, 1981), and hemodialysis membranes (Lyman, Seare, & Albo, 1977). Hydrophobic surfaces are essentially water repellent and provoke adverse reactions in blood contact. Many studies have shown that the blood compatibility of polyurethanes can be improved by making the surface more hydrophilic (Takahara, Tashita, & Kajiyama, 1985). A number of in-vivo and in-vitro studies have been carried out to assess the cellular and tissue responses of PU either subcutaneously, intramuscularly, or intraperitoneally (Akiyama et al., 1997; Bakker et al., 1990; Bruin et al., 1993; Han et al., 1992; Marois et al., 1989, 1993, 1996; Okoshi et al., 1992; van der Giessen et al., 1996; Watkinson et al., 1995; Wu et al., 2012). PU-based microchip electrophoresis has also been tested with various analytes to evaluate its separation performance (Piccin et al., 2007). Due to its excellent hardness, high aspect ratio (~ 3.5) microstructure made from PU can be easily fabricated and bonded while microstructures made from PDMS are too soft to stand their own weight. These microstructures were then used as microfluidic filters to separate or concentrate the targeted particles or cells (Kuo et al., 2009). The other main advantage of PU over other polymers is its feasibility to be chemically tailored for specific applications, thus it has been widely used in applications like cell culture, tissue scaffolds (Folch, Mezzour, & Du, 2000; Moraes et al., 2009; Shen et al., 2006; Vermette et al., 2001).

1.3.3.3 Thermoplastic polymers

Thermoplastic polymers are polymers that can be easily molded using thermoforming processes such as hot embossing, injection molding, extrusion, etc, and can be easily recast into a new shape by reheating to a temperature above the glass transition temperature. As a result, these polymers tend to have low temperature stability but allow easier machinability and mass production. The common thermoplastic polymers used in microfluidic devices are PMMA, polycarbonate, and cyclic olefin polymers/co-polymers (COC/COP).

PMMA

PMMA is a rigid transparent thermoplastic material that undergoes phase transition to a viscoelastic state above $T_g = 105°C$ (Ucar, Akova, & Aysan, 2012). Accordingly, it is well suited for mass industrial production and due to its excellent chemical, mechanical, and optical properties (Table 1.1), it has recently attracted considerable attention in the medical (orthopedics (Jaeblon, 2010)) and biological (Chen, Svec, & Knapp, 2008) applications for the analysis of DNA (Chen & Chen, 2000; Sassi, Paulus, Cruzado, Bjornson, & Hooper, 2000); amino acids, peptides, and proteins (Wainright et al., 2002; Xue, Wainright, Gangakhedkar, & Gibbons, 2001); saccharine (Dang et al., 2006); pollutants and explosives (Wang, Pumera, Collins, & Mulchandani, 2002); and ions and organic acids (Pumera et al., 2002). Some review papers (Becker & Gartner, 2000; Chen, Svec, & Knapp, 2008; Fiorini & Chiu, 2005; Jaeblon, 2010) have been published with more elaborate information on PMMA fabrication methods, bonding, and applications.

Fabrication of microfluidic devices using PMMA The cost of manufacturing PMMA-based products is relatively low as compared to silicon and glass. Various methods described in microfabrication methods section have been used to develop single layer PMMA parts bonded to other materials or PMMA itself for the purpose of forming microfluidic devices. These methods include hot embossing (Martynova et al., 1997), room-temperature imprinting (Xu, Locascio, Gaitan, & Lee, 2000), injection molding (McCormick, Nelson, Alonso-Amigo, Benvegnu, & Hooper, 1997; Piotter, Hanemann, Ruprecht, & Hausselt, 1997), laser ablation (Chen, Li, & Shen, 2016; Sun, Kwok, & Nguyen, 2006), in situ polymerization (Chen et al., 2003, 2008), solvent etching (Chen, Lin, & Chen, 2007) thoroughly reviewed by Chen, Svec, & Knapp (2008). In the hot embossing method, a substrate containing the microfluidic network design as protruded features is used, and a PMMA plate is embossed against it at elevated temperatures ($>T_g = 105°C$) and pressures. Fig. 1.15 illustrates a high surface area PMMA-based microfluidic device fabricated by X-ray lithography and used for extraction of DNA by testing various postfeatures in a microchannel (Reedy et al., 2011).

Some of the smallest feature sizes and highest aspect ratios achieved in fabrication of PMMA microdevices are listed in Table 1.6.

PMMA interconnection and bonding In addition to conventional interconnection methods described in other sections, world-to-chip interfacing into PMMA microfluidic devices has been achieved through an adhesive-free in-plane interconnection method (Sabourin, Dufva, Jensen, Kutter, & Snakenborg, 2010). The connection is made by press-fit interconnection of oversized deformable tubes into PMMA and their UV-assisted bonding. Capillaries and optical fibers have also been interconnected with

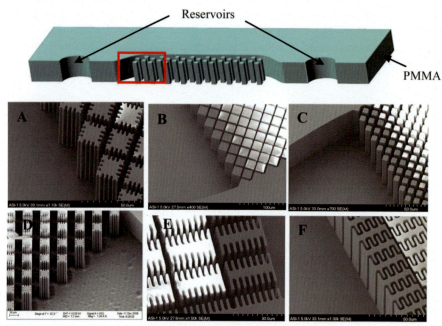

Figure 1.15 Schematic of the Poly(methyl methacrylate) (PMMA) microchannel for DNA extraction (Dimensions: 1 cm long channel, 800 μm wide, and 50 μm deep) with various post designs shown (Scanning electron microscope (SEM) images of the red box) in A-F. (a) 14 μm square posts with ∼3 μm extensions with 4 μm distance between posts. (b) 22 μm square posts with 4 μm distance between posts. (c) 8 μm square posts with 4 μm distance between posts. (d) similar to design (a) but with 17 μm between each post. (e) 6 μm × 30 μm posts with 8 μm extensions. (f) 6 μm × 30 μm posts with 5 μm extensions.
Permission Reedy et al. (2011).

Table 1.6 Minimum feature sizes (MFS) and maximum aspect ratios (AR) fabricated in PMMA.

Fabrication method	MFS (μm)	AR	References
E-beam lithography	0.16	7	Gorelick, Guzenko, Vila-Comamala, and David (2010)
Lithographie, Galvanoformung, Abformung (LIGA)	5	10	Reedy et al. (2011)
LIGA	8	19	Becker and Heim (2000)
LIGA	24	24	Zhang et al. (2018)

PMMA channels (Hartmann et al., 2008) by in-plane insertion into the channel and usage of UV-curable glues to fix them on the device.

Direct and indirect bonding methods have been used for fabricating enclosed PMMA microdevices. Direct bonding includes thermal fusion bonding (Martynova et al., 1997), local welding by ultrasonic (Truckenmuller, Ahrens, Cheng, Fischer, & Saile, 2006) or microwave energy (Lei, Ahsan, Budraa, Li, & Mai, 2004), and solvent bonding (Shah et al., 2006; Wang et al., 2002). Bond strength as high as 23.5 MPa has been reported for PMMA using the solvent bonding method (Hsu & Chen, 2007). In the indirect bonding method which is simpler, an additional glue or epoxy layer is required to facilitate bonding of PMMA to itself or to other materials (Becker & Gartner, 2000; Chen et al., 2005). However, the challenge is not to clog the microchannels with the gluing material which has been avoided by techniques to control wetting tension between the UV-curable adhesive and the surface of substrate such as screen printing (Han, 2003), or microcontact printing (Dang, 2005). PMMA bonding to PDMS and parylene have already been discussed in PDMS and parylene sections. Other bonding methods for PMMA have been summarized in the two review articles (Chen, Svec, & Knapp, 2008; Tsao & DeVoe, 2009).

PMMA is low cost and easy to form for developing microfluidic devices with exceptional mechanical, optical, and chemical properties (Table 1.1). Extreme hydrophobicity due to the lack of ionizable functional groups in PMMA has limited its application and led to the development of various surface modification processes. They have been categorized (Chen, Svec, & Knapp, 2008) into covalent modifications for the formation of amine-terminated surfaces (Henry et al., 2000), dynamic coating with charged surfactants or hydrophilic neutral polymers (Dang, Zhang, Hagiwara, Mishina, & Baba, 2003), and bulk modification (Wang et al., 2005) of the polymer during the fabrication process by copolymerization of monomers. Postfabrication modification by coating the surface with silicon nanoparticles followed by silanization has been shown to form a superhydrophilic layer that enables long-term surfactant free operation of the device (Ortiz, Chen, Stuckey, & Steele, 2017).

Polycarbonate

PCs are one of the thermoplastic polymers which can be easily molded using thermoforming processes. The major advantages of PC over other plastics are its ultimate strength (~ 2.0 GPa) and transparency throughout the visible spectrum down until 400 nm. It is not as chemically inert as plastics. For instance, organic solvents like acetone and ammonia are not compatible with PC. Its high refractive index ($n = 1.58$) make it attractive for optical applications. PC has a glass transition temperature of 145°C which is usually sufficient for most biological microfluidic applications such as PCR thermal cycling (Fig. 1.16).

Microfabrication methods for PC can be categorized as direct structuring like laser ablation (Lin, Wen, Fan, Matson, & Smith, 1999; Suriyage, Ghantasala, Iovenitti, &

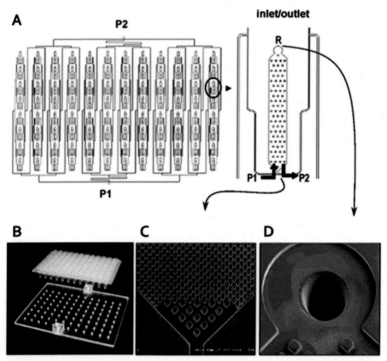

Figure 1.16 Layout of the polycarbonate plate-based microfluidic platform. (a) Schematics of the microfluidic device, P1 and P2 are the control ports and R is the sample inlet/outlet reservoirs. (b) Photography of the polycarbonate microfluidic plate and a commercial 96-well titer plate. (c−d) Scanning electron microscope (SEM) images at the entrance and exit section with a 150 μm bed entrance hole drilled using laser.
(Witek et al., 2008)—Reproduced by permission of Journal of Analytical chemistry.

Harvey, 2004; Waddell, 2002) with a width over 50 μm and an aspect ratio up to 10, and micromilling (Ogonczyk et al., 2010) with a diameter over 30 μm and an aspect ratio up to 1, or replication methods such as injection molding (Attia et al., 2009; Becker & Locascio, 2002; Chang, Chang, Chau, & Chen, 2005; Gottschlich, 2004; Griffiths, Dimov, Brousseau, & Hoyle, 2007; Ruprecht et al., 1995), and hot embossing (Liu et al., 2001; Ye, Yin, & Fang, 2005) with a width over 40 μm and an aspect ratio up to 2. An extensive review of microfabrication methods for PC can be found elsewhere (Attia et al., 2009; Becker and Gärtner, 2008; Becker & Locascio, 2002; Jensen et al., 2004).

Various bonding methods have been used in the fabrication of PC microfluidic devices, and they can be classified into thermal, chemical, and adhesive methods. Thermal processes (Chen et al., 2005; Ogonczyk et al., 2010; Park, Hupert et al., 2008; Park, Lee et al., 2008; Yang et al., 2002) use compression under a temperature around its glass transition temperature for bonding slabs or thin foils and results in an average bonding strength of 0.55 MPa. Chemical bonding induced by the modification of surface chemistry can be achieved by the plasma treatment (Klintberg et al., 2003;

Wang et al., 2008) or the introduction of active surface groups (Lee & Ram, 2009), and shows a highest bonding strength of over 6.8 MPa. Alternatively, there are some commercial glues or adhesives that can be used to create a strong bonding as well.

Due to its higher glass transition temperature and low manufacturing cost, PC is an ideal material for fabrication of disposal devices and has been used in several biomedical and bioanalytical applications such as PCR (Chan et al., 2008; Cooney, 2012; Hashimoto, 2004; Liu et al., 2001; Peham, 2012; Yang et al. 2002).

COC/COP

Both COCs and COPs are amorphous polymers produced by chain copolymerization of cyclic monomers. Typically, COC and COP have glass-like transparency (>90%) in near UV, high tensile strength (46–63 MPa), high moisture resistance (<0.01%), good chemical resistance to acids, bases, and polar solvents (Topas Advanced Polymers, 2012), and high dielectric constant (30 kV/mm) (Lamonte & Mcnally, 2001). They are commercially available either in pellet, solution, or sheet forms from various manufacturers (Fig. 1.17).

Similar to other polymers, fabrication methods for COC/COP can be categorized as direct structuring methods such as laser ablation (Bundgaard, Perozziello, & Geschke, 2006; Cai et al., 2017; Jensen et al., 2004; Sabbert, Bauer, & Ehrfeld, 1999, pp. 185–189) and micromilling (Bundgaard et al., 2006; Grumann et al., 2006) or replication methods such as injection molding (Angelov & Coulter, 2008; Appasamy et al., 2005; Ito, Kazama, & Kikutani, 2007; Kalima, 2007; Lee, 2005; Pakkanen et al., 2002; Schütte et al., 2010; Steigert et al., 2007), hot embossing (Aghvami et al., 2017; Bhattacharyya

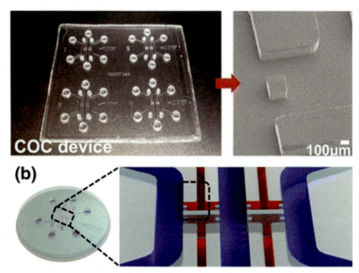

Figure 1.17 (a) Photograph of 4 cyclic olefin copolymers (COC) device array and scanning electron microscope (SEM) of the post (left) and channel structure of a device (right). (b) A single device schematic with the gel area expanded shows the SEM image area outlined . Jeon et al., 2011—Reproduced by permission of Journal of Biomedical Microdevices.

& Klapperich, 2006; Faure, 2008; Fredrickson et al., 2006; Illa et al., 2009; Kameoka et al., 2001; Liu et al., 2007; Park, Hupert et al., 2008; Park, Lee et al., 2008; Yang et al., 2005), and nanoimprint lithography (Bilenberg et al., 2005; Gourgon et al., 2005; Gustafsson, Mogensen, & Kutter, 2008; Nilsson, Balslev, & Kristensen, 2005).

A bonding step is essential for the fabrication of microfluidic systems which usually require sealed microchannels to prevent sample contamination and evaporation. Use of adhesives or glues is one of the most common bonding techniques for polymers. UV adhesives (Do & Ahn, 2008) have been demonstrated to bond COP parts together at room temperature to form a microfluidic chip with a bonding strength of 2 MPa. Thermal bonding is also commonly used for thermoplastic polymers such as COP (Bedair & Oleschuk, 2006; Bhattacharyya & Klapperich, 2006; Choi, Kim, & Kwon, 2008; Gustafsson, Mogensen, & Kutter, 2008; Kameoka et al., 2001; Kim et al., 2006; Mair, Geiger, Albert, Fréchet, & Svec, 2006; Nilsson et al., 2005; Yang et al., 2005; Wallow, 2007) which is heated above its glass transition temperature to allow the polymer chains to diffuse between the mating surfaces thus promoting adhesion. No quantitative study of the bonding strength had been investigated due to the low surface energy of thermoplastics. Oxygen plasma (Kettner et al., 2006) and UV/ozone (Tsao, Hromada, Liu, Kumar, & DeVoe, 2007) treatments were then used to activate surfaces and improve the bonding strength of COP substrates up to 0.8 mJ/cm^2 under specific bonding conditions (Tsao et al., 2007). Solvent bonding, also known as solvent welding, can also be used to temporarily dissolve the surfaces of COP, enable the mobility of polymer chains across the bonding interface, and thus results in the highest bonding strength of 10 MPa (Aghvami et al., 2017; Chen, Svec, & Knapp, 2008; Faure, 2008; Kettner et al., 2006; Liu et al., 2007; Ro, Liu, & Knapp, 2006; Tsao et al., 2007; Tsao, Liu, & DeVoe, 2008; Wallow, 2007).

Due to its surface properties and optical transparency, COP-based microchip electrophoresis provides faster separations and easier integration of sample preparation (Blas, Delaunay, & Rocca, 2008; Sueyoshi, Kitagawa, & Otsuka, 2008) and optical detection (Bliss et al., 2007; Hurth, Lenigk, & Zenhausern, 2008; Mogensen et al., 2001), than traditional capillary electrophoresis. Compared to other polymers, COP-based microchips usually have lower background fluorescence and higher electrophoretic efficiency (Yi, Xiaodong, & Fan, 2008). COP-based microchannels have also been used in solid phase extraction where either the interested analytes or the undesired impurities are retained by the stationary phase (Gustafsson, Mogensen, & Kutter, 2008; Illa et al., 2009). Moreover, COP-based electrospray emitters have been used for mass spectrometry where the ionized analytes are separated depending on their interaction with external electric and/or magnetic fields (Kameoka et al., 2002; Yang et al., 2004; Yang, Li, & Lee, 2005; Park, Lee, & Craighead, 2008; Shinohara et al., 2008). Since COP is relatively transparent compared to other polymers at shorter wavelengths (240–360 nm), it can be used as optical components such as microlenses (Appasamy et al., 2005), photonic crystals (Bilenberg et al., 2004), and optical waveguides (Okagbare, 2010). Because of its moisture resistance and adhesion to metallic films, COP can be applied as substrates for blood contacting (Choi et al., 2008; Grumann et al., 2006; Jang et al., 2006; Kim et al., 2006) and DNA analysis applications (Bhattacharyya & Klapperich, 2006; Castaño-Alvarez, Fernández-Abedul, &

Materials and methods for microfabrication of microfluidic devices

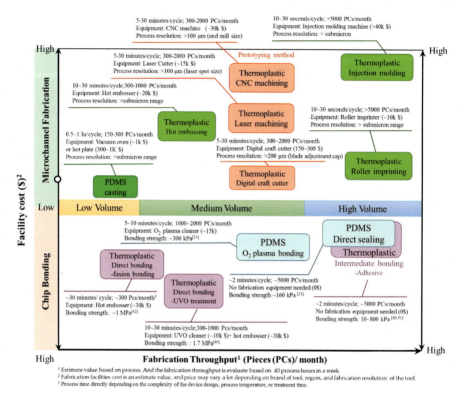

Figure 1.18 Fabrication and bonding techniques for mass fabrication (Tsao, 2016).

Costa-García, 2007; Gulliksen et al., 2005; Hurth et al., 2008; Larsen, Poulsen, Birgens, Martin, & Kristensen, 2008).

A summary of different fabrication and bonding methods for use with thermoplastics and their rates of production when scaling up for mass fabrication are shown in Fig. 1.18.

1.3.4 Paper

Paper, usually as a cellulose fiber network, can spontaneously generate the capillary flow to transport aqueous liquids due to its porosity and hydrophilicity. This self-pumping/priming mechanism makes it an attractive substrate for use in low cost microfluidic devices for diagnostic applications if a method to direct and control the flow of fluid can be devised. The velocity of motions in the paper-based microfluidic channels are determined by many factors such as the pore size, porosity, surface energy of paper as well as the viscosity of liquid and can be estimated by the well-known Lucas—Washburn equation (Anbuhi et al., 2012). The first paper based microfluidic device was presented by Muller and coworkers who patterned paraffin boundary on paper to speed up the elution of a pigment mixture (Müller & Clegg, 1949). Recently, with the advancement of micromachining technologies, Whitesides Group of Harvard University has developed many novel patterning strategies with more delicately controlling of flowing path and flow rate (Martinez, Phillips, Butte, & Whitesides, 2007). Following these early works, many other channel patterning technologies have been investigated which can be categorized as follows: (i) photolithography (Martinez, Phillips, & Whitesides, 2008); (ii) plotting (Bruzewicz, Reches, & Whitesides, 2008); (iii) wax printing (Lu, Shi, Jiang, Qin, & Lin, 2009; Noiphung et al., 2013; de Tarso Garcia, Garcia Cardoso, Diego Garcia, Carrilho, & Tomazelli Coltro, 2014); (iv) surface treatments (Li, Tian, Nguyen, & Shen, 2008); (v) paper cutting (Wang, Wu, & Zhu, 2010), and most commonly inkjet printing/etching (Abe, Suzuki, & Citterio, 2008; Carrilho, Martinez, & Whitesides, 2009; Dixon, Ng, Ryan, Miltenburg, & Wheeler, 2016; Maejima, Tomikawa, Suzuki, & Citterio, 2013; Wang et al., 2014).

Except for cutting where the individual regions on the substrate are physically separated from each other, the fundamental mechanism for directing flow in paper has been through the creation of difference of hydrophobicity between channels (hydrophilic) and boundaries (hydrophobic) by patterning. Generally, the patterning can be accomplished by three different principles: (i) printing the hydrophobic materials (wax and PDMS) on paper as boundaries (photolithography and plotting); (ii) uniformly coating paper with hydrophobic materials (SU-8 and polystyrene) then used solvents to dissolve those materials and making channels and (iii) Applying chemicals to modify the surface hydroxide group on designed area of paper to make the hydrophobic boundaries. Table 1.7 lists some important performance parameters of each patterning technologies:

Most of the applications of paper-based microfluidic devices have been on developing low cost diagnostic devices. The ability to use patterning to fabricate microfluidic channels in paper to perform parallel analysis of various analytes was first demonstrated by Whitesides and coworkers (Martinez et al., 2007). Here, wax printing was used to pattern microfluidic channel network which enabled a urine sample at the inlet reservoir to be split into three segments for simultaneous analysis of glucose and proteins. Other reactants were patterned at the end of the respective microchannel

Table 1.7 The selected factors of paper micropatterning technologies.

Methods	Channel size (μm)	Barrier size (μm)	Reagents
Photolithography	186 ± 13	248 ± 13	SU-8
Inkjet etching	420 ± 50	N/A	Polystyrene
Plotting	1000	1000	Polydimethylsiloxane
Wax printing	561 ± 45	850 ± 50	Wax
Surface treatments	1500	N/A	Alkyl ketene dimer
Paper cutting	400[a]	N/A	N/A

[a]laser cutting; resolution depended on the type of paper Nie, 2012.

which produced a colorimetric assay when the sample arrived at that location due to capillary flow. The colorimetric paper based analytical devices have been extensively reviewed by Chao in 2008 (Zhao & van der Berg, 2008), Whitesides in 2010 (Martinez, Phillips, Whitesides, & Carrilho, 2009), and later by Cate et al. (Cate, Adkins, Mettakoonpitak, & Henry, 2015), and Carrell et al. (2019). Other than colorimetric detection, electrochemical (EC) (Dungchai, Chailapakul, & Henry, 2009), electrochemiluminescence (ECL) (Delaney, Hogan, Tian, & Shen, 2011), differential pulse voltammetry (DPV) (Ge et al., 2013), amperometric (Adkins, Noviana, & Henry, 2016) and electroimpedance spectroscopy (EIS) (Ge et al., 2013) have been used for detection in paper-based microfluidic devices. These sensing methods provide lower detecting limit (down to 0.2 nM (Ge et al., 2013)), higher accuracy, and shorter detection time than colorimetric methods. Recent developments in EC and ECL detection in paper-based microfluidic devices are reviewed by Li et al. in 2012 (Li, Ballerini, & Shen, 2012) and an overview of the different EC detection methods used was reviewed by Mettakoonpitak et al. (2016). Various unit operations such as hydrodynamic focusing (Fu, Lutz, Kauffman, & Yager, 2010), mixing (Rezk et al., 2012), dilution (Osborn et al., 2010), and separation (Osborn et al., 2010) have also been demonstrated in paper-based microfluidic devices. In addition, power sources on-chip that could power the unit operation have also been developed (Thom, Yeung, Pillion, & Phillips, 2012). Recently, paper-based devices have also been shown to be used for 3D cell culture (Li et al. 2012).

Paper is superior to other materials for making analytical microfluidic devices because of its properties of (1) low cost, (2) porous structure (for both self-driven capillary flow and reagent immobilization), (3) flexible (easy to pack and carry). However, the nonuniform nature of this cellulose fiber network and the time it takes to transport the sample in the microfluidic network combined with the inherent challenges of reproducibility and stability are the current challenges that are being worked on.

1.3.5 Thread

Threads made from cotton, silk, nylon, and polyester have been used as an alternative low cost microfluidic device with many of the same advantages as paper microfluidic devices such as using capillary forces to passively drive fluid motion through the device resulting in a low cost, portable package. While paper devices require patterning to direct motion of fluid and have a low wet strength, threads have a much higher wet strength and have been used both directly threaded through a plastic frame and as a patterned substrate. However, since they were first demonstrated by two different groups within months of each other (Reches et al., 2010; Li, Tian, & Shen, 2010), there was limited interest compared to paper microfluidic devices due to the larger number of variables that affect flow in threads. Flow in threads is governed by the Lucas—Washburn equation and is affected by pore size, porosity, surface energy, and viscosity of the fluid (Das, Das, Kothari, & Fangueiro, 2011). However, the pore size is nonuniform and is affected by the physical condition of the thread such as the tension it is under, the number of strings in the thread, and the number of twists of the string per inch of thread (tpi). The larger variety of materials available results in a wider range of surface energies to tune the thread to specific applications and to vary flow profiles within the thread (Berthier, Brakke, Gosselin, Berthier, & Navarro, 2017).

1.3.5.1 Patterning threads

Thread devices can broadly be classified into 1-D and 2-D devices depending on whether the thread is used by itself or after it has been woven into a plane.

A 1-D thread consists of numerous strings twisted together to drive capillary flow through the interstring space. Patterning of 1-D paper devices to act as valves was demonstrated using knots to modulate the pore size and porosity of the threads and hence alter fluid resistance (Safavieh, Zhou, & Juncker, 2011). This was used to control motion through a network of threads and control mixing of fluids in the network by reducing or redirecting flow through individual threads.

2-D thread based devices consist of threads interwoven among each other to create a flat plane. They have been patterned using several of the methods used in paper devices including photolithography (Wu & Zhang, 2015), wax screen printing (Liu, Zhang, & Liu, 2015), laser machining (Yang et al., 2017) and cutting. In addition, by leveraging the choice of materials available, devices have been patterned using a combination of hydrophobic and hydrophilic silk (Bhandari, Narahari, & Dendukuri, 2011) to create channels within the device that are hydrophilic and bounded by hydrophobic threads and to control flow rate by modulating channel resistance. Table 1.8 lists the variety of patterning methods and materials used for fabricating thread devices.

Table 1.8 Fabrication methods used for thread devices.

Patterning method	Material	Barrier to flow	Dimensions
Knots	Cotton	High hydraulic resistance knots	1D
Drop casting	Cotton	Wax	1D
Photolithography	Cotton	PVC (polyvinyl chloride) photoresist	2D
Weaving	Polyester	Hydrophobic threads	2D
Weaving	Silk	Hydrophobic threads	2D
Laser machining	Cellulose/Polyester blend Nylon	Fluoropolymer-coated thread	2D
Screen printing	Cotton	Wax	2D

1.3.5.2 Applications

The most common applications are in the detection of analytes for diagnostics or water quality monitoring using colorimetric sensing. Colorimetric sensing uses a testing reagent which senses the presence of a specific analyte in solution and responds with a visible color change. The degree of change in color is used as a marker for the concentration of the analyte in solution and is often measured using a paired camera or scanner. This was first using a 1D threads sewed into a plastic frame for simultaneous detection of ketone, nitrite, and bovine serum albumin (BSA) and for identification of glucose and alkaline phosphate in artificial urine (Safavieh et al., 2011). Similar detection methods were shown in 2D devices using photolithographically patterned devices for detection of glucose and BSA (Wu & Zhang, 2015). Full fledged immunoassays have been demonstrated on 1D threads for the detection of C-reactive protein (CRP) in buffers (Zhou, Safavieh, Mao, & Juncker, 2010); Rabbit IgG, CRP's, leptin, and osteopontin in diluted serum (Zhou, Mao, & Juncker, 2012); and carcinoembryonic antigen (CEA) (Jia, Song, Liu, Meng, & Mao, 2017).

Other sensing modalities that have been used on threads include EC sensing which has better resolution than colorimetric sensing led to the development of electrodes made using threads (Gaines, Gonzalez-Guerrero, Uchida, & Gomez, 2018) and devices that use cyclic voltammograms (CV's) and multiple pulse amperometry (MPA) for detection of acetaminophen (ACT) and diclofenac (DCF) (Agustini, Bergamini, & Marcolino-Junior, 2016). Capacitive contactless sensing which showed the combination of capillary electrophoresis with capacitive sensing on threads for separation of potassium, sodium, and lithium in solution (Quero, Bressan, Alberto Fracassi da Silva, & Pereira de Jesus, 2019). Flow rate sensing using a patterned 2D thread (Yang et al., 2017), strain, and pH sensors were also demonstrated (Mostafalu et al., 2016).

Threads are a versatile medium for low cost, multiplexed diagnostics due to the wide range of materials and formats possible, self-driving capillary flow, and easy transport. However, the large number of tuneable parameters has made it a challenging platform to work with compared with paper devices. Recent reviews by Weng, Kang, Guo, Peng, and Jiang (2019) and Farajikhah, Paull, Innis, Cabot, & Wallace (2019) provide excellent overviews of the sensing methods and fabrication techniques used on threads.

1.3.6 Pressure sensitive adhesives

PSAs were used to make fabrication of microfluidic devices more simple, faster, and inexpensive (Greer, Scott, Wittwer, & Gale, 2007; Serra et al., 2017; Shen, Chen, Guo, & Cheng, 2005) by eliminating most of the current microfabrication steps such as photolithography, etching, and bonding (Nath et al., 2010). However, particle absorption into the adhesive was found to be a challenge in some applications (Gale et al., 2018).

Adhesive are broadly categorized based on their backbone as acrylic, rubber, and silicone adhesives. The first PSAs were made from rubber. They are the cheapest adhesives and also have the simplest formulation (Creton, 2003). As natural rubber does not provide sufficient adhesion, it was blended with tackifier resins such as aliphatic or aromatic hydrocarbons and polyterpenes (Khan & Poh, 2011). Acrylic PSAs are mostly copolymers of a long side-chain acrylic such as n-butyl acrylate or 2-ethylhexyl acrylate with low glass transition temperature (Tg), a short side-chain acrylic like methyl acrylate and vinyl acetate for adjusting the T_g, and acrylic acid to provide better adhesion. A crosslinking step is generally done to improve the creep and resistance to cold flow (Creton, 2003). Silicone PSAs are typically composed of a polysiloxane (silicone) polymer and a silicate resin. The silicone polymer and silicate resin are dissolved in a nonpolar hydrocarbon solvent such as hexane (Tan & Pfister, 1999). Silicone PSAs have a variety of applications due to their high thermal stability, high oxidative stability, low surface energy, permeability to many gases, and biocompatibility (Melancon et al., 2004).

PSAs used in microfluidic fabrication are available in three types: transfer, one-sided, and double-sided tapes (Mohammadzadeh et al., 2018) and can be selected from companies such as 3M and Adhesives Research. Fig. 1.19 shows the cross section of these adhesive tapes. Transfer adhesives are completely made from adhesive material while double-sided tapes have a layer coated with adhesive on both sides. Transfer tapes are usually more suitable for thinner application such as biochemical and cellular assays but for thicker applications such as cell culture, double-sided tapes are better suited due to the slower perfusion of media needed over cells. In addition, several other parameters affect the choice of tape, such as the fabrication method, tape thickness, material properties, cost, and availability of the adhesive tape (Walsh III et al., 2017).

Cutting tools such as cutting plotter (i.e., xurography) and laser cutters are used for patterning PSA's (Walsh III et al., 2017; Yuen & Goral, 2010). An example of this process is shown in the work by Weigl et al. who fabricated a low-cost complex 3D microfluidic flow structure using laser cutter and lamination (Weigl, Bardell, Schulte, Battrell, & Hayenga, 2001). In another work, sheets of PSA coated mylar were used for fabricating a microfluidic mixer. They were cut using a 25 W CO_2 laser, and after cutting, the layers were laminated (Munson & Yager, 2003). By using xurography, Atencia et al. made a diffusion-based gradient generator for biochemical assays (Atencia, Cooksey, & Locascio, 2012). Pessoa de Santana et al. used xurography to manufacture microchannels on glass slides for electrophoresis application (de Santana et al., 2013). In another work, xurography was used for development of a low cost microfluidic technology for point-of-care micromixing devices (Martínez-López, Mojica, Rodríguez, & Siller, 2016).

1.4 Conclusion and future trends

Materials and manufacturing techniques used in microelectronic semiconductor industry were adopted to develop the first MEMS and microfluidic devices. Silicon and glass were initially utilized because their fabrication techniques already existed and were highly developed. Some properties of these materials such as their solvent

Materials and methods for microfabrication of microfluidic devices 47

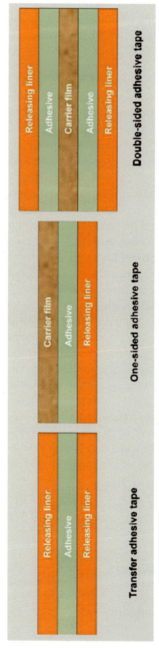

Figure 1.19 Different types of pressure sensitive adhesive tapes (Mohammadzadeh et al., 2018).

resistance, stiffness, and durability still make them the material of choice in many microfluidic applications. However, to lower the cost and enhance the functionality of these devices, other materials have been investigated extensively in the past few decades. Polymers have attracted widespread attention among academic researchers as well as commercial companies due to their extraordinary range of mechanical, chemical, and optical properties. They exist in highly elastic or stiff forms (highly dependent on their polymer chain size and length) with chemical inertness and biocompatibility. Their surface properties can be modified physically (plasma, corona, mechanical roughening, etc.) or chemically (monolayer deposition, grafting, etc.). A wide range of conventional optical (photolithography) or micromechanical (microinjection molding, hot embossing, laser micromachining, micromilling, casting, stereolithography, and inkjet printing), and xurography-based fabrication methods have been applied to develop prototyping and mass manufacturing techniques for polymeric materials. This lowers the cost of the devices significantly and enables the development of disposable devices which is necessary for biomedical applications. Most of the microfabrication techniques in polymers take advantage of the temperature, heat, or light-dependent phase transition behavior of polymers and the ability to form them into the required shape. Using these techniques, a wide range of microfluidic devices composed of silicon, glass, PDMS, parylene, polyimide, polyurethane, polycarbonate, PMMA, COC/COP, paper, thread, and PSA laminates have been developed. These devices have been used in a wide range of applications such as biological studies, tissue manufacturing, medical diagnostics, drug delivery, drug discovery, analytical chemistry, and molecular diagnosis. Although it is still not clear which of the materials introduced above will be dominant in the development of lab-on-a-chip devices, but from the cost, ease of fabrication, scalability, and accessibility point of view, paper, xurographic, and COC-based devices demonstrate extraordinary potential to be adapted in the near future. Glass and silicon devices continue to dominate in commercial production of microfluidic components and in biochemical applications. The existence of the extensive level of research on PDMS and the emergence of 3D printed molds enhancing its suitability for rapid prototyping have made it the material of choice for research and development. As a result, polymeric materials will continue to lead the progress of lab-on-a-chip devices as the field advances.

1.5 Acronyms

APTES	3-aminopropyltriethoxysilan
COC	Cyclic Olefin Copolymers
COP	Cyclic Olefin Polymers
DNA	Deoxyribonucleic Acid
DRIE	Deep Reactive-Ion Etching
EC	Electrochemical
ECL	Electrochemiluminescence
EDM	Electrode Discharge Machining
GPTES	3-glycidoxypropyltriethoxysilane

HF	Hydrofluoric Acid
ICP	Inductively Coupled Plasma
LDPE	Low Density Polyethylene
LIGA	Lithographie, Galvanoformung, Abformung
MEMS	Microelectromechanical Systems
MFS	Minimum Feature Size
PC	Polycarbonate
PCB	Printed Circuit Board
PCR	Polymerase Chain Reaction
PDMS	Polydimethylsiloxane
PETG	Polyethylene Terephthalate Glycol
PI	Polyimide
PMMA	Poly(methyl methacrylate)
PP	Polypropylene
PR	Photoresist
PS	Polystyrene
PSG	Phosphosilicate Glass
PTFE	Polytetrafluoroethylene
PU	Polyurethane
RIE	Reactive-Ion Etching
SCCM	Standard Cubic Centimeters per Minute
USG	Undoped Silicate Glass
UV	Ultraviolet

References

Abe, K., Suzuki, K., & Citterio, D. (2008). Inkjet-printed microfluidic multianalyte chemical sensing paper. *Analytical Chemistry, 80*(18), 6928−6934. https://doi.org/10.1021/ac800604v

Adkins, J. A., Noviana, E., & Henry, C. S. (2016). Development of a quasi-steady flow electrochemical paper-based analytical device. *Analytical Chemistry, 88*(21), 10639−10647. https://doi.org/10.1021/acs.analchem.6b03010

Aghvami, S. A., Opathalage, A., Zhang, Z. K., Ludwig, M., Heymann, M., Norton, M., et al. (2017). Rapid prototyping of cyclic olefin copolymer (COC) microfluidic devices. *Sensors and Actuators B: Chemical, 247*(August), 940−949. https://doi.org/10.1016/j.snb.2017.03.023

Agirregabiria, M., et al. (2005). Fabrication of SU-8 multilayer microstructures based on successive CMOS compatible adhesive bonding and releasing steps. *Lab on a Chip, 5*(5), 545−552. https://doi.org/10.1039/B500519A

Agustini, D., Bergamini, M. F., & Marcolino-Junior, L. H. (2016). Low cost microfluidic device based on cotton threads for electroanalytical application. *Lab on a Chip, 16*(2), 345−352. https://doi.org/10.1039/c5lc01348h

Akiyama, N., et al. (1997). A comparison of CORVITA and expanded polytetrafluoroethylene vascular grafts implanted in the abdominal aortas of dogs. *Surgery Today, 27*(9), 840−845. Available at http://www.ncbi.nlm.nih.gov/pubmed/9306607. (Accessed 11 October 2011).

Alexandrov, S. E., Lipovskii, A. A., Osipov, A. A., Reduto, I. V., & Tagantsev, D. K. (2017). Plasma-etching of 2D-poled glasses: A route to dry lithography. *Applied Physics Letters, 111*(11), 111604.

Anbuhi, S., Chavan, P., Clemence Sicard, Leung, V., Zakir Hossain, S. M., Pelton, R. H., et al. (2012). Creating fast flow channels in paper fluidic devices to control timing of sequential reactions. *Lab on a Chip, 12*(23), 5079−5085. https://doi.org/10.1039/C2LC41005B

Angelov, A., & Coulter, J. (2008). The development and characterization of polymer microinjection molded gratings. *Polymer Engineering and Science, 48*(11), 2169−4346. https://doi.org/10.1002/pen.21162

Anoop, R., & Sen, A. K. (2015). Capillary flow enhancement in rectangular polymer microchannels with a deformable wall. *Physical Review E, 92*(1), 013024. https://doi.org/10.1103/PhysRevE.92.013024

Appasamy, S., et al. (2005). High-throughput plastic microlenses fabricated using microinjection molding techniques. *Optical Engineering, 44*, 123401. Available at http://link.aip.org/link/opegar/v44/i12/p123401/s1/html.

Armani, D. K., & Liu, C. (2000). Microfabrication technology for polycaprolactone, a biodegradable polymer. *Journal of Micromechanics and Microengineering, 10*, 80−84.

Armani, D., Liu, C. & Aluru, N. (1999). Re-configurable fluid circuits by PDMS elastomer micromachining. In: Twelfth IEEE international conference on micro electro mechanical systems, MEMS '99, 1999, 222−227.

Assael, M. J., Botsios, S., Gialou, K., & Metaxa, I. N. (2005). Thermal conductivity of polymethyl methacrylate (PMMA) and borosilicate crown glass BK7. *International Journal of Thermophysics*, 261595−261605.

Atencia, J., Cooksey, G. A., & Locascio, L. E. (2012). A robust diffusion-based gradient generator for dynamic cell assays. *Lab on a Chip, 12*(2), 309−316.

Attia, U. M., & Alcock, J. R. (2011). A review of micro-powder injection moulding as a microfabrication technique. *Journal of Micromechanics and Microengineering, 21*(4), 043001. Available at http://stacks.iop.org/0960-1317/21/i=4/a=043001. (Accessed 27 September 2012).

Attia, U. M., Marson, S., & Alcock, J. R. (2009). Micro-injection moulding of polymer microfluidic devices. *Microfluidics and Nanofluidics, 7*(1), 1−28. Available at http://www.springerlink.com/content/942q72w1g938816x/. (Accessed 20 August 2012).

Bagolini, A., et al. (2002). Polyimide sacrificial layer and novel materials for post-processing surface micromachining. *Journal of Micromechanics and Microengineering, 12*(4), 385. Available at http://stacks.iop.org/0960-1317/12/i=4/a=306.

Bakker, D., et al. (1990). Biocompatibility of a polyether urethane, polypropylene oxide, and a polyether polyester copolymer. A qualitative and quantitative study of three alloplastic tympanic membrane materials in the rat middle ear. *Journal of Biomedical Materials Research, 24*(4), 489−515. Available at http://www.ncbi.nlm.nih.gov/pubmed/2347874. (Accessed 11 October 2011).

Balagadde, F. K., You, L., Hansen, C. L., Arnold, F. H., & Quake, S. R. (2005). Long-term monitoring of bacteria undergoing programmed population control in a microchemostat. *Science, 309*, 137−140.

Bartholomeusz, D. A., Boutté, R. W., & Andrade, J. D. (2005). Xurography: Rapid prototyping of microstructures using a cutting plotter. *Journal of Microelectromechanical Systems, 14*(6), 1364−1374.

Becker, H. (2000). Hot embossing as a method for the fabrication of polymer high aspect ratio structures. *Sensors and Actuators A: Physical, 83*(1−3), 130−135. https://doi.org/10.1016/S0924-4247(00)00296-X. Available at . (Accessed 11 October 2011).

Becker, H., & Gartner, C. (2000). Polymer microfabrication methods for microfluidic analytical applications. *Electrophoresis, 21*, 12−26.

Becker, H., & Gärtner, C. (2008). Polymer microfabrication technologies for microfluidic systems. *Analytical and Bioanalytical Chemistry, 390*(1), 89−111. https://doi.org/10.1007/s00216-007-1692-2

Becker, E. W., Ehrfeld, W., Hagmann, P., Maner, A., & Münchmeyer, D. (1986). Fabrication of microstructures with high aspect ratios and great structural heights by synchrotron radiation lithography, galvanoforming, and plastic moulding (LIGA process). *Microelectronic Engineering, 4*(1), 35−56. https://doi.org/10.1016/0167-9317(86)90004-3

Becker, H., & Heim, U. (2000). Hot embossing as a method for the fabrication of polymer high aspect ratio structures. *Sensors and Actuators, 83*, 130−135.

Becker, H., & Locascio, L. E. (2002). Polymer microfluidic devices. *Talanta, 56*(2), 267−287. Available at http://www.ncbi.nlm.nih.gov/pubmed/18968500.

Bedair, M., & Oleschuk, R. (2006). Fabrication of porous polymer monoliths in polymeric microfluidic chips as an electrospray emitter for direct coupling to mass spectrometry. *Analytical Chemistry, 78*(4), 1130−1138. https://doi.org/10.1021/ac0514570

Bell, T. E., Wise, K. D., & Anderson, D. J. (1997). Flexible micromachined electrode array for a cochlear prosthesis. *Proc. of International Conference on Solid-State Sensors and Actuators (Tranducers '97), 2*, 1315−1318. https://doi.org/10.1109/SENSOR.1997.635478

Belloy, E., Thurre, S., Walckiers, E., Sayah, A., & Gijs, M. A. M. (2000). The introduction of powder blasting for sensor and microsystem applications. *Sensors and Actuators A: Physical, 84*(3), 330−337. https://doi.org/10.1016/S0924-4247(00)00390-3

Berthier, J., Brakke, K. A., Gosselin, D., Berthier, E., & Navarro, F. (2017). Thread-based microfluidics: Flow patterns in homogeneous and heterogeneous microfiber bundles. *Medical Engineering and Physics, 48*, 55−61. https://doi.org/10.1016/j.medengphy.2017.08.004

Bertsch, A., et al. (2002). Microstereolithography: A review. *MRS Proceedings, 758*(-1). Available at http://journals.cambridge.org/abstract_S1946427400153357. (Accessed 27 September 2012).

Bhagat, A. A. S., Jothimuthu, P., Pais, A., & Papautsky, I. (2007). Re-useable quick-release interconnect for characterization of microfluidic systems. *Journal of Micromechanics and Microengineering, 17*, 42−49.

Bhandari, P., Narahari, T., & Dendukuri, D. (2011). Fab-chips: A versatile, fabric-based platform for low-cost, rapid and multiplexed diagnostics. *Lab on a Chip, 11*(15), 2493−2499. https://doi.org/10.1039/c1lc20373h

Bhattacharya, S., Datta, A., Berg, J. M., & Gangopadhyay, S. (2005). Studies on surface wettability of poly(dimethyl) siloxane (PDMS) and glass under oxygen-plasma treatment and correlation with bond strength. *Journal of Microelectromechanical Systems, 14*, 590−597.

Bhattacharyya, A., & Klapperich, C. (2006). Thermoplastic microfluidic device for on-chip purification of nucleic acids for disposable diagnostics. *Analytical Chemistry, 78*(3), 788−880. https://doi.org/10.1021/ac051449j

Bilenberg, B., et al. (2004). PMMA to SU-8 bonding for polymer based lab-on-a-chip systems with integrated optics. *Journal of Micromechanics and Microengineering, 14*, 814. Available at http://iopscience.iop.org/0960-1317/14/6/008.

Bilenberg, B., Hansen, M., Johansen, D., Özkapici, V., Jeppesen, C., Szabo, P., et al. (2005). Topas-based lab-on-a-chip microsystems fabricated by thermal nanoimprint lithography. *Journal of Vacuum Science and Technology B: Microelectronics and Nanometer Structures, 23*, 2944.

Biron, M. (2007). Thermoplastics and Thermoplastic Composites: Technical Information for Plastics Users (Google eBook) (p. 944). Elsevier. Available at: http://books.google.com/books?id=g_11KTQ-RjYC&pgis=1.

Blas, M., Delaunay, N., & Rocca, J.-L. (2008). Electrokinetic-based injection modes for separative microsystems. *Electrophoresis, 29*(1), 20−52. https://doi.org/10.1002/elps.200700389

Bliss, C. L., McMullin, J. N., & Backhouse, C. J. (2007). Rapid fabrication of a microfluidic device with integrated optical waveguides for DNA fragment analysis. *Lab on a Chip, 7*(10), 1280−1287. https://doi.org/10.1039/b708485d

Boger, A., Bisig, A., Bohner, M., Heini, P., & Schneider, E. (2008). Variation of the mechanical properties of PMMA to suit osteoporotic cancellous bone. *Journal of Biomaterials Science, Polymer Edition, 19*, 1125−1142.

Boretos, J. W., & Pierce, W. S. (1968). Segmented polyurethane: A polyether polymer. An initial evaluation for biomedical applications. *Journal of Biomedical Materials Research, 2*(1), 121−130. https://doi.org/10.1002/jbm.820020109

Brahmasandra, S. N., Johnson, B. N., Webster, J. R., Burke, D. T., Mastrangelo, C. H., & Burns, M. A. (1998). In *On-chip DNA band detection in microfabricated separation systems Proc. of the SPIE Conference on Microfluidic Devices and Systems*.

Brash, J. L., Fritzinger, B. K., & Bruck, S. D. (1973). Development of block copolyetherurethane intra-aortic balloons and other medical devices. *Journal of Biomedical Materials Research, 7*(4), 313−334. https://doi.org/10.1002/jbm.820070405

Brook, M. (2000). *Silicon in organic, organometallic and polymer chemistry*. New York. USA: John Wiley and Sons.

Bruin, P., et al. (1993). Autoclavable highly cross-linked polyurethane networks in ophthalmology. *Biomaterials, 14*(14), 1089−1097. Available at http://www.ncbi.nlm.nih.gov/pubmed/7508760. (Accessed 11 October 2011).

Bruzewicz, D. A., Reches, M., & Whitesides, G. M. (2008). Low-cost printing of poly(dimethylsiloxane) barriers to define microchannels in paper. *Analytical Chemistry, 80*(9), 3387−3392. https://doi.org/10.1021/ac702605a

Bu, M., Melvin, T., Ensell, G. J., Wilkinson, J. S., & Evans, A. G. R. (2004). A new masking technology for deep glass etching and its microfluidic application. *Sensors and Actuators A: Physical, 115*(2−3), 476−482. https://doi.org/10.1016/j.sna.2003.12.013

Bundgaard, F., Perozziello, G., & Geschke, O. (2006). Rapid prototyping tools and methods for all-Topas® cyclic olefin copolymer fluidic microsystems. *Proceedings of the Institution of Mechanical Engineers − Part C: Journal of Mechanical Engineering Science, 220*(11), 1625−1632. Available at http://pic.sagepub.com/lookup/doi/10.1243/09544062JMES295. (Accessed 6 April 2012).

Burns, M. A., et al. (1998). An integrated nanoliter DNA analysis device. *Science, 282*(5388), 484−487. Available at http://www.sciencemag.org/cgi/doi/10.1126/science.282.5388.484.

Burshtein, N., Chan, S. T., Toda-Peters, K., Shen, A. Q., & Haward, S. J. (October 2019). 3D-Printed glass microfluidics for fluid dynamics and rheology. *Current Opinion in Colloid & Interface Science, 43*, 1−14. https://doi.org/10.1016/j.cocis.2018.12.005

Bustillo, J. M., Howe, R. T., Muller, R. S., & Fellow, L. (1998). *Surface micromachining for microelectromechanical systems* (Vol. 86), 8.

Cai, J., Jiang, J., Gao, F., Jia, G., Zhuang, J., Tang, G., et al. (2017). Rapid prototyping of cyclic olefin copolymer based microfluidic system with CO_2 laser ablation. *Microsystem Technologies, 23*(10), 5063−5069. https://doi.org/10.1007/s00542-017-3282-3

Campbell, D. J., Beckman, K. J., Calderon, C. E., Doolan, P. W., Ottosen, R. M., Ellis, A. B., et al. (1999). Replication and compression of bulk and surface structures with polydimethylsiloxane elastomer. *Journal of Chemical Education, 76*, 537−541.

Carlen, E. T., & Mastrangelo, C. H. (2002). Electrothermally activated paraffin microactuators. *Journal of Microelectromechanical Systems, 11*, 165−174.

Carrell, C., Kava, A., Nguyen, M., Menger, R., Munshi, Z., Call, Z., et al. (February 2019). Beyond the lateral flow assay: A review of paper-based microfluidics. *Microelectronic Engineering, 206*, 45−54. https://doi.org/10.1016/j.mee.2018.12.002

Carrilho, E., Martinez, A. W., & Whitesides, G. M. (2009). Understanding wax printing: A simple micropatterning process for paper-based microfluidics. *Analytical Chemistry, 81*(16), 7091−7095. https://doi.org/10.1021/ac901071p

Castaño-Alvarez, M., Fernández-Abedul, M., & Costa-García, A. (2007). Electroactive intercalators for DNA analysis on microchip electrophoresis. *Electrophoresis, 28*(24), 4679−4768. https://doi.org/10.1002/elps.200700160

Cate, D. M., Adkins, J. A., Mettakoonpitak, J., & Henry, C. S. (2015). Recent developments in paper-based microfluidic devices. *Analytical Chemistry, 87*(1), 19−41. https://doi.org/10.1021/ac503968p

Chan, C.-H., Chen, J.-K., & Chang, F.-C. (2008). Specific DNA extraction through fluid channels with immobilization of layered double hydroxides on polycarbonate surface. *Sensors and Actuators B: Chemical, 133*(1), 327−332. https://doi.org/10.1016/j.snb.2008.02.041

Chang, J. A., Chang, Y. J., Chau, S. W., & Chen, S. C. (2005). Micro injection molding of micro fluidic platform. In *ANTEC-conference proceedings-* (Vol. 2, p. 136).

Chang, T. Y., Yadav, V. G., De Leo, S., Mohedas, A., Rajalingam, B., Chen, C. L., et al. (2007). Cell and protein compatibility of parylene-C surfaces. *Langmuir, 23*, 11718−11725.

Chen, P. J. (2007). Surface-micromachined parylene dual valves for on-chip unpowered microflow regulation. *Journal of Microelectromechanical Systems, 16*, 223−231.

Chen, Y. H., & Chen, S. H. (2000). Analysis of DNA fragments by microchip electrophoresis fabricated on poly(methyl methacrylate) substrates using a wire-imprinting method. *Electrophoresis, 21*, 165−170.

Chen, G., Svec, F., & Knapp, D. (2008). Light-actuated high pressure-resisting microvalve for on-chip flow control based on thermo-responsive nanostructured polymer. *Lab on a Chip, 8*(7), 1198−1402. https://doi.org/10.1039/b803293a

Chen, H. Y., Elkasabi, Y., & Lahann, J. (2006). Surface modification of confined microgeometries via vapordeposited polymer coatings. *Journal of the American Chemical Society, 128*, 374−380.

Chen, Z., Gao, Y., Su, R., Li, C., & Lin, J. (2003). Fabrication and characterization of poly(methyl methacrylate) microchannels by in situ polymerization with a novel metal template. *Electrophoresis, 24*, 3246−3252.

Chen, H. Y., & Lahann, J. (2005). Fabrication of discontinuous surface patterns within microfluidic channels using photodefinable vapor-based polymer coatings. *Analytical Chemistry, 77*, 6909−6914.

Chen, H. Y., & Lahann, J. (2007). Vapor-assisted micropatterning in replica structures: A solventless approach towards topologically and chemically designable surfaces. *Advanced Materials, 19*, 3801−3808.

Chen, J., Lin, Y., & Chen, G. (2007). Fabrication of poly(methyl methacrylate) microfluidic chips by redox-initiated polymerization. *Electrophoresis, 28*, 2897−2903.

Chen, X., Li, T., & Shen, J. (2016). CO_2 laser ablation of microchannel on PMMA substrate for effective fabrication of microfluidic chips. *International Polymer Processing, 31*(2), 233−238. https://doi.org/10.3139/217.3184

Chen, P. J., Shih, C. Y., & Tai, Y. C. (2006). Design, fabrication and characterization of monolithic embedded parylene microchannels in silicon substrate. *Lab on a Chip, 6*, 803−810.

Chen, Y., Zhang, L., & Chen, G. (2008). Fabrication, modification, and application of poly(methyl methacrylate) microfluidic chips. *Electrophoresis, 29*, 1801−1814.

Chen, J., Wabuyele, M., Chen, H., Patterson, D., Hupert, M., Shadpour, H., et al. (2005). Electrokinetically synchronized Polymerase chain reaction microchip fabricated in polycarbonate. *Analytical Chemistry, 77*(2), 658–666. https://doi.org/10.1021/ac048758e

Choi, S. H., Kim, D. S., & Kwon, T. H. (2008). Microinjection molded disposable microfluidic lab-on-a-chip for efficient detection of agglutination. *Microsystem Technologies, 15*(2), 309–316. https://doi.org/10.1007/s00542-008-0689-x

Chow, W. W. Y., Lei, K. F., Shi, G. Y., Li, W. J., & Huang, Q. (2006). Microfluidic channel fabrication by PDMS-interface bonding. *Smart Materials and Structures, 15*, S112–S116.

Christensen, A. M., Chang-Yen, D. A., & Gale, B. K. (2005). Characterization of interconnects used in PDMS microfluidic systems. *Journal of Micromechanics and Microengineering, 15*, 928–934.

Chuang, H. S., & Wereley, S. (2009). Design, fabrication and characterization of a conducting PDMS for microheaters and temperature sensors. *Journal of Micromechanics and Microengineering, 19*, 045010.

Chung, A. J., Kim, D., & Erickson, D. (2008). Electrokinetic microfluidic devices for rapid, low power drug delivery in autonomous microsystems. *Lab on a Chip, 8*(2), 330–338. https://doi.org/10.1039/b713325a

Ciftlik, A. T., & Gijs, M. A. (2011). A low-temperature parylene-to-silicon dioxide bonding technique for high-pressure microfluidics. *Journal of Micromechanics and Microengineering, 21*, 035011.

Ciftlik, A. T., & Gijs, M. A. (2012). Parylene to silicon nitride bonding for post-integration of high pressure microfluidics to CMOS devices. *Lab on a Chip, 12*, 396–400.

Clarson, S. J., & Semlyen, J. A. (1993). *Siloxane Polymers*. Englewood Cliffs, NJ: Prentice-Hall.

Cooney, C., et al. (2012). A plastic, disposable microfluidic flow cell for coupled on-chip PCR and microarray detection of infectious agents. *Biomedical Microdevices, 14*(1), 45–53. https://doi.org/10.1007/s10544-011-9584-9

Creton, C. (2003). Pressure-sensitive adhesives: An introductory Course. *MRS Bulletin, 28*(6), 434–439.

Dabaghi, M., Saraei, N., Fusch, G., Rochow, N., Brash, J. L., Fusch, C., et al. (2019). An ultrathin, all PDMS-based microfluidic lung assist device with high oxygenation capacity. *Biomicrofluidics, 13*(3), 034116. https://doi.org/10.1063/1.5091492

Dang, F. Q., Kakehi, K., Cheng, J. J., Tabata, O., Kurokawa, M., & Nakajima, K. (2006). Hybrid dynamic coating with n-dodecyl beta-D-maltoside and methyl cellulose for high-performance carbohydrate analysis on poly(methyl methacrylate) chips. *Analytical Chemistry, 78*, 1452–1458.

Dang, F., et al. (2005). Replica multichannel polymer chips with a network of sacrificial channels sealed by adhesive printing method. *Lab on a Chip, 5*(4), 472–478.

Dang, F., Zhang, L., Hagiwara, H., Mishina, Y., & Baba, Y. (2003). Ultrafast analysis of oligosaccharides on microchip with light-emitting diode confocal fluorescence detection. *Electrophoresis, 24*, 714–721.

Das, B., Das, A., Kothari, V. K., & Fangueiro, R. (2011). Development of mathematical model to predict vertical wicking behaviour. Part I: Flow through yarn. *Journal of the Textile Institute, 102*(11), 957–970. https://doi.org/10.1080/00405000.2010.529281

Delaney, J. L., Hogan, C. F., Tian, J., & Shen, W. (2011). Electrogenerated chemiluminescence detection in paper-based microfluidic sensors. *Analytical Chemistry, 83*(4), 1300–1306. https://doi.org/10.1021/ac102392t

Delivopoulos, E., Murray, A. F., Macleod, N. K., & Curtis, J. C. (2009). Guided growth of neurons and glia using microfabricated patterns of parylene-c on a SiO$_2$ background. *Biomaterials, 30*, 2048−2058.

Devanathan, T., Sluetz, J. E., & Young, K. A. (1980). In vivo thrombogenicity of implantable cardiac pacing leads. *Biomaterials Medical Devices and Artificial Organs, 8*(4), 369−379. Available at http://www.ncbi.nlm.nih.gov/pubmed/7272410. (Accessed 11 October 2011).

Dietrich, T. R., Ehrfeld, W., Lacher, M., Kramer, M., & Speit, B. (1996). Fabrication technologies for microsystems utilizing photoetchable glass. *Microelectronic Engineering, 30*(1−4), 497−504.

Dixon, C., Ng, A. H. C., Ryan, F., Miltenburg, M. B., & Wheeler, A. R. (2016). An inkjet printed, roll-coated digital microfluidic device for inexpensive, miniaturized diagnostic assays. *Lab on a Chip, 16*(23), 4560−4568. https://doi.org/10.1039/C6LC01064D

Do, J., & Ahn, C. (2008). A polymer lab-on-a-chip for magnetic immunoassay with on-chip sampling and detection capabilities. *Lab on a Chip, 8*(4), 542−551. https://doi.org/10.1039/b715569g

Dubey, A. K., & Yadava, V. (2008). Laser beam machining—a review. *International Journal of Machine Tools and Manufacture, 48*(6), 609−628. https://doi.org/10.1016/j.ijmachtools.2007.10.017. Available at . (Accessed 10 August 2012).

Duffy, D. C., Mcdonald, J. C., Schueller, O. J. A., & Whitesides, G. M. (1998). Rapid prototyping of microfluidic systems in poly(dimethylsiloxane). *Analytical Chemistry, 70*, 4974−4984.

Dungchai, W., Chailapakul, O., & Henry, C. S. (2009). Electrochemical detection for paper-based microfluidics. *Analytical Chemistry, 81*(14), 5821−5826. https://doi.org/10.1021/ac9007573

Dykes, J. M., et al. (2007). Creation of embedded structures in SU-8. *Proceedings of SPIE, 6465*. 64650N−64650N−12. Available at http://link.aip.org/link/PSISDG/v6465/i1/p64650N/s1&Agg=doi. (Accessed 13 August 2012).

Eddings, M. A., Johnson, M. A., & Gale, B. K. (2008). Determining the optimal PDMS−PDMS bonding technique for microfluidic devices. *Journal of Micromechanics and Microengineering, 18*, 1−4.

Effenhauser, C. S., Bruin, G. J. M., Paulus, A., & Ehrat, M. (1997). Integrated capillary electrophoresis on flexible silicone microdevices: Analysis of DNA restriction fragments and detection of single DNA molecules on microchips. *Analytical Chemistry, 69*, 3451−3457.

Egashira, K., Mizutani, K., & Nagao, T. (2002). Ultrasonic vibration drilling of Microholes in glass. *CIRP Annals − Manufacturing Technology, 51*(1), 339−342.

Ehrfeld, W., Lehr, H., Frank, M., Wolf, A., Gruber, H.-P., & Bertholds, A. (1996). Microelectro discharge machining as a technology in micromachining. In S. W. Pang, P. M. Edward Motamedi, K. H. Chau, R. M. Roop, W. Bailey, C. R. Friedrich, et al. (Eds.), *Micromachining and microfabrication '96* (pp. 332−337). https://doi.org/10.1117/12.251221

Erickson, D., & Li, D. (2004). Integrated microfluidic devices. *Analytica Chimica Acta, 507*(1), 11−26. https://doi.org/10.1016/j.aca.2003.09.019

Erickson, J., Tooker, A., Tai, Y. C., & Pine, J. (2008). Caged neuron MEA: A system for long-term investigation of cultured neural network connectivity. *Journal of Neuroscience Methods, 175*, 1−16.

Fallahi, H., Zhang, J., Phan, H.-P., & Nguyen, N.-T. (2019). Flexible microfluidics: Fundamentals, recent developments, and applications. *Micromachines, 10*(12), 830. https://doi.org/10.3390/mi10120830

Fan, Z., Ludi, H., & Widmers, H. M. (1992). Capillary electrophoresis and sample injection systems integrated on a planar glass chip. *Analytical Chemistry, 64*(17), 1926−1932. https://doi.org/10.1021/ac00041a030

Fan, X., & White, I. M. (2011). Optofluidic microsystems for chemical and biological analysis. *Nature Photonics, 5*(10), 591–597. https://doi.org/10.1038/nphoton.2011.206

Farajikhah, S., Paull, B., Innis, P. C., Cabot, J. M., & Wallace, G. G. (2019). Life-saving threads; advances in textile-based analytical devices. *ACS Combinatorial Science, 21*(4), 229–240. https://doi.org/10.1021/acscombsci.8b00126

Faure, K., et al. (2008). Development of an acrylate monolith in a cyclo-olefin copolymer microfluidic device for chip electrochromatography separation. *Electrophoresis, 29*(24), 4948–5003. https://doi.org/10.1002/elps.200800235

Faustino, V., Catarino, S. O., Lima, R., & Minas, G. (2016). Biomedical microfluidic devices by using low-cost fabrication techniques: A review. *Journal of Biomechanics, 49*(11), 2280–2292. https://doi.org/10.1016/j.jbiomech.2015.11.031

Fiorini, G. S., & Chiu, D. T. (2005). Disposable microfluidic devices: Fabrication, function, and application. *Biotechniques, 38*, 429–446.

Fiorini, G. S., et al. (2007). Fabrication improvements for thermoset polyester (TPE) microfluidic devices. *Lab on a Chip, 7*(7), 923–926. Available at http://www.ncbi.nlm.nih.gov/pubmed/17594014.

Flaherty, M. (1995). In *Conformal polymer film protects circuits, stabilizes solder joints Proc. of the Int. Electronics Packaging Conf.*

Folch, A., Mezzour, S., & Du, M. (2000). Stacks of microfabricated structures as scaffolds for cell culture and tissue engineering. *Tissue Engineering*, 207–214.

Fredrickson, C., Xia, Z., Das, C., Ferguson, R., Tavares, F., & Fan, Z. H. (2006). Effects of fabrication process parameters on the properties of cyclic olefin copolymer microfluidic devices. *Journal of Microelectromechanical Systems, 15*(5), 1060–1068. Available at http://ieeexplore.ieee.org/xpls/abs_all.jsp?arnumber=1707765.

Fredrickson, C. K., & Fan, Z. H. (2004). Macro-to-micro interfaces for microfluidic devices. *Lab on a Chip, 4*, 526–533.

Freire, S. L. S., Yang, H., Luk, V. N., & O'brien, B. (2011). Characterizing electro-osmotic flow in parylene microchannels. *Polymer-Plastics Technology and Engineering, 50*, 931–936.

Fu, Y. Q., et al. (2009). Deep reactive ion etching as a tool for nanostructure fabrication. *Journal of Vacuum Science & Technology B: Microelectronics and Nanometer Structures, 27*(3), 1520–1526.

Fu, P. F., Glover, S., King, R. K., Lee, C. L., Pretzer, M. R., & Tomalia, M. K. (2003). Polypropylene-polysiloxane block copolymers via hydrosilation of mono-vinylidene capped isotactice polypropylene. *Abstracts of Papers American Chemical Society, 225*, U575–U576.

Fu, E., Lutz, B., Kauffman, P., & Yager, P. (2010). Controlled reagent transport in disposable 2D paper networks. *Lab on a Chip, 10*(7), 918–920. https://doi.org/10.1039/b919614e

Gad-El-Hak, M. (2002). *The MEMS Handbook (Google eBook)*. CRC Press. Available at http://books.google.com/books?id=g0v3r6WNaBkC&pgis=1. (Accessed 27 September 2012).

Gaines, M., Gonzalez-Guerrero, M. J., Uchida, K., & Gomez, F. A. (2018). A microfluidic glucose sensor incorporating a novel thread-based electrode system. *Electrophoresis*, 1–5. https://doi.org/10.1002/elps.201800010

Gale, B. K., Jafek, A. R., Lambert, C. J., Goenner, B. L., Moghimifam, H., Nze, U. C., et al. (2018). A review of current methods in microfluidic device fabrication and future commercialization prospects. *Inventions, 3*(3), 60.

de Tarso Garcia, P., Garcia Cardoso, T. M., Diego Garcia, C., Carrilho, E., & Tomazelli Coltro, W. K. (2014). A handheld stamping process to fabricate microfluidic paper-based analytical devices with chemically modified surface for clinical assays. *RSC Advances, 4*(71), 37637–37644. https://doi.org/10.1039/C4RA07112C

Gartner, C., Klemm, R., & Becker, H. (2007). Methods and instruments for continuous-flow PCR on a chip. *Polymer, 6465*. https://doi.org/10.1117/12.713797, 646502-646502−8.

Gattass, R. R., & Mazur, E. (2008). Femtosecond laser micromachining in transparent materials. *Nature Photonics, 2*(4), 219−225. https://doi.org/10.1038/nphoton.2008.47. Available at . (Accessed 29 July 2012).

Gawad, S., Schild, L., & Renaud, P. (2001). Micromachined impedance spectroscopy flow cytometer for cell analysis and particle sizing. *Lab on a Chip, 1*(1), 76−82. https://doi.org/10.1039/B103933B

Ge, L., Wang, S., Yu, J., Li, N., Ge, S., & Yan, M. (2013). Molecularly imprinted polymer grafted porous Au-paper electrode for an microfluidic electro-analytical origami device. *Advanced Functional Materials, 23*(24), 3115−3123. https://doi.org/10.1002/adfm.201202785

Giselbrecht, S., Gietzelt, T., Gottwald, E., Guber, A. E., Trautmann, C., Truckenmüller, R., et al. (2004). Microthermoforming as a novel technique for manufacturing scaffolds in tissue engineering (CellChips). *IEE Proceedings − Nanobiotechnology, 151*(4), 151−157. https://doi.org/10.1049/ip-nbt:20040824

Glasgow, I. K., Beebe, D. J., & White, V. E. (1999). Design rules for polyimide solvent bonding. *Sensors and Materials, 11*(5), 269−278.

Goldstein, Y., Grover, N. B., Chang, C., Jelli, A., Andre, J., Mark, P., et al. (1979). *A gas chromatographic air analyzer fabricated*, 12: 1880−86.

Gorelick, S., Guzenko, V. A., Vila-Comamala, J., & David, C. (2010). Direct e-beam writing of dense and high aspect ratio nanostructures in thick layers of PMMA for electroplating. *Nanotechnology, 21*, 1−8.

Gorham, W. F. (1966). A new, general synthetic method for the preparation of linear poly-p-xylylenes. *Journal of Polymer Science, 4*, 3027−3039.

Gösele, U., & Tong, Q.-Y. (1998). Semiconductor wafer bonding. *Annual Review of Materials Science, 28*(1), 215−241. https://doi.org/10.1146/annurev.matsci.28.1.215

Gottschlich, N. (2004). Production of plastic components for microfluidic applications. *Business in Brief: Future Drug Discovery*, 1−4. Available at http://www.touchbriefings.com/pdf/855/fdd041_greiner_tech.pdf. (Accessed 11 July 2012).

Gourgon, C., et al. (2005). Uniformity across 200 mm silicon wafers printed by nanoimprint lithography. *Journal of Physics D: Applied Physics, 38*, 70. Available at http://iopscience.iop.org/0022-3727/38/1/012.

Greer, J., Scott, O. S., Wittwer, C. T., & Gale, B. K. (2007). Comparison of glass etching to xurography prototyping of microfluidic channels for DNA melting analysis. *Journal of Micromechanics and Microengineering, 17*(12), 2407.

Griffiths, C. A., Dimov, S. S., Brousseau, E. B., & Hoyle, R. T. (2007). The effects of tool surface quality in micro-injection moulding. *Journal of Materials Processing Technology, 189*(1), 418−427.

Grover, W. H., Skelley, A. M., Liu, C. N., Lagally, E. T., & Mathies, R. A. (2003). Monolithic membrane valves and diaphragm pumps for practical large-scale integration into glass microfluidic devices. *Sensors and Actuators B: Chemical, 89*(3), 315−323. https://doi.org/10.1016/S0925-4005(02)00468-9

Grumann, M., Steigert, J., Riegger, L., Moser, I., Enderle, B., Riebeseel, K., et al. (2006). Sensitivity enhancement for colorimetric glucose assays on whole blood by on-chip beam-guidance. *Biomedical Microdevices, 8*(3), 209−214. https://doi.org/10.1007/s10544-006-8172-x

Gulliksen, A., Solli, L., Drese, K., Sörensen, O., Frank, K., Rogne, H., et al. (2005). Parallel nanoliter detection of cancer markers using polymer microchips. *Lab on a Chip, 5*(4), 416−436. https://doi.org/10.1039/b415525d

Guo, L. J. (2007). Nanoimprint lithography: Methods and material requirements. *Advanced Materials, 19*(4), 495−513. Available at http://doi.wiley.com/10.1002/adma.200600882. (Accessed 16 July 2012).

Gustafsson, O., Mogensen, K., & Kutter, J. (2008). Underivatized cyclic olefin copolymer as substrate material and stationary phase for capillary and microchip electrochromatography. *Electrophoresis, 29*(15), 3145−3197. https://doi.org/10.1002/elps.200800131

Han, D. K., Lee, K. B., Park, K. D., Kim, C. S., Jeong, S. Y., Kim, Y. H., et al. (1992). In vivo canine studies of a Sinkhole valve and vascular graft coated with biocompatible PU-PEO-SO3. *ASAIO Journal (American Society for Artificial Internal Organs), 39*(3). M537−41. Available at http://www.ncbi.nlm.nih.gov/pubmed/8268593. (Accessed 11 October 2011).

Han, J., et al. (2003). UV adhesive bonding techniques at room temperature for plastic lab-on-a-chip. In *7th international conference of miniaturized chemical and biochemical analysis systems*. California, USA: Squaw Valley.

Haraldsson, K. T., Hutchison, J. B., Sebra, R. P., Good, B. T., Anseth, K. S., & Bowman, C. N. (2006). 3D polymeric microfluidic device fabrication via contact liquid photolithographic polymerization (CLiPP). *Sensors and Actuators B: Chemical, 113*(1), 454−460. https://doi.org/10.1016/j.snb.2005.03.096

Harendt, C., et al. (1992). Silicon fusion bonding and its characterization. *Journal of Micromechanics and Microengineering, 2*(3), 113−116. Available at http://www.iop.org/EJ/abstract/0960-1317/2/3/001.

Hartmann, D. M., Nevill, J. T., Pettigrew, K. I., Votaw, G., Kung, P., & Crenshaw, H. C. (2008). A low-cost, manufacturable method for fabricating capillary and optical fiber interconnects for microfluidic devices. *Lab on a Chip, 8*, 609−616.

Hashimoto, M., et al. (2004). Rapid PCR in a continuous flow device. *Lab on a Chip, 4*(6), 638−645. https://doi.org/10.1039/B406860B

Hassler, C., Metzen, R. P., Ruther, P., & Stieglitz, T. (2010). Characterization of parylene C as an encapsulation material for implanted neural prostheses. *Journal of Biomedical Materials Research Part B: Applied Biomaterials, 93*, 266−274.

Heckele, M., & Schomburg, W. K. (2004). Review on micro molding of thermoplastic polymers. *Journal of Micromechanics and Microengineering, 14*(3), R1−R14. Available at http://stacks.iop.org/0960-1317/14/i=3/a=R01. (Accessed 27 September 2012).

Henry, A. C., Tutt, T. J., Galloway, M., Davidson, Y. Y., Mcwhorter, C. S., Soper, S. A., et al. (2000). Surface modification of poly(methyl methacrylate) used in the fabrication of microanalytical devices. *Analytical Chemistry, 72*, 5331−5337.

Hillborg, H., Ankner, J. F., Gedde, U. W., Smith, G. D., Yasuda, H. K., & Wikstrom, K. (2000). Crosslinked polydimethylsiloxane exposed to oxygen plasma studied by neutron reflectometry and other surface specific techniques. *Polymer, 41*, 6851−6863.

Hof, L. A., & Abou Ziki, J. (2017). Micro-Hole drilling on glass substrates—a review. *Micromachines, 8*(2), 53.

Hoffmann, M., & Voges, E. (2002). Bulk silicon micromachining for MEMS in optical communication systems. *Journal of Micromechanics and Microengineering, 12*(4), 349−360. https://doi.org/10.1088/0960-1317/12/4/301

Hori, R., & Wada, M. (2005). The thermal expansion of wood cellulose crystals. *Cellulose, 12*(5), 479−484.

Hsu, Y. C., & Chen, T. Y. (2007). Applying Taguchi methods for solvent assisted PMMA bonding technique for static and dynamic micro-TAS devices. *Biomedical Microdevices, 9*, 513−522.

Hua, F., Gaur, A., Sun, Y., Word, M., Jin, N., Adesida, I., et al. (2006). Processing dependent behavior of soft imprint lithography on the 1−10-nm scale. *IEEE Transactions on Nanotechnology, 5*(3), 301−308. https://doi.org/10.1109/TNANO.2006.874051

Hupert, M. L., Jason Guy, W., Llopis, S. D., Shadpour, H., Rani, S., Nikitopoulos, D. E., et al. (2006). Evaluation of micromilled metal mold masters for the replication of microchip electrophoresis devices. *Microfluidics and Nanofluidics, 3*(1), 1−11. https://doi.org/10.1007/s10404-006-0091-x

Hurth, C., Lenigk, R., & Zenhausern, F. (2008). A compact LED-based module for DNA capillary electrophoresis. *Applied Physics B, 93*(2−3), 693−699. https://doi.org/10.1007/s00340-008-3218-9

Hwang, D. J., Choi, T. Y., & Grigoropoulos, C. P. (2004). Liquid-assisted femtosecond laser drilling of straight and three-dimensional microchannels in glass. *Applied Physics A: Materials Science and Processing, 79*(3), 605−612.

Hwang, K. S., Park, J. H., Lee, J. H., Yoon, D. S., Kim, T. S., Han, I., et al. (2004). Effect of atmospheric-plasma treatments for enhancing adhesion of Au on parylene-c-coated protein chips. *Journal of the Korean Physical Society, 44*, 1168−1172.

Ilic, B., & Craighead, H. G. (2000). Topographical patterning of chemically sensitive biological materials using a polymer-based dry lift off. *Biomedical Microdevices, 2*, 317−322.

Ilic, B., Czaplewski, D., Zalalutdinov, M., Schmidt, B., & Craighead, H. G. (2002). Fabrication of flexible polymer tubes for micro and nanofluidic applications. *Journal of Vacuum Science and Technology B, 20*, 2459−2465.

Illa, X., De Malsche, W., Bomer, J., Han, G., Jan, E., Morante, J., et al. (2009). An array of ordered pillars with retentive properties for pressure-driven liquid chromatography fabricated directly from an unmodified cyclo olefin polymer. *Lab on a Chip, 9*(11), 1511−1517. https://doi.org/10.1039/b818918h

Ito, H., Kazama, K., & Kikutani, T. (2007). Effects of process conditions on surface replication and higher order Structure Formation in micromolding. *Macromolecular Symposia, 249*(1), 628−1262. https://doi.org/10.1002/masy.200750447

Ito, T., Soubue, K., & Ohya, S. (2002). Water glass bonding for Micro total analysis systems. *Sensors and Actuators B: Chemical, 81*, 187−195.

Jacobson, S. C., Roland, H., Koutny, L. B., & Ramsey, J. M. (1994). High-speed separations on a microchip. *Analytical Chemistry, 66*(7), 1114−1118. https://doi.org/10.1021/ac00079a029

Jaeblon, T. (2010). Polymethylmethacrylate: Properties and contemporary uses in orthopaedics. *Journal of the American Academy of Orthopaedic Surgeons, 18*, 297−305.

Jang, W. I., et al. (2006). Self-operated blood plasma separation using micropump in polymer-based microfluidic device. *Proceedings of SPIE, 6415*, 641511. Available at http://cat.inist.fr/?aModele=afficheN&cpsidt=18866544.

Jang, Y., Lee, M., Kim, H., Cha, C., Jung, J., & Oh, J. (2019). Comprehensive tuning of bioadhesive properties of polydimethylsiloxane (PDMS) membranes with controlled porosity. *Biofabrication, 11*(3), 035021. https://doi.org/10.1088/1758-5090/ab1da9

Jang, A., Zou, Z., Lee, K. K., Ahn, C. H., & Bishop, P. L. (2011). State-of-the-art lab chip sensors for environmental water monitoring. *Measurement Science and Technology, 22*(3), 032001. https://doi.org/10.1088/0957-0233/22/3/032001

Jedrkiewicz, O., Bonanomi, S., Selva, M., & Di Trapani, P. (2015). Experimental investigation of high aspect ratio tubular microstructuring of glass by means of picosecond Bessel Vortices. *Applied Physics A, 120*(1), 385−391.

Jensen, M. F., McCormack, J. E., Helbo, B., Christensen, L. H., Christensen, T. R., & Oliver, G. (2004). Rapid prototyping of polymer microsystems via excimer laser ablation of polymeric moulds. *Lab on a Chip, 4*(4), 391−395. https://doi.org/10.1039/b403037k

Jeon, J. S., Chung, S., Kamm, R. D., & Charest, J. L. (2011). Hot embossing for fabrication of a microfluidic 3D cell culture platform. *Biomedical Microdevices, 13*(2), 325–333. https://doi.org/10.1007/s10544-010-9496-0

Jia, X., Song, T., Liu, Y., Meng, L., & Mao, X. (2017). An immunochromatographic assay for carcinoembryonic antigen on cotton thread using a composite of carbon nanotubes and gold nanoparticles as reporters. *Analytica Chimica Acta, 969*, 57–62. https://doi.org/10.1016/j.aca.2017.02.040

Jinno, S., Moeller, H. C., Chen, C. L., Rajalingam, B., Chung, B. G., Dokmeci, M. R., et al. (2008). A. Microfabricated multilayer parylene-c stencils for the generation of patterned dynamic co-cultures. *Journal of Biomedical Materials Research, 86A*, 278–288.

Jin, J.-Y., Yoo, S., Bae, J.-S., & Kim, Y.-K. (2013). Deep wet etching of borosilicate glass and fused silica with dehydrated AZ4330 and a Cr/Au mask. *Journal of Micromechanics and Microengineering, 24*(1), 015003.

Judy, J. W. (2001). Microelectromechanical systems (MEMS): Fabrication, design and applications. *Smart Materials and Structures, 10*(6), 1115–1134. Available at http://stacks.iop.org/0964-1726/10/i=6/a=301. (Accessed 27 September 2012).

Kalima, V., et al. (2007). Transparent thermoplastics: Replication of diffractive optical elements using micro-injection molding. *Optical Materials, 30*(2), 285–291. Available at http://www.sciencedirect.com/science/article/pii/S092534670600437X.

Kameoka, J., et al. (2001). A polymeric microfluidic chip for CE/MS determination of small molecules. *Analytical Chemistry, 73*(9), 1935–1976. Available at http://toxnet.nlm.nih.gov/cgi-bin/sis/search/r?dbs+hsdb:@term+@rn+541-15-1.

Kameoka, J., et al. (2002). An electrospray ionization source for integration with microfluidics. *Analytical Chemistry, 74*(22), 5897–6798. Available at http://toxnet.nlm.nih.gov/cgi-bin/sis/search/r?dbs+hsdb:@term+@rn+50-49-7.

Kartalov, E. P., Anderson, W. F., & Scherer, A. (2006). The analytical approach to polydimethylsiloxane microfluidic technology and its biological applications. *Journal of Nanoscience and Nanotechnology, 6*, 2265–2277.

Kato, Y. X., Furukawa, S., Samejima, K., Hironaka, N., & Kashino, M. (June 2012). Photosensitive-polyimide based method for fabricating various neural electrode architectures. *Frontiers in Neuroengineering, 5*, 11. https://doi.org/10.3389/fneng.2012.00011

Ke, K., Hasselbrink, E. F., & Hunt, A. J. (2005). Rapidly prototyped three-dimensional nanofluidic channel networks in glass substrates. *Analytical Chemistry, 77*(16), 5083–5088. https://doi.org/10.1021/ac0505167

Keohane, K., Brennan, D., Galvin, P., & Griffin, B. T. (2014). Silicon microfluidic flow focusing devices for the production of size-controlled PLGA based drug loaded microparticles. *International Journal of Pharmaceutics, 467*(1–2), 60–69.

Kettner, P., et al. (2006). New results on plasma activated bonding of imprinted polymer features for bio MEMS applications. *Journal of Physics: Conference Series, 34*, 65. Available at http://iopscience.iop.org/1742-6596/34/1/011.

Khan Malek, C. G. (2006). Laser processing for bio-microfluidics applications (part I). *Analytical and Bioanalytical Chemistry, 385*(8), 1351–1361. Available at https://pubmed.ncbi.nlm.nih.gov/16773304/.

Khan, I., & Poh, B. T. (2011). Natural rubber-based pressure-sensitive adhesives: A review. *Journal of Polymers and the Environment, 19*(3), 793.

Kim, T. N., Campbell, K., Groisman, A., Kleinfeld, D., & Schaffer, C. B. (2005). Femtosecond laser-drilled capillary integrated into a microfluidic device. *Applied Physics Letters, 86*(20), 201106. https://doi.org/10.1063/1.1926423

Kim, S., Kim, J., Joung, Y.-H., Ahn, S., Choi, J., & Koo, C. (2019). Optimization of selective laser-induced etching (SLE) for fabrication of 3D glass microfluidic device with multi-layer micro channels. *Micro and Nano Systems Letters, 7*(1), 15. https://doi.org/10.1186/s40486-019-0094-5

Kim, D. S., Lee, S. H., Ahn, C. H., Lee, J. Y., & Kwon, T. H. (2006). Disposable integrated microfluidic biochip for blood typing by plastic microinjection moulding. *Lab on a Chip, 6*(6), 794−802. https://doi.org/10.1039/b516495h

Kim, Y. S., Lee, H. H., & Hammond, P. T. (2003). High density nanostructure transfer in soft molding using polyurethane acrylate molds and polyelectrolyte multilayers. *Nanotechnology, 14*(10), 1140−1144. Available at http://stacks.iop.org/0957-4484/14/i=10/a=312?key=crossref.255e51eab33e6bb6c94003fc84adee1e.

Kim, H., & Najafi, K. (2005). Characterization of low-temperature wafer bonding using thin-film parylene. *Journal of Microelectromechanical Systems, 14*, 1347−1355.

Kim, K., Park, S., Lee, J. B., Manohara, H., Desta, Y., Murphy, M., et al. (2002). Rapid replication of polymeric and metallic high aspect ratio microstructures using PDMS and LIGA technology. *Microsystem Technologies, 9*, 5−10.

Kim, Y.-M., Son, S.-U., Choi, J.-Y., Byun, D.-Y., & Lee, S.-H. (2008). Design and fabrication of electrostatic inkjet head using silicon micromachining technology. *JSTS:Journal of Semiconductor Technology and Science, 8*(2), 121−127. https://doi.org/10.5573/JSTS.2008.8.2.121

Klintberg, L., et al. (2003). Fabrication of a paraffin actuator using hot embossing of polycarbonate. *Sensors and Actuators A: Physical, 103*(3), 307−316. Available at http://www.sciencedirect.com/science/article/pii/S092442470200403X.

Kohlmann, M., & Vogel, W. (1979). Stochastic control theory and stochastic differential systems: Proceedings of a Workshop of the 'Sonderforschungsbereich 72. In *Bonn' which Took Place January 1979 at*. Der Deutschen Forschungsgemeinschaft an Der Universit{ä} tBad Honnef, Springer-Verlag.

Kolew, A., et al. (2010). Hot embossing of micro and sub-micro structured inserts for polymer replication. *Microsystem Technologies, 17*(4), 609−618. Available at http://www.springerlink.com/index/10.1007/s00542-010-1182-x.

Korte, F., Serbin, J., Koch, J., Egbert, A., Fallnich, C., Ostendorf, A., et al. (2003). Towards nanostructuring with femtosecond laser pulses. *Applied Physics A: Materials Science & Processing, 77*(2), 229−235.

Kovacs, G. T. A., Maluf, N. I., & Petersen, K. E. (1998). Bulk micromachining of silicon. *Proceedings of the IEEE, 86*(8), 1536−1551.

Ko, J. S., Yoon, H. C., Yang, H. S., Pyo, H. B., Chung, K. H., Kim, S. J., et al. (2003). A polymer-based microfluidic device for immunosensing biochips. *Lab on a Chip, 3*, 106−113.

Kudryashov, S. I., Mourou, G., Joglekar, A., Herbstman, J. F., & Hunt, A. J. (2007). Nanochannels fabricated by high-intensity femtosecond laser pulses on dielectric surfaces. *Applied Physics Letters, 91*(14), 141111. https://doi.org/10.1063/1.2790741

Kuo, J. S., Zhao, Y., Ng, L., Yen, G. S., Lorenz, R. M., Lim, D. S. W., et al. (2009). Microfabricating high-aspect-ratio structures in polyurethane-methacrylate (PUMA) disposable microfluidic devices. *Lab on a Chip, 9*(13), 1951−1956. https://doi.org/10.1039/b902124h

Kuoni, A., et al. (2003). Polyimide membrane with ZnO piezoelectric thin film pressure transducers as a differential pressure liquid flow sensor. *Journal of Micromechanics and Microengineering, 13*(4), S103. Available at http://stacks.iop.org/0960-1317/13/i=4/a=317.

Kutchoukov, V. G., Laugere, F., Van Der Vlist, W., Pakula, L., Garini, Y., Alkemade, P. F. A., & Bossche, A. (2003). Fabrication of nanochannels using glass to glass anodic bonding. In *Transducers 03 12th international conference on solidstate sensors actuators and microsystems digest of technical papers cat No03TH8664* (Vol. 2). https://doi.org/10.1109/SENSOR.2003.1217018

Lagally, E. T., Simpson, P. C., & Mathies, R. A. (2000). Monolithic integrated microfluidic DNA amplification and capillary electrophoresis analysis system. *Sensors and Actuators B: Chemical, 63*(3), 138–146. https://doi.org/10.1016/S0925-4005(00)00350-6

Lahann, J., Balcells, M., Lu, H., Rodon, T., Jensen, K. F., & Langer, R. (2003). Reactive polymer coatings: A first step toward surface engineering of microfluidic devices. *Analytical Chemistry, 75*, 2117–2122.

Lake, J. H., Cambron, S. D., Walsh, K. M., & McNamara, S. (2011). Maskless grayscale lithography using a positive-tone photodefinable polyimide for MEMS applications. *Microelectromechanical Systems, 20*(6), 1483–1488. https://doi.org/10.1109/JMEMS.2011.2167664

Lakshminarayanan, S. (2018). Micro/nano patterning on polymers using soft lithography technique. *Micro/Nanolithography: A Heuristic Aspect on the Enduring Technology, 69*.

Lamonte, R. R., & Mcnally, D. (March 2001). *Cyclic olefin copolymers*.

Lang, W. (1996). Silicon microstructuring technology. *Materials Science and Engineering: Reports, 17*(1), 1–55. https://doi.org/10.1016/0927-796X(96)00190-8

Larsen, A., Poulsen, L., Birgens, H., Martin, D., & Kristensen, A. (2008). Pinched flow fractionation devices for detection of single nucleotide polymorphisms. *Lab on a Chip, 8*(5), 818–839. https://doi.org/10.1039/b802268b

Laser, D. J., & Santiago, J. G. (2004). A review of micropumps. *Journal of Micromechanics and Microengineering, 14*(6), R35–R64. https://doi.org/10.1088/0960-1317/14/6/R01

Lee, W. G., Kim, Y.-G., Chung, B. G., Demirci, U., & Ali, K. (2010). Nano/microfluidics for diagnosis of infectious diseases in developing countries. *Advanced Drug Delivery Reviews, 62*(4–5), 449–457. https://doi.org/10.1016/j.addr.2009.11.016

Lee, K. Y., Labianca, N., Zolgharnain, S., Rishton, S. A., Gelorme, J. D., Shaw, J. M., et al. (1995). Micromachining applications of a high resolution ultrathick photoresist. *Journal of Vacuum Science and Technology, B 13*, 3012–3016.

Lee, D.-S., et al. (2005). Wafer-scale fabrication of polymer-based microdevices via injection molding and photolithographic micropatterning protocols. *Analytical Chemistry, 77*(16), 5414–5434. https://doi.org/10.1021/ac050286w

Lee, J.-Y., Lee, S.-W., Lee, S.-K., & Park, J.-H. (2013). Through-glass copper via using the glass reflow and seedless electroplating processes for wafer-level RF MEMS packaging. *Journal of Micromechanics and Microengineering, 23*(8), 085012.

Lee, K. S., & Ram, R. J. (2009). Plastic-PDMS bonding for high pressure hydrolytically stable active microfluidics. *Lab on a Chip, 9*(11), 1618–1624. Available at http://www.rsc.org/Publishing/Journals/article.asp?doi=b820924c.

Le, N. N., Huynh, K. K., Hue Phan, T. C., Dung Dang, T. M., & Dang, M. C. (2017). Fabrication of 25 Mm-filter microfluidic chip on silicon substrate. *Advances in Natural Sciences: Nanoscience and Nanotechnology, 8*(1), 015003.

Lei, K. F., Ahsan, S., Budraa, N., Li, W. J., & Mai, J. D. (2004). Microwave bonding of polymer-based substrates for potential encapsulated micro/nanofluidic device fabrication. *Sensors and Actuators A, 114*, 340–346.

Lei, Y. H., Liu, Y. P., Wang, W., Wu, W. G., & Li, Z. H. (2011). *Fabrication and characterization of parylene C-caulked PDMS for low-permeable microfluidics*. Mexico: MEMS Cancun.

Li, X., Abe, T., & Esashi, M. (2001). *Deep reactive ion etching of Pyrex glass using SF 6 plasma* (Vol. 87, pp. 139−145).

Liao, Y., Cheng, Y., Liu, C., Song, J., He, F., Shen, Y., et al. (2013). Direct laser writing of sub-50 Nm nanofluidic channels buried in glass for three-dimensional micro-nanofluidic integration. *Lab on a Chip, 13*(8), 1626. https://doi.org/10.1039/c3lc41171k

Li, X., Ballerini, D. R., & Shen, W. (2012). A perspective on paper-based microfluidics: Current status and future trends. *Biomicrofluidics, 6*(1). https://doi.org/10.1063/1.3687398, 11301−1130113.

Li, S., & Chen, S. (2003). Polydimethylsiloxane fluidic interconnects for microfluidic systems. *IEEE Transactions on Advanced Packaging, 26*, 242−247.

Lin, C.-H., Lee, G.-B., Chang, B.-W., & Chang, G.-L. (2002). A new fabrication process for ultra-thick microfluidic microstructures utilizing SU-8 photoresist. *Journal of Micromechanics and Microengineering, 12*(5), 590−597. https://doi.org/10.1088/0960-1317/12/5/312

Lin, C.-H., Lee, G.-B., Lin, Y.-H., & Chang, G.-L. (2001). A fast prototyping process for fabrication of microfluidic systems on soda-lime glass. *Journal of Micromechanics and Microengineering, 11*(6), 726−732. https://doi.org/10.1088/0960-1317/11/6/316

Lin, Y., Wen, J., Fan, X., Matson, D. W., & Smith, R. D. (1999). Laser micromachined isoelectric focusing devices on polymer substrate for electrospray mass spectrometry. In *Proceedings of SPIE* (Vol. 3877, pp. 28−35). The International Society for Optical Engineering. https://doi.org/10.1117/12.359351.

Lin, A. W., & Wong, C. P. (1992). Encapsulant for nonhermetic multichip packaging applications. *IEEE Transactions on Components, Packaging, and Manufacturing Technology, 15*, 510−518.

Lion, N., Rohner, T. C., Dayon, L., Arnaud, I. L., Damoc, E., Youhnovski, N., et al. (2003). Microfluidic systems in proteomics. *Electrophoresis, 24*(21), 3533−3562. https://doi.org/10.1002/elps.200305629

Li, X., Tian, J., Nguyen, T., & Shen, W. (2008). Paper-based microfluidic devices by plasma. *Analytical Chemistry, 80*, 9131−9134. https://doi.org/10.1039/b811135a.10.1021/ac801729t, 2008903553.

Li, X., Tian, J., & Shen, W. (2010). Thread as a versatile material for low-cost microfluidic diagnostics. *ACS Applied Materials and Interfaces, 2*(1), 1−6. https://doi.org/10.1021/am9006148

Liu, J., et al. (2007). Monolithic column plastic microfluidic device for peptide analysis using electrospray from a channel opening on the edge of the device. *International Journal of Mass Spectrometry, 259*(1), 65−137. Available at http://www.sciencedirect.com/science/article/pii/S1387380606004143.

Liu, Y., Fanguy, J. C., Bledsoe, J. M., & Henry, C. S. (2000). Dynamic coating using polyelectrolyte multilayers for chemical control of electroosmotic flow in capillary electrophoresis microchips. *Analytical Chemistry, 72*, 5939−5944.

Liu, Y., Ganser, D., Schneider, A., Liu, R., Grodzinski, P., & Kroutchinina, N. (2001). Microfabricated polycarbonate CE devices for DNA analysis. *Analytical Chemistry, 73*(17), 4196−4201. https://doi.org/10.1021/ac010343v

Liu, M. C., Ho, D., & Tai, Y. C. (2008). Monolithic fabrication of three-dimensional microfluidic networks for constructing cell culture array with an integrated combinatorial mixer. *Sensors and Actuators B: Chemical, 129*, 826−833.

Liu, M., Zhang, C., & Liu, F. (2015). Understanding wax screen-printing: A novel patterning process for microfluidic cloth-based analytical devices. *Analytica Chimica Acta, 891*, 234−246. https://doi.org/10.1016/j.aca.2015.06.034

Lo, R., & Meng, E. (2011). Reusable, adhesiveless and arrayed in-plane microfluidic interconnects. *Journal of Micromechanics and Microengineering, 21*, 054021.

Lu, Y., Shi, W., Jiang, L., Qin, J., & Lin, B. (2009). Rapid prototyping of paper-based microfluidics with wax for low-cost, portable bioassay. *Electrophoresis, 30*(9), 1497–1500. https://doi.org/10.1002/elps.200800563

Lyman, D. J., et al. (1971). The development and implantation of a polyurethane hemispherical artificial heart. *Transactions – American Society for Artificial Internal Organs, 17*, 456–463. Available at http://www.ncbi.nlm.nih.gov/pubmed/5158130. (Accessed 11 October 2011).

Lyman, D., Seare, W., & Albo, D. (1977). Polyurethane elastomers in surgery. *International Journal of Polymeric Materials, 5*, 211–229.

Maejima, K., Tomikawa, S., Suzuki, K., & Citterio, D. (2013). Inkjet printing: An integrated and green chemical approach to microfluidic paper-based analytical devices. *RSC Advances, 3*(24), 9258. https://doi.org/10.1039/c3ra40828k

Mair, D., Geiger, E., Albert, P., Fréchet, J., & Svec, F. (2006). Injection molded microfluidic chips featuring integrated interconnects. *Lab on a Chip, 6*(10), 1346–1400. https://doi.org/10.1039/b605911b

Malecha, K., Gancarz, I., & Golonka, L. J. (2009). A PDMS/LTCC bonding technique for microfluidic application. *Journal of Micromechanics and Microengineering, 19*, 1–8.

Malek, C. K., & Saile, V. (2004). Applications of LIGA technology to precision manufacturing of high-aspect-ratio micro-components and -systems: A review. *Microelectronics Journal, 35*(2), 131–143. https://doi.org/10.1016/j.mejo.2003.10.003. Available at . (Accessed 20 July 2012).

Ma, G.-C., Lin, W.-H., Huang, C.-E., Chang, T.-Y., Liu, J.-Y., Yang, Y.-J., et al. (2019). A silicon-based coral-like nanostructured microfluidics to isolate rare cells in human circulation: Validation by SK-BR-3 cancer cell line and its utility in circulating fetal nucleated red blood cells. *Micromachines, 10*(2), 132.

Maluf, N. (2002). An introduction to microelectromechanical systems engineering. *Measurement Science and Technology, 13*(2), 229.

Mangriotis, M. D., et al. (1999). Flexible microfluidic polyimide channels. In *The 10th international conference on solid-state sensors and actuators. Sendai, Japan* (pp. 772–775).

Man, P. F., Jones, D. K., & Mastrangelo, C. H. (1997). Microfluidic plastic interconnects for multibioanalysis chip modules. In K. H. Chau, & P. J. French (Eds.), *Micromachined devices and components III* (Vol. 3224, pp. 196–200). SPIE. https://doi.org/10.1117/12.284516.

Manz, A., Miyahara, Y., Miura, J., Watanabe, Y., Miyagi, H., & Sato, K. (1990). Design of an open-tubular column liquid chromatograph using silicon chip technology. *Sensors and Actuators B: Chemical, 1*(1–6), 249–255.

Manz, A.,D. J. H., Verpoorte, E. M. J., Fettinger, J. C., Ludi, H., & Widmer, H. M. (1991). Miniaturization of chemical-analysis systems – a look into next century technology or just a fashionable craze. *Chimia, 45*(4), 103–105.

Mark, J.E. (2007). Physical Properties of Polymers Handbook (Google eBook) (p. 1076). Springer. Available at: http://books.google.com/books?id=fZl7q7UgEXkC&pgis=1

Marois, Y., et al. (1993). A novel microporous polyurethane vascular graft: in vivo evaluation of the UTA prosthesis implanted as infra-renal aortic substitute in dogs. *Journal of Investigative Surgery: The Official Journal of the Academy of Surgical Research, 6*(3), 273–288. Available at http://www.ncbi.nlm.nih.gov/pubmed/8398999. (Accessed 11 October 2011).

Mark, R. E., et al. (2001). *Handbook of Physical Testing of Paper* (2nd edition). Burien, Washington, USA: CRC Press.

Marois, Y., et al. (1989). In vivo evaluation of hydrophobic and fibrillar microporous polyetherurethane urea graft. *Biomaterials, 10*(8), 521−531. Available at http://www.ncbi.nlm.nih.gov/pubmed/2605286. (Accessed 11 October 2011).

Marois, Y., et al. (1996). Vascugraft microporous polyesterurethane arterial prosthesis as a thoraco-abdominal bypass in dogs. *Biomaterials, 17*(13), 1289−1300. Available at http://www.ncbi.nlm.nih.gov/pubmed/8805976. (Accessed 11 October 2011).

Martínez-López, J., Mojica, M., Rodríguez, C., & Siller, H. (2016). Xurography as a rapid fabrication alternative for point-of-care devices: Assessment of passive Micromixers. *Sensors, 16*(5), 705.

Martinez, P. R., Basit, A. W., & Gaisford, S. (2018). The history, developments and Opportunities of stereolithography. *In 3D Printing of Pharmaceuticals*, 55−79 (Springer).

Martinez, A. W., Phillips, S. T., J Butte, M., & Whitesides, G. M. (2007). Patterned paper as a platform for inexpensive, low-volume, portable bioassays. *Angewandte Chemie (International Ed. in English), 46*(8), 1318−1320. https://doi.org/10.1002/anie.200603817

Martinez, A. W., Phillips, S. T., & Whitesides, G. M. (2008). Three-dimensional microfluidic devices fabricated in layered paper and tape. *Proceedings of the National Academy of Sciences of the United States of America, 105*(50), 19606−19611. https://doi.org/10.1073/pnas.0810903105

Martinez, A. W., Phillips, S. T., Whitesides, G. M., & Carrilho, E. (2009). Diagnostics for the developing world: Microfluidic paper-based analytical devices. *Analytical Chemistry, 82*(1), 3−10. https://doi.org/10.1021/ac9013989

Martynova, L., Locascio, L. E., Gaitan, M., Kramer, G. W., Christensen, R. G., & Maccrehan, W. A. (1997). Fabrication of plastic microfluid channels by imprinting methods. *Analytical Chemistry, 69*, 4783−4789.

Masuda, M., Sugioka, K., Cheng, Y., Aoki, N., Kawachi, M., Shihoyama, K., et al. (2003). 3-D microstructuring inside photosensitive glass by femtosecond laser excitation. *Applied Physics A: Materials Science & Processing, 76*(5), 857−860. https://doi.org/10.1007/s00339-002-1937-z

Mata, A., Fleischman, A. J., & Roy, S. (2005). Characterization of polydimethyl-siloxane (PDMS) properties for biomedical micro/nanosystems. *Biomedical Microdevices*, 7281−7293.

Mccormick, R. M., Nelson, R. J., Alonso-Amigo, M. G., Benvegnu, D. J., & Hooper, H. H. (1997). Microchannel electrophoretic separations of DNA in injection-molded plastic substrates. *Analytical Chemistry, 69*, 2626−2630.

Mcdonald, J. C., Duffy, D. C., Anderson, J. R., Chiu, D. T., Wu, H., Schueller, O. J., et al. (2000). Fabrication of microfluidic systems in poly(dimethylsiloxane). *Electrophoresis, 21*, 27−40.

McDonald, J. C., Metallo, S. J., & Whitesides, G. M. (2001). Fabrication of a configur able, single-use microfluidic device. *Analytical Chemistry*, 735645−735650.

McDonald, J. C., & Whitesides, G. M. (2002). Poly(dimethylsiloxane) as a material for fabricating microfl uidic devices. *Accounts of Chemical Research*, 35491−35499.

Mehta, G., Lee, J., Cha, W., Tung, Y. C., Linderman, J. J., & Takayama, S. (2009). Hard top soft bottom microfluidic devices for cell culture and chemical analysis. *Analytical Chemistry, 81*, 3714−3722.

Melancon, K. C., Kremer, A. M., Sherman, A. A., Zhou, Z., Tumey, M. L., & Lunsford, D. A. (May 2004). *Silicone pressure sensitive adhesives, articles and methods*.

Melchels, F. P. W., Feijen, J., & Grijpma, D. W. (2010). A review on stereolithography and its applications in biomedical engineering. *Biomaterials, 31*(24), 6121−6130. https://doi.org/10.1016/j.biomaterials.2010.04.050

Mettakoonpitak, J., Boehle, K., Nantaphol, S., Teengam, P., Jaclyn, A., Adkins, et al. (2016). Electrochemistry on paper-based analytical devices: A review. *Electroanalysis, 28*(7), 1420–1436. https://doi.org/10.1002/elan.201501143

Metz, S., Bertsch, A., Bertrand, D., & Renaud, P. (2004). Flexible polyimide probes with microelectrodes and embedded microfluidic channels for simultaneous drug delivery and multi-channel monitoring of bioelectric activity. *Biosensors and Bioelectronics, 19*(10), 1309–1318. https://doi.org/10.1016/j.bios.2003.11.021

Metz, S., Jiguet, S., Bertsch, A., & Renaud, P. (2004). Polyimide and SU-8 microfluidic devices manufactured by heat-depolymerizable sacrificial material technique. *Lab on a Chip, 4*(2), 114–120. https://doi.org/10.1039/B310866J

Metz, S., Trautmann, C., et al. (2004). Polyimide microfluidic devices with integrated nanoporous filtration areas manufactured by micromachining and ion track technology. *Journal of Micromechanics and Microengineering, 14*(3), 324–331. Available at http://stacks.iop.org/0960-1317/14/i=3/a=002. (Accessed 31 July 2012).

Metz, S., Holzer, R., & Renaud, P. (2001). Polyimide-based microfluidic devices. *Lab on a Chip, 1*(1), 29–34. Available at http://www.ncbi.nlm.nih.gov/pubmed/15100886.

Microchem. (2012). *SU-8 negative epoxy series resists*. http://www.microchem.com/Prod-SU8_KMPR.htm.

Miki, N. (2005). Wafer bonding techniques for MEMS. *Sensor Letters, 3*(4), 11. Available at http://www.ingentaconnect.com/content/asp/senlet/2005/00000003/00000004/art00001. (Accessed 27 September 2012).

Mimoun, B., Pham, H. T. M., Vincent, H., & Dekker, R. (2013). Residue-free plasma etching of polyimide coatings for small pitch vias with improved step coverage. *Journal of Vacuum Science and Technology B, Nanotechnology and Microelectronics: Materials, Processing, Measurement, and Phenomena, 31*(2), 021201. https://doi.org/10.1116/1.4788795

Minges, M.L. (1989). Electronic Materials Handbook: Packaging (p. 1224). ASM International. Available at: http://books.google.com/books?id=c2YxCCaM9RIC&pgis=1.

Mogensen, K. B., et al. (2001). Monolithic integration of optical waveguides for absorbance detection in microfabricated electrophoresis devices. *Electrophoresis, 22*(18), 3930–3938. Available at http://www.ncbi.nlm.nih.gov/pubmed/11700723. (Accessed 2 July 2012).

Mohammadzadeh, A., Fox-Robichaud, A. E., & Ravi Selvaganapathy, P. (2018). Rapid and inexpensive method for fabrication of multi-material multi-layer microfluidic devices. *Journal of Micromechanics and Microengineering, 29*(1), 015013.

Mohammadzadeh, A., Robichaud, A. E. F., & Ravi Selvaganapathy, P. (2019). Rapid and inexpensive method for fabrication and integration of electrodes in microfluidic devices. *Journal of Microelectromechanical Systems, 28*(4), 597–605.

Moraes, C., Kagoma, Y. K., Beca, B. M., Tonelli-Zasarsky, R. L. M., Sun, Y., & Simmons, C. A. (2009). Integrating polyurethane culture substrates into poly(dimethylsiloxane) microdevices. *Biomaterials, 30*(28), 5241–5250. https://doi.org/10.1016/j.biomaterials.2009.05.066

Morimoto, Y., Tan, W.-H., & Takeuchi, S. (2009). Three-dimensional axisymmetric flow-focusing device using stereolithography. *Biomedical Microdevices, 11*(2), 369–377. Available at http://www.ncbi.nlm.nih.gov/pubmed/19009352.

Mostafalu, P., Akbari, M., Alberti, K. A., Xu, Q., Ali, K., Sameer, R., et al. (April 2016). A toolkit of thread-based microfluidics, sensors, and electronics for 3D tissue embedding for medical diagnostics. *Microsystems and Nanoengineering, 2*, 16039. https://doi.org/10.1038/micronano.2016.39

Müller, R. H., & Clegg, D. L. (1949). Automatic paper chromatography. *Analytical Chemistry, 21*(9), 1123–1125. https://doi.org/10.1021/ac60033a032

Munson, M. S., & Yager, P. (2003). A novel microfluidic mixer based on successive lamination. *In*, 495−498.

Natarajan, S., Chang-Yen, D. A., & Gale, B. K. (2008). Large-area, high-aspect-ratio SU-8 molds for the fabrication of PDMS microfluidic devices. *Journal of Micromechanics and Microengineering, 18*, 045021.

Nath, P., Fung, D., Kunde, Y. A., Zeytun, A., Branch, B., & Goddard, G. (2010). Rapid prototyping of robust and versatile microfluidic components using adhesive transfer tapes. *Lab on a Chip, 10*(17), 2286−2291.

Ng, J. M. K., Gitlin, I., Stroock, A. D., & Whitesides, G. M. (2002). Components for integrated poly(dimethylsiloxane) microfluidic systems. *Electrophoresis, 23*, 3461−3473.

Ngoi, B. K. A., & Sreejith, P. S. (2000). Ductile regime finish machining − a review. *International Journal of Advanced Manufacturing Technology, 16*(8), 547−550. https://doi.org/10.1007/s001700070043

Nguyen, T. N. T., & Lee, N.-E. (2007). Deep reactive ion etching of polyimide for microfluidic applications. *Journal of the Korean Physical Society, 51*(3), 984. Available at http://www.kps.or.kr/jkps/abstract_view.asp?articleuid=A8A3FF79-647E-4A84-AA25-48C2D0B0BF1B.

Nicholson, J. (1997). *The Chemistry of Polymers*. The Royal Society of Chemistry. https://doi.org/10.1039/9781847552075.

Nie, J., et al. (2012). Low-cost fabrication of paper-based microfluidic devices by one-step plotting. *Analytical Chemistry, 84*(15), 6331−6335.

Nikumb, S., et al. (2005). Precision glass machining, drilling and profile cutting by short pulse lasers. *Thin Solid Films, 477*(1−2), 216−221. https://doi.org/10.1016/j.tsf.2004.08.136. Available at . (Accessed 6 August 2012).

Nilsson, D., Balslev, S., & Kristensen, A. (2005). A microfluidic dye laser fabricated by nanoimprint lithography in a highly transparent and chemically resistant cyclo-olefin copolymer (COC). *Journal of Micromechanics and Microengineering, 15*(2), 296−300. Available at http://stacks.iop.org/0960-1317/15/i=2/a=008. (Accessed 2 July 2012).

Noh, H.-S., Huang, Y. S., & Hesketh, P. J. (2004a). Parylene micromolding, a rapid and low-cost fabrication method for parylene microchannel. *Sensors and Actuators B: Chemical, 102*, 78−85.

Noh, H.-S., Moon, K. S., Cannon, A., Hesketh, P. J., & Wong, C. P. (2004b). Wafer bonding using microwave heating of parylene intermediate layers. *Journal of Micromechanics and Microengineering*, 14625−14631.

Noiphung, J., Songjaroen, T., Dungchai, W., Henry, C. S., Chailapakul, O., & Laiwattanapaisal, W. (2013). Electrochemical detection of glucose from whole blood using paper-based microfluidic devices. *Analytica Chimica Acta, 788*, 39−45. https://doi.org/10.1016/j.aca.2013.06.021

Nosal, A., Zydorczyk, A., Sobczyk-Guzenda, A., Głuchowski, L., Szymanowski, H., & Gazicki-Lipman, M. (2009). Parylene coatings on biological specimens. *Journal of Achievements in Materials and Manufacturing Engineering, 37*, 442−447.

Ogonczyk, D., et al. (2010). Bonding of microfluidic devices fabricated in polycarbonate. *Lab on a Chip, 10*(10), 1324−1327. Available at http://www.rsc.org/Publishing/Journals/article.asp?doi=b924439e.

Oh, K. W., & Ahn, C. H. (2006). A review of microvalves. *Journal of Micromechanics and Microengineering, 16*(5), R13−R39. https://doi.org/10.1088/0960-1317/16/5/R01

Okagbare, P., et al. (2010). Fabrication of a cyclic olefin copolymer planar waveguide embedded in a multi-channel poly(methyl methacrylate) fluidic chip for evanescence excitation. *Lab on a Chip, 10*(1), 66−139. https://doi.org/10.1039/b908759a

Okoshi, T., et al. (1992). Penetrating micropores increase patency and achieve extensive endothelialization in small diameter polymer skin coated vascular grafts. *ASAIO Journal (American Society for Artificial Internal Organs), 42*(5), M398−M401. Available at http://www.ncbi.nlm.nih.gov/pubmed/8944915. (Accessed 11 October 2011).

Olson, R. (1989). Parylene conformal coatings and their applications for electronics. In *Proc. In 19th electrical electronics insulation conference*.

Ortiz, R., Chen, J. L., Stuckey, D. C., & Steele, T. W. J. (2017). Poly(Methyl methacrylate) surface modification for surfactant-free real-time toxicity assay on droplet microfluidic platform. *ACS Applied Materials and Interfaces, 9*(15), 13801−13811. https://doi.org/10.1021/acsami.7b02682

Osborn, J. L., Lutz, B., Fu, E., Kauffman, P., Stevens, D. Y., & Yager, P. (2010). Microfluidics without pumps: Reinventing the T-sensor and H-filter in paper networks. *Lab on a Chip, 10*(20), 2659−2665. https://doi.org/10.1039/c004821f

Rihakova, L., & Chmelickova, H. (2015). Laser micromachining of glass, silicon, and ceramics. *Advances in Materials Science and Engineering 2015*. https://doi.org/10.1155/2015/584952

Pakkanen, T. T., Hietala, J., Pääkkönen, E. J., Pääkkönen, P., Jääskeläinen, T., & Kaikuranta, T. (2002). Replication of sub micron features using amorphous thermoplastics. *Polymer Engineering and Science, 42*(7), 1600−3208. https://doi.org/10.1002/pen.11055

Pal, P., & Sato, K. (2015). A comprehensive review on convex and concave corners in silicon bulk micromachining based on anisotropic wet chemical etching. *Micro and Nano Systems Letters, 3*(1), 6.

Paoletti, F., Roth, S., & De Rooij, N. F. (2007). *A new fabrication method for borosilicate glass capillary tubes with lateral inlets and outlets inlets- access holes outlet*.

Papra, A., Bernard, A., Juncker, D., Larsen, N. B., Michel, B., & Delamarche, E. (2001). Microfluidic networks made of poly(dimethylsiloxane), Si, and Au coated with polyethylene glycol for patterning proteins onto surfaces. *Langmuir, 17*, 4090−4095.

Park, D., Hupert, M., Witek, M., You, B., Datta, P., Guy, J., et al. (2008). A titer plate-based polymer microfluidic platform for high throughput nucleic acid purification. *Biomedical Microdevices, 10*(1), 21−33.

Park, S.-M., Lee, K., & Craighead, H. (2008). On-chip coupling of electrochemical pumps and an SU-8 tip for electrospray ionization mass spectrometry. *Biomedical Microdevices, 10*(6), 891−898. https://doi.org/10.1007/s10544-008-9203-6

Park, S., Lee, J., Yoon, H., Kim, B., Sim, S., Chae, H., et al. (2008). Fabrication and testing of a PDMS multi-stacked hand-operated LOC for use in portable immunosensing systems. *Biomedical Microdevices, 10*(6), 859−927. https://doi.org/10.1007/s10544-008-9200-9

Peham, J., et al. (2012). Disposable microfluidic chip for rapid pathogen identification with DNA microarrays. *Microsystem Technologies, 18*(3), 311−318. https://doi.org/10.1007/s00542-011-1401-0

Pekas, N., Zhang, Q., Nannini, M., & Juncker, D. (2010). Wet-etching of structures with straight facets and adjustable taper into glass substrates. *Lab on a Chip, 10*(4), 494−498. https://doi.org/10.1039/b912770d

Pelton, R. (2009). Bioactive paper provides a low-cost platform for diagnostics. *Trends in Analytical Chemistry, 28*(8), 925−942.

Petersen, K. E. (1979). Fabrication of an integrated, planar silicon ink-jet structure. *IEEE Transactions on Electron Devices, 26*(12), 1918−1920. https://doi.org/10.1109/T-ED.1979.19796

Petersen, K. E. (1982). Silicon as a mechanical material. *Proceedings of the IEEE, 70*(5), 420−457. https://doi.org/10.1109/PROC.1982.12331

Phan, H.-P., Zhong, Y., Nguyen, T.-K., Park, Y., Dinh, T., Song, E., et al. (2019). Long-lived, transferred crystalline silicon carbide nanomembranes for implantable flexible electronics. *ACS Nano, 13*(10), 11572−11581. https://doi.org/10.1021/acsnano.9b05168

Piccin, E., et al. (2007). Polyurethane from biosource as a new material for fabrication of microfluidic devices by rapid prototyping. *Journal of Chromatography A, 1173*(1−2), 151−158. Available at http://www.ncbi.nlm.nih.gov/pubmed/17964580.

Pinto, V. C., Sousa, P. J., Cardoso, V. F., & Minas, G. (2014). Optimized SU-8 processing for low-cost microstructures fabrication without cleanroom facilities. *Micromachines, 5*(3), 738−755.

Piotter, V., Hanemann, T., Ruprecht, R., & Hausselt, J. (1997). Injection molding and related techniques for fabrication of microstructures. *Microsystem Technologies, 3*, 129−133.

Pumera, M., Wang, J., Opekar, F., Jelinek, I., Feldman, J., Lowe, H., et al. (2002). Contactless conductivity detector for microchip capillary electrophoresis. *Analytical Chemistry, 74*, 1968−1971.

Qin, D., Xia, Y. N., & Whitesides, G. M. (1996). Rapid prototyping of complex structures with feature sizes larger than 20 mu m. *Advanced Materials, 8*, 917−&.

Qin, D., Xia, Y., & Whitesides, G. M. (2010). Soft lithography for micro- and nanoscale patterning. *Nature Protocols, 5*(3), 491−502. https://doi.org/10.1038/nprot.2009.234. Available at . (Accessed 24 July 2012).

Qiu, X., Zhu, J., Oiler, J., Yu, C., Wang, Z., & Yu, H. (2009). Localized Parylene-C bonding with reactive multilayer foils. *Journal of Physics D-Applied Physics, 42*, 1−6.

Quaglio, M., Canavese, G., Giuri, E., Marasso, S. L., Perrone, D., Cocuzza, M., et al. (2008). Evaluation of different PDMS interconnection solutions for silicon, Pyrex and COC microfluidic chips. *Journal of Micromechanics and Microengineering, 18*, 055012.

Quero, R. F., Bressan, L. P., Alberto Fracassi da Silva, J., & Pereira de Jesus, D. (February 2019). A novel thread-based microfluidic device for capillary electrophoresis with capacitively coupled contactless conductivity detection. *Sensors and Actuators B: Chemical, 286*, 301−305. https://doi.org/10.1016/j.snb.2019.01.168

Rabek, J.F. (1995). Polymer Photodegradation: Mechanisms and Experimental Methods (Google eBook) (p. 664). Springer. Available at: http://books.google.com/books?id=dXwbS128lXoC&pgis=1.

Rai-Choudhury, P. (1997). *Handbook of microlithography, micromachining, and microfabrication* (Vol. 1). IET. Available at http://books.google.com/books?hl=en&lr=&id=-kbT328H1XQC&pgis=1. (Accessed 27 September 2012).

Rangsten, P., Hedlund, C., & Katardjiev, I. V. (1998). *"Etch rates of crystallographic planes in Z -cut quartz — experiments and simulation" 1.*

Razi-ul, M. H., & Wise, K. D. (2013). A glass-in-silicon reflow process for three-dimensional microsystems. *Journal of Microelectromechanical Systems, 22*(6), 1470−1477.

Reches, M., Mirica, K. A., Dasgupta, R., Dickey, M. D., Butte, M. J., & Whitesides, G. M. (2010). Thread as a matrix for biomedical assays. *ACS Applied Materials and Interfaces, 2*(6), 1722−1728. https://doi.org/10.1021/am1002266

Reedy, C. R., Price, C. W., Sniegowski, J., Ferrance, J. P., Begley, M., & Landers, J. P. (2011). Solid phase extraction of DNA from biological samples in a post-based, high surface area poly(methyl methacrylate) (PMMA) microdevice. *Lab on a Chip, 11*, 1603−1611.

Rezai, P., Selvaganapathy, P. R., & Rwohl, G. (2011). Plasma enhanced bonding of polydimethylsiloxane with parylene and its optimization. *Journal of Micromechanics and Microengineering, 21*.

Rezk, A. R., Qi, A., R Friend, J., Li, W. H., & Yeo, L. Y. (2012). Uniform mixing in paper-based microfluidic systems using surface acoustic waves. *Lab on a Chip, 12*(4), 773—779. https://doi.org/10.1039/c2lc21065g

Rich, C. A., & Wise, K. D. (1999). An 8-bit microflow controller using pneumatically actuated microvalves. In *Proc. Of the IEEE micro electro mechanical systems (MEMS)*.

Rigden, J. S. (1996). *Macmillan Encyclopedia of Physics*. New York: Simon & Schuster Macmillan.

Rihakova, L., & Chmelickova, H. (2015). Laser micromachining of glass, silicon and ceramics. A review. *European International Journal of Science and Technology, 4*(7), 41—49.

Rival, A., Jary, D., Delattre, C., Fouillet, Y., Castellan, G., Bellemin-Comte, A., et al. (2014). An EWOD-based microfluidic chip for single-cell isolation, MRNA purification and subsequent multiplex QPCR. *Lab on a Chip, 14*(19), 3739—3749.

Rizvi, N. H. (2003). *Femtosecond laser micromachining: Current status and applications* (Vol. 50, pp. 107—112) (50).

Rogers, J. A., & Nuzzo, R. G. (2005). Recent progress in soft lithography. *Materials Today, 8*(2), 50—56. https://doi.org/10.1016/S1369-7021(05)00702-9. Available at . (Accessed 27 September 2012).

Ro, K., Liu, J., & Knapp, D. (2006). Plastic microchip liquid chromatography-matrix-assisted laser desorption/ionization mass spectrometry using monolithic columns. *Journal of Chromatography A, 1111*(1), 40—47. https://doi.org/10.1016/j.chroma.2006.01.105

Roman, G. T., Hlaus, T., Bass, K. J., Seelhammer, T. G., & Culbertson, C. T. (2005). Sol-gel modified poly(dimethylsiloxane) microfluidic devices with high electroosmotic mobilities and hydrophilic channel wall characteristics. *Analytical Chemistry, 77*, 1414—1422.

Ronggui, S. (1991). Characterization of reactive ion etching of glass and its applications in integrated optics. *Journal of Vacuum Science and Technology A: Vacuum, Surfaces, and Films, 9*(5), 2709. https://doi.org/10.1116/1.577229

Roos, N., Schulz, H., Bendfeldt, L., Fink, M., Pfeiffer, K., & Scheer, H. (2002). First and second generation purely thermoset stamps for hot embossing. *Engineering Conference, 62*(1—3), 399—405. https://doi.org/10.1016/S0167-9317(02)00512-9

Rossier, J. S., Vollet, C., Carnal, A., Lagger, G., Gobry, V., H Girault, H., et al. (2002). Plasma etched polymer microelectrochemical systems. *Lab on a Chip, 2*(3), 145—150. https://doi.org/10.1039/b204063h

Ruprecht, R., et al. (1995). In K. W. Markus (Ed.), *Injection molding of LIGA and LIGA-similar microstructures using filled and unfilled thermoplastics* (pp. 146—157). Available at http://adsabs.harvard.edu/cgi-bin/nph-bib_query?bibcode=1995SPIE.2639.146R.

Saarela, V., Franssila, S., Tuomikoski, S., Marttila, S., Ostman, P., Sikanen, T., et al. (2006). Re-useable multi-inlet PDMS fluidic connector. *Sensors and Actuators B: Chemical, 114*, 552—557.

Sabbert, D., Bauer, H., & Ehrfeld, W. (1999). *ArF-excimer laser ablation experiments on Cycloolefin copolymer ž COC/*.

Sabourin, D., Dufva, M., Jensen, T., Kutter, J., & Snakenborg, D. (2010). One-step fabrication of microfluidic chips with in-plane, adhesive-free interconnections. *Journal of Micromechanics and Microengineering, 20*, 1—7.

Safavieh, R., Zhou, G. Z., & Juncker, D. (2011). Microfluidics made of yarns and knots: From fundamental properties to simple networks and operations. *Lab on a Chip, 11*(15), 2618—2624. https://doi.org/10.1039/c1lc20336c

de Santana, P. P., Segato, T. P., Carrilho, E., Sousa Lima, R., Dossi, N., Kamogawa, M. Y., et al. (2013). Fabrication of glass microchannels by xurography for electrophoresis applications. *Analyst, 138*(6), 1660—1664.

Sasaki, H., Onoe, H., Osaki, T., Kawano, R., & Takeuchi, S. (2010). Parylene-coating in PDMS microfluidic channels prevents the absorption of fluorescent dyes. *Sensors and Actuators B: Chemical, 150*, 478−482.

Sassi, A. P., Paulus, A., Cruzado, I. D., Bjornson, T., & Hooper, H. H. (2000). Rapid, parallel separations of d1S80 alleles in a plastic microchannel chip. *Journal of Chromatography A, 894*, 203−217.

Sastri, V.R. (2010). Plastics in Medical Devices: Properties, Requirements and Applications (Google ebook) (p. 352). Elsevier. Available at: http://books.google.com/books?id=WX4MW1GU3bMC&pgis=1.

Schift, H., David, C., Gabriel, M., Gobrecht, J., Heyderman, L., Kaiser, W., et al. (2000). Nanoreplication in polymers using hot embossing and injection molding. *Microelectronic Engineering, 53*(1−4), 171−174. https://doi.org/10.1016/S0167-9317(00)00289-6

Schlautmann, S., Wensink, H., Schasfoort, R., Elwenspoek, M., & Van Den Berg, A. (2001). Powder-blasting technology as an alternative tool for microfabrication of capillary electrophoresis chips with integrated conductivity sensors. *Journal of Micromechanics and Microengineering, 11*(4), 386−389. https://doi.org/10.1088/0960-1317/11/4/318

Schmidt, M.a. (1998). Wafer-to-Wafer bonding for microstructure formation. *Proceedings of the IEEE, 86*(8), 1575−1585. https://doi.org/10.1109/5.704262

Schröder, A., & Bensarsa, D. (2002). The Young's modulus of wet paper. *Journal of Pulp and Paper Science, 28*(12), 410−415.

Schultz, G. A., Corso, T. N., Prosser, S. J., & Zhang, S. (2000). *Electrospray Device for Mass Spectrometry, 72*(17), 4058−4063.

Schütte, J., Freudigmann, C., Benz, K., Jan, B., Gebhardt, R., & Martin, S. (2010). A method for patterned in situ biofunctionalization in injection-molded microfluidic devices. *Lab on a Chip, 10*(19), 2551−2559. https://doi.org/10.1039/c005307d

Search, H., et al. (1994). *Three-dimensional micro flow manifolds for miniaturized chemical analysis systems*.

Seethapathy, S., & Górecki, T. (2012). Applications of polydimethylsiloxane in analytical chemistry: A review. *Analytica Chemica Acta*, 48−62.

Selbrede, S. C., & Zucker, M. L. (1997). *Characterization of parylene-n thin films for low-k vlsi applications Low-Dielectric Constant Materials III Materials society symposium*.

Selvarasah, S., Chao, S. H., Chen, C. L., Sridhar, S., Busnaina, A., Khademhosseini, A., et al. (2008). A reusable high aspect ratio parylene-C shadow mask technology for diverse micropatterning applications. *Sensors and Actuators A: Physical*, 306−315, 145-146.

Serra, M., Pereiro, I., Yamada, A., Viovy, J.-L., Descroix, S., & Ferraro, D. (2017). A simple and low-cost chip bonding solution for high pressure, high temperature and biological applications. *Lab on a Chip, 17*(4), 629−634.

Shah, J. J., Geist, J., Locascio, L. E., Gaitan, M., Rao, M. V., & Vreeland, W. N. (2006). Capillarity induced solvent-actuated bonding of polymeric microfluidic devices. *Analytical Chemistry, 78*, 3348−3353.

Sharma, A. K., & Yasuda, H. (1982). Effect of glow-discharge treatment of substrates on parylene-substrate adhesion. *Journal of Vacuum Science and Technology, 21*, 994−998.

Shen, K., Chen, X., Guo, M., & Cheng, J. (2005). A microchip-based PCR device using flexible printed circuit technology. *Sensors and Actuators B: Chemical, 105*(2), 251−258.

Shen, J.-Y., Chan-Park, M. B.-E., Feng, Z.-Q., Chan, V., & Feng, Z.-W. (2006). UV-embossed microchannel in biocompatible polymeric film: Application to control of cell shape and orientation of muscle cells. *Journal of Biomedical Materials Research Part B: Applied Biomaterials, 77*(2), 423–430. https://doi.org/10.1002/jbm.b.30449

Shin, J. Y. (2005). Chemical Structure and Physical Properties of Cyclic Olefin Copolymers: IUPAC Technical Report (p. 14). International Union of Pure and Applied Chemistry. Available at: http://books.google.com/books?id=9gTnPgAACAAJ&pgis=1.

Shin, Y. S., Cho, K., Lim, S. H., Chung, S., Park, S., Chung, C., ... Chang, J. K. (2003). PDMS-based micro PCR chip with Parylene coating. *Journal of Micromechanics and Microengineering*, 13768.

Shinohara, H., et al. (2008). Polymer microchip integrated with nano-electrospray tip for electrophoresis-mass spectrometry. *Sensors and Actuators B: Chemical, 132*(2), 368–741. Available at http://www.sciencedirect.com/science/article/pii/S0925400507007927.

Shiu, P. P., et al. (2008). Rapid fabrication of tooling for microfluidic devices via laser micromachining and hot embossing. *Journal of Micromechanics and Microengineering, 18*(2), 025012. Available at http://stacks.iop.org/0960-1317/18/i=2/a=025012. (Accessed 27 September 2012).

Shiu, P., Knopf, G. K., & Ostojic, M. (2010). Fabrication of metallic micromolds by laser and electro-discharge micromachining. *Microsystem Technologies, 16*, 477–485.

Sia, S. K., & Whitesides, G. M. (2003). Microfluidic devices fabricated in poly(dimethylsiloxane) for biological studies. *Electrophoresis, 24*, 3563–3576.

Sidorova, J. M., Li, N., Schwartz, D. C., Folch, A., & Monnat, R. J. (2009). Microfluidic-assisted analysis of replicating DNA molecules. *Nature Protocols, 4*(6), 849–861. https://doi.org/10.1038/nprot.2009.54

Sikanen, T., et al. (2005). Characterization of SU-8 for electrokinetic microfluidic applications. *Lab on a Chip, 5*(8), 888–896. Available at http://www.ncbi.nlm.nih.gov/pubmed/16027941.

Silverio, V., & Cardoso de Freitas, S. (2018). Microfabrication techniques for microfluidic devices. *In Complex Fluid-Flows in Microfluidics*, 25–51 (Springer).

Spectrometry, I., et al. (October 2010). *Low-cost microfluidic emitters for nano-electrospray.*

Spierings, G. A. C. M. (1993). Wet chemical etching of silicate glasses in hydrofluoric acid based solutions. *Journal of Materials Science, 28*(23), 6261–6273. https://doi.org/10.1007/BF01352182

Steigert, J., et al. (2007). Rapid prototyping of microfluidic chips in COC. *Journal of Micromechanics and Microengineering, 17*, 333. Available at http://iopscience.iop.org/0960-1317/17/2/020.

Sticker, D., Rothbauer, M., Lechner, S., Hehenberger, M.-T., & Ertl, P. (2015). Multi-layered, membrane-integrated microfluidics based on replica molding of a thiol–ene epoxy thermoset for organ-on-a-chip applications. *Lab on a Chip, 15*(24), 4542–4554.

Stokes, C., & Palmer, P. J. (2006). *3D micro-fabrication processes: A review.*

Sueyoshi, K., Kitagawa, F., & Otsuka, K. (2008). Recent progress of online sample preconcentration techniques in microchip electrophoresis. *Journal of Separation Science, 31*(14), 2650–2716. https://doi.org/10.1002/jssc.200800272

Sugioka, K., Xu, J., Wu, D., Hanada, Y., Wang, Z., Cheng, Y., et al. (2014). Femtosecond laser 3D micromachining: A powerful tool for the fabrication of microfluidic, optofluidic, and electrofluidic devices based on glass. *Lab on a Chip, 14*(18), 3447–3458. https://doi.org/10.1039/C4LC00548A

Suh, H.-J., Bharathi, P., Beebe, D. J., & Moore, J. S. (2000). Dendritic material as a dry-release sacrificial layer. *Journal of Microelectromechanical Systems, 9*(2), 198–205. https://doi.org/10.1109/84.846700

Sun, Y., Kwok, Y. C., & Nguyen, N. T. (2006). Low-pressure, high-temperature thermal bonding of polymeric microfluidic devices and their applications for electrophoretic separation. *Journal of Micromechanics and Microengineering, 16*, 1681–1688.

Suriyage, N. U., Ghantasala, M. K., Iovenitti, P., & Harvey, E. C. (2004). Fabrication, measurement, and modeling of electro-osmotic flow in micromachined polymer microchannels. In *Proceedings of SPIE* (Vol. 5275, pp. 149–160). The International Society for Optical Engineering. https://doi.org/10.1117/12.521576.

Suzuki, Y., & Tai, Y. C. (2003). Micromachined high-aspect-ratio parylene beam and its application to low-frequency seismometer. In *Proc. Int. Conf. MEMS'03. (Kyotom Japan)*.

Suzuki, Y., & Tai, Y. C. (2006). Micromachined high-aspect-ratio parylene spring and its application to low-frequency accelerometers. *Journal of Microelectromechanical Systems, 15*, 1364–1370.

Tacito, R. D., & Steinbruchel, C. (1996). Fine-line patterning of parylene-n by reactive ion etching for application as an interlayer dielectric. *Journal of the Electrochemical Society, 143*, 1973–1977.

Takahara, A., Tashita, J. I., & Kajiyama, T. (1985). Microphase separated structure, surface composition and blood compatibility of segmented poly(urethaneureas) with various soft segment components. *Polymer, 26*, 987–996.

Tan, C. P., Cipriany, B. R., Lin, D. M., & Craighead, H. G. (2010). Nanoscale resolution, multicomponent biomolecular arrays generated by aligned printing with parylene peel-off. *Nano Letters, 10*, 719–725.

Tan, C. P., & Craighead, H. G. (2010). Surface engineering and patterning using parylene for biological applications. *Materials, 3*, 1803–1832.

Tang, L., & Lee, N. Y. (2010). A facile route for irreversible bonding of plastic-PDMS hybrid microdevices at room temperature. *Lab on a Chip, 10*, 1274–1280.

Tang, K. C., Liao, E., Ong, W. L., Wong, J. D. S., Agarwal, A., Nagarajan, R., et al. (2006). Evaluation of bonding between oxygen plasma treated polydimethyl siloxane and passivated silicon. *Journal of Physics: Conference Series MEMS 2006, 34*, 155–161.

Tan, H. S., & Pfister, W. R. (1999). Pressure-sensitive adhesives for transdermal drug delivery systems. *Pharmaceutical Science and Technology Today, 2*(2), 60–69.

Tay, F. E. H., et al. (2001). A novel micro-machining method for the fabrication of thick-film SU-8 embedded micro-channels. *Journal of Micromechanics and Microengineering, 11*(1), 27–32. Available at http://iopscience.iop.org/0960-1317/11/1/305.

Terry, S. C., Jerman, J. H., & Angell, J. B. (1979). A gas chromatographic air analyzer fabricated on a silicon wafer. *IEEE Transactions on Electron Devices, 26*(12), 1880–1886. Available at http://ieeexplore.ieee.org/lpdocs/epic03/wrapper.htm?arnumber=1480369.

Thompson, K., Gianchandani, Y. B., Booske, J., & Cooper, R. F. (2002). Direct silicon-silicon bonding by electromagnetic induction heating. *Journal Of Microelectromechanical Systems, 11*. https://doi.org/10.1109/JMEMS.2002.800929

Thom, N. K., Yeung, K., Pillion, M. B., & Phillips, S. T. (2012). 'Fluidic batteries' as low-cost sources of power in paper-based microfluidic devices. *Lab on a Chip, 12*(10), 1768–1770. https://doi.org/10.1039/c2lc40126f

Thorsen, T., et al. (2001). Dynamic pattern formation in a vesicle-generating microfluidic device. *Physical Review Letters, 86*(18), 4163–4166. Available at http://prl.aps.org/abstract/PRL/v86/i18/p4163_1. (Accessed 13 June 2011).

Tian, H., Hühmer, A. F., & Landers, J. P. (2000). Evaluation of silica resins for direct and efficient extraction of DNA from complex biological matrices in a miniaturized format. *Analytical Biochemistry, 283*(2), 175–191. https://doi.org/10.1006/abio.2000.4577

Todo, A., & Kashiwa, N. (1996). Structure and properties of new olefin polymers. *Macromolecular Symposia, 101*, 301–308. https://doi.org/10.1002/masy.19961010134.

Tong, Q. Y., Schmidt, E., Gösele, U., & Reiche, M. (1994). Hydrophobic silicon wafer bonding. *Applied Physics Letters, 64*(5), 625. https://doi.org/10.1063/1.111070

Tooker, A., Meng, E., Erickson, J., Tai, Y. C., & Pine, J. (2005). Biocompatible parylene neurocages. Developing a robust method for live neural network studies. *IEEE Engineering in Medicine and Biology Magazine, 24*, 30−33.

Topas Advanced Polymers. (2012). *Topas advanced polymers.* Available at http://www.topas.com/products-topas_coc. (Accessed 2 July 2012).

Traub, M. C., Longsine, W., & Truskett, Van N. (2016). Advances in nanoimprint lithography. *Annual Review of Chemical and Biomolecular Engineering, 7*, 583−604.

Truckenmuller, R., Ahrens, R., Cheng, Y., Fischer, G., & Saile, V. (2006). An ultrasonic welding based process for building up a new class of inert fluidic microsensors and -actuators from polymers. *Sensors and Actuators A, 132*, 385−392.

Truckenmuller, R., et al. (2002). Low-cost thermoforming of micro fluidic analysis chips. *Journal of Micromechanics and Microengineering, 12*(4), 375−379. Available at http://stacks.iop.org/0960-1317/12/i=4/a=304. (Accessed 3 October 2012).

Tsao, C.-W. (2016). Polymer microfluidics: Simple, low-cost fabrication process bridging academic lab research to commercialized production. *Micromachines, 7*(12), 225. https://doi.org/10.3390/mi7120225

Tsao, C. W., & Devoe, D. L. (2009). Bonding of thermoplastic polymer microfluidics. *Microfluidics and Nanofluidics, 6*, 1−16.

Tsao, C., Hromada, L., Liu, J., Kumar, P., & DeVoe, D. (2007). Low temperature bonding of PMMA and COC microfluidic substrates using UV/ozone surface treatment. *Lab on a Chip, 7*(4), 499−1004. https://doi.org/10.1039/b618901f

Tsao, C. W., Liu, J., & DeVoe, D. L. (2008). Droplet formation from hydrodynamically coupled capillaries for parallel microfluidic contact spotting. *Journal of Micromechanics and Microengineering, 18*, 25013. Available at http://iopscience.iop.org/0960-1317/18/2/025013.

Tse, L. A., et al. (2003). Stereolithography on silicon for microfluidics and microsensor packaging. *Microsystem Technologies, 9*(5), 319−323. Available at http://www.springerlink.com/Index/10.1007/s00542-002-0254-y.

Tsutsui, T., Imamura, E., & Kayanagi, H. (1981). The development of nonstended trileaflet valve prosthesis. Artif organs. *Artificial Organs, 10*, 590−593.

Ucar, Y., Akova, T., & Aysan, I. (2012). Mechanical properties of polyamide versus different PMMA denture base materials. *Journal of Prosthodontics, 21*, 173−176.

Unger, M. A., Chou, H. P., Thorsen, T., Scherer, A., & Quake, S. R. (2000). Monolithic microfabricated valves and pumps by multilayer soft lithography. *Science, 288*, 113−116.

Utracki, L.A. (2002). Polymer Blends Handbook (Google eBook) (p. 1442). Springer. Available at: http://books.google.com/books?id=VSmgMoUNBV4C&pgis=1.

Van Kan, J. A., Wang, L. P., Shao, P. G., Bettiol, A. A., & Watt, F. (2007). High aspect ratio PDMS replication through proton beam fabricated Ni masters. *Nuclear Instruments and Methods in Physics Research B, 260*, 353−356.

Van der Giessen, W. J., et al. (1996). Marked inflammatory sequelae to implantation of biodegradable and nonbiodegradable polymers in porcine coronary arteries. *Circulation, 94*(7), 1690−1697. Available at http://www.ncbi.nlm.nih.gov/pubmed/8840862. (Accessed 11 October 2011).

Vermette, P., et al. (2001). *Biomedical applications of polyurethanes, Landes bioscience Austin, TX.* Available at http://asterix.msp.univie.ac.at/.Chemistry eBooks Collection/Polymers/Biomedical applications of polyurethanes 2001 - Vermette.pdf. (Accessed 30 November 2010).

Verpoorte, E., A Manz, H. L., Bruno, A. E., Maystre, F., Krattiger, B., Widmer, H. M., et al. (1992). A silicon flow cell for optical detection in miniaturized total chemical analysis systems. *Sensors and Actuators B: Chemical, 6*(1−3), 66−70.

Verpoorte, E., & De Rooij, N. F. (2003). Microfluidics meets MEMS. *Proceedings of the IEEE, 91*(6), 930−953. https://doi.org/10.1109/JPROC.2003.813570

Veselov, D. S., Bakun, A. D., & Voronov, Y. A. (2016). *Reactive ion etching of silicon using low-power plasma etcher*. IOP Publishing. In , 748:012017.

Vlachopoulou, M. E., Tserepi, A., Pavli, P., Argitis, P., Sanopoulou, M., & Misiakos, K. (2009). A low temperature surface modification assisted method for bonding plastic substrates. *Journal of Micromechanics and Microengineering, 19*, 1−6.

Vo-Dinh, T., & Cullum, B. (2000). Biosensors and biochips: Advances in biological and medical diagnostics. *Fresenius' Journal of Analytical Chemistry, 366*(6), 540−551.

Waddell, E. (2002). UV laser micromachining of polymers for microfluidic applications. *Journal of the Association for Laboratory Automation, 7*(1), 78−82. https://doi.org/10.1016/S1535-5535(04)00179-0

Wainright, A., Williams, S. J., Ciambrone, G., Xue, Q., Wei, J., & Harris, D. (2002). Sample pre-concentration by isotachophoresis in microfluidic devices. *Journal of Chromatography A, 979*, 69−80.

Wallow, T., et al. (2007). Low-distortion, high-strength bonding of thermoplastic microfluidic devices employing case-II diffusion-mediated permeant activation. *Lab on a Chip, 7*(12), 1825−1856. https://doi.org/10.1039/b710175a

Walsh, D. I., III, Kong, D. S., Murthy, S. K., & Carr, P. A. (2017). Enabling microfluidics: From clean rooms to makerspaces. *Trends in Biotechnology, 35*(5), 383−392.

Wang, Y., Chen, H., He, Q., & Soper, S. A. (2008). A high-performance polycarbonate electrophoresis microchip with integrated three-electrode system for end-channel amperometric detection. *Electrophoresis, 29*(9), 1881−1888. https://doi.org/10.1002/elps.200700377

Wang, H. Y., Foote, R. S., Jacobson, S. C., Schneibel, J. H., & Ramsey, J. M. (1997). Temperature bonding for microfabrication of chemical analysis devices. *Sensors and Actuators B: Chemical, 45*, 199−207.

Wang, X., Lin, Q., & Tai, Y. C. (1999). Parylene micro check valve. In *Proc. Of the IEEE micro electro mechanical systems (MEMS)*.

Wang, J., Monton, M. R. N., Zhang, X., Carlos, D., Filipe, M., Pelton, R., et al. (2014). Hydrophobic sol−gel channel patterning strategies for paper-based microfluidics. *Lab on a Chip, 14*(4), 691−695. https://doi.org/10.1039/C3LC51313K

Wang, J., Muck, J. A., Chatrathi, M. P., Chen, G., Mittal, N., Spillman, S. D., et al. (2005). Bulk modification of polymeric microfluidic devices. *Lab on a Chip, 5*, 226−230.

Wang, J., Pumera, M., Chatrathi, M. P., Escarpa, A., Konrad, R., Griebel, A., et al. (2002). Towards disposable lab-on-a-chip: poly(methylmethacrylate) microchip electrophoresis device with electrochemical detection. *Electrophoresis, 23*, 596−601.

Wang, J., Pumera, M., Collins, G. E., & Mulchandani, A. (2002). Measurements of chemical warfare agent degradation products using an electrophoresis microchip with contactless conductivity. *Analytical Chemistry, 74*, 6121−6125.

Wang, W., Wu, W.-Y., & Zhu, J.-J. (2010). Tree-shaped paper strip for semiquantitative colorimetric detection of protein with self-calibration. *Journal of Chromatography A, 1217*(24), 3896−3899. https://doi.org/10.1016/j.chroma.2010.04.017

Watkinson, A. F., et al. (1995). Esophageal carcinoma: Initial results of palliative treatment with covered self-expanding endoprostheses. *Radiology, 195*(3), 821–827. Available at http://www.ncbi.nlm.nih.gov/pubmed/7538682. (Accessed 11 October 2011).

Webster, J. R., Burke, D. T., Burns, M. A., & Mastrangelo, C. H. (1998). An inexpensive plastic technology for microfabricated capillary electrophoresis chips. In *Proc. of the μTAS '98 Workshop* (pp. 249–252). Springer.

Webster, J. R., & Mastrangelo, C. H. (1997). Large-volume integrated capillary electrophoresis stage fabricated using micromachining of plastics on silicon substrates. In *International conference on solid- state sensors and actuators (tranducers)*.

Weerakoon-Ratnayake, K. M., O'Neil, C. E., Uba, F. I., & Soper, S. A. (2017). Thermoplastic nanofluidic devices for biomedical applications. *Lab on a Chip, 17*(3), 362–381.

Weigl, B. H., Bardell, R., Schulte, T., Battrell, F., & Hayenga, J. (2001). Design and rapid prototyping of thin-film laminate-based microfluidic devices. *Biomedical Microdevices, 3*(4), 267–274.

Weng, X., Kang, Y., Guo, Q., Peng, B., & Jiang, H. (2019). Recent advances in thread-based microfluidics for diagnostic applications. *Biosensors and Bioelectronics, 132*, 171–185. https://doi.org/10.1016/J.BIOS.2019.03.009

Westwood, S. M., Jaffer, S., & Gray, B. L. (2008). Enclosed SU-8 and PDMS microchannels with integrated interconnects for chip-to-chip and world-to-chip connections. *Journal of Micromechanics and Microengineering, 18*, 064014.

Wiedemeier, S., Römer, R., Wächter, S., Staps, U., Kolbe, C., & Gastrock, G. (2017). Precision moulding of biomimetic disposable chips for droplet-based applications. *Microfluidics and Nanofluidics, 21*(11), 167.

Witek, M. A., Hupert, M. L., Park, D. S.-W., Fears, K., Murphy, M. C., & Soper, S. A. (2008). 96-well polycarbonate-based microfluidic titer plate for high-throughput purification of DNA and RNA. *Analytical Chemistry, 80*(9), 3483–3491. https://doi.org/10.1021/ac8002352

Worgull, M. (2009). *Hot embossing: Theory and technology of microreplication (google eBook)*, William Andrew. Available at http://books.google.com/books?hl=en&lr=&id=Ycg-fKKf_s4C&pgis=1. (Accessed 27 September 2012).

Worgull, M., Heckele, M., & Schomburg, W. K. (2005). Large-scale hot embossing. *Microsystem Technologies, 12*(1–2), 110–115. https://doi.org/10.1007/s00542-005-0012-z

Wright, D., Rajalingam, B., Karp, J. M., Selvarasah, S., Ling, Y., Yeh, J., et al. (2008). Reusable, reversibly sealable parylene membranes for cell and protein patterning. *Journal of Biomedical Materials Research Part A, 85*, 530–538.

Wright, D., Rajalingam, B., Selvarasah, S., Dokmeci, M. R., & Khademhosseini, A. (2007). Generation of static and dynamic patterned co-cultures using microfabricated parylene-c stencils. *Lab on a Chip, 7*, 1272–1279.

Wu, W.-I., et al. (2012). Polyurethane-based microfluidic devices for blood contacting applications. *Lab on a Chip, 12*(5), 960–970. Available at http://www.ncbi.nlm.nih.gov/pubmed/22273592. (Accessed 12 March 2012).

Wu, W.-I., Sask, K. N., Brash, J. L., & Ravi Selvaganapathy, P. (2012). Polyurethane-based microfluidic devices for blood contacting applications. *Lab on a Chip, 12*(5), 960–970. https://doi.org/10.1039/c2lc21075d

Wu, P., & Zhang, C. (2015). Low-cost, high-throughput fabrication of cloth-based microfluidic devices using a photolithographical patterning technique. *Lab on a Chip, 15*(6), 1598–1608. https://doi.org/10.1039/c4lc01135j

Xiao, D., Zhang, H., & Wirth, M. (2002). Chemical modification of the surface of poly(dimethylsiloxane) by atom-transfer radical polymerization of acrylamide. *Langmuir, 18*, 9971−9976.

Xia, Y., & Whitesides, G. M. (1998). Soft lithography. *Angewandte Chemie International Edition, 37*(5), 550−575. https://doi.org/10.1002/(SICI)1521-3773(19980316)37:5<550::AID-ANIE550>3.0.CO;2-G

Xu, J., Locascio, L., Gaitan, M., & Lee, C. S. (2000). Room-temperature imprinting method for plastic microchannel fabrication. *Analytical Chemistry, 72*(8), 1930−1933. https://doi.org/10.1021/ac991216q. Available at. (Accessed 11 October 2011).

Xue, Q., Wainright, A., Gangakhedkar, S., & Gibbons, I. (2001). Multiplexed enzyme assays in capillary electrophoretic single-use microfluidic devices. *Electrophoresis, 22*, 4000−4007.

Yadavali, S., Lee, D., & Issadore, D. (2019). Robust microfabrication of highly parallelized three-dimensional microfluidics on silicon. *Scientific Reports, 9*(1), 1−10.

Yang, L. (2004). Fabrication of SU-8 embedded microchannels with circular cross-section. *International Journal of Machine Tools and Manufacture, 44*(10), 1109−1114. https://doi.org/10.1016/j.ijmachtools.2004.02.021

Yang, Y., Li, C., Kameoka, J., Lee, K., & Craighead, H. (2005). A polymeric microchip with integrated tips and in situ polymerized monolith for electrospray mass spectrometry. *Lab on a Chip, 5*(8), 869−945. https://doi.org/10.1039/b503025k

Yang, Y., et al. (2004). Quantitative mass spectrometric determination of methylphenidate concentration in urine using an electrospray ionization source integrated with a polymer microchip. *Analytical Chemistry, 76*(9), 2568−2642. https://doi.org/10.1021/ac0303618

Yang, J., Liu, Y., Rauch, C. B., Stevens, R. L., Liu, R. H., Lenigk, R., et al. (2002). High sensitivity PCR assay in plastic micro reactors. *Lab on a Chip, 2*(4), 179−187. https://doi.org/10.1039/B208405H

Yang, Y., Li, C., Lee, K., et al. (2005). Coupling on-chip solid-phase extraction to electrospray mass spectrometry through an integrated electrospray tip. *Electrophoresis, 26*(19), 3622−3652. https://doi.org/10.1002/elps.200500121

Yang, Y., Xing, S., Fang, Z., Li, R., Koo, H., & Pan, T. (2017). Wearable microfluidics: Fabric-based digital droplet flowmetry for perspiration analysis. *Lab on a Chip, 17*(5), 926−935. https://doi.org/10.1039/c6lc01522k

Yang, X., Yang, J. M., Wang, X. Q., Meng, E., Tai, Y. C., & Ho, C. M. (1998). Micromachined membrane particle filters. In *Proceedings of the IEEE micro electro mechanical systems (MEMS)*.

Ye, M.-Y., Yin, X.-F., & Fang, Z.-L. (2005). DNA separation with low-viscosity sieving matrix on microfabricated polycarbonate microfluidic chips. *Analytical and Bioanalytical Chemistry, 381*(4), 820−827. https://doi.org/10.1007/s00216-004-2988-0

Yin, H., et al. (2004). Microfluidic chip for peptide analysis with an integrated HPLC column, sample enrichment column, and nanoelectrospray tip. *Analytical Chemistry, 77*(2), 527−533. https://doi.org/10.1021/ac049068d

Yin, H., et al. (2005). Microfluidic chip for peptide analysis with an integrated HPLC column, sample enrichment column, and nanoelectrospray tip. *Analytical Chemistry, 77*(2), 527−533. Available at http://www.ncbi.nlm.nih.gov/pubmed/15649049.

Yi, L., Xiaodong, W., & Fan, Y. (2008). Microfluidic chip made of COP (cyclo-olefin polymer) and comparion to PMMA (polymethylmethacrylate) microfluidic chip. *Journal of Materials Processing Technology, 208*(1−3), 63−69. https://doi.org/10.1016/j.jmatprotec.2007.12.146. Available at . (Accessed 7 March 2012).

Youn, S.-W., et al. (2008). Dynamic mechanical thermal analysis, forming and mold fabrication studies for hot-embossing of a polyimide microfluidic platform. *Journal of Micromechanics and Microengineering, 18*(4), 45025. Available at http://stacks.iop.org/0960-1317/18/i=4/a=045025.

Yuen, P. K., & Goral, V. N. (2010). Low-cost rapid prototyping of flexible microfluidic devices using a desktop digital craft cutter. *Lab on a Chip, 10*(3), 384−387.

Zafar Razzacki, S., Thwar, P. K., Yang, M., Ugaz, V. M., & Burns, M. A. (2004). Integrated microsystems for controlled drug delivery. *Advanced Drug Delivery Reviews, 56*(2), 185−198.

Zhang, J., Tan, K. L., Hong, G. D., Yang, L. J., & Gong, H. Q. (2001). Polymerization optimization of SU-8 photoresist and its applications in microfluidic systems and MEMS. *Journal of Micromechanics and Microengineering, 11*(1), 20−26. https://doi.org/10.1088/0960-1317/11/1/304

Zhang, T., Yi, F., Wang, B., Liu, J., Wang, Y., & Zhou, Y. (2018). A method to fabricate high-aspect-ratio microstructures using PMMA photoresist. *Microsystem Technologies, 24*(2), 1223−1226. https://doi.org/10.1007/s00542-017-3490-x

Zhao, W., & Van der Berg, A. (2008). Lab on paper. *Lab on a Chip, 8*(12), 1988−1991.

Zhou, G., Mao, X., & Juncker, D. (2012). Immunochromatographic assay on thread. *Analytical Chemistry, 84*(18), 7736−7743. https://doi.org/10.1021/ac301082d

Zhou, G. Z., Safavieh, R., Mao, X., & Juncker, D. (October 2010). Immunoassay on cotton yarn for low-cost diagnostics. *Mtas*, 1−3.

Ziaie, B. (2004). Hard and soft micromachining for BioMEMS: Review of techniques and examples of applications in microfluidics and drug delivery. *Advanced Drug Delivery Reviews, 56*(2), 145−172. https://doi.org/10.1016/j.addr.2003.09.001. Available at . (Accessed 12 July 2012).

Zoumpoulidis, T., Bartek, M., Graaf, P. D., & Dekker, R. (2009). High-aspect-ratio through-wafer parylene beams for stretchable silicon electronics. *Sensors and Actuators A: Physical, 156*, 257−264.

Zulfiqar, A., Pfreundt, A., Svendsen, W. E., & Dimaki, M. (2015). Fabrication of polyimide based microfluidic channels for biosensor devices. *Journal of Micromechanics and Microengineering, 25*(3), 035022. https://doi.org/10.1088/0960-1317/25/3/035022

Surface coatings for microfluidic biomedical devices

2

M. Sonker[1,2], B.G. Abdallah[1], A. Ros[1,2]
[1]School of Molecular Sciences, Arizona State University, Tempe, AZ, United States; [2]Center for Applied Structural Discovery, The Biodesign Institute, Tempe, AZ, United States

Guided reading questions:

1. What are the major types of surface modifications available for most common microfluidic device materials?
2. What are the most commonly used strategies for immobilizing biomolecules on surfaces?
3. What kind of applications can be enabled using different surface modification strategies discussed in this chapter?

2.1 Introduction

Microfluidic devices have attracted interest in the medical and diagnostic fields as they have the potential to perform many of the current large-scale applications at a much smaller scale so as to reduce sample consumption and instrument size. Some applications, especially electrophoretic separations, have demonstrated excellent performance such as rapid separations on the order of seconds and efficient separations of diagnostically relevant species (Li & Kricka, 2006; Pagaduan, Sahore, & Woolley, 2015; Reyes, Iossifidis, Auroux, & Manz, 2002; Verpoorte, 2002). For example, rapid DNA sequencing has been demonstrated in a high throughput format (Paegel, Emrich, Wedemayer, Scherer, & Mathies, 2002), and microfluidic-based protein and DNA separations, similar in working principle to gel electrophoresis techniques, have now been commercialized for over a decade (Panaro et al., 2000). A further advantage of swift analysis is also appreciated in time-critical situations such as during surgery or for analytes that change composition over time. Another intriguing advantage of microfluidic devices is their portability and potential for point-of-care diagnostics (Yager et al., 2006), which has been demonstrated via a variety of marketed applications (Chin, Linder, & Sia, 2012). Additionally, as most microfluidic devices only require sample volumes in the microliter to nanoliter range or below for analyses, they are further suited for situations when sample amount is limited, such as in minimally invasive diagnosis. As the medical and diagnostic applications of microfluidic devices focus on the qualitative or quantitative determination of biomolecules, the biocompatibility of these devices becomes critical.

The latter refers to several requirements for microfluidic devices: First, microchannel surfaces should resist nonspecific adsorption of biomolecules (see Fig. 2.1) and provide a stable and nonaltering composition over the course of an analysis. Due to the high surface-to-volume ratio apparent in microchannels, there is a high potential for surface adsorption and deterioration, especially in combination with diagnostic samples such as body fluids (Sonker, Sahore, & Woolley, 2017). Consequently, microfluidic applications strongly depend on the tailoring and controlling of surface properties in such devices. Second, for cell-based assays, the microfluidic environment has to be adapted so that cells can adhere to surfaces if required and that intra- and intercellular processes proceed regularly which poses an important requirement for the matrices used to embed or hold specific cells (Knob, Sahore, Sonker, & Woolley, 2016). Third, several other specific surface conditions arising from the particular application at hand have to be considered such as temperature compatibility, stability under flow and applied electric fields, and solvent compatibility. Considering these guidelines and requirements, most microfluidic applications require some sort of surface pretreatment prior to analysis. Treatments can involve passivation strategies to prevent nonspecific adsorption or unwanted changes in surface properties during the course of an analysis. Furthermore, if the sensing element in a microfluidic application is a biomolecule, immobilization strategies rendering a high yield of active biomolecules on a surface are required. The control of specific biomolecule immobilization is, thus, another important requirement in many microfluidic applications (Kim & Herr, 2013).

Microfluidic devices can be created with a variety of materials; thus, surface treatment strategies strongly depend on the properties of the material (Nge, Rogers, & Woolley, 2013). Covalent immobilization schemes require specific active surface groups which vary from material to material deeming such strategies specific for a given microfluidic device. Bifunctional linker molecules may also be used which allow for specific linkage to a surface reactive group but also react specifically with functional groups on biomolecules. In contrast to covalent immobilization schemes, adsorptive coatings may present an alternative, less complex route to coat microfluidic surfaces for various purposes. The knowledge of the noncovalent interactions driving

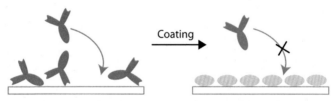

Figure 2.1 Schematic representing the prevention of non-specific adsorption to surfaces via adequate coating strategies. Left: proteins (here an IgG molecule is shown schematically) can adsorb to the untreated surface. Right: Due to coating with a blocking agent (i.e., another protein as specified in Section 2.4.1) the IgG molecules are hindered from nonspecific adsorption. Coatings can be of other non-covalent type or covalently bound to the surface

an adsorptive coating is important for the quality of the coating. In general, such interactions are determined by electrostatic, van der Waals, and/or hydrophobic interactions. The functionality of the coating can be tuned similarly to covalent strategies, and nonspecific adsorption can be suppressed in most cases. Functional groups of the adsorptive coating material can also be used for further specific biomolecule immobilization. The ease of use of adsorptive strategies and often diverse applicability to various materials has led to their widespread recognition in microfluidics.

The objective of this chapter is to provide an overview of the various strategies used to accomplish surface coating procedures for medically related microfluidic devices. First, covalent strategies are described in sections based on various substrate material properties and, thus, surface functional groups. Next, adsorptive coatings are discussed based on the specific class of coating materials. Finally, selected microfluidic applications for medical research are detailed, and future perspectives on coating procedures are discussed.

2.2 Covalent immobilization strategies: polymer devices

Covalent strategies are characterized by a chemical bond formed between a functional group of the substrate surface, i.e., the microfluidic channel walls, and a functional group of the coating agent (see Fig. 2.2). The chemical reactivity of the functional group of the coating agents is specifically chosen based on the functional group on the substrate. Covalent coatings are usually characterized by their excellent stability during microfluidic manipulations; however, they have to be adapted to the available surface functionality of the microfluidic material. This makes universal strategies between different microfluidic device materials difficult compared to other surface treatment methods. Covalent strategies for the most popular microfluidic device materials are outlined in this section separated into subsections based on the substrates.

2.2.1 Polydimethylsiloxane devices

Microfluidic systems fabricated with polydimethylsiloxane (PDMS) represent a significant portion of microfluidic devices, especially those used for important bioanalytical

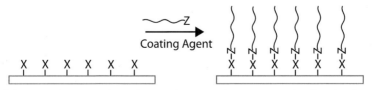

Figure 2.2 General scheme of covalent coating strategies. (X = reactive functional group of substrate surface, Z = reactive functional group of coating agent).

and medical applications (Gross, Kartalov, Scherer, & Weiner, 2007; Ni et al., 2009; Nisar, Afzulpurkar, Mahaisavariya, & Tuantranont, 2008; Sung & Shuler, 2010; Wu, Huang, & Lee, 2010). A major advantage of this material arises due to its widely ranging optical transparency in the visible light region down into the ultraviolet (UV) range with adequate pretreatment which makes it amenable for many fluorescence-based applications (Hellmich, Greif, Pelargus, Anselmetti, & Ros, 2006; Hellmich et al., 2005). Additionally, PDMS is gas permeable which accommodates cell culturing within microfluidic devices fabricated with this material; a considerable advantage for cell-based studies. Moreover, PDMS devices can be fabricated from a prestructured master exhibiting the negative relief of a desired microdevice. The prestructured master can be obtained via standard photolithography techniques, and minimal clean room infrastructure is further required for PDMS chip assembly. PDMS devices, thus, provide a suitable route for prototyping techniques which have led to the widespread adoption of its use in microfluidics research (Eduok, Faye, & Szpunar, 2017; Gokaltun, Yarmush, Asatekin, & Usta, 2017).

One issue with PDMS devices—as for many other microfluidic devices—is an inconsistent surface composition over the time course of an analytical measurement. Due to its polymeric character and long chain polymer reorientation effects on the surface, strategies need to be developed in order to maintain a given surface composition. The various strategies reported for bioanalytical and biomedical applications are described in the following sections as well as suitable techniques for stable surface functionalization.

2.2.1.1 Silanization strategies

One of the most commonly used covalent attachment strategies involves the linkage of alkoxysilane derivatives via hydroxyl group bearing surfaces resulting in siloxane linkages (see Fig. 2.3(a)). This method has not only been extensively used with glass and silica surfaces (see Section 2.3.1) but has also found widespread use for its application in PDMS-based microfluidic devices. A considerable advantage of this technique is the fact that the linkage can be mediated via one to three alkoxy groups of the reacting silane, providing a means for proper orientation and stable cross-linking to the surface. Furthermore, the functionality of the silane can be adjusted to obtain a desired chemical reactivity. As a result, hydrophobic or hydrophilic side chains can be introduced, but also various chemical functionalities become accessible for further cross-linking if desired. This is a key benefit of PDMS as a variety of chemical functionalities can be established on PDMS microchannel surfaces in contrast to other polymers which are more limited toward generalized surface functionalization. It is important to understand that silanization strategies are only successful with a considerable amount of hydroxide groups on the surface. Hydroxyl groups can be created on microchannel walls via oxidative treatments including oxygen plasma, air plasma (McDonald et al., 2000), or UV irradiation (Efimenko, Wallace, & Genzer, 2002) in an oxygen-rich atmosphere. This pretreatment step is not a covalent immobilization

Surface coatings for microfluidic biomedical devices

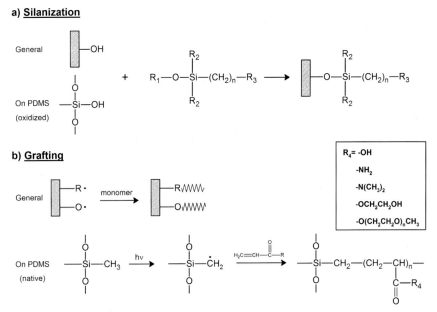

Figure 2.3 Schematics for selected covalent immobilization schemes: (a) Silanization refers to the condensation reaction of alkoxysilanes with hydroxyl groups on surfaces. This reaction can generally be used on hydroxylated surfaces, but has also found application on oxidized PDMS. (R2 = alkyl or alkoxy, R3 = functional end-group such as -NH2 or -COOH). (b) Grafting is a widespread method for immobilizing a variety of polymers. After activation and radical formation on the surface, reaction with monomers results in covalent polymer immobilization on a surface. Also shown is the activation scheme for UV activated grafting of acrylamides on native PDMS surfaces.

strategy but merely provides necessary functional groups on the substrate surface (see Section 2.5 for more details). PDMS surfaces treated with these techniques are hydrophilic and exhibit contact angles on the order of <20 degrees in contrast to native PDMS which exhibits a contact angle on the order of ~120 degrees (Hellmich et al., 2005). Although the mentioned treatments are very effective, PDMS devices need to be stored in aqueous solutions or used immediately after oxidative treatment due to the hydrophobic recovery phenomenon (Fritz & Owen, 1995); an effect that renders a hydrophilic PDMS surface hydrophobic with a half life of 1 day due to the reorganization of surface polymer chains when exposed to air.

Probably, the most utilized silane molecules are amino derivatives usually in the triethoxysilane or trimethoxysilane form. The amino group serves as the linker molecule for well-known amide bond formations with carboxylic groups mediated by carbodiimide (Miyaki, Zeng, Nakagama, & Uchiyama, 2007). For example, aminopropyltriethoxysilane (APTES) has been used for antibody attachment and cell adhesion to PDMS (Misiakos, Kakabakos, Petrou, & Ruf, 2004; Zhang, Crozatier, Le Berre, & Chen, 2005). Furthermore, Yu et al. (2009) reported improved covalent immobilization of proteins due to increased hydrophilicity after APTES treatment. This was achieved by binding an aldehyde modified dextran to APTES immobilized on a PDMS surface. With this covalent strategy, a PDMS-based device could be used to detect various biomarkers via an enzyme-linked immunosorbent assay (ELISA). Other silanization examples consist of the use of trimethoxymethylsilane to suppress nonspecific protein adsorption and attach biomolecules to microchannel walls after a silanization procedure (Sui et al., 2006). Silane-based coatings have also been demonstrated that significantly reduce nonspecific protein adsorption and improve cell adhesion to PDMS surfaces (Jon et al., 2003). This silanization process was applied via a patterning procedure consisting of a silane-copolymer anchor bound to a functional polyethylene glycol (PEG). A similar silane-based PEG coating of PDMS was also reported by Kovach, Capadona, Gupta, and Potkay (2014) to reduce fibrinogen adsorption in microchannels for long-term compatibility with blood samples. Control of electroosmotic flow (EOF) in a microchannel is also critical in many types of electrokinetic experiments to improve reproducibility between trials and substrate types and to increase analysis times. In addition to its use for immobilization purposes, a methoxysilane can be used to link a highly ionizable carboxyl-polymer to PDMS to introduce a high EOF (Miyaki et al., 2007).

Another strategy for attaching silanes has been demonstrated via the self-assembly of thiolated-silanes on gold surfaces. After coating PDMS microfluidic devices with a thin gold layer, the attachment of the thiolated silanes is accomplished via the self-assembly and stable linkage of thiols to gold. This approach is very popular in surface derivatization applications and has been applied to render surfaces hydrophilic via PEGylated thiols in microfluidic networks (Papra et al., 2001) as well as in microcontact printing applications (Delamarche et al., 2003). Furthermore, 3-mercaptopropyl trimethoxysilane has been employed as a coating procedure in a PDMS device to detect CD4+ T cells using an ester-based coupling agent functionalized to the surface followed by the immobilization of avidin and a biotinylated CD4 antibody to the surface (Cheng et al., 2009). CD4 cells could then be isolated from whole blood and counted, which is necessary when monitoring the stages of a disease such as human immunodeficiency virus (HIV) in positively tested patients. Similarly, an optical real-time affinity biosensor developed using a PDMS-based channel for multianalyte detection was also reported using thiolated silanes and biotin/avidin immobilization (Misiakos et al., 2004).

Derivatized silanes can also be exploited to covalently attach a wider variety of molecules to PDMS surfaces. A combination of UV activation with silanization to covalently pattern polyacrylamide to the surface of PDMS has been explored by Xiao, Le, and Wirth (2004), Xiao, Zhang, and Wirth (2002). An initial UV exposure oxidizes the PDMS which allows silanes to self-assemble on the surface. In this case, a trichlorosilane was adhered to the surface due to its capability of initiating atom-transfer radical polymerization of polyacrylamide. The resulting formation of a polyacrylamide layer on the PDMS surface reduces nonspecific adsorption and maintains hydrophilicity, two important improvements critical for efficient and highly sensitive biomolecule separation and diagnostics. Kreider et al. (2013) reported a strategy for coupling horseradish peroxidase enzyme on PDMS mixed with polyurethane. An atmospheric plasma was used to introduce silanol groups on the surface which were further treated with (3-aminopropyl)trimethoxysilane (APTMS) to render amine group functionality, and finally the enzyme was immobilized using glutaraldehyde as a crosslinker. This surface treatment strategy showed a more stable enzyme coating compared to physically adsorbed enzyme coating. In a different report, the surface of PDMS was hydrophilized with poly(acrylic acid) via surface initiated atomic transfer radical polymerization using a trichlorosilane as initiator (Shahsavan, Quinn, d'Eon, & Zhao, 2015). Nagahashi, Teramura, and Takai (2015) reported a highly stable polymer membrane immobilized on PDMS surfaces using various organosilanes to reduce protein adsorption for medical devices in contact with blood. In addition, β-glucosidase was immobilized very recently on a PDMS surface using APTES treatment and glutaraldehyde as a crosslinker (Hernández-Maya & Cañizares-Macías, 2018) to evaluate enzyme activity. This immobilization strategy was found to be very stable, and only 30% decrease in enzyme activity was reported after 30 days of initial immobilization.

2.2.1.2 Other immobilization schemes on PDMS

An effective and commonly used alternative method to silanization is photoinitiated UV grafting to facilitate the covalent linkage of polymers to PDMS surfaces (see Fig. 2.3(b)) (Eduok et al., 2017; Gokaltun et al., 2017; Hu et al., 2002). A major motivation for this approach is its ability to increase surface hydrophilicity while reducing protein adsorption on the substrate. Additionally, stabilization of EOF can be achieved using this surface treatment which results in a significant increase in the resolution of electrophoretic separations. In the follow-up work, the dynamics of this approach were studied by examining the ability to differentially pattern various regions on a PDMS surface using UV-initiated grafting which proved to be feasible (Hu et al., 2004). In terms of biomedical applications, UV grafting can be used to selectively micropattern PDMS in specific regions to direct cell attachment and growth as well as to immobilize antibodies for immunoassays (Hu et al., 2004). In a recent study, a hydrophilic PDMS surface was achieved using polyvinyl alcohol (PVA) as a surface coating. Oxygen plasma treated PDMS surfaces were used to covalently bond PVA molecules, and the device was used for droplet microfluidics and generating emulsions (Trantidou, Elani, Parsons, & Ces, 2017).

Another alternative to silanization is to coat PDMS with poly-xylylenes via a chemical vapor deposition (CVD) method (Lahann et al., 2003). Such polymer coatings can be employed to immobilize molecules, facilitate antibody/biotin binding assays, and improve cell adhesion assays for pharmacology studies. Follow-up studies of this approach also employed CVD to discontinuously pattern bio-inert species and reduce nonspecific protein adsorption (Chen & Lahann, 2005; Chen, McClelland, Chen, & Lahann, 2008). Zhang, Cheng, Hong, Yang, and Lin (2015) covalently modified

PDMS with carboxybetaine to render a biocompatible and antifouling coating. A Si—H functionalized PDMS film was fabricated first, and then allyl carboxybetaine was grafted to the PDMS surface via a hydrosilylation reaction. Another polymerization strategy utilizing cerium-catalyzed polymerization of various monomeric compounds can be employed for polymer coatings. The exploited Ce-catalytic action originates from the formation of siloxane radicals which further react with selected monomers resulting in their immobilization. When applied to electrochromatography studies, an increased separation efficiency and selectivity can be realized (Slentz, Penner, & Regnier, 2002). Martin and Bhushan (2017) reported a superhydrophobic and superoleophobic PDMS coating using spray coating of SiO_2 nanoparticles followed by vapor deposition of fluorosilane. Very recently, biofunctional PDMS devices were fabricated using CO_2 plasma to introduce both carboxylic and hydroxyl groups on the surface. This device was used to immobilize fibronectin on the channels walls to culture cells as a proof of concept (Shakeri et al., 2019). Such novel surface coatings on PDMS may lead to robust, stable, inexpensive and biocompatible microfluidic devices for biomedical applications and point-of-care diagnostics.

2.2.2 Thermoplastic devices

Thermoplastics constitute a wide range of polymer materials that can be molded into required geometry and features by the application of heat and pressure. Thermoplastics have gained tremendous attention in microfluidics due to their inexpensiveness, inertness to chemicals and biomolecules, optical clarity, gas impermeability and available surface chemistries (Nge et al., 2013; Zilio, Sola, Damin, Faggioni, & Chiari, 2014). This section describes the recent advances in surface coating methods specific to widely used thermoplastic polymers.

2.2.2.1 Polymethyl methacrylate

Polymethyl methacrylate (PMMA) is a very popular material for microfluidic applications. A variety of different surface activation and coupling procedures addressing a broad range of functionalities have been reported for PMMA. Several of these methods are aimed at introducing amine functionalities on PMMA surfaces (see Fig. 2.4). One example of this is a poly(ethyleneimine) (PEI) coating which is an amine-bearing polymer that can enhance antibody binding to the surface of PMMA (Bai et al., 2006). An improved antibody surface coverage with up to a ten-fold increase in overall binding was demonstrated with this immobilization strategy, leading to significant improvements in immunoassay performance. Another antibody immobilization on PMMA involved oxygen plasma treatment followed by deposition of PEI as an amine-bearing polymer and glutaraldehyde as a crosslinker using inkjet printing technology. The layer with exposed amine groups was used to crosslink anti-C-reactive protein (CRP) antibodies using glutaraldehyde as a crosslinker. A device was reported to detect CRP in a range of 10—500 ng/mL in a fluorescence-based immunoassay (Feyssa et al., 2013).

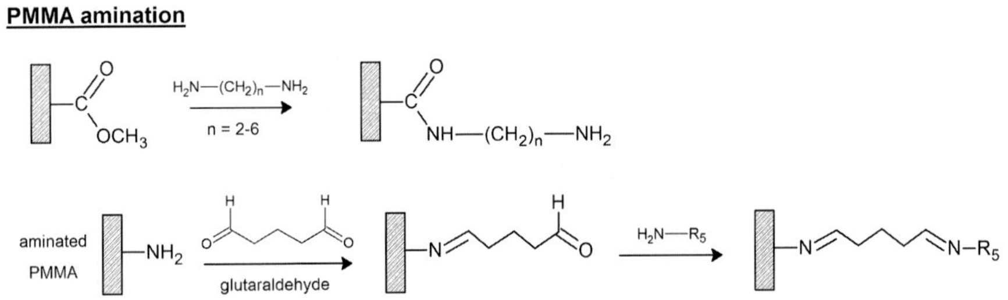

PMMA amination

Figure 2.4 Amination on PMMA is shown via activation of a short bifunctional amine. Other methods exist to create aminated PMMA, as discussed in the text. Amine groups can further be used to link other functional molecules, such as that shown in the reaction with the bifunctional glutaraldehyde and subsequent immobilization of amine-bearing molecules, such as proteins.

Another example to surface treat PMMA with amine functionalities is based on an activation procedure with lithiated diamines to link alkyl cyanates to PMMA (Henry et al., 2000). This method was further employed by Hashimoto, Barany, and Soper (2006), Hashimoto et al. (2005) for improved detection of single DNA base mutations. Similar activation strategies can be used to detect low abundance mutations in DNA using a microarray (Wang et al., 2003). Primers are linked to a PMMA surface functionalized with amines, followed by a ligase detection reaction with immobilized primers to induce hybridization detection. Additionally, PMMA can be silanized to incorporate a larger variety of functional groups to the surface such as specialized amines for the immobilization of biomolecules. A procedure using lithium aluminum hydride (LAH) to expose hydroxyl groups on the PMMA surface can be applied for further functionalization with organosilanes that facilitate the immobilization of DNA oligomers for DNA microarray analysis (Cheng, Wei, Hsu, & Young, 2004). Chehimi, Lamouri, Picot, and Pinson (2014) recently reported surface grafting of PMMA by reduction of diazonium salts. The PMMA surface was irradiated by atmospheric plasma to obtain oxygen-containing polar functional groups, and then benzenediazonium salts with various functional groups were used to modify it. This procedure was used to produce grafted PMMA surfaces with various hydrophilic/hydrophobic characteristics resulting in contact angles ranging from 60 to ∼110 degrees.

Oxidation for carboxylic acid functionality has also been reported as a suitable covalent immobilization strategy for PMMA. For example, McCarley et al. (2005) discussed a device to capture and concentrate cells and proteins using treatments for patterning polymers to substrate surfaces. For this purpose, carboxylic acid groups can be patterned on a PMMA surface with UV treatment in an oxygen-rich environment onto which antibodies are immobilized for the detection of cells (for example, MCF-7 breast cancer cells) and other proteins in solution. Antibody linkage for immunoassays has also been reported via a sol—gel immobilization strategy (Wang et al., 2008). Sol—gel films are first adsorbed to substrate surfaces in which biomolecules can be immobilized within the gel networks. The mildness of this procedure is beneficial in that bioreactivity is preserved, nonspecific adsorption is reduced, and effective immobilization of target analytes can be achieved for immunosensing with low detection limits. For example, this method has been applied in a microreactor for proteolysis via trypsin immobilization on a sol—gel coated PMMA microchannel surface (Huang et al., 2006).

An indirect approach to immobilize antibodies within a PMMA/polycarbonate microfluidic device to perform an ELISA is also possible using functionalized carbon nanotubes (CNTs) (Sun, Yang, Kostov, & Rasooly, 2010). In this example, a pressure-driven device was used, and antibody immobilization was achieved via linkage onto CNTs functionalized with poly(diallyldimethylammonium) chloride. This functionalization step renders a positive charge on the coated CNTs; therefore, immobilization is achieved via electrostatic interactions with a negatively charged antibody. The developed ELISA was used to detect bacterial toxins such as Staphylococcal Enterotoxin B (SEB) with detection limits comparable to conventional ELISA leading to a point-of-care device performing with high sensitivity.

Various other coating procedures based on commercial coating agents have been reported including the chemical SurModics (a company specializing in surface coatings for medical applications) and Reacti-Bind procedures (Liu & Rauch, 2003). These methods and the cetrimonium bromide (CTAB) surfactant were tested in the development of microfluidic hybridization array (MHAC) devices in which DNA probe attachment is a crucial step. It was shown that the Reacti-Bind method is the least effective of the three whereas the CTAB method provides improved immobilization of amine-modified DNA oligomers, and the SurModics procedure is the most effective in producing high-quality spots along the array with the least amount of surface pretreatment. As a whole, all of these methods can improve DNA-oligomer immobilization and consequently chip efficiencies, hybridization kinetics, and detection limits.

2.2.2.2 Cyclic olefin polymers and copolymers

Cyclic olefin polymer (COP) and cyclic olefin polymer (COC) are another example of commonly used thermoplastic materials offering similar properties to PMMA. Compared to PMMA, COC and COP also exhibit better compatibility to biomolecules, are chemically resistant to a wider range of organic solvents, have glass-like optical transparency, and are highly transparent to X-rays. Due to these properties, COC and COP have found applications in a wide range of microfluidic devices in the past 2 decades (Echelmeier, Sonker, & Ros, 2019; Novak, Ranu, & Mathies, 2013; Nunes, Ohlsson, Ordeig, & Kutter, 2010; Sanjay et al., 2015). However, the bare COC/COP surface is very hydrophobic and may be prone to nonspecific adsorption. Thus, many reports have surfaced in the past decade tuning the hydrophilicity of COC and COP surfaces.

The most common surface functionalization methods involve grafting of an inert hydrophilic polymer like PEG on COC surfaces. Lee and coworkers (Jeong, Hong, Kang, Choi, & Lee, 2013) reported a poly(oligo(ethylene glycol) methacrylate) coating using UV-photografting for site-selective patterning of biotin-streptavidin in COC microchannels, as shown in Fig. 2.5(a). Roy, Yue, Venkatraman, and Ma (2013) compared various polymers for surface modification of COC in terms of

Surface coatings for microfluidic biomedical devices 89

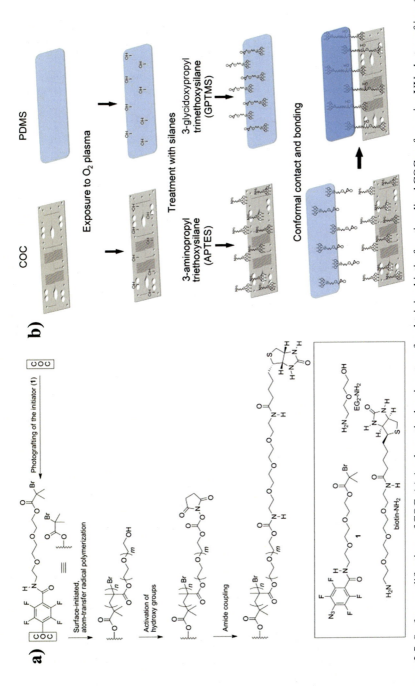

Figure 2.5 Surface modifications of COC; (a) A schematic showing steps for obtaining biotin-functionalized COC surface using UV-photografting. (b) A schematic showing steps for silanization of COC and PDMS surfaces to enable room-temperature bonding.

hydrophilicity, biocompatibility, optical clarity, and bond strength. Out of acrylic acid, acrylamide, 2-hydroxyethyl methacrylate and N-vinylpyrrolidone (NVP) monomers, NVP was found to provide the best surface coating in terms of optical clarity and biocompatibility for COC-based microfluidic devices. Woolley and coworkers (Nielsen et al., 2018, 2019; Sonker, Knob, Sahore, & Woolley, 2017; Sonker, Parker, Nielsen, Sahore, & Woolley, 2018; Sonker, Yang, Sahore, Kumar, & Woolley, 2016) recently reported several COC/COP microfluidic devices with UV-photografted polyethylene glycol diacrylate (PEGDA) layer to produce hydrophilic and nonadsorptive microchannels. These devices were used for solid-phase extraction (using reactive monoliths) and microchip electrophoretic separations of various biomarkers implicated in preterm births.

Other than photografting approaches, many other novel surface treatments have also been reported for COC/COP substrates. Similar to PMMA, COC/COP can also be functionalized using silanes to introduce various desirable surface functional groups for immobilizing biomolecules or improving bonding to another substrate such as PDMS and PMMA (Cortese, Mowlem, & Morgan, 2011). An example of such silanization-based room-temperature bonding of PDMS and COC is shown in Fig. 2.5(b). Ladner et al. (2013) described a plasma polymerization deposition method for producing a brominated COC surface using 1-bromopropane. The brominated COC surface was then used for functionalization of fluorinated alkynes using click chemistry. A hydrophobic coating of fluorocarbon or spin-coated Teflon on nanotextured COP surfaces was also reported as stable and protective layer reducing plastic deformation (Dragatogiannis et al., 2015). Another covalent grafting method for functionalization of COC surfaces was reported by Brisset et al. (2015) using aryl diazonium salts. Combined with UV irradiation, reduction of various diazonium salts produced a stable coating for wide range functional groups that can be used for biomolecule immobilization on COC surfaces. In a recent report (Wang, Wang, Zheng, & Lam, 2015), superhydrophilic and superhydrophobic COP surfaces were achieved using direct femtosecond laser irradiation. Based on the laser power deposition rate, COP surfaces with variable surface wettability (showing water contact angle of 0−163 degrees) were produced. El Fissi, Vandormael, Houssiau, and Francis (2016) reported a hybrid TiO_2/COC material obtained by physical vapor deposition of TiO_2 film on COC substrates. The hybrid material showed higher chemical resistance to polar solvents and acidic or basic solutions and may offer potential as a biocompatible material. Gleichweit et al. (2018) investigated UV/Ozone treatment of COC surfaces for optimizing bonding parameters for elastomeric COC material below the glass transition temperature. The UV/ozone treatment duration was optimized, and resulting bond strength was studied for developing doormat type microfluidic valves. Very recently, corona discharge was also exploited for functionalization of COC/COP surfaces. A decrease in water contact angle from the bare substrate was reported indicating an increase in hydrophilicity due to incorporation of oxygen-containing functional groups on the surface that may lead to development of novel biomedical devices in the future.

2.2.3 Other polymer devices

2.2.3.1 Polycarbonate

A successful approach to covalent linkage on polycarbonate involves the creation of carboxylic groups on the surface. Accordingly, several of the previously described reaction schemes can be employed. For example, UV/ozone treatment can be used to create carboxyl groups for the linkage of amino groups via carbodiimide activation (Li, Wang, Ou, & Yu, 2007). Subsequently, DNA probes can be attached within a polycarbonate DNA microarray coupled to PDMS microchannels for hybridization assays. Complementary DNA fluorescence assays carried out in such a device show great selectivity against mismatched pairs, giving them great potential to be used for portable plastic biochips. For the attachment of antibodies and other proteins, carboxylic groups can be patterned as described above for PMMA. This approach is applicable for mammalian cell capture such as capturing MCF-7 breast cancer cells in addition to protein capture by immobilizing various amide polymers (McCarley et al., 2005). Another approach that has been successful on PMMA can also be exploited for polycarbonate (Hashimoto et al., 2005, 2006). Surface activation with lithiated diamines can also be used with polycarbonate for the coupling of DNA on microfluidic surfaces to detect single base pair mutations in addition to improving polymerase chain reaction (PCR) applications. Furthermore, spraying a photosensitive polymer ("3D" link blocking solution of SurModics brand "TRIDIA") as a thin film followed by UV polymerization can also successfully derivatize polycarbonate surfaces. TRIDIA coatings utilize a hydrophilic polymer containing *N*-hydroxysuccinimide ester reactive groups which promotes binding of amine modified DNA while suppressing nonspecific adsorption Surmodics, 2020. This approach can also be used to treat DNA microarrays coupled to PCR experiments (Lenigk et al., 2002). An improvement of hybridization kinetics (efficiency of the process increasing hybridization velocity) was reported with this approach for the purpose of studying single nucleotide polymorphisms using a patterned TRIDIA coated array.

Recently, the abundance of carboxylic functional groups on polycarbonate surfaces has also been exploited for introducing novel surface chemistries for cell cultures, DNA purification, and new device bonding strategies as demonstrated by Lee and coworkers (Jang, Park, & Lee, 2014a, 2014b). A surface coating without plasma treatment was realized by modification with aminosilanes through urethane linkages to introduce silanol groups that were later used for thermal bonding of two polycarbonate surfaces and selective patterning of *E. coli* for cell culture studies. Following a similar approach, polycarbonate surfaces with variable hydrophilic and hydrophobic characteristics were also reported using various silanes. The same group later demonstrated a room-temperature process for producing a glass-like, sol–gel coating on polycarbonate surfaces using aminosilanes (Zhang, Trinh, Yoo, & Lee, 2014). This surface modification enabled a single-step polycarbonate bonding that was later adopted for adsorbing DNA for purification and amplification studies. Jankowski and Garstecki (2016) also reported surface modification of polycarbonate to produce a stable hydrophilic carboxylic acid—rich surface required for biomolecular immobilization. Polyethyleneimine was used for initial modification leading to primary amines on the polycarbonate surface followed by treatment with another reagent named poly(ethylene-alt-maleic anhydride), resulting in reduction of the maleic anhydride groups to produce the hydrophilic carboxylic acid—rich surface. Due to the available versatile surface treatment options, polycarbonate devices have also recently gained attention for droplet microfluidics (Su et al., 2019) and studying crystal nucleation (Selzer, Spiegel, & Kind, 2018) as an alternative device material to widely used thermoplastics and PDMS.

2.2.3.2 Polystyrene

Although it is the least common polymer used in medical microfluidics, polystyrene can also be used as a microfluidic device material. One well-received example utilizes a gold coating and thiol linker with a carboxylic acid head group for self-assembly on polystyrene surfaces (Darain, Gan, & Tjin, 2009). In this example, carbodiimide activation was employed to covalently bind to the amino-groups of immunoglobulin G (IgG) molecules, and the device was tested with a surface-coated antibody/antigen assay to detect IgG via fluorescence microscopy. Detection limits were in the range of typical microfluidic detection assays with a wide linear response for the immunosensor. In comparison to conventional immunoassay-based detection methods such as ELISA, this method provided a significantly lower time requirement on the order of 25 min (compared to several hours for competing methods) and had a more conservative sample volume requirement. Recently, a simple prototyping method to fabricate perfusable polystyrene-based microfluidic devices using standard lithography techniques for applications in cell cultures was demonstrated (Tran et al., 2014). This device was successfully used to culture endothelial cells under controlled hydrodynamic and physiological conditions. Another biocompatible polystyrene surface coating was recently reported by Guo et al. (2015) for label-free protein biosensing applications. Polystyrene solution was spin-coated on a glass/gold substrate, baked, and plasma etched prior to protein immobilization. The treated polystyrene film showed a significant improvement (up to 300%) in protein adhesion compared to bare glass or gold substrates.

2.3 Covalent immobilization strategies: glass devices

Silicon dioxide (SiO_2) surfaces are likely the most studied surfaces for microfluidic applications. Their surface properties are suitable for a variety of applications not only in microfluidics but also in capillary chromatography and capillary electrophoresis. Glass, fused silica, and quartz materials can all be derivatized via the same coupling chemistry. By far, the most used derivatization strategy is silanization via silanol groups generated on SiO_2 surfaces. Activation schemes involve reactive oxygen treatment, preactivation with acids such as Piranha acid or other strong acids, and treatment with strong bases such as NaOH.

2.3.1 Silanization

As discussed in Section 2.2.1.1, silanol groups on SiO_2 surfaces react with alkoxysilanes forming a stable covalent bond. Silanes similar to those used with PDMS are employed for SiO_2, and subsequent covalent reactions to bind other entities may be exploited depending on the employed silane head group. The applications of silanization on glass are multifarious, and several examples of this are given in the following paragraphs.

Proteins such as antibodies can be immobilized to glass microchannel substrates for the detection of bacteria via a biosensor using APTES. APTES is used to create an amine reactive surface to bind carboxyl groups for antibody attachment. A device of this type operates with a continuous flow of a bacterial suspension through a microchannel to facilitate specific immobilization of bacteria to an antibody-derivatized channel wall for sensitive detection (Boehm, Gottlieb, & Hua, 2007). Silanization can also be employed for bilayer lipid membrane (BLM) attachment on glass surfaces to reconstitute membrane proteins for electrophysiological and single molecule studies. For example, perfluorooctyl-trichlorosilane (PF-TCS) can be used to render glass hydrophobic followed by an injection of a lipid-based solution to facilitate the formation of BLMs. The incorporation of a spark-assisted chemical engraving method to develop the glass microstructures makes the complete device fabrication process simple and quick for easy integration (Sandison, Zagnoni, Abu-Hantash, & Morgan, 2007).

A slightly different application of silanization can be used to immobilize antibodies on glass beads to detect pathogens within a microchannel (Lee, Yang, Kim, & Park, 2006). Initially, the glass beads are coated with an aminosilane (APTMS) and functionalized with aldehydes to form a carboxy terminus for covalent immobilization with the primary amines of various antibodies. The channel is then packed with the functionalized beads and in this example was used to specifically bind with IgG as well as *E. coli* using their respective antibodies. Highly specific binding to the target analyte can be achieved with this method, and the use of glass beads provides a greater functionalized surface area thus a higher antibody concentration resulting in improved detection sensitivity compared to devices where only channel walls are treated. Application of this method in a glass microfluidic channel is also possible to covalently attach enzymes for biocatalysis studies (Lee, Srinivasan, Ku, & Dordick, 2003). Another antibody immobilization technique via silanization in a glass microchannel involves a protein A surface coating following a necessary presilanization step for IgG attachment (Dodge, Fluri, Verpoorte, & de Rooij, 2001). Coating channels with protein A for antibody binding reduces antibody denaturation and provides a higher binding affinity compared to direct glass immobilization resulting in increased antibody preconcentration and assay sensitivity. Additionally, protein A bound antibodies are oriented correctly for efficient antigen binding resulting in an even greater increase in immunoassay efficiency.

Bifunctional silanization of a glass substrate can also be applied to microfluidic PCR (Shoffner, Cheng, Hvichia, Kricka, & Wilding, 1996) or capillary electrophoresis (CE) (Hjertén, 1985) coupled with a secondary treatment using various polymers. Untreated or not properly treated devices have the potential to inhibit PCR making it important to develop devices with optimal surface chemistries. Possible PCR compatible silanes include SurfaSil and SigmaCote coated with the polymers polyglycine and polyadenylic acid. It has been shown that higher yields of amplified product are obtained from channels coated with SurfaSil and polyglycine, with results comparable, and in some cases exceeding, those obtained from a conventional PCR experiment. In terms of capillary electrophoresis, polydimethylacrylamide can be immobilized to glass capillary walls with trimethoxysilane via a well-known coating procedure to reduce EOF (high EOF reduces resolution by causing the sample plug to broaden) and nonspecific adsorption of analytes (which leads to a heterogeneous spatial distribution of the analyte thus poor separation). This method has been applied extensively for the aforementioned benefits, namely in lab-on-a-chip devices that incorporate cell lysis, DNA amplification by PCR, and analysis by CE (Waters et al., 1998).

Silanization strategies are also used for flow-through DNA microarray devices (Wei, Cheng, Huang, Yen, & Young, 2005). One distinct example is a glass/PMMA hybrid device in which a PMMA microfluidic channel is used to deliver sample to a microarray patterned on glass via "shuttle hybridization." As mentioned previously, PMMA can be silanized and functionalized with organosilanes for DNA immobilization (Cheng et al., 2004). To immobilize DNA on the glass portion of the device, the surface is silanized with triethoxysilane and then functionalized with an aldehyde derivative for immobilization of amine-functionalized DNA oligo probes. Overall, the continuous flow mechanism within the device significantly reduces DNA hybridization time. Similar silanization methods are employed within three-dimensional DNA microarray devices that connect glass microfluidic channels perpendicular to a 2D glass surface. In these devices, channel walls are silanized and functionalized to immobilize amine-derivatized DNA oligos on the glass channel surface onto which injected analyte can be hybridized. Using this surface treatment method, high-density immobilization is successfully attained compared to traditional two-dimensional array patterning methods (Benoit et al., 2001; Cheek, Steel, Torres, Yu, & Yang, 2001).

Recently, borosilicate glass and silica surfaces were modified using hexamethyldisilazane (HMDS) and dodecyltriethoxysilane to obtain similar surface hydrophobic characteristics (Grate et al., 2013). The authors reported that treating glass surface with boiling concentrated nitric acid prior to silanization produces similar surface characteristics as silanized silica surfaces. Silane treatment can also lead to uniform surface charge characteristics often required in microfluidics for electrophoretic applications. Ramsey and coworkers used the coating homogeneity of silanized glass surfaces for improving electrophoretic separation efficiency of cationic species. Microchip electrophoresis devices, fabricated from glass, were coated with (3-aminopropyl) di-isopropylethoxysilane (APDIPES) and APTES using a CVD method. The treated device surfaces exhibited uniform electroosmotic mobility over a pH range of 2.8−7.5. These silanized glass devices were then reported for fast and efficient CE integrated with electrospray ionization (ESI)-mass spectrometry (MS) of peptides and proteins (Batz, Mellors, Alarie, & Ramsey, 2014). In another recent study, 3-mercaptopropyl trimethoxysilane was used to modify the surface of glass microfluidic devices fabricated by direct laser writing. This surface was used for immobilization of epithelial cell adhesion molecule (EpCAM) antibody (biotinylated) using streptavidin-biotin interaction. The device was used for capturing circulating tumor cells with ∼75% capture efficiency (Nieto et al., 2015).

2.3.2 Other strategies

Other than silanization, immobilization of polymers like PVA has also been used extensively for applications related to electrophoresis on glass surfaces. Generally, PVA-based coatings increase device efficiency by reducing nonspecific adsorption which improves separations due to reduced analyte-wall interactions. PVA coatings are further stable in a broad pH range and facilitate the suppression of EOF while concomitantly increasing the resolution of the applied separation. To demonstrate PVA-based coatings and illustrate its advantages, several groups have coated glass microfluidic devices for electrophoresis (Belder, Deege, Kohler, & Ludwig, 2002; Ludwig & Belder, 2003). The PVA coating procedure is very simple and chemically noncomplex as a 1% aqueous solution of PVA is simply flushed through microchannels to coat them. Thermal bonding is then used to covalently attach the polymer to channel walls. PVA coated devices versus noncoated devices exhibit controllable and suppressed EOF, reduced nonspecific adsorption of analyte fluorophores, and a three-fold increase in separation efficiency. Furthermore, sensitivity is increased, and the need to wash or etch devices for reuse is unnecessary thus improving robustness. To potentially increase separation efficiency even further, PVA coatings coupled with an organic background electrolyte solution can be used (Varjo, Ludwig, Belder, & Riekkola, 2004). The use of a lower conductivity buffer solution allows for stronger electric fields to be applied thus increasing sensitivity. Under these conditions, a similar comparison of PVA versus non-PVA coated channels showed that PVA coated channels improved the resolution of a complex separation while noncoated channels could not even achieve baseline resolution. The same PVA coating procedure can also be applied to a PDMS-based device to achieve similar improvements in overall electrophoretic separation (Wu, Luo, Zhou, Dai, & Lin, 2005).

Xu et al. (2013) reported a space-selective metallization method for "electroless" plating of the internal surface of a glass microfluidic device using copper and gold plating solutions. Laser ablation was used to fabricate the microstructures and increase the roughness of the surface in the glass microfluidic device. The metal atoms in the plating solution were found to be anchored on the rough surface only. These plated surfaces were then used for applications in microreactors, microheaters, and manipulation of microorganisms and cells.

2.4 Adsorption strategies

In contrast to covalent attachment techniques, adsorption strategies rely on intramolecular interactions between the coating material and the substrate surface. They can be mediated via electrostatic interactions, van der Waals forces, and/or hydrophobic interactions. A major characteristic of these coatings is their ease of use, since microchannels generally have to be incubated with a solution containing the coating agent for a certain length of time. Subsequent use for biomedical applications is straightforward and advantageous as minimal washing procedures are required. In some cases, the coating agent can even be added to the solution during specific analyses which is referred to as dynamic coating. In contrast, coating of the substrate prior to the actual analyses is termed static coating.

Adsorptive coatings have been widely adopted and can perform similarly to covalent strategies in terms of preventing biofouling and nonspecific adsorption as well as to serve as linker molecules for further biomolecular attachment. Due to their noncovalent nature, strategies for adsorptive coatings vary from material to material and are also based on previous surface treatment steps. Adsorptive coating agents can be classified into four major groups which are characterized by multivalent interactions with the substrate surface, strong electrostatic interactions, or a combination of the two. In the following sections, polymer, polyelectrolyte, surfactant, and protein adsorptive coatings are described which constitute the majority of noncovalent coating strategies for microfluidic applications as schematically depicted in Fig. 2.6.

2.4.1 Proteins

Protein coatings represent a very popular approach to coat microfluidic channel surfaces. For example, coating with the protein bovine serum albumin (BSA) has been used in molecular biology for several decades to block surface sites from nonspecific adsorption. BSA is a soluble protein with a high tendency to adsorb to hydrophobic

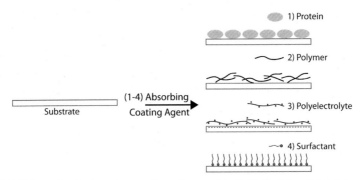

Figure 2.6 Schematic of adsorptive coatings discussed in 2.4.1 Proteins, 2.4.2 Adsorptive polymer coatings, 2.4.3 Polyelectrolyte multilayers, 2.4.4 Surfactants

surfaces such as wax-coated, paper-based microfluidic immunoassay devices where it can be used as a surface coating to reduce nonspecific adsorption (Lu, Shi, Qin, & Lin, 2010). Despite this characteristic, BSA surface treatments are not only limited to hydrophobic surfaces but can also be applied to hydrophilic surfaces, a contributing factor to its widespread use. A representative application of BSA coating applied to PDMS has been described by Eteshola and Leckband (2001) who reported background reduction by reducing the nonspecific adsorption of analytes in a sensor detecting IgG molecules for immunohistochemical analysis. BSA was not only employed to directly suppress nonspecific adsorption but also as a linker to covalently bind protein A for subsequent directed immobilization of IgG. A detection limit in the nanomolar range was reported in the employed sensor performing an ELISA. Further discussion of BSA as an advantageous medical device surface coating can be found in Section 2.6.2.

The tetrameric protein streptavidin has also been employed extensively as a linker molecule by taking advantage of its very high binding affinity to biotin. Biotin-streptavidin binding is nearly covalent in strength, and the small molecule biotin can be readily derivatized with other linker molecules or proteins. As a result, this binding pair has found widespread application in the physical and life sciences and can also be employed in adsorptive strategies for microfluidic surface coatings. Utilizing multilayers of biotin and NeutrAvidin, a derivative of streptavidin with similar binding characteristics to biotin, is one method to accomplish this on PDMS (Linder, Verpoorte, Thormann, de Rooij, & Sigrist, 2001). The multilayer approach consists of sandwiched layers of biotinylated IgG, followed by NeutrAvidin and biotinylated dextran. This three-layer sandwich has the ability to reduce nonspecific protein adsorption and maintain stable EOF for electrophoresis applications. The same strategy can also be used to immobilize other biomolecular probes to biotinylated surfaces. There are other less complex protein-based dynamic coatings to reduce nonspecific adsorption and control EOF, as demonstrated in PMMA-based microfluidic devices, but likely compatible with a variety of substrates (Naruishi, Tanaka, Higashi, & Wakida, 2006). Protein blocking agents commonly found in ELISA procedures such as Block Ace and UltraBlock as well as lysozyme can be used for this purpose. Depending on the protein coating employed, EOF can be enhanced or reduced, and its direction can be changed depending on buffer pH and charge on the protein.

For cell-based assays, other strategies mimicking extracellular matrices are commonly pursued. The matrices can be applied with an adsorptive strategy that allows for embedding biological cells for subsequent in vitro studies. A key point is to provide biocompatible surfaces in which cell studies can be performed in optimized and nonhazardous environments. An example for a cell-based assay with potential in tissue engineering, cell-matrix interactions, and cellular communication studies within a patterned microfluidic PDMS device has been demonstrated by Hou et al. (2008). PDMS in its native state resists cell adhesion and growth which is necessary in cell-based assays thus motivating the need for an appropriate surface coating procedure. An extracellular matrix mixture consisting of collagen, fibronectin, and hyaluronic acid can be coated onto PDMS to facilitate cell adhesion and growth with sufficient biocompatibility. Furthermore, a technique for layer-by-layer deposition of extracellular matrix has also been developed to micropattern cell cocultures as a future tissue engineering tool to study cell-cell communication and cell-matrix interactions (Fukuda et al., 2006). Others have also suggested complete fabrication processes using alternate substrates such as polystyrene to overcome some of the potential disadvantages of PDMS in cell-based assays such as gas permeability, substrate deterioration, small molecule adsorption, and hydrophobic recovery (Young et al., 2011). Cell assays including cell culture and blood neutrophil migration detection have been successfully performed with a polystyrene device surface coated using similar extracellular matrix proteins to promote cell adhesion. Gubala et al. (2013) described a microfluidic device for studying the biomolecule adsorption on variously treated COP channels. Adsorption of anti-human IgG and DNA was studied on differently charged COP surfaces after treatment with APTES, BSA, and PEG. Recently, Khnouf, Karasneh, and Albiss (2016) also evaluated various methods for protein (BSA) immobilization on PDMS and PMMA surfaces including passive adsorption, adsorption using glutaraldehyde as crosslinker, silanization followed by glutaraldehyde or 1-ethyl-3-(3-dimethylaminopropyl) carbodiimide hydrochloride as crosslinkers, and PEI treatment. The authors concluded that for PDMS, carbodiimide hydrochloride as crosslinker yielded highest BSA binding, while for PMMA, PEI resulted in highest BSA binding. Another interesting conclusion from this study was that room temperature−cured PDMS exhibited less nonspecific binding compared to oven-cured PDMS.

2.4.2 Adsorptive polymer coatings

Adsorptive polymer coatings have proven to be a versatile method for a variety of adsorptive coating strategies; however, the choice of the coating polymer depends strongly on the microfluidic surface due to variations in surface interactions among materials. Because glass, silica, and PDMS exhibit a similar surface chemistry, similar polymer-based coating strategies can be applied.

In Section 2.3.2, PVA immobilization was discussed; however, dynamic coating of this polymer is also possible and advantageous for electrophoretic applications. The dynamic coating method can be more stable than static immobilization due to constantly replenishing the substrate surface with coating material. Furthermore, a variety of polymer microfluidic materials have been subjected to dynamic coating procedures. On PMMA, dynamic adsorptive coating of cellulose was reported to enable long-term use (100+ runs) of a single microfluidic device used for DNA electrophoresis. Devices with this type of coating can last on the order of 1 month where the only requirement is to replenish the coating agent daily. The application of gel electrophoresis was performed multiple times in which consistently high and reproducible separation efficiencies were realized for the duration of the device's lifetime (Du & Fang, 2005). An added benefit in this case is that the same medium containing the coating agent also contains the sieving medium that drives the separation which simplifies their integration.

An additional dynamic coating of PDMS with poly(dimethylacrylamide) (PDMA) can be applied to electrophoresis applications. The coating procedure is simple in that 0.01% PDMA is added to the normal running buffer solution which is then injected into a microchannel in the same manner as conventional capillary electrophoresis. In a study of this procedure, PDMA surface adsorption was confirmed with contact angle measurements and infrared spectroscopy indicating a successful and stable surface coating when applied (Chen, Ren, Bi, & Chen, 2004). PDMA-coated channels show a reversal in EOF to a negative polarity which allows for improved injection of negatively charged samples. Additionally, a suppression of EOF occurs which improves sensitivity, and a hydrophilic surface is maintained within the microchannel which increases substrate robustness and reproducibility. Recently, Lasave, Borisov, Ehgartner, and Mayr (2015) reported an oxygen sensor in a glass-based microfluidic device by physical adsorption of polymeric nanoparticles. The nanoparticles were covalently grafted with oxygen indicators such as Pt(II) meso-di(pentafluorophenyl)diphenylporphyrin or Pt(II) benzoporphyrin which exhibit oxygen-dependent luminescence in red or near-infrared (NIR) region of the spectrum, respectively. A fast and reproducible luminescent response to gaseous and aqueous oxygen was detected using this adsorbed nanoparticle layer on the glass substrate. These devices were further developed for packed-bed microreactors using enzyme-immobilized silica beads along with oxygen-sensing nanoparticles. More recently, silica nanoparticles were physically adsorbed on PMMA to create a superhydrophilic surface (Ortiz, Chen, Stuckey, & Steele, 2017). This surface was then spatially silanized by n-dodecyltrichlorosilane (DTS) to obtain a superhydrophobic surface. This device was used for reproducible droplet generation and bacterial viability assays for toxicity monitoring.

2.4.3 Polyelectrolyte multilayers

Polyelectrolyte multilayers (PEMs) represent another adsorptive approach that has been widely used for a variety of applications. The interaction forces between the coating and substrate surface are mediated via electrostatic interactions which contribute to the stability of such coatings. Compared to the short lifetime of many physical adsorption strategies, PEMs can offer a more robust solution. Additionally, in electrophoretic applications, PEMs have the potential to control EOF in that they can reduce or even reverse EOF according to the polyelectrolyte charge characteristics of the exposed layer. This resulting EOF stabilization is a key player in increasing separation efficiency and resolution. For example, CE coupled to ESI-MS benefits from the use of PEMs such as polyamine-coated glass surfaces in which ESI-MS can be performed without an external pressure source or spray tip (Mellors, Gorbounov, Ramsey, & Ramsey, 2008). The reduction of nonspecific adsorption and control of EOF contributed to this efficient, stable, and sensitive microfluidic mass spectrometric approach for protein detection. On glass and silica as well as polymers, PEM coatings are able to change the direction of and control EOF due to differing surface charges in the employed polyelectrolyte solution (Katayama, Ishihama, & Asakawa, 1998a, 1998b).

PEM coating procedures called successive multiple ionic-polymer layer (SMIL) coatings can also be applied by placing a cationic polybrene solution between the anionic polymer dextran sulfate and the channel wall. These types of coatings maintain stability across a wide pH range, show robustness against strong acids and bases, and improve device reproducibly. Another PEM example of the many available utilizes a positively charged poly(allylamine hydrochloride) layer electrostatically self-assembled to a negatively charged silicon surface (Hau, Trau, Sucher, Wong, & Zohar, 2003). A similar approach can be applied to a PDMS microfluidic electrophoresis device to attain EOF control and improve overall stability (Liu, Fanguy, Bledsoe, & Henry, 2000).

It becomes apparent that the large variety of polyelectrolytes and their simple administration as a surface treatment makes this method versatile for a diverse set of applications and microfluidic substrates. More extensive methods for further fine tuning can be employed as well. To further study the stabilization PEMs provide, devices made of various substrates have been compared for consistency in separation performance (Currie et al., 2009). In this study, PMMA and glass microchannels were coated with poly(diallyldimethylammonium) chloride and polystyrene sulfonate (PSS) and compared to noncoated glass channels to show that PEM coated glass had a stable EOF that was independent of solution pH. Additionally, PMMA coated with PEMs provide comparable, and in some cases better, separation efficiency than glass devices which is generally not the case due to fabrication inconsistencies with polymer-based substrates. Polystyrene and poly(ethylene terephthalate) glycol (PETG) substrates have also been studied due to their significantly different polymer surface chemistries and EOF mobilities in relation to more popular polymers. With these polymers, similar results can be realized with alternating layers of cationic poly(allylamine hydrochloride) and anionic PSS that give either negative or positive surface charges, respectively, for directional control of EOF (Barker, Ross, Tarlov, Gaitan, & Locascio, 2000; Barker, Tarlov, Canavan, Hickman, & Locascio, 2000). EOF mobilities of this system in both polymers were measured and demonstrated the ability to bring the dissimilar EOF characteristics of the untreated polymers into close proximity of one another with a uniform PEM coating. This overall increase in performance and reduced variation between substrate materials as a result of PEM surface coatings opens up the possibility to confidently use cheaper and easier to fabricate polymeric-based substrates to improve many biomedical microfluidic applications.

PEMs can also be employed as a stable surface coating procedure that can be combined with subsequent immobilization of analytes. The polyelectrolytes PEI and poly(acrylic acid) can improve specific protein binding as well as long-term stability and bioreactivity due to an increase in the hydrophilicity of a coated PDMS substrate (Sung, Chang, Makamba, & Chen, 2008). A slightly more complex multistep protein modification of PDMS can also be accomplished with PEM coating, gold nanoparticle patterning, and protein patterning. An example application of such a device illustrated the ability to separate a group of neurotransmitters as well as environmental pollutants with high separation efficiency, reproducibility, and stability (Wang, Xu, & Chen, 2006).

Cell immobilization can also be undertaken using PEM coatings. Poly(diallylimethylammonium chloride) and PSS have been shown to improve cell adhesion due to increasing the wettability of PDMS (Kidambi et al., 2007). Using this method to treat PDMS, the degree of adhesion of various cell types with dissimilar cellular morphologies has been examined in which an overall improvement in cell culturing capability was realized regardless of cell type. The importance of this PEM method becomes apparent in tissue engineering applications where cell proliferation and adhesion are imperative and require a cell-friendly substrate material.

2.4.4 Surfactants

Surfactant molecules are generally amphiphilic consisting of a hydrophobic tail and hydrophilic head moiety and have the potential to combine these two unique properties into an effective surface coating. First, the hydrophilic, often charged moiety, can be employed for electrostatic attachment. Second, the hydrophobic moiety can be employed to further control surface properties such as reducing nonspecific protein adsorption or to control EOF velocity and direction. It has to be noted that depending on substrate surface properties, these two properties of the surfactant can be interchanged such that the more hydrophobic entity interacts with the surface more strongly.

A commonly employed surfactant in traditional protein analyses is sodium dodecyl sulfate (SDS) which has also been adapted and employed as an adsorptive coating agent in a variety of microfluidic applications. For example, the influence of SDS on the separation of hydrophobic species by micellar electrokinetic chromatography in PDMS devices has been studied (Roman, McDaniel, & Culbertson, 2006). Notably, SDS forms a pseudo-chromatographic phase eliminating protein adsorption and increasing EOF, consequently resulting in a rapid, highly resolved and efficient separation. Mixed coatings with other polymers can also be employed with SDS to tune the degree of adsorption to PDMS surfaces based on the concentration of SDS in solution (Berglund, Przybycien, & Tilton, 2003).

The nonionic polyoxyethylene Brij-35 and cetyltrimethylammonium bromide (CTAB) surfactants are also candidates for the reduction of nonspecific binding and EOF control in electrophoretic separations. Usually, these surfactants are employed as dynamic coating agents and are added to an electrophoresis running buffer; however, cross-linked PDMS layers on silica capillaries and glass devices in conjunction with a Brij-35 adsorptive surface treatment can also decrease EOF in addition to reducing buffer pH dependence (Youssouf Badal, Wong, Chiem, Salimi-Moosavi, & Harrison, 2002). Furthermore, CTAB and SDS were shown to work as alternative adsorptive surface coating agents for additional control of EOF. An even simpler Brij-35 coating only involving the incubation of PDMS channels with the surfactant can be used to improve separation efficiency by increasing wettability and significantly reducing nonspecific adsorption and EOF for a wide solution pH range (Dou, Bao, Xu, Meng, & Chen, 2004).

The majority of nonionic surfactants are block copolymers consisting of long chains of ethylene oxide (or PEGs) and propylene oxide, commercialized under the trademark "Pluronic." Good resistance to protein adsorption on PDMS surfaces was demonstrated with Pluronic F108 under dynamic coating conditions (Viefhues et al., 2011). Triton X-100, another amphiphilic Pluronic polyethylene oxide can also be used as a coating agent that yields an acceptable reduction in protein adsorption as well as improved performance in capillary-based electrophoretic applications in PDMS/glass devices (Kang et al., 2005). In addition to dynamic coating, nonionic surfactants can also be successfully applied as surface coating agents statically. Various Pluronics on PDMS surfaces have been reported to reduce EOF as well as maintain long term stability when statically coated (Hellmich et al., 2005).

A final and slightly different surfactant that has gained popularity is based on phospholipid bilayer systems which form by injecting lipid vesicles into a microchannel that spontaneously fuse with channel walls made of substrates such as PDMS or glass (Yang, Baryshnikova, Mao, Holden, & Cremer, 2003). These systems can be employed for ligand binding assays in which ligand-receptor binding can be measured under simulated membrane conditions along a microchannel, for example with dinitrophenyl conjugated lipids and corresponding antibodies. Additionally, fluorescence assays can be used to rapidly construct complete binding curves in one experiment, thus using less protein sample compared to traditional methods (Yang, Jung, Mao, & Cremer, 2001). Controlled bilayer environments also open up new possibilities for biosensors in cell signaling studies in which key cellular functionalities stem from cell membrane ligand-receptor mechanisms.

2.5 Other strategies utilizing surface treatments

The coating strategies discussed thus far function either by covalently binding suitable molecules to various substrates or by an adsorptive coating to form surface layers, mostly based on organic molecules. Although these two categories encompass many of the surface treatments available for microfluidic devices, there remain other approaches that can be used to change the surface properties of biomedical microfluidic devices. For instance, exposure to reactive plasma gases can produce radicals that change the chemical composition of a surface, or physical sputtering techniques can be used to deposit thin layers on surfaces. One common example of this involves the use of reactive oxygen species to alter PDMS and glass surfaces via UV or plasma treatment in oxygen or ozone atmospheres. While these treatments may be required as a precursor to subsequent covalent strategies such as silanization (discussed in Section 2.2), they can also be used as a stand-alone method to alter surface properties as desired.

UV and UV/ozone exposure has been shown to increase surface wettability with UV/ozone treatment resulting in a greater change in surface chemistry and, therefore, increased surface wettability (Efimenko et al., 2002). Polycarbonate that has been irradiated with UV shows a similar increase in wettability in addition to EOF changes that are pH independent after treatment unlike with glass substrates (Liu et al., 2001). Increasing the wettability of substrates such as PDMS improves performance in bioanalytical applications, a possible example being DNA electrophoresis in a UV-treated device yielding high resolution and reproducibility. UV/Ozone treatment can be taken a step further to form porous polymer monoliths by adsorbing a UV-activated photoinitiator and monomers to channel walls followed by polymerization to noncovalently adhere the polymer to the surface. The durability and robustness of this attachment has been shown to withstand high pressures, despite its adsorptive nature (Burke & Smela, 2012).

Oxygen plasma treatment is a considerably widespread surface modification method for microfluidic devices, namely PDMS-based, but can also be used with other substrates. A short treatment on the order of 1 min produces hydroxyl groups on the PDMS surface allowing for the formation of covalent siloxane bonds (Si−O−Si) with other substrates including itself, glass, silicon, polystyrene, and others. This adhesion is irreversible, and bond strengths between PDMS and other substrates have been shown to increase linearly with the degree of plasma exposure (Bhattacharya, Datta, Berg, & Gangopadhyay, 2005). This high correlation between bond strength and plasma exposure can be used to develop optimized plasma treatment parameters based on the degree of bonding needed. Concomitantly, an increase in surface wettability occurs due to the creation of silanol groups (Si−OH), rendering negatively charged channel walls for electroosmosis (Duffy, McDonald, Schueller, & Whitesides, 1998). Changes in PDMS wettability after plasma treatment and after exposure to several chemicals has also been studied (Mata, Fleischman, & Roy, 2005). While plasma treatment increases the wettability of PDMS, treatment with several different acids and bases including strong acids such as H_2SO_4 revert the contact angle of plasma-treated PDMS to a more native hydrophobic and less wettable state. This opens up the possibility of differentially patterning hydrophobic and hydrophilic regions on the same substrate in a lab-on-a-chip microfluidic device depending on the surface properties needed at each zone.

Metal sputtering methods can also be utilized in surface treatment schemes, for example sputtering and evaporation of gold on microchannel surfaces. The gold-coated surfaces serve as templates for self-assembled monolayers (SAMs) to which a variety of coupling schemes can be applied with an adequate choice of thiol head groups (see also Section 2.2.1a). One example of this involves binding collagen to SAMs using Schiff base chemistry for the development of cell analysis arrays with improved cell adhesion and attraction to treated channel walls (Leong, Boardman, Ma, & Jen, 2009). Other metals can also be coated on microfluidic devices, for example aluminum sputtering and plasma treatment to create a biocompatible surface for increased cell adhesion and proliferation (Patrito, McCague, Norton, & Petersen, 2007). The metal is then etched in areas designated by a mask to expose a hydrophilic and reactive PDMS surface that favors cell adhesion. The novelty of this inexpensive and simple method over others discussed is that only a single-component substrate is used without the need for surfactants or extracellular matrix protein adsorption methods previously described.

2.6 Examples of applications

The majority of the microfluidic surface modifications mentioned in this chapter have a specific focus in terms of application. While popular surface modifications were discussed, the applications they are tuned for were only briefly mentioned. In this section, three diagnostic applications are looked at in further detail to demonstrate the great potential of microfluidics in the medical sciences as well as to further emphasize the necessity of adequate surface coatings for successful analyses. The applications selected are those that are highly regarded in their respective fields and take proof-of-concept surface treatment studies and apply them to biological and medically focused applications. The microfluidic devices discussed herein are considered to be complete lab-on-a-chip devices in that they are fully integrated analysis systems capable of complete diagnostics-based studies.

2.6.1 Lab-on-a-chip drug analysis of blood serum

Throughout this chapter, a significant number of the surface treatments discussed were applied to bioanalysis assays using microfluidic capillary electrophoresis. Two major issues with CE in a microfluidic device are sample adsorption to capillary walls and unstable, high EOF. Both of these effects reduce resolution and efficiency and, therefore, need to be addressed to attain a high-quality separation. As presented in many of the previous sections, a variety of channel wall surface treatments have been shown to significantly reduce EOF as well as nonspecific adsorption. There are benefits and drawbacks of different surface coatings based on invasiveness, difficulty, and durability in which an ideal coating would be easy to apply, not interfere with sample analytes, and be robust throughout multiple trials over time using the same device.

A lab-on-a-chip device with complete drug analysis capabilities including sample mixing, immunoreaction, separation using capillary electrophoresis, and analysis has been realized using a glass microfluidic device (see Fig. 2.7(a)) (Chiem & Harrison, 1998). The automatability and positive results achieved with this device have opened new possibilities to further develop such devices for clinical use. Specifically in this study, the detection and analysis of the asthma drug theophylline (Th) from a blood serum sample was demonstrated. The mixing portion involved the labeling of diluted blood serum with a tracer and immunoreaction with a specific antibody, anti-Th. The free Th was then separated from antibody-bound Th for quantitative analysis (see Fig. 2.7(b)). The performance of the device was comparable to traditional, nonintegrated methods with great detection limits, and analysis times were significantly shortened due to the microscale nature of the device.

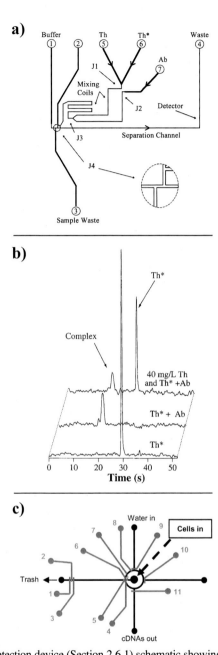

Figure 2.7 (a) Drug detection device (Section 2.6.1) schematic showing the various operating regions. Mixing of the antigen (Th) with the tracer (Th*) is performed between J1 and J3. Antibody (Ab) is then mixed with antigen and tracer in the J3-J4 immunoassay region. J4 shows the injection point into the electrophoresis region followed by detection. (b) A representative electropherogram showing actual results from a complete experiment. The bottom-most plot represents a control containing only tracer in buffer. The middle plot represents a mixture of antibody and tracer and the top plot represents a sample immunoassay with tracer and antibody. The Ab-Th* complex shows a distinct peak that is high when only tracer is present (middle) but decreases when This added due to competitive binding to Ab. A comparison of the two is used to quantify Th concentration. (c) Schematic of the single cell transcriptome device (Section 2.6.2). Numbers 1−11 represent independently controlled valves and the center 'cells in' region is used for sample injection. Initially, valves 1−3 are used to pump sample and cell trapping occurred at closed valves 4−7. Valves 8 and 10 were used to add cell lysis reagents and reverse transcriptase for PCR.

Because surface treatments are the focus of this chapter, it is important to mention the contribution of a surface treatment to the success of this integrated device. Similar devices without surface treatment showed low efficiency, tailing of analytes, and background fluorescence due to adsorption (Nielsen, Rickard, Santa, Sharknas, & Sittampalam, 1991). Dynamic coating using the nonionic surfactant Tween 20 was utilized to reduce nonspecific adsorption for a variety of reasons including ease of application compared to covalent methods and biocompatibility (Tween 20 is a common immunoassay washing agent that prevents nonspecific antibody binding). Additionally, this surface coating contributed to stable sample migration times due to a stabilization of EOF (Chiem & Harrison, 1997). In this specific experiment, Tween 20 was shown to be beneficial; however, as mentioned throughout this chapter, a multitude of different surface coatings have been utilized for capillary electrophoresis. When selecting a surface coating for your application, it is important to consider all aspects of the experiment and choose one that meets the requirements of the experiment (substrate, analyte, etc). Recently, Picher et al. developed a lab-on-a-chip device for continuous glucose monitoring using whole blood (Picher et al., 2013). The device surface was coated with crystalline surface protein (SbpA) monolayers that acted as antifouling coating and was also used as an immobilization matrix for glucose oxidase. This enzyme modified surface was used for bioelectrochemical measurements of glucose concentrations ranging from 500 μM to 50 mM.

2.6.2 Single cell transcriptome analysis with microfluidic PCR

Gene expression is a highly studied area to improve our understanding of organisms including their regulatory pathways, growth, etc. To investigate complete genetic expression or the transcriptome, single cell analysis is appropriate. Due to small sample volume availability in these types of studies, microfluidics is an excellent platform to employ, especially since there is the potential for complete lab-on-a-chip development. Similar to the analysis of proteins examined in Section 2.6.1, DNA analysis poses similar obstacles in terms of substrate/analyte interactions that can impede successful analysis, exemplifying the need for surface treatments. Advancements in microfluidics have led to the development of a PDMS device that can capture and lyse cells followed by reverse transcriptase polymerase chain reaction (RT-PCR) amplification and analysis to study gene expression in mouse brain (Bontoux et al., 2008). The layout of this device is schematically depicted in Fig. 2.7(c). Injection of individual neuronal cells into the device and subsequent processing and analysis allowed for an average detection of 5000 genes per cell, the expected number in a single cell of this type. This exceptional sensitivity and ability to study a cell's transcriptome is a significant clinical advancement toward rapid and more complete genetic analysis to understand the pathology and physiology of an organism.

A necessary and common surface treatment was used in this device: dynamic channel coating with the protein BSA. Due to its biocompatibility and ease of use, BSA surface passivation has been commonly used in microfluidic PCR to reduce adsorption

(Zhang, Xu, Ma, & Zheng, 2006) in addition to other applications discussed in Section 2.4.1. It has been reported that *Taq* polymerase adsorption is significant and contributes the most to poor PCR performance compared to DNA adsorption which still occurs but to a lesser extent (Erill, Campoy, Erill, Barbé, & Aguiló, 2003). BSA has found widespread use due to its competitive adsorption to substrate walls with *Taq* and DNA, effectively reducing unwanted analyte adsorption. A potential explanation of this phenomenon is that BSA has similar charge characteristics as DNA under microfluidic PCR conditions and, therefore, has similar attraction to substrate channel walls (Nagai, Murakami, Morita, Yokoyama, & Tamiya, 2001). An added benefit of BSA is that it acts as a stabilizing agent of polymerase enzymes in solution. Similar to the Tween 20 CE surface coating, an appropriate surface coating for DNA PCR was applied with multiple benefits to ensure increased performance while remaining simple to apply without introducing detrimental side effects to the sample.

Recently, a cost-effective COP-based PCR chip was developed for quantitative detection of pathogenic microorganisms (Tachibana et al., 2015). The device surface was rendered hydrophilic by dynamic coatings using different polymers and surfactants like carboxymethyl cellulose, sodium cocoyl sarcosinate, and Tween 20 to facilitate capillary-based flow of samples. This chip was further used for quantitative real-time PCR with DNA concentrations as low as 2 fg/µL using human and *E. coli* genomic DNA. Another gene amplification PCR chip was reported by Qin, Lv, Xing, Li, and Deng (2016) using a NOA81 optical adhesive. Various BSA based dynamic coatings were tested to provide the essential channel hydrophilicity required for gene amplification. Successful amplification was demonstrated for HLA-DRB1 and AEB-HV genes with an on-chip PCR method. Trinh et al. (2016) reported a PMMA-based PCR chip for rapid diagnoses of foodborne pathogens. The PMMA surface was treated with APTES to incorporate a thin epoxy-PDMS layer which was used to improve bond strength between two PMMA sheets to encapsulate a microfluidic channel. This device was used for microscale PCR using *E. coli* and *C. condimenti* DNA within 25 min. Following a common theme, a vast number of surface treatments have been developed for microfluidic PCR in addition to the selected example, and it is recommended to the interested reader to review Section 2.8 for more resources and other potential surface treatments applicable for PCR.

2.6.3 Immunosensor to detect pathogenic bacteria

Immunoassays such as ELISA are very common diagnostic tools in the health sciences due to their high specificity, sensitivity, and versatility to detect a wide range of target analytes. Traditional immunoassays involve an antibody coated on a substrate such as a standard titer plate to which a sample is applied. If target antigens are present, they bind to the immobilized antibodies and can be detected by a variety of readout methods. One can imagine that bound antibodies required in immunoassays could also be coated to the surface of a microfluidic device as discussed in Section 2.2 for a variety of substrate materials.

An important real world health application for immunoassays is the detection of pathogens such as *E. coli* in the food industry due to the health risks associated with foodborne pathogens. Consequently, rapid analysis of low sample volumes is needed which makes microfluidics favorable over complex, labor intensive immunoassays such as conventional ELISA. This has led to the development of simpler detection methods using impedance measurements, classified as immunosensors. One such example based on immunosensing is a PDMS micro-immunosensor that can detect dangerous foodborne pathogens such as *E. coli* and *S. aureus*. The device utilizes an integrated nanoporous alumina membrane to which bacterial antibodies are covalently immobilized to a self-assembled, epoxy-functionalized trimethoxysilane monolayer (Tan et al., 2011). As described in other silanization procedures, reactive hydroxyl groups on the substrate surface are needed (in this case formed with H_2O_2 treatment) to react with silane methoxy groups to silanize the surface. Amino groups on the antibodies then react with an open epoxy group functionalized to the silane which provides a covalent linkage between the antibody and the substrate surface. When a sample flows into the membrane, sensing is accomplished when bacteria attach to the antibodies and begin to block a nanopore, effectively increasing the impedance through the device (see Fig. 2.8(a)).

Similar surface chemistry has also been applied to a glass microfluidic bacterial immunosensor (Boehm et al., 2007). Instead of an integrated membrane, the immunoassay takes place in a chamber within the glass chip silanized to immobilize antibodies (Fig. 2.8(b)). As sample flows into the chamber, bacteria bind to antibodies and act as insulators by replacing equal volumes of conducting solution, thus altering the impedance of the system. In both of the aforementioned examples, analysis times are very rapid and high sensitivity is attained, illustrating the capability of microfluidics as a platform for immunosensing. Furthermore, the versatility of silanization and covalent immobilization of antibodies is illustrated with the ability to apply this surface treatment to multiple substrates and device designs. Despite these differences, the treatment remains effective in driving the immunoassay and maintaining high sensitivity. Further versatility can be realized by considering the ability to immobilize a variety of antibodies to various surfaces to detect complex bacterial samples or other biological analytes.

2.7 Conclusions and future trends

It is apparent that surface coatings are essential for the success of many medical microfluidic devices for a variety of applications whether applied to sensitive diagnosis or as research tools in the field of medicinal biology and chemistry. As was demonstrated throughout this chapter, the variety of materials and coating strategies for microfluidic materials is enormous. Among those, silicon dioxide—based devices are the best characterized, and their covalent surface chemistry can be well adapted to a specific problem. It is, therefore, not astonishing that glass devices are used in many commercial microfluidic devices, such as in the cartridges used for the Bioanalyzer instrument

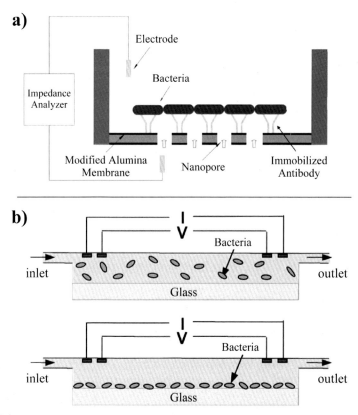

Figure 2.8 (a) Immunosensor schematic showing the capture of bacteria as it passes through a nanopore membrane. Antibodies immobilized to the surface trap bacteria which block the pores leading to an increase in impedance through the system. (b) Another example of an impedance based immunosensor using a simpler two chamber design in which glass is silanized to immobilize antibodies. As bacteria flow from the inlet into the large chamber (top), they are captured by the antibodies (bottom) which alters the electrical properties of the chamber. Bacterial sensing is accomplished by observing a change in impedance.

from Agilent, for example. On the other hand, most polymer devices are flexible; a property that could become advantageous for point-of-care devices, implantation, and continuous monitoring. Additionally, most polymer devices can be fabricated with mass replication tools such as injection molding which allows for economical and mass production. Nowadays, such replication tools can even be generated with nanometer-sized features allowing for versatile integration and parallelization.

Despite advancements in microfluidics, the surface chemistry of polymer devices strongly depends on the chemical composition of the polymer employed making general surface treatment schemes, such as that provided by the silanization of glass, not available. Consequently, the application of polymer devices greatly depends on the choice of the polymer material; thus, available immobilization strategies will have to be adapted to novel polymer materials. A large variety of successful usages of polymer devices has been demonstrated and discussed throughout this chapter illustrating that adequate surface coatings can be developed for polymers to compete with glass devices in various applications. A specific advantage of polymer materials over glass devices arises due to their gas permeability, which becomes important for cell-based studies and diagnosis. PDMS, for example, has shown excellent gas permeability and cell culturing capability in tandem with appropriate surface treatments. In summary, one can expect the continuation of silicon dioxide–based devices for high sensitivity applications and where reproducibility is greatly influenced by covalent and stable coatings. Polymer devices have great potential for point-of-care and single use applications where within-chip reproducibility is not a stringent requirement but cost effectiveness is essential.

2.8 Sources of further information and advice

In this chapter, a general overview of covalent and adsorptive surface coatings for microfluidic applications was given for the most common strategies used. For other materials and detailed protocols, the reader is referred to the literature cited in this chapter. Moreover, some review articles provide a useful source on coating strategies and their applications. For example, one of the most common materials used in the field is PDMS (Section 2.2.1) and the properties and general handling procedures of PDMS are described by Mata et al. (2005) and Lee, Park, and Whitesides (2003). Moreover, various common surface modifications for PDMS are summarized in references Makamba, Kim, Lim, Park, and Hahn (2003), Wong and Ho (2009), Zhou, Ellis, and Voelcker (2010), Zhou, Khodakov, Ellis, and Voelcker (2012), Gokaltun et al. (2017), and Eduok et al. (2017). Surface modifications of other polymers, specifically PMMA and PC, were reviewed by Soper et al. (2002) and by Kitsara and Ducrée (2013). Additionally, various strategies for protein immobilization in microfluidic assays were recently reviewed by Kim and Herr (2013).

Other than surface modification, integration of monolithic and other porous support material and structures have also gained immense interest in microfluidics recently. The integrated material can offer increased surface area and versatile range of surface modifications for proteins, antibodies, and enzyme attachment in applications for microreactors, biomarker extractions, or separations. These topics were recently reviewed by Knob et al. (2016), Tetala and Vijayalakshmi (2016), and Sonker, Sahore et al. (2017). The interested reader is further referred to reviews in the clinically important field of tissue engineering and PCR analysis. Surface treatments and procedures regarding tissue engineering were outlined by Park et al. (2007). In relation to miniaturized PCR analysis, various substrates were discussed by Zhang et al. (2006) including PDMS, PMMA, and polycarbonate. Static and dynamic passivation as we as well as coupled surface chemistries were outlined including protein coatings, surfactants, silanization, and polymer coatings, etc. This review covers a vast majority of papers published covering on-chip PCR as well as methods to develop such devices including aspects of fabrication, surface chemistry, implementation, etc., and specific applications such as microbial detection and disease diagnosis. Finally, surface treatments for microchip electrophoresis have also been extensively reviewed in Doherty, Meagher, Albarghouthi, and Barron (2003) and Dolnik (2004).

References

Bai, Y., Koh, C. G., Boreman, M., Juang, Y. J., Tang, I. C., Lee, L. J., et al. (2006). Surface modification for enhancing antibody binding on polymer-based microfluidic device for enzyme-linked immunosorbent assay. *Langmuir, 22*(22), 9458−9467. https://doi.org/10.1021/la0611231.

Barker, S. L., Ross, D., Tarlov, M. J., Gaitan, M., & Locascio, L. E. (2000). Control of flow direction in microfluidic devices with polyelectrolyte multilayers. *Analytical Chemistry, 72*(24), 5925−5929. https://doi.org/10.1021/ac0008690.

Barker, S. L., Tarlov, M. J., Canavan, H., Hickman, J. J., & Locascio, L. E. (2000). Plastic microfluidic devices modified with polyelectrolyte multilayers. *Analytical Chemistry, 72*(20), 4899−4903. https://doi.org/10.1021/ac000548o.

Batz, N. G., Mellors, J. S., Alarie, J. P., & Ramsey, J. M. (2014). Chemical vapor deposition of aminopropyl silanes in microfluidic channels for highly efficient microchip capillary electrophoresis-electrospray ionization-mass spectrometry. *Analytical Chemistry, 86*(7), 3493−3500. https://doi.org/10.1021/ac404106u.

Belder, D., Deege, A., Kohler, F., & Ludwig, M. (2002). Poly(vinyl alcohol)-coated microfluidic devices for high-performance microchip electrophoresis. *Electrophoresis, 23*(20), 3567−3573. https://doi.org/10.1002/1522-2683(200210)23:20<3567::AID-ELPS3567>3.0.CO;2-3.

Benoit, V., Steel, A., Torres, M., Yu, Y.-Y., Yang, H., & Cooper, J. (2001). Evaluation of three-dimensional microchannel glass biochips for multiplexed nucleic acid fluorescence hybridization assays. *Analytical Chemistry, 73*(11), 2412−2420. https://doi.org/10.1021/ac000946r.

Berglund, K. D., Przybycien, T. M., & Tilton, R. D. (2003). Coadsorption of sodium dodecyl sulfate with hydrophobically modified nonionic cellulose polymers. 1. Role of polymer hydrophobic modification. *Langmuir, 19*(7), 2705−2713. https://doi.org/10.1021/la026429g.

Bhattacharya, S., Datta, A., Berg, J. M., & Gangopadhyay, S. (2005). Studies on surface wettability of poly(dimethyl) siloxane (PDMS) and glass under oxygen-plasma treatment and correlation with bond strength. *Journal of Microelectromechanical Systems, 14*(3), 590−597. https://doi.org/10.1109/JMEMS.2005.844746.

Boehm, D. A., Gottlieb, P. A., & Hua, S. Z. (2007). On-chip microfluidic biosensor for bacterial detection and identification. *Sensors and Actuators, B: Chemical, 126*(2), 508−514. https://doi.org/10.1016/j.snb.2007.03.043.

Bontoux, N., Dauphinot, L., Vitalis, T., Studer, V., Chen, Y., Rossier, J., et al. (2008). Integrating whole transcriptome assays on a lab-on-a-chip for single cell gene profiling. *Lab on a Chip, 8*(3), 443–450. https://doi.org/10.1039/b716543a.

Brisset, F., Vieillard, J., Berton, B., Morin-Grognet, S., Duclairoir-Poc, C., & Le Derf, F. (2015). Surface functionalization of cyclic olefin copolymer with aryldiazonium salts: A covalent grafting method. *Applied Surface Science, 329*, 337–346. https://doi.org/10.1016/j.apsusc.2014.12.060.

Burke, J. M., & Smela, E. (2012). A novel surface modification technique for forming porous polymer monoliths in poly(dimethylsiloxane). *Biomicrofluidics, 6*(1). https://doi.org/10.1063/1.3693589ER, 016506.

Cheek, B. J., Steel, A. B., Torres, M. P., Yu, Y.-Y., & Yang, H. (2001). Chemiluminescence detection for hybridization assays on the flow-thru chip, a three-dimensional microchannel biochip. *Analytical Chemistry, 73*(24), 5777–5783. https://doi.org/10.1021/ac0108616.

Chehimi, M. M., Lamouri, A., Picot, M., & Pinson, J. (2014). Surface modification of polymers by reduction of diazonium salts: Polymethylmethacrylate as an example. *Journal of Materials Chemistry C, 2*(2), 356–363. https://doi.org/10.1039/C3TC31492H.

Cheng, X., Gupta, A., Chen, C., Tompkins, R. G., Rodriguez, W., & Toner, M. (2009). Enhancing the performance of a point-of-care CD4+ T-cell counting microchip through monocyte depletion for HIV/AIDS diagnostics. *Lab on a Chip, 9*(10), 1357–1364. https://doi.org/10.1039/B818813K.

Cheng, J.-Y., Wei, C.-W., Hsu, K.-H., & Young, T.-H. (2004). Direct-write laser micromachining and universal surface modification of PMMA for device development. *Sensors and Actuators, B: Chemical, 99*(1), 186–196. https://doi.org/10.1016/j.snb.2003.10.022.

Chen, H.-Y., & Lahann, J. (2005). Fabrication of discontinuous surface patterns within microfluidic channels using photodefinable vapor-based polymer coatings. *Analytical Chemistry, 77*(21), 6909–6914. https://doi.org/10.1021/ac050964e.

Chen, H. Y., McClelland, A. A., Chen, Z., & Lahann, J. (2008). Solventless adhesive bonding using reactive polymer coatings. *Analytical Chemistry, 80*(11), 4119–4124. https://doi.org/10.1021/ac800341m.

Chen, L., Ren, J., Bi, R., & Chen, D. (2004). Ultraviolet sealing and poly(dimethylacrylamide) modification for poly(dimethylsiloxane)/glass microchips. *Electrophoresis, 25*(6), 914–921. https://doi.org/10.1002/elps.200305766.

Chiem, N., & Harrison, D. J. (1997). Microchip-based capillary electrophoresis for immunoassays: Analysis of monoclonal antibodies and theophylline. *Analytical Chemistry, 69*(3), 373–378. https://doi.org/10.1021/ac9606620.

Chiem, N. H., & Harrison, D. J. (1998). Microchip systems for immunoassay: An integrated immunoreactor with electrophoretic separation for serum theophylline determination. *Clinical Chemistry, 44*(3), 591–598. https://doi.org/10.1093/clinchem/44.3.591.

Chin, C. D., Linder, V., & Sia, S. K. (2012). Commercialization of microfluidic point-of-care diagnostic devices. *Lab on a Chip, 12*(12), 2118–2134. https://doi.org/10.1039/c2lc21204h.

Cortese, B., Mowlem, M. C., & Morgan, H. (2011). Characterisation of an irreversible bonding process for COC–COC and COC–PDMS–COC sandwich structures and application to microvalves. *Sensors and Actuators, B: Chemical, 160*(1), 1473–1480. https://doi.org/10.1016/j.snb.2011.07.040.

Currie, C. A., Shim, J. S., Lee, S. H., Ahn, C., Limbach, P. A., Halsall, H. B., et al. (2009). Comparing polyelectrolyte multilayer-coated PMMA microfluidic devices and glass microchips for electrophoretic separations. *Electrophoresis, 30*(24), 4245−4250. https://doi.org/10.1002/elps.200900403.

Darain, F., Gan, K. L., & Tjin, S. C. (2009). Antibody immobilization on to polystyrene substrate−on-chip immunoassay for horse IgG based on fluorescence. *Biomedical Microdevices, 11*(3), 653−661. https://doi.org/10.1007/s10544-008-9275-3.

Delamarche, E., Donzel, C., Kamounah, F. S., Wolf, H., Geissler, M., Stutz, R., et al. (2003). Microcontact printing using poly(dimethylsiloxane) stamps hydrophilized by poly(ethylene oxide) silanes. *Langmuir, 19*(21), 8749−8758. https://doi.org/10.1021/la034370n.

Dodge, A., Fluri, K., Verpoorte, E., & de Rooij, N. F. (2001). Electrokinetically driven microfluidic chips with surface-modified chambers for heterogeneous immunoassays. *Analytical Chemistry, 73*(14), 3400−3409. https://doi.org/10.1021/ac0015366.

Doherty, E. A., Meagher, R. J., Albarghouthi, M. N., & Barron, A. E. (2003). Microchannel wall coatings for protein separations by capillary and chip electrophoresis. *Electrophoresis, 24*(1−2), 34−54. https://doi.org/10.1002/elps.200390029.

Dolnik, V. (2004). Wall coating for capillary electrophoresis on microchips. *Electrophoresis, 25*(21−22), 3589−3601. https://doi.org/10.1002/elps.200406113.

Dou, Y.-H., Bao, N., Xu, J.-J., Meng, F., & Chen, H.-Y. (2004). Separation of proteins on surface-modified poly(dimethylsiloxane) microfluidic devices. *Electrophoresis, 25*(17), 3024−3031. https://doi.org/10.1002/elps.200405986.

Dragatogiannis, D. A., Koumoulos, E., Ellinas, K., Tserepi, A., Gogolides, E., & Charitidis, C. A. (2015). Nanoscale mechanical and tribological properties of plasma nanotextured COP surfaces with hydrophobic coatings. *Plasma Processes and Polymers, 12*(11), 1271−1283. https://doi.org/10.1002/ppap.201500023.

Du, X. G., & Fang, Z. L. (2005). Static adsorptive coating of poly(methyl methacrylate) microfluidic chips for extended usage in DNA separations. *Electrophoresis, 26*(24), 4625−4631. https://doi.org/10.1002/elps.200500274.

Duffy, D. C., McDonald, J. C., Schueller, O. J. A., & Whitesides, G. M. (1998). Rapid prototyping of microfluidic systems in poly(dimethylsiloxane). *Analytical Chemistry, 70*(23), 4974−4984. https://doi.org/10.1021/ac980656z. M3: doi: 10.1021/ac980656z; 25. 10.1021/ac980656z.

Echelmeier, A., Sonker, M., & Ros, A. (2019). Microfluidic sample delivery for serial crystallography using XFELs. *Analytical and Bioanalytical Chemistry, 411*(25), 6535−6547. https://doi.org/10.1007/s00216-019-01977-x.

Eduok, U., Faye, O., & Szpunar, J. (2017). Recent developments and applications of protective silicone coatings: A review of PDMS functional materials. *Progress in Organic Coatings, 111*, 124−163. https://doi.org/10.1016/j.porgcoat.2017.05.012.

Efimenko, K., Wallace, W. E., & Genzer, J. (2002). Surface modification of Sylgard-184 poly(dimethyl siloxane) networks by ultraviolet and ultraviolet/ozone treatment. *Journal of Colloid and Interface Science, 254*(2), 306−315. https://doi.org/10.1006/jcis.2002.8594.

El Fissi, L., Vandormael, D., Houssiau, L., & Francis, L. A. (2016). Surface functionalization of cyclic olefin copolymer (COC) with evaporated TiO_2 thin film. *Applied Surface Science, 363*, 670−675. https://doi.org/10.1016/j.apsusc.2015.11.234.

Erill, I., Campoy, S., Erill, N., Barbé, J., & Aguiló, J. (2003). Biochemical analysis and optimization of inhibition and adsorption phenomena in glass−silicon PCR-chips. *Sensors and Actuators, B: Chemical, 96*(3), 685−692. https://doi.org/10.1016/S0925-4005(03)00522-7.

Eteshola, E., & Leckband, D. (2001). Development and characterization of an ELISA assay in PDMS microfluidic channels. *Sensors and Actuators, B: Chemical, 72*(2), 129−133. https://doi.org/10.1016/S0925-4005(00)00640-7.

Feyssa, B., Liedert, C., Kivimaki, L., Johansson, L.-S., Jantunen, H., & Hakalahti, L. (2013). Patterned immobilization of antibodies within roll-to-roll hot embossed polymeric microfluidic channels. *PLoS One, 8*(7), e68918. https://doi.org/10.1371/journal.pone.0068918.

Fritz, J. L., & Owen, M. J. (1995). Hydrophobic recovery of plasma-treated polydimethylsiloxane. *The Journal of Adhesion, 54*(1−4), 33−45. https://doi.org/10.1080/00218469508014379.

Fukuda, J., Khademhosseini, A., Yeh, J., Eng, G., Cheng, J., Farokhzad, O. C., et al. (2006). Micropatterned cell co-cultures using layer-by-layer deposition of extracellular matrix components. *Biomaterials, 27*(8), 1479−1486. https://doi.org/10.1016/j.biomaterials.2005.09.015.

Gleichweit, E., Baumgartner, C., Diethardt, R., Murer, A., Sallegger, W., Werkl, D., et al. (2018). UV/Ozone surface treatment for bonding of elastomeric COC-based microfluidic devices. *Proceedings, 2*(13), 943. https://doi.org/10.3390/proceedings2130943.

Gokaltun, A., Yarmush, M. L., Asatekin, A., & Usta, O. B. (2017). Recent advances in nonbiofouling PDMS surface modification strategies applicable to microfluidic technology. *Technology, 05*(01), 1−12. https://doi.org/10.1142/s2339547817300013.

Grate, J. W., Warner, M. G., Pittman, J. W., Dehoff, K. J., Wietsma, T. W., Zhang, C., et al. (2013). Silane modification of glass and silica surfaces to obtain equally oil-wet surfaces in glass-covered silicon micromodel applications. *Water Resources Research, 49*(8), 4724−4729. https://doi.org/10.1002/wrcr.20367.

Gross, P. G., Kartalov, E. P., Scherer, A., & Weiner, L. P. (2007). Applications of microfluidics for neuronal studies. *Journal of the Neurological Sciences, 252*(2), 135−143. https://doi.org/10.1016/j.jns.2006.11.009.

Gubala, V., Siegrist, J., Monaghan, R., O'Reilly, B., Gandhiraman, R. P., Daniels, S., et al. (2013). Simple approach to study biomolecule adsorption in polymeric microfluidic channels. *Analytica Chimica Acta, 760*, 75−82. https://doi.org/10.1016/j.aca.2012.11.030.

Guo, B., Li, S., Song, L., Yang, M., Zhou, W., Tyagi, D., et al. (2015). Plasma-treated polystyrene film that enhances binding efficiency for sensitive and label-free protein biosensing. *Applied Surface Science, 345*, 379−386. https://doi.org/10.1016/j.apsusc.2015.03.070.

Hashimoto, M., Barany, F., & Soper, S. A. (2006). Polymerase chain reaction/ligase detection reaction/hybridization assays using flow-through microfluidic devices for the detection of low-abundant DNA point mutations. *Biosensors and Bioelectronics, 21*(10), 1915−1923. https://doi.org/10.1016/j.bios.2006.01.014.

Hashimoto, M., Hupert, M. L., Murphy, M. C., Soper, S. A., Cheng, Y. W., & Barany, F. (2005). Ligase detection reaction/hybridization assays using three-dimensional microfluidic networks for the detection of low-abundant DNA point mutations. *Analytical Chemistry, 77*(10), 3243−3255. https://doi.org/10.1021/ac048184d.

Hau, W. L. W., Trau, D. W., Sucher, N. K., Wong, M., & Zohar, Y. (2003). Surface-chemistry technology for microfluidics. *Journal of Micromechanics and Microengineering, 13*(2), 272.

Hellmich, W., Greif, D., Pelargus, C., Anselmetti, D., & Ros, A. (2006). Improved native UV laser induced fluorescence detection for single cell analysis in poly(dimethylsiloxane) microfluidic devices. *Journal of Chromatography A, 1130*(2), 195−200. https://doi.org/10.1016/j.chroma.2006.06.008.

Hellmich, W., Regtmeier, J., Duong, T. T., Ros, R., Anselmetti, D., & Ros, A. (2005). Poly(oxyethylene) based surface coatings for poly(dimethylsiloxane) microchannels. *Langmuir: The ACS Journal of Surfaces and Colloids, 21*(16), 7551–7557. https://doi.org/10.1021/la0510432.

Henry, A. C., Tutt, T. J., Galloway, M., Davidson, Y. Y., McWhorter, C. S., Soper, S. A., et al. (2000). Surface modification of poly(methyl methacrylate) used in the fabrication of microanalytical devices. *Analytical Chemistry, 72*(21), 5331–5337. https://doi.org/10.1021/ac000685l.

Hernández-Maya, F. M., & Cañizares-Macías, M. P. (2018). Evaluation of the activity of β-glucosidase immobilized on polydimethylsiloxane (PDMS) with a microfluidic flow injection analyzer with embedded optical fibers. *Talanta, 185*, 53–60. https://doi.org/10.1016/j.talanta.2018.03.038.

Hjertén, S. (1985). High-performance electrophoresis: Elimination of electroendosmosis and solute adsorption. *Journal of Chromatography A, 347*(0), 191–198. https://doi.org/10.1016/S0021-9673(01)95485-8.

Hou, S., Yang, K., Qin, M., Feng, X.-Z., Guan, L., Yang, Y., et al. (2008). Patterning of cells on functionalized poly(dimethylsiloxane) surface prepared by hydrophobin and collagen modification. *Biosensors and Bioelectronics, 24*(4), 912–916. https://doi.org/10.1016/j.bios.2008.07.045.

Huang, Y., Shan, W., Liu, B., Liu, Y., Zhang, Y., Zhao, Y., et al. (2006). Zeolite nanoparticle modified microchip reactor for efficient protein digestion. *Lab on a Chip, 6*(4), 534–539. https://doi.org/10.1039/B517590A.

Hu, S., Ren, X., Bachman, M., Sims, C. E., Li, G. P., & Allbritton, N. (2002). Surface modification of poly(dimethylsiloxane) microfluidic devices by ultraviolet polymer grafting. *Analytical Chemistry, 74*(16), 4117–4123. https://doi.org/10.1021/ac025700w.

Hu, S., Ren, X., Bachman, M., Sims, C. E., Li, G. P., & Allbritton, N. L. (2004). Surface-directed, graft polymerization within microfluidic channels. *Analytical Chemistry, 76*(7), 1865–1870. https://doi.org/10.1021/ac049937z.

Jang, M., Park, C. K., & Lee, N. Y. (2014a). Modification of polycarbonate with hydrophilic/hydrophobic coatings for the fabrication of microdevices. *Sensors and Actuators, B: Chemical, 193*, 599–607. https://doi.org/10.1016/j.snb.2013.11.121.

Jang, M., Park, S., & Lee, N. Y. (2014b). Polycarbonate bonding assisted by surface chemical modification without plasma treatment and its application for the construction of plastic-based cell arrays. *Sensors and Actuators, A: Physical, 206*, 57–66. https://doi.org/10.1016/j.sna.2013.11.022.

Jankowski, P., & Garstecki, P. (2016). Stable hydrophilic surface of polycarbonate. *Sensors and Actuators, B: Chemical, 226*, 151–155. https://doi.org/10.1016/j.snb.2015.11.100.

Jeong, S. P., Hong, D., Kang, S. M., Choi, I. S., & Lee, J. K. (2013). Polymeric functionalization of cyclic olefin copolymer surfaces with nonbiofouling poly(oligo(ethylene glycol) methacrylate). *Asian Journal of Organic Chemistry, 2*(7), 568–571. https://doi.org/10.1002/ajoc.201300078.

Jon, S., Seong, J., Khademhosseini, A., Tran, T.-N. T., Laibinis, P. E., & Langer, R. (2003). Construction of nonbiofouling surfaces by polymeric self-assembled monolayers. *Langmuir, 19*(24), 9989–9993. https://doi.org/10.1021/la034839e.

Kang, J., Yan, J., Liu, J., Qiu, H., Yin, X.-B., Yang, X., et al. (2005). Dynamic coating for resolving rhodamine B adsorption to poly(dimethylsiloxane)/glass hybrid chip with laser-induced fluorescence detection. *Talanta, 66*(4), 1018–1024. https://doi.org/10.1016/j.talanta.2005.01.002.

Katayama, H., Ishihama, Y., & Asakawa, N. (1998a). Stable capillary coating with successive multiple ionic polymer layers. *Analytical Chemistry, 70*(11), 2254–2260. https://doi.org/10.1021/ac9708755.

Katayama, H., Ishihama, Y., & Asakawa, N. (1998b). Stable cationic capillary coating with successive multiple ionic polymer layers for capillary electrophoresis. *Analytical Chemistry, 70*(24), 5272–5277. https://doi.org/10.1021/ac980522l.

Khnouf, R., Karasneh, D., & Albiss, B. A. (2016). Protein immobilization on the surface of polydimethylsiloxane and polymethyl methacrylate microfluidic devices. *Electrophoresis, 37*(3), 529–535. https://doi.org/10.1002/elps.201500333.

Kidambi, S., Udpa, N., Schroeder, S. A., Findlan, R., Lee, I., & Chan, C. (2007). Cell adhesion on polyelectrolyte multilayer coated polydimethylsiloxane surfaces with varying topographies. *Tissue Engineering, 13*(8), 2105–2117. https://doi.org/10.1089/ten.2006.0151.

Kim, D., & Herr, A. E. (2013). Protein immobilization techniques for microfluidic assays. *Biomicrofluidics, 7*(4), 041501. https://doi.org/10.1063/1.4816934.

Kitsara, M., & Ducrée, J. (2013). Integration of functional materials and surface modification for polymeric microfluidic systems. *Journal of Micromechanics and Microengineering, 23*(3), 033001. https://doi.org/10.1088/0960-1317/23/3/033001.

Knob, R., Sahore, V., Sonker, M., & Woolley, A. T. (2016). Advances in monoliths and related porous materials for microfluidics. *Biomicrofluidics, 10*(3), 032901. https://doi.org/10.1063/1.4948507.

Kovach, K. M., Capadona, J. R., Gupta, A. S., & Potkay, J. A. (2014). The effects of PEG-based surface modification of PDMS microchannels on long-term hemocompatibility. *Journal of Biomedical Materials Research Part A, 102*(12), 4195–4205. https://doi.org/10.1002/jbm.a.35090.

Kreider, A., Richter, K., Sell, S., Fenske, M., Tornow, C., Stenzel, V., et al. (2013). Functionalization of PDMS modified and plasma activated two-component polyurethane coatings by surface attachment of enzymes. *Applied Surface Science, 273*, 562–569. https://doi.org/10.1016/j.apsusc.2013.02.080.

Ladner, Y., d'Orlyé, F., Perréard, C., Da Silva, B., Guyon, C., Tatoulian, M., et al. (2013). Surface functionalization of COC microfluidic materials by plasma and click chemistry processes. *Plasma Processes and Polymers, 10*(11), 959–969. https://doi.org/10.1002/ppap.201300066.

Lahann, J., Balcells, M., Lu, H., Rodon, T., Jensen, K. F., & Langer, R. (2003). Reactive polymer coatings: A first step toward surface engineering of microfluidic devices. *Analytical Chemistry, 75*(9), 2117–2122. https://doi.org/10.1021/ac020557s.

Lasave, L. C., Borisov, S. M., Ehgartner, J., & Mayr, T. (2015). Quick and simple integration of optical oxygen sensors into glass-based microfluidic devices. *RSC Advances, 5*(87), 70808–70816. https://doi.org/10.1039/C5RA15591F.

Lee, J. N., Park, C., & Whitesides, G. M. (2003). Solvent compatibility of poly(dimethylsiloxane)-based microfluidic devices. *Analytical Chemistry, 75*(23), 6544–6554. https://doi.org/10.1021/ac0346712.

Lee, M.-Y., Srinivasan, A., Ku, B., & Dordick, J. S. (2003). Multienzyme catalysis in microfluidic biochips. *Biotechnology and Bioengineering, 83*(1), 20–28. https://doi.org/10.1002/bit.10642.

Lee, N. Y., Yang, Y., Kim, Y. S., & Park, S. (2006). Microfluidic immunoassay platform using antibody-immobilized glass beads and its application for detection of *Escherichia coli* O157 : H7. *Bulletin of the Korean Chemical Society, 27*(4), 479−483. https://doi.org/10.5012/bkcs.2006.27.4.479.

Lenigk, R., Liu, R. H., Athavale, M., Chen, Z., Ganser, D., Yang, J., et al. (2002). Plastic biochannel hybridization devices: A new concept for microfluidic DNA arrays. *Analytical Biochemistry, 311*(1), 40−49. https://doi.org/10.1016/S0003-2697(02)00391-3.

Leong, K., Boardman, A. K., Ma, H., & Jen, A. K. Y. (2009). Single-cell patterning and adhesion on chemically engineered poly(dimethylsiloxane) surface. *Langmuir, 25*(8), 4615−4620. https://doi.org/10.1021/la8037318.

Li, S. F. Y., & Kricka, L. J. (2006). Clinical analysis by microchip capillary electrophoresis. *Clinical Chemistry, 52*(1), 37−45. https://doi.org/10.1373/clinchem.2005.059600.

Linder, V., Verpoorte, E., Thormann, W., de Rooij, N. F., & Sigrist, H. (2001). Surface biopassivation of replicated poly(dimethylsiloxane) microfluidic channels and application to heterogeneous immunoreaction with on-chip fluorescence detection. *Analytical Chemistry, 73*(17), 4181−4189. https://doi.org/10.1021/ac010421e.

Liu, Y., Fanguy, J. C., Bledsoe, J. M., & Henry, C. S. (2000). Dynamic coating using polyelectrolyte multilayers for chemical control of electroosmotic flow in capillary electrophoresis microchips. *Analytical Chemistry, 72*(24), 5939−5944. https://doi.org/10.1021/ac000932l.

Liu, Y., Ganser, D., Schneider, A., Liu, R., Grodzinski, P., & Kroutchinina, N. (2001). Microfabricated polycarbonate CE devices for DNA analysis. *Analytical Chemistry, 73*(17), 4196−4201. https://doi.org/10.1021/ac010343v.

Liu, Y., & Rauch, C. B. (2003). DNA probe attachment on plastic surfaces and microfluidic hybridization array channel devices with sample oscillation. *Analytical Biochemistry, 317*(1), 76−84. https://doi.org/10.1016/S0003-2697(03)00051-4.

Li, Y., Wang, Z., Ou, L. M. L., & Yu, H.-Z. (2007). DNA detection on plastic: Surface activation protocol to convert polycarbonate substrates to biochip platforms. *Analytical Chemistry, 79*(2), 426−433. https://doi.org/10.1021/ac061134j.

Ludwig, M., & Belder, D. (2003). Coated microfluidic devices for improved chiral separations in microchip electrophoresis. *Electrophoresis, 24*(15), 2481−2486. https://doi.org/10.1002/elps.200305498.

Lu, Y., Shi, W., Qin, J., & Lin, B. (2010). Fabrication and characterization of paper-based microfluidics prepared in nitrocellulose membrane by wax printing. *Analytical Chemistry, 82*(1), 329−335. https://doi.org/10.1021/ac9020193;10.1021/ac9020193.

Makamba, H., Kim, J. H., Lim, K., Park, N., & Hahn, J. H. (2003). Surface modification of poly(dimethylsiloxane) microchannels. *Electrophoresis, 24*(21), 3607−3619. https://doi.org/10.1002/elps.200305627.

Martin, S., & Bhushan, B. (2017). Transparent, wear-resistant, superhydrophobic and superoleophobic poly(dimethylsiloxane) (PDMS) surfaces. *Journal of Colloid and Interface Science, 488*, 118−126. https://doi.org/10.1016/j.jcis.2016.10.094.

Mata, A., Fleischman, A. J., & Roy, S. (2005). Characterization of polydimethylsiloxane (PDMS) properties for biomedical micro/nanosystems. *Biomedical Microdevices, 7*(4), 281−293. https://doi.org/10.1007/s10544-005-6070-2.

McCarley, R. L., Vaidya, B., Wei, S., Smith, A. F., Patel, A. B., Feng, J., et al. (2005). Resistfree patterning of surface architectures in polymer-based microanalytical devices. *Journal of the American Chemical Society, 127*(3), 842−843. https://doi.org/10.1021/ja0454135.

McDonald, J. C., Duffy, D. C., Anderson, J. R., Chiu, D. T., Wu, H., Schueller, O. J., et al. (2000). Fabrication of microfluidic systems in poly(dimethylsiloxane). *Electrophoresis, 21*(1), 27−40. https://doi.org/10.1002/(SICI)1522-2683(20000101)21:1<27::AID-ELPS27>3.0.CO;2-C.

Mellors, J. S., Gorbounov, V., Ramsey, R. S., & Ramsey, J. M. (2008). Fully integrated glass microfluidic device for performing high-efficiency capillary electrophoresis and electrospray ionization mass spectrometry. *Analytical Chemistry, 80*(18), 6881−6887. https://doi.org/10.1021/ac800428w.

Misiakos, K., Kakabakos, S. E., Petrou, P. S., & Ruf, H. H. (2004). A monolithic silicon optoelectronic transducer as a real-time affinity biosensor. *Analytical Chemistry, 76*(5), 1366−1373. https://doi.org/10.1021/ac0353334.

Miyaki, K., Zeng, H.-L., Nakagama, T., & Uchiyama, K. (2007). Steady surface modification of polydimethylsiloxane microchannel and its application in simultaneous analysis of homocysteine and glutathione in human serum. *Journal of Chromatography A, 1166*(1−2), 201−206. https://doi.org/10.1016/j.chroma.2007.08.030.

Nagahashi, K., Teramura, Y., & Takai, M. (2015). Stable surface coating of silicone elastomer with phosphorylcholine and organosilane copolymer with cross-linking for repelling proteins. *Colloids and Surfaces B: Biointerfaces, 134*, 384−391. https://doi.org/10.1016/j.colsurfb.2015.07.040.

Nagai, H., Murakami, Y., Morita, Y., Yokoyama, K., & Tamiya, E. (2001). Development of a microchamber array for picoliter PCR. *Analytical Chemistry, 73*(5), 1043−1047. https://doi.org/10.1021/ac000648u.

Naruishi, N., Tanaka, Y., Higashi, T., & Wakida, S.-i. (2006). Highly efficient dynamic modification of plastic microfluidic devices using proteins in microchip capillary electrophoresis. *Journal of Chromatography A, 1130*(2), 169−174. https://doi.org/10.1016/j.chroma.2006.07.005.

Nge, P. N., Rogers, C. I., & Woolley, A. T. (2013). Advances in microfluidic materials, functions, integration, and applications. *Chemical Reviews, 113*(4), 2550−2583. https://doi.org/10.1021/cr300337x.

Nielsen, J. B., Nielsen, A. V., Carson, R. H., Lin, H.-J. L., Hanson, R. L., Sonker, M., et al. (2019). Analysis of thrombin-antithrombin complex formation using microchip electrophoresis and mass spectrometry. *Electrophoresis, 40*(21), 2853−2859. https://doi.org/10.1002/elps.201900235.

Nielsen, A. V., Nielsen, J. B., Sonker, M., Knob, R., Sahore, V., & Woolley, A. T. (2018). Microchip electrophoresis separation of a panel of preterm birth biomarkers. *Electrophoresis, 0*(0). https://doi.org/10.1002/elps.201800078.

Nielsen, R. G., Rickard, E. C., Santa, P. F., Sharknas, D. A., & Sittampalam, G. S. (1991). Separation of antibody−antigen complexes by capillary zone electrophoresis, isoelectric focusing and high-performance size-exclusion chromatography. *Journal of Chromatography A, 539*(1), 177−185. https://doi.org/10.1016/S0021-9673(01)95371-3.

Nieto, D., Couceiro, R., Aymerich, M., Lopez-Lopez, R., Abal, M., & Flores-Arias, M. T. (2015). A laser-based technology for fabricating a soda-lime glass based microfluidic device for circulating tumour cell capture. *Colloids and Surfaces B: Biointerfaces, 134*, 363−369. https://doi.org/10.1016/j.colsurfb.2015.07.007.

Nisar, A., Afzulpurkar, N., Mahaisavariya, B., & Tuantranont, A. (2008). MEMS-based micropumps in drug delivery and biomedical applications. *Sensors and Actuators, B: Chemical, 130*(2), 917−942. https://doi.org/10.1016/j.snb.2007.10.064.

Ni, M., Tong, W. H., Choudhury, D., Rahim, N. A., Iliescu, C., & Yu, H. (2009). Cell culture on MEMS platforms: A review. *International Journal of Molecular Sciences, 10*(12), 5411−5441. https://doi.org/10.3390/ijms10125411;10.3390/ijms10125411.

Novak, R., Ranu, N., & Mathies, R. A. (2013). Rapid fabrication of nickel molds for prototyping embossed plastic microfluidic devices. *Lab on a Chip, 13*(8), 1468−1471. https://doi.org/10.1039/C3LC41362D.

Nunes, P. S., Ohlsson, P. D., Ordeig, O., & Kutter, J. P. (2010). Cyclic olefin polymers: Emerging materials for lab-on-a-chip applications. *Microfluidics and Nanofluidics, 9*(2), 145−161. https://doi.org/10.1007/s10404-010-0605-4.

Ortiz, R., Chen, J. L., Stuckey, D. C., & Steele, T. W. J. (2017). Poly(methyl methacrylate) surface modification for surfactant-free real-time toxicity assay on droplet microfluidic platform. *ACS Applied Materials and Interfaces, 9*(15), 13801−13811. https://doi.org/10.1021/acsami.7b02682.

Paegel, B. M., Emrich, C. A., Wedemayer, G. J., Scherer, J. R., & Mathies, R. A. (2002). High throughput DNA sequencing with a microfabricated 96-lane capillary array electrophoresis bioprocessor. *Proceedings of the National Academy of Sciences of the United States of America, 99*(2), 574−579. https://doi.org/10.1073/pnas.012608699.

Pagaduan, J. V., Sahore, V., & Woolley, A. T. (2015). Applications of microfluidics and microchip electrophoresis for potential clinical biomarker analysis. *Analytical and Bioanalytical Chemistry, 407*(23), 6911−6922. https://doi.org/10.1007/s00216-015-8622-5.

Panaro, N. J., Yuen, P. K., Sakazume, T., Fortina, P., Kricka, L. J., & Wilding, P. (2000). Evaluation of DNA fragment sizing and quantification by the agilent 2100 bioanalyzer. *Clinical Chemistry, 46*(11), 1851−1853. https://doi.org/10.1093/clinchem/46.11.1851.

Papra, A., Bernard, A., Juncker, D., Larsen, N. B., Michel, B., & Delamarche, E. (2001). Microfluidic networks made of poly(dimethylsiloxane), Si, and Au coated with polyethylene glycol for patterning proteins onto surfaces. *Langmuir, 17*(13), 4090−4095. https://doi.org/10.1021/la0016930.

Park, H., Cannizzaro, C., Vunjak-Novakovic, G., Langer, R., Vacanti, C. A., & Farokhzad, O. C. (2007). Nanofabrication and microfabrication of functional materials for tissue engineering. *Tissue Engineering, 13*(8), 1867−1877. https://doi.org/10.1089/ten.2006.0198.

Patrito, N., McCague, C., Norton, P. R., & Petersen, N. O. (2007). Spatially controlled cell adhesion via micropatterned surface modification of poly(dimethylsiloxane). *Langmuir, 23*(2), 715−719. https://doi.org/10.1021/la062007l.

Picher, M. M., Küpcü, S., Huang, C.-J., Dostalek, J., Pum, D., Sleytr, U. B., et al. (2013). Nanobiotechnology advanced antifouling surfaces for the continuous electrochemical monitoring of glucose in whole blood using a lab-on-a-chip. *Lab on a Chip, 13*(9), 1780−1789. https://doi.org/10.1039/C3LC41308J.

Qin, K., Lv, X., Xing, Q., Li, R., & Deng, Y. (2016). A BSA coated NOA81 PCR chip for gene amplification. *Anal. Methods, 8*(12), 2584−2591. https://doi.org/10.1039/C5AY03233D.

Reyes, D. R., Iossifidis, D., Auroux, P. A., & Manz, A. (2002). Micro total analysis systems. 1. Introduction, theory, and technology. *Analytical Chemistry, 74*(12), 2623−2636. https://doi.org/10.1021/ac0202435.

Roman, G. T., McDaniel, K., & Culbertson, C. T. (2006). High efficiency micellar electrokinetic chromatography of hydrophobic analytes on poly(dimethylsiloxane) microchips. *Analyst, 131*(2), 194−201. https://doi.org/10.1039/B510765B.

Roy, S., Yue, C. Y., Venkatraman, S. S., & Ma, L. L. (2013). Fabrication of smart COC chips: Advantages of N-vinylpyrrolidone (NVP) monomer over other hydrophilic monomers. *Sensors and Actuators, B: Chemical, 178*, 86−95. https://doi.org/10.1016/j.snb.2012.12.058.

Sandison, M. E., Zagnoni, M., Abu-Hantash, M., & Morgan, H. (2007). Micromachined glass apertures for artificial lipid bilayer formation in a microfluidic system. *Journal of Micromechanics and Microengineering, 17*(7), S189−S196. https://doi.org/10.1088/0960-1317/17/7/S17.

Sanjay, S. T., Fu, G., Dou, M., Xu, F., Liu, R., Qi, H., et al. (2015). Biomarker detection for disease diagnosis using cost-effective microfluidic platforms. *Analyst, 140*(21), 7062−7081. https://doi.org/10.1039/C5AN00780A.

Selzer, D., Spiegel, B., & Kind, M. (2018). A generic polycarbonate based microfluidic tool to study crystal nucleation in microdroplets. *Journal of Crystallization Process and Technology, 8*(1), 1−17. https://doi.org/10.4236/jcpt.2018.81001.

Shahsavan, H., Quinn, J., d'Eon, J., & Zhao, B. (2015). Surface modification of polydimethylsiloxane elastomer for stable hydrophilicity, optical transparency and film lubrication. *Colloids and Surfaces A: Physicochemical and Engineering Aspects, 482*, 267−275. https://doi.org/10.1016/j.colsurfa.2015.05.024.

Shakeri, A., Imani, S. M., Chen, E., Yousefi, H., Shabbir, R., & Didar, T. F. (2019). Plasma-induced covalent immobilization and patterning of bioactive species in microfluidic devices. *Lab on a Chip, 19*(18), 3104−3115. https://doi.org/10.1039/C9LC00364A.

Shoffner, M. A., Cheng, J., Hvichia, G. E., Kricka, L. J., & Wilding, P. (1996). Chip PCR. I. Surface passivation of microfabricated silicon-glass chips for PCR. *Nucleic Acids Research, 24*(2), 375−379. https://doi.org/10.1093/nar/24.2.375.

Slentz, B. E., Penner, N. A., & Regnier, F. E. (2002). Capillary electrochromatography of peptides on microfabricated poly(dimethylsiloxane) chips modified by cerium(IV)-catalyzed polymerization. *25th International Symposium on High Performance Liquid Phase Separations and Related Techniques, 948*(1−2), 225−233. https://doi.org/10.1016/S0021-9673(01)01319-X.

Sonker, M., Knob, R., Sahore, V., & Woolley, A. T. (2017). Integrated electrokinetically driven microfluidic devices with pH-mediated solid-phase extraction coupled to microchip electrophoresis for preterm birth biomarkers. *Electrophoresis, 38*(13−14), 1743−1754. https://doi.org/10.1002/elps.201700054.

Sonker, M., Parker, E. K., Nielsen, A. V., Sahore, V., & Woolley, A. T. (2018). Electrokinetically operated microfluidic devices for integrated immunoaffinity monolith extraction and electrophoretic separation of preterm birth biomarkers. *Analyst, 143*(1), 224−231. https://doi.org/10.1039/C7AN01357D.

Sonker, M., Sahore, V., & Woolley, A. T. (2017). Recent advances in microfluidic sample preparation and separation techniques for molecular biomarker analysis: A critical review. *Analytica Chimica Acta, 986*, 1−11. https://doi.org/10.1016/j.aca.2017.07.043.

Sonker, M., Yang, R., Sahore, V., Kumar, S., & Woolley, A. T. (2016). On-chip fluorescent labeling using reversed-phase monoliths and microchip electrophoretic separations of selected preterm birth biomarkers. *Analytical Methods, 8*(43), 7739−7746. https://doi.org/10.1039/C6AY01803C.

Soper, S. A., Henry, A. C., Vaidya, B., Galloway, M., Wabuyele, M., & McCarley, R. L. (2002). Surface modification of polymer-based microfluidic devices. *Immobilization of Functional Biomolecules and Cells, 470*(1), 87−99. https://doi.org/10.1016/S0003-2670(02)00356-2.

Sui, G., Wang, J., Lee, C.-C., Lu, W., Lee, S. P., Leyton, J. V., et al. (2006). Solution-phase surface modification in intact poly(dimethylsiloxane) microfluidic channels. *Analytical Chemistry, 78*(15), 5543−5551. https://doi.org/10.1021/ac060605z.

Su, S., Jing, G., Zhang, M., Liu, B., Zhu, X., Wang, B., et al. (2019). One-step bonding and hydrophobic surface modification method for rapid fabrication of polycarbonate-based droplet microfluidic chips. *Sensors and Actuators, B: Chemical, 282,* 60−68. https://doi.org/10.1016/j.snb.2018.11.035.

Sung, W.-C., Chang, C.-C., Makamba, H., & Chen, S.-H. (2008). Long-term affinity modification on poly(dimethylsiloxane) substrate and its application for ELISA analysis. *Analytical Chemistry, 80*(5), 1529−1535. https://doi.org/10.1021/ac7020618.

Sung, J. H., & Shuler, M. L. (2010). In vitro microscale systems for systematic drug toxicity study. *Bioprocess and Biosystems Engineering, 33*(1), 5−19. https://doi.org/10.1007/s00449-009-0369-y;10.1007/s00449-009-0369-y.

Sun, S., Yang, M., Kostov, Y., & Rasooly, A. (2010). ELISA-LOC: Lab-on-a-chip for enzyme-linked immunodetection. *Lab on a Chip, 10*(16), 2093−2100. https://doi.org/10.1039/C003994B.

Surmodics (2020). *[TRIDIA (TM) activated slides].* Surmodics. https://shop.surmodics.com. (Accessed 19 November 2020).

Tachibana, H., Saito, M., Shibuya, S., Tsuji, K., Miyagawa, N., Yamanaka, K., et al. (2015). On-chip quantitative detection of pathogen genes by autonomous microfluidic PCR platform. *Biosensors and Bioelectronics, 74,* 725−730. https://doi.org/10.1016/j.bios.2015.07.009.

Tan, F., Leung, P. H. M., Liu, Z.-b., Zhang, Y., Xiao, L., Ye, W., et al. (2011). A PDMS microfluidic impedance immunosensor for *E. coli* O157:H7 and *Staphylococcus aureus* detection via antibody-immobilized nanoporous membrane. *Sensors and Actuators, B: Chemical, 159*(1), 328−335. https://doi.org/10.1016/j.snb.2011.06.074.

Tetala, K. K. R., & Vijayalakshmi, M. A. (2016). A review on recent developments for biomolecule separation at analytical scale using microfluidic devices. *Analytica Chimica Acta, 906,* 7−21. https://doi.org/10.1016/j.aca.2015.11.037.

Tran, R., Ahn, B., Myers, D. R., Qiu, Y., Sakurai, Y., Moot, R., et al. (2014). Simplified prototyping of perfusable polystyrene microfluidics. *Biomicrofluidics, 8*(4), 046501. https://doi.org/10.1063/1.4892035.

Trantidou, T., Elani, Y., Parsons, E., & Ces, O. (2017). Hydrophilic surface modification of PDMS for droplet microfluidics using a simple, quick, and robust method via PVA deposition. *Microsystems and Nanoengineering, 3*(1), 16091. https://doi.org/10.1038/micronano.2016.91.

Trinh, K. T. L., Zhang, H., Kang, D.-J., Kahng, S.-H., Tall, B. D., & Lee, N. Y. (2016). Fabrication of polymerase chain reaction plastic lab-on-a-chip device for rapid molecular diagnoses. *International Neurourology Journal, 20*(Suppl. 1), S38−S48. https://doi.org/10.5213/inj.1632602.301.

Varjo, S. J., Ludwig, M., Belder, D., & Riekkola, M. L. (2004). Separation of fluorescein isothiocyanate-labeled amines by microchip electrophoresis in uncoated and polyvinyl alcohol-coated glass chips using water and dimethyl sulfoxide as solvents of background electrolyte. *Electrophoresis, 25*(12), 1901−1906. https://doi.org/10.1002/elps.200405914.

Verpoorte, E. (2002). Microfluidic chips for clinical and forensic analysis. *Electrophoresis, 23*(5), 677−712. https://doi.org/10.1002/1522-2683(200203)23:5<677::AID-ELPS 677>3.0.CO;2-8.

Viefhues, M., Manchanda, S., Chao, T. C., Anselmetti, D., Regtmeier, J., & Ros, A. (2011). Physisorbed surface coatings for poly(dimethylsiloxane) and quartz microfluidic devices. *Analytical and Bioanalytical Chemistry, 401*(7), 2113–2122. https://doi.org/10.1007/s00216-011-5301-z.

Wang, H., Meng, S., Guo, K., Liu, Y., Yang, P., Zhong, W., et al. (2008). Microfluidic immunosensor based on stable antibody-patterned surface in PMMA microchip. *Electrochemistry Communications, 10*(3), 447–450. https://doi.org/10.1016/j.elecom.2008.01.005.

Wang, Y., Vaidya, B., Farquar, H. D., Stryjewski, W., Hammer, R. P., McCarley, R. L., et al. (2003). Microarrays assembled in microfluidic chips fabricated from poly(methyl methacrylate) for the detection of low-abundant DNA mutations. *Analytical Chemistry, 75*(5), 1130–1140. https://doi.org/10.1021/ac020683w.

Wang, B., Wang, X., Zheng, H., & Lam, Y. C. (2015). Surface wettability modification of cyclic olefin polymer by direct femtosecond laser irradiation. *Nanomaterials, 5*(3), 1442–1453. https://doi.org/10.3390/nano5031442.

Wang, A.-J., Xu, J.-J., & Chen, H.-Y. (2006). Proteins modification of poly(dimethylsiloxane) microfluidic channels for the enhanced microchip electrophoresis. *Journal of Chromatography A, 1107*(1–2), 257–264. https://doi.org/10.1016/j.chroma.2005.12.040.

Waters, L. C., Jacobson, S. C., Kroutchinina, N., Khandurina, J., Foote, R. S., & Ramsey, J. M. (1998). Microchip device for cell lysis, multiplex PCR amplification, and electrophoretic sizing. *Analytical Chemistry, 70*(1), 158–162. https://doi.org/10.1021/ac970642d.

Wei, C. W., Cheng, J. Y., Huang, C. T., Yen, M. H., & Young, T. H. (2005). Using a microfluidic device for 1 microl DNA microarray hybridization in 500 s. *Nucleic Acids Research, 33*(8), e78. https://doi.org/10.1093/nar/gni078.

Wong, I., & Ho, C. M. (2009). Surface molecular property modifications for poly(dimethylsiloxane) (PDMS) based microfluidic devices. *Microfluidics and Nanofluidics, 7*(3), 291–306. https://doi.org/10.1007/s10404-009-0443-4.

Wu, M. H., Huang, S. B., & Lee, G. B. (2010). Microfluidic cell culture systems for drug research. *Lab on a Chip, 10*(8), 939–956. https://doi.org/10.1039/b921695b.

Wu, D., Luo, Y., Zhou, X., Dai, Z., & Lin, B. (2005). Multilayer poly(vinyl alcohol)-adsorbed coating on poly(dimethylsiloxane) microfluidic chips for biopolymer separation. *Electrophoresis, 26*(1), 211–218. https://doi.org/10.1002/elps.200406157.

Xiao, D., Le, T. V., & Wirth, M. J. (2004). Surface modification of the channels of poly(dimethylsiloxane) microfluidic chips with polyacrylamide for fast electrophoretic separations of proteins. *Analytical Chemistry, 76*(7), 2055–2061. https://doi.org/10.1021/ac035254s.

Xiao, D., Zhang, H., & Wirth, M. (2002). Chemical modification of the surface of poly(dimethylsiloxane) by atom-transfer radical polymerization of acrylamide. *Langmuir, 18*(25), 9971–9976. https://doi.org/10.1021/la205553.

Xu, J., Wu, D., Hanada, Y., Chen, C., Wu, S., Cheng, Y., et al. (2013). Electrofluidics fabricated by space-selective metallization in glass microfluidic structures using femtosecond laser direct writing. *Lab on a Chip, 13*(23), 4608–4616. https://doi.org/10.1039/C3LC50962A.

Yager, P., Edwards, T., Fu, E., Helton, K., Nelson, K., Tam, M. R., et al. (2006). Microfluidic diagnostic technologies for global public health. *Nature, 442*(7101), 412–418. https://doi.org/10.1038/nature05064.

Yang, T., Baryshnikova, O. K., Mao, H., Holden, M. A., & Cremer, P. S. (2003). Investigations of bivalent antibody binding on fluid-supported phospholipid membranes: The effect of hapten density. *Journal of the American Chemical Society, 125*(16), 4779−4784. https://doi.org/10.1021/ja029469f.

Yang, T., Jung, S.-y., Mao, H., & Cremer, P. S. (2001). Fabrication of phospholipid bilayer-coated microchannels for on-chip immunoassays. *Analytical Chemistry, 73*(2), 165−169. https://doi.org/10.1021/ac000997o.

Young, E. W., Berthier, E., Guckenberger, D. J., Sackmann, E., Lamers, C., Meyvantsson, I., et al. (2011). Rapid prototyping of arrayed microfluidic systems in polystyrene for cell-based assays. *Analytical Chemistry, 83*(4), 1408−1417. https://doi.org/10.1021/ac102897h.

Youssouf Badal, M., Wong, M., Chiem, N., Salimi-Moosavi, H., & Harrison, D. J. (2002). Protein separation and surfactant control of electroosmotic flow in poly(dimethylsiloxane)-coated capillaries and microchips. *Journal of Chromatography A, 947*(2), 277−286. https://doi.org/10.1016/S0021-9673(01)01601-6.

Yu, L., Li, C. M., Liu, Y., Gao, J., Wang, W., & Gan, Y. (2009). Flow-through functionalized PDMS microfluidic channels with dextran derivative for ELISAs. *Lab on a Chip, 9*(9), 1243−1247. https://doi.org/10.1039/b816018j.

Zhang, A., Cheng, L., Hong, S., Yang, C., & Lin, Y. (2015). Preparation of anti-fouling silicone elastomers by covalent immobilization of carboxybetaine. *RSC Advances, 5*(107), 88456−88463. https://doi.org/10.1039/C5RA17206C.

Zhang, Z. L., Crozatier, C., Le Berre, M., & Chen, Y. (2005). In situ bio-functionalization and cell adhesion in microfluidic devices. In *Proceedings of the 30th international conference on micro- and nano-engineering* (Vols. 78−79, pp. 556−562). https://doi.org/10.1016/j.mee.2004.12.071.

Zhang, Y., Trinh, K. T. L., Yoo, I.-S., & Lee, N. Y. (2014). One-step glass-like coating of polycarbonate for seamless DNA purification and amplification on an integrated monolithic microdevice. *Sensors and Actuators, B: Chemical, 202*, 1281−1289. https://doi.org/10.1016/j.snb.2014.06.078.

Zhang, C., Xu, J., Ma, W., & Zheng, W. (2006). PCR microfluidic devices for DNA amplification. *Biotechnology Advances, 24*(3), 243−284. https://doi.org/10.1016/j.biotechadv.2005.10.002.

Zhou, J., Ellis, A. V., & Voelcker, N. H. (2010). Recent developments in PDMS surface modification for microfluidic devices. *Electrophoresis, 31*(1), 2−16. https://doi.org/10.1002/elps.200900475.

Zhou, J., Khodakov, D. A., Ellis, A. V., & Voelcker, N. H. (2012). Surface modification for PDMS-based microfluidic devices. *Electrophoresis, 33*(1), 89−104. https://doi.org/10.1002/elps.201100482;10.1002/elps.201100482.

Zilio, C., Sola, L., Damin, F., Faggioni, L., & Chiari, M. (2014). Universal hydrophilic coating of thermoplastic polymers currently used in microfluidics. *Biomedical Microdevices, 16*(1), 107−114. https://doi.org/10.1007/s10544-013-9810-8.

Actuation mechanisms for microfluidic biomedical devices

A. Rezk, J. Friend, L. Yeo
RMIT University, Melbourne, Australia

Revised by: Yu Zhou
R&D, Siemens, Tarrytown, NY, United States

Reading Questions

1. What are the current actuation mechanisms in microfluidic systems?
2. What are the advantages and limitations of electrokinetics and acoustics mechanisms and their roles for actuation of fluids and particles in microfluidic devices?
3. What are the main challenges for research and development of microscale fluid actuation?

3.1 Introduction

Actuating and manipulating fluids and particles at microscale dimensions poses a considerable challenge, primarily due to the surface area to volume ratio as the characteristic system dimension is reduced, which reflects the increasing dominance of surface and viscous forces in retarding fluid flow. This is captured by the characteristically small Reynolds numbers (Re $\equiv \rho U L/\mu \leq 1$) in microfluidic systems, wherein ρ and μ are the density and viscosity of the fluid, and U and L are the characteristic velocity and length scales, respectively. Laminarity of the flow is also inherent in these low Re systems, thereby highlighting further challenges with regards to fluid mixing, especially in diffusion-limited systems.

To date, external syringe pumps have been widely utilized to induce flow and mixing in microfluidic systems. Although these are precise and reliable, they are fairly large and hence confined to laboratory benchtops, thereby proving difficult to integrate with other operations on the microfluidic device comprising a miniaturized handheld platform for portable operations, for example, for use at the point of need (Yeo, Chang, Chan, & Friend, 2011). This is further complicated by the inlet and outlet tubing and ancillary connections required for fluid transfer between the pump and the chip, which requires careful handling by a skilled user, therefore making their use considerably challenging for adoption by patients, for example, in diagnostic testing. The majority of medical testing also involves molecular and bioparticle manipulation, which require additional microfluidic capability for fast and sensitive preconcentration, sorting, and detection.

In this chapter, we summarize the various mechanisms for microfluidic actuation within two subcategories: mechanical and nonmechanical actuation mechanisms (Table 3.1). This is followed by a brief overview of two mechanisms, namely electrokinetics and acoustics, which we believe constitute the most promising and practical methods for driving fluid and particle motion in microfluidic devices, as reflected by recent growing interest and popularity in their use.

3.2 Electrokinetics

To date, electrokinetics, which concerns the use of electric fields to manipulate fluid flow, is one of the most preferred and widely used methods for microfluidic actuation. This is because electrodes are cheaply and easily fabricated and can be integrated without much difficulty in microfluidic devices, and they have the ability to provide high electroosmotic flow rates, efficient electrophoretic separation, and precise dielectrophoretic particle positioning. Here, we provide an overview of the basic principles underlying these flows and a brief summary of their use for microfluidic actuation. The reader is referred to a more comprehensive treatise on the subject in Chang and Yeo (2010) and Ramos and Morgan (2016).

3.2.1 The electric double layer

A channel surface in contact with an electrolyte solution tends to acquire a net charge through various surface-charging mechanisms (Hunter, 1987). Consequently, free ions in the bulk with opposite charge to that on the surface (counterions) are attracted to the channel surface, while ions with like charge (coions) are repelled. A thin polarized layer rich in counterions, known as the Debye double layer, therefore arises adjacent to the channel surface, as depicted in Fig. 3.1a and b.

The electric potential field φ in the double layer can be described via a solution of Gauss' Law $\nabla^2 \varphi = -\rho_e/\varepsilon$ governing charge conservation. For planar systems of symmetrical binary electrolytes, the volume charge density ρ_e can be specified by the Poisson–Boltzmann distribution; in the limit of small surface potentials $\varphi_s \ll RT/zF$ $\sim$ 25.7 mV(298K), linearization of the resultant Poisson equation together with boundary conditions prescribed by the surface potential $\varphi = \varphi_s = \lambda_D E_s(y=0)$ and a potential and electric field $E = -d\varphi/dy$ that decays away from the surface to the bulk ($y \to \infty$) permit an approximate analytical solution in the form:

$$\varphi = \varphi_s e^{-y/\lambda_D}, \tag{3.1}$$

where,

$$\lambda_D = \sqrt{\frac{\varepsilon RT}{2F^2 z^2 C_\infty}} \tag{3.2}$$

Table 3.1 Summary of the main mechanical and nonmechanical actuation mechanisms for microfluidic actuation.

Mechanical	Principal/Notes	References
Piezoelectric	A diaphragm comprising a piezoelectric disc, or a stack, that deforms when subject to an electric field to induce fluid motion by peristaltic (i.e., sequential contraction and relaxation) action along the length of the channel.	Jang et al. (2007); Koch, Harris, Evans, White, and Brunnschweiler (1998); Schabmueller et al. (2002)
Pneumatic/Thermopneumatic	Air is employed to actuate and relax a diaphragm to create a pressure difference that pumps the fluid; often combined with diffusers. Heated and cooled air are used in thermopneumatic versions.	Grover, Ivester, Jensen, and Mathies (2006); Jeong and Yang (2000); Kim, Na, Kang, and Kim (2005); Pol, Lintel, Elwenspoek, and Fluitman (1990)
Rotary/Centrifugal (e.g., rotary gears, Lab-on-a-CD)	Reservoirs, valves, and channels are patterned on a compact disc (CD). Fluid actuation within these structures arising from centrifugal forces is achieved upon rotation using a laboratory micromotor. A thermopneumatic addition combines this with heating of the reservoir to allow bidirectional pumping.	Abi-Samra et al. (2011); Gorkin. Clime. Madou, and Kido (2010)
Shape-memory alloys (SMAs)	SMAs are thin films, and more recently wires, used as valves, pumps, latches, and multiplexers due to their ability to exert large strains on soft elastomers such as PDMS under an electric field.	Benard, Kahn, Heuer, and Huff (1998); Vyawahare, Sitaula, Martin, Adalianb, and Scherer (2008); Xu et al. (2001)

Continued

Table 3.1 Continued

Mechanical	Principal/Notes	References
Electromagnetic	Fluid actuation is achieved by applying an oscillating magnetic field with the use of magnetic elements strategically embedded in a soft polymeric structure, resulting in its vibration. This is combined with diffuser and nozzle elements close to the inlets and outlets to achieve net flow direction.	Al-Halhouli, Kilanib, and Büttgenb (2010); Khoo and Liu (2000); Zhou and Amirouche (2011)
Electrostatic	Coulombic attraction force between oppositely charged plates drives the deflection of a soft membrane when an appropriate voltage is applied. The deflected membrane returns to its initial position upon relaxation of the field. The alternating deflection results in a pressure difference that, in turn, pumps the fluid.	Bae, Han, Masel, and Shannon (2007); Machauf, Nemirovsky, and Dinnar (2005); Zengerle, Richter et al. (1992)
Acoustic (e.g., flexural waves, bubble streaming, and surface acoustic waves (SAWs))	Flexural Waves: Bulk vibration of a thin piezoelectric film that generates an acoustic field, which, in turn, causes fluid to flow (acoustic streaming). Bubble streaming: Acoustic streaming driven via excitation of bubbles attached at strategic positions on a channel using a piezoelectric transducer. Typically used for fluid mixing and recently for particle sorting and trapping. SAW: MHz order frequency electromechanical surface waves that generate a direct acoustic force on particles or a momentum that generates fluid flow (acoustic streaming) for fluidic actuation and micro/nano particle and biomolecule manipulation.	Luginbuhl et al. (1997); Meng et al. (2000); Moroney et al. (1991) Ahmed, Mao, Juluri, and Huang (2009a), Ahmed, Mao, Shi, Juluria, and Huang (2009b); Hashmi, Yua, Reilly-Collette, Heiman, and Xu (2012); Wang, Jalikop, and Hilgenfeldt 2012) Friend and Yeo (2011); Yeo et al. (2011)

Nonmechanical	Principal/Notes	References
Capillary (e.g., pressure and surface tension gradients)	Pressure gradient: Flow induced by a pressure difference across an interface that drives wetting of fluids in channels or in paper-based substrates. Attractive because it offers a passive actuation mechanism without requiring active pumping.	Gervais and Delamarche (2009); Ichikawa, Hosokawa, and Maeda (2004); Martinez, Phillips, and Whitesides (2010)
	Surface tension gradient: Generation of interfacial flow due to chemical (e.g., surfactant) concentration, thermal (thermocapillary), electrical (electrocapillary), or optical (optocapillary) gradients.	Basu and Gianchandani (2008); Darhuber and Troian (2005)
Electrokinetics (e.g., electroosmosis, electrophoresis, dielectrophoresis, and electrowetting)—Chang and Yeo (2010)	Electroosmosis: Bulk motion of aqueous solution along a fixed solid boundary due to an external electric field.	Lazar and Karger (2002); Takamura, Onoda, Inokuchi, Adachi, Oki and Horiike (2003); Wang et al. (2009)
	Electrophoresis: Use of an applied electric field to move charged particles or ions in a stationary fluid.	Kenyon, Meighan and Haye (2011); Wu et al. (2008)
	Dielectrophoresis: Motion of dielectric particles suspended in a medium due to the application of a *nonuniform* electric field.	Pethig, 2010; Menachery, Graham, Messerli, Pethig & Smith (2010)
	Electrowetting: Control of the wettability of a drop or film through an applied electric field by the generation of a Maxwell force at the contact line or a Maxwell pressure along the interface (depending on electrode configuration).	Mugele and Baret (2005); Yeo and Chang (2005); Wheeler (2008)

Continued

Table 3.1 Continued

Nonmechanical	Principal/Notes	References
Optics (optofluidics) (e.g., laser microfluidic actuation, optical tweezing, and optical chromatography)—Fainman, Lee, Psaltis, and Yang (2010)	Laser microfluidic actuation: The momentum carried by incident propagating light gives rise to a radiation pressure at the fluid interface due to the difference in refractive index, resulting in interfacial deformation or even jetting. In addition, localization of the laser beam induces thermocapillary forces leading to fluid flow (see also *Capillary entry*).	Baroud, Vincent and Delville (2007); Delville et al. (2009); Dixit, Kim, Vasilyev, Eid and Faris (2010); Grigoriev (2005)
	Optical tweezers: Dielectric particles can be trapped and moved due to the optical gradient within the tightly focused laser beam. Alternatively, birefringence can be exploited in which a particle can be rotated in a standard optical trap simply by manipulating the polarization of the light beam.	Chiou, Ohta and Wu (2005); Dholakia, MacDonald and Spalding (2002); Grier (1997); Neale, Macdonald, Dholakia, and Krauss (2005)
	Optical chromatography: Use of a focused laser beam to trap particles along its axis of propagation, where the beam is positioned against the fluid flow and the particles' trapped location is a balance between fluid drag and optical pressure.	Imasaka (1998); Hart and Terray (2003); Hart, Terray, Arnold and Leski (2007)
Magnetohydrodynamic	Use of a Lorentz force to pump conducting fluids, perpendicular to both the electric and the magnetic field.	Bau, Zhong and Yi, (2001); Eijel, Dalton, Hayden, Burt and Manz (2003); Jang and Lee (2000); Lemoff and Lee (2000)
Microbubbles	Generated either electrochemically (e.g., via electrolysis) or thermally (e.g., cavitation). The bubble oscillation is used to drive pumping in microchannels, often by pushing on diaphragms.	Kabata, Suzuki, Kishigami & Haga (2005); Suzuki and Yoneyama (2002); Yoshimi, Shinoda, Mishima, Nakao and Munekane (2004); Yin and Prosperetti (2005)

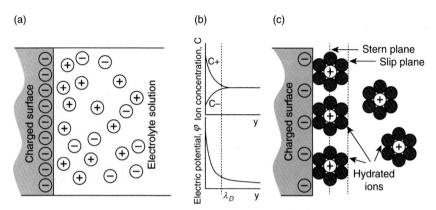

Figure 3.1 (a) Schematic depiction of, and (b) concentration profile (top) and electric potential variation (bottom) in the Debye double layer of thickness λD that arises as a consequence of an electrolyte solution in contact with charged surface, showing the enrichment in counterions and depletion in coions. (c) Stern layer that comprises hydrated counterions bound by water molecules.

is the Debye screening length or double layer thickness. The above is known as the *Debye–Hückel approximation* (Debye & Hückel, 1923), wherein y is the coordinate normal to the surface, ε the permittivity, R the molar gas constant, T the absolute temperature, z' the ionic valency, F the Faraday constant, and C the bulk ion concentration. We note the inverse relationship between the Debye length and the ion concentration (and hence conductivity) in Eq. (3.2): strong electrolytes lead to thin double layers ($\sim 0.1–10$ nm), whereas weaker electrolytes give rise to thicker double layers (~ 10 nm–1 μm).

The Debye–Hückel approximation, which assumes that the counterions are mobile point charges distributed by rapid and random thermal motion in the *diffuse* double layer, nevertheless fails to account for hydration or solvation effects due to the finite ion size. These effects were later taken into account by allowing for a *Stern* layer comprising hydrated counterions that are bound by water molecules, whose local screening effect permits their adsorption onto the surface (Fig. 3.1c) (Stern, 1924). A slip plane, therefore, must exist between the rigid and stationary Stern layer and the mobile diffuse layer, along which the potential, more specifically known as the zeta potential ζ, can be experimentally measured (in contrast to the difficulty in characterizing the actual potential on the surface). For weak to moderate electrolytes, in keeping with the small potential limit in the Debye–Hückel approximation, $\zeta \sim \lambda_D E_s \sim \lambda_D \sigma_s/\varepsilon$.

Electrokinetic phenomena, therefore, arise as a consequence of slippage of the diffuse double layer over the charged surface upon the application of an applied electric field to generate bulk flow (*electroosmosis* in the case of stationary charged surfaces) or particle motion (*electrophoresis* in the case of a stationary medium), or an applied external force to produce an electric potential (*streaming potential* in the case of flow over a stationary surface or *sedimentation potential* in the case of charged particles moving in a stationary medium). Given their relevance to microfluidic actuation, we briefly highlight the first two cases in the discussion to follow.

3.2.2 Electroosmosis

3.2.2.1 Electroosmotic slip

In its most general case, electroosmosis comprises the bulk motion of electrolyte that arises when a tangential electric field is applied across the *equilibrium* double layer that forms when the electrolyte is in contact with a solid boundary that acquires surface charge as a consequence. As depicted in Fig. 3.2, counterions in the diffuse layer are attracted to the electrode with opposite polarity, their net charge giving rise to a Maxwell (Lorentz) force $p_e E$ and hence momentum transfer on the liquid, which drives an electrokinetic slip at the slip plane. This slip can be derived from a balance between the hydrodynamic viscous and Maxwell stresses, assuming that the double layer is sufficiently thin compared to the channel radius/width such that the flow is unidirectional along the channel and that the pressure gradient only arises as a consequence of the tangential gradient in the normal surface field. Details of the derivation can be found in Chang and Yeo (2010); here, it suffices to quote the result, known as the *Smoluchowski slip velocity*:

$$u_s = -\frac{\varepsilon \zeta E_x}{\mu}, \tag{3.3}$$

where E_x is the applied tangential field and μ is the viscosity. Typically, $\zeta \sim$ 10–100 mV, and hence slip velocities up to around 1 mm/s can be generated with fields of approximately 100 V/cm.

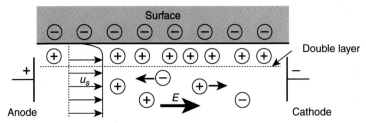

Figure 3.2 Counterions within the diffuse double layer are attracted toward the electrode with the opposite polarity upon application of a tangential electric field, giving rise to a net Maxwell force and hence bulk motion of the fluid known as electroosmosis. Given the double layer is thin relative to most microchannel dimensions, the flow velocity profile is essentially flat across the channel.

3.2.2.2 Electroosmotic pumping

The velocity, therefore, increases from its zero value (i.e., no-slip) at the channel wall to the maximum value given in Eq. (3.3) at the slip plane. Consequently, the slip drags the rest of the liquid in the channel along, giving rise to bulk electroosmotic flow. Given the asymptotically small Debye length, the bulk flow can be considered to arise from slip at the channel walls, and hence the velocity profile is essentially flat across the channel. This plug flow is convenient and particularly advantageous over pressure-driven flow from many perspectives, especially for microfluidic applications, since it minimizes hydrodynamic dispersion that leads to sample band broadening. Moreover, the independence of the slip velocity on the channel dimension then suggests that the volumetric flow rate, which is proportional to the channel cross-sectional area, scales as the square of the characteristic channel dimension H^2. This is a considerable advantage over the H^4 scaling of the volumetric flow rate arising from pressure-driven flows, which sharply diminishes with miniaturization of the channel dimension as H decreases. Together with the benefits of on-chip electrode integration—therefore removing the need for cumbersome fluid transfer from large mechanical or syringe pumps onto the microfluidic device, the elimination of mechanically moving parts, the ease of changing the flow direction upon reversal of the electrode polarity, and the constant pulse-free fluid motion—electroosmotic pumps, thus, constitute a very attractive mechanism for microfluidic actuation.

It can further be shown from simple scaling arguments that a channel dimension H close to λ_D optimizes the power efficiency of the electroosmotic pump (Chang & Yeo, 2010)—in larger channels, power is wasted in the large electroneutral bulk region outside the double layer where there is no net momentum transfer due to the absence of net charge, whereas in smaller channels, the flow is suppressed by increased viscous dissipation. As such, and given that the volumetric flow rate scales with cross-sectional area, it is expedient to employ a parallel bundle of thin channels (e.g., nanopores) whose dimensions are comparable to the double layer thickness—an example being that in packed capillaries or porous silica monoliths (Chen, Wang, & Chang, 2005; Wang, Chen, & Chang, 2006). For cylindrical pore geometries, and neglecting the tortuosity of the pore networks, the maximum pressure that can be developed in such pumps, taking into account the hydrodynamic load that imposes a back pressure within a channel, can be expressed by:

$$\Delta p_{\max} = \frac{8\mu Q_{eo}}{\left(A_p R_p^2/L_p\right) = \left(A_l R_l^2/L_l\right)}, \quad (3.4)$$

where $Q_{eo} = u_s A_p = n\pi R_p^2 u_s$ is the electroosmotic flow rate of the pump comprising n cylindrical pores of radius R_p and length L_p, i.e., the maximum flow rate when there is no pressure-driven flow ($\Delta p = 0$), and $A_l = \pi R_l^2$ the effective cross-sectional area of the hydrodynamic load section with radius R_l and length L_l, whose flow rate is specified by the Hagen–Poiseuille equation:

$$Q = \frac{A_l R_l^2}{8\mu} \frac{\Delta p_{\max}}{L_l}. \tag{3.5}$$

Substituting Eq. (3.4) into Eq. (3.5),

$$Q = Q_{eo}\left(1 - \frac{\Delta p}{\Delta p_{\max}}\right), \tag{3.6}$$

indicating the linear relationship between the back pressure and flow rate, and from which the efficiency of the pump can be obtained:

$$\eta = \frac{Q}{Q_{eo}} = 1 - \frac{\Delta p}{\Delta p_{\max}}. \tag{3.7}$$

The pump becomes more efficient therefore as $\Delta p_{\max}$ increases, which, from Eq. (3.4), can be obtained by reducing R_p/R_l such that Q approaches Q_{eo}. This is, however, constrained, since decreasing R_p below λ_D results in overlapping double layers and hence diminishing slip velocities. The pump operation is, therefore, optimal when $R_p \sim \lambda_D$, as suggested above, noting from Eq. (3.4) that Q_{eo}, and hence Q, can be compensated by increasing the applied field strength, although this, on the other hand, is limited by undesirable effects of bubble generation as a consequence of the increased current, which can cause blockage of the channel and whose large capillary pressures could cancel out any increase in the flow rate.

The theory above, nevertheless, breaks down for nanochannels when the channel dimension becomes comparable to the Debye length, such that an electroneutral ohmic region in the bulk no longer exists and the entire channel consists of a polarized region due to double layer overlap. In addition, entrance, resistive, pore neck charge storage, and electroviscous effects may also become important in these cases (Chang & Yeo, 2010). There are several analytical models as well as molecular simulations dedicated to nanochannel electroosmosis (see, for example, Petsev (2010) and Qiao and Aluru (2003)); we refer the reader to these, as the subject is beyond the scope of the present overview.

3.2.2.3 Electroosmotic mixing

Given the irrotationality of the electric field, the similarity between the hydrodynamic streamlines and the electric field—i.e., both velocity and electric fields are governed by the same divergence-free conditions—renders the electroosmotic flow an irrotational potential flow (hence the flat velocity profiles observed in Fig. 3.2) in the absence of an externally applied pressure gradient (Chang & Yeo, 2010). An unfortunate consequence of this result, which is quite unexpected for microfluidic flows where viscous stresses are usually dominant, is the absence of flow vortices to induce mixing in the microfluidic device, which, although advantageous in minimizing sample dispersion as discussed earlier, can be problematic given the typically low biomolecular diffusivities that result in long reaction times in transport-limited cases. Various strategies have, therefore, been adopted to increase mixing efficiency in electroosmotic flows. For example, it is possible to revoke the field and streamline similarity by generating a back pressure gradient in the channel through the introduction of surface charge, or bulk pH or electrolyte concentration (and hence ζ-potential) gradients along the channel (Ajdari, 1995; Herr et al., 2000; Minerick, Ostafin, & Chang, 2002). Alternatively, interfacial instabilities can be introduced in the case of two coflowing electrolytes with differences in their conductivities (Lin, Storey, Oddy, Chen, & Santiago, 2004; Pan, Ren, & Yang, 2007), as illustrated in Fig. 3.3, although the electric fields required to drive such transverse electrokinetic instabilities are often fairly large.

3.2.3 Electrophoresis

Electrophoresis refers to the application of electric fields to move charged particles or ions in a stationary fluid. Two asymptotic limits for the particle size a can be

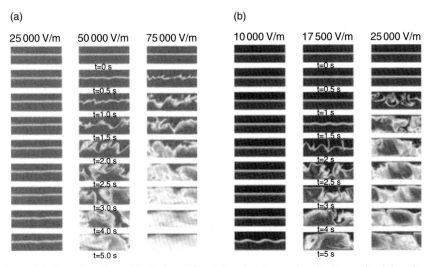

Figure 3.3 Transient electrokinetic instability driven by the gradient in the conductivity of two coflowing electrolyte solutions under an applied longitudinal electric field. (a) Experimental results and (b) numerical simulation.
Reprinted with permission from Lin et al. (2004). Copyright 2004, American Institute of Physics.

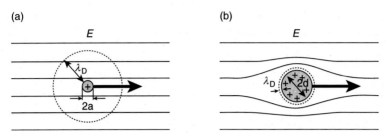

Figure 3.4 (a) The electric field lines around a particle remain undistorted around a charged particle if its size a is small compared to the Debye double layer thickness ($a \ll \lambda_D$). (b) On the other hand, the double layer screens the external field when the particle size is large compared to the double layer thickness ($a \gg \lambda_D$).

considered (Chang & Yeo, 2010). In the small particle size limit (Fig. 3.4a), i.e., $a \ll \lambda_D$, the particle can be assumed to be a point charge, and hence double layer screening effects can be neglected. In this case, the presence of the point charge does not influence and hence distort the field lines, and simply translates under electromigration effects in the absence of electrokinetic slip in the double layer around the particle. A balance between the Coulomb force exerted by the point charge q and the viscous drag force then leads to the Hückel equation for the electrophoretic mobility of the particle:

$$v_{ep} = \frac{2\varepsilon\zeta}{3\mu}, \qquad (3.8)$$

which is related to the electrophoretic velocity through $u_{ep} = v_{ep}E$.

In the large particle size limit (Fig. 3.4b), i.e., $a \gg \lambda_D$, the double layer screens the external field, and hence the Maxwell force only acts in the double layer to drive an electrokinetic slip flow and not on the particle itself. In this case, the Smoluchowski slip velocity in Eq. (3.3) can be used along the particle surface such that the electrophoretic velocity has the same dependency as the electroosmotic slip velocity but with opposite sign:

$$u_s = \frac{\varepsilon\zeta E_x}{\mu}. \qquad (3.9)$$

The discrimination in the electrophoretic mobility and hence migration velocity based on charge (more specifically, the surface charge density and hence the ζ-potential) in Eqs. (3.8) and (3.9) provides the underlying basis for electrophoretic separation technology. We note, however, the absence of the dependence on particle size or shape (although the former is implicit in the ζ-potential in the point charge theory). More common, however, is the use of gels or polymer (i.e., gel electrophoresis), which provides a medium that acts as a molecular sieve to facilitate steric and reptation effects, thus permitting size-based discrimination (i.e., smaller molecules migrate more quickly in the gel compared to larger molecules with the same electrophoretic mobility under the same electric field). More recently, a powerful technique has been proposed as an alternative to gel electrophoresis, in which the ends of polyelectrolyte molecules are tagged with a large uncharged monodispersed protein or polymer that exerts a large drag on the molecule while leaving its net charge intact. This technique, known as end labelled free-solution electrophoresis (Meagher et al., 2005), has been demonstrated as a fast and efficient method for the separation of gene fragments in DNA sequencing. Other methods for multiplex DNA sequencing using capillary array electrophoresis in microfluidic platforms (Paegel, Emrich, Wedemayer, Scherer, & Mathies, 2002), as well as electrophoretic detection of DNA sequence variations in microfluidic devices, have also been proposed—for the latter, see, for example, the work on single nucleotide polymorphism detection using restriction fragment length polymorphism (Footz, Somerville, Tomaszewski, Elyas, & Backhouse, 2004) and single-strand conformation polymorphism (Szántai & Guttman, 2006). The reader is also referred to the review by Wu, Qin, and Lin (2008) and Yeo et al. (2011).

We note that the buffer solution also moves due to electroosmosis, and hence the electroosmotic velocity must be taken into account. Defining an electroosmotic mobility $v_{eo} = u_s/E$, the apparent mobility and hence the apparent velocity of the charged particle moving through the buffer solution under combined electrophoresis and electroosmosis is simply the sum of the electrophoretic and electroosmotic mobilities. When the charged particles have the same polarity as that of the ions in the buffer solution, the apparent mobility, therefore, exceeds the electrophoretic mobility, whereas the converse is true if the charged species has the opposite polarity to the ions in solution. Interestingly then, the charged particles can be trapped when the electrophoretic and electroosmotic mobilities are equal, which can be exploited to reduce the length required for electrophoretic separation.

To date, several extensions to the above electrophoretic theories have been proposed with more sophisticated theories to account for electroviscous effects—including that for nonspherical (Chen & Koch, 1996) and porous particles (Natraj & Chen, 2002), tangential surface conduction (Camp & Capitano, 2005), counterion condensation (Chang & Yeo, 2010), as well as conducting Stern layer and convective currents effects (Shubin, Hunter, & O'Brien, 1993).

3.2.4 AC electrokinetics

The use of direct current (DC) electric fields is not without inherent disadvantages. High DC field intensities can sustain large currents that cause molecular and cellular degradation, and particle aggregation, as well as bubble and ion contamination generation. These problems can, however, be circumvented with the use of high frequency (>10 kHz) alternating current (AC) fields. The polarization mechanism and hence flow dynamics associated with AC electrokinetics are, however, fundamentally different from its DC or low frequency AC counterpart. Above frequencies associated with time scales that are below the double layer charge relaxation time scale $\lambda_D^2/D = \varepsilon/\sigma$, wherein D is the ionic diffusivity and σ the conductivity, there is insufficient time to polarize the double layer. As such, AC electrokinetics utilizes the electric field itself to induce polarization on the electrode surface in place of polarization due to the natural surface charges on the channel surface, as in DC electrokinetics (Chang & Yeo, 2010). Correspondingly, the induced polarization is nonuniform, given the double layer is no longer in equilibrium; as a result, the ζ-potential is now field-dependent, and thus it can be seen, for example, from the slip velocity given by Eq. (3.3), that AC electrokinetic phenomena are nonlinear. Moreover, at these high frequencies, electrochemical reactions at the electrodes are usually absent at the root mean square (RMS) voltages typically employed, and hence problems associated with bubble and ion generation are nonexistent. Further, the AC current is localized in the double layer, therefore minimizing penetration and, thus, damage in molecular and cellular structures. Below, we provide only a very brief summary of this subject in the context of AC electroosmosis; for a more in-depth discourse on nonlinear and nonequilibrium electrokinetics, the reader may wish to consult the text by Chang and Yeo (2010). It is worth noting that it is possible to drive similar field-induced double layer polarization using DC fields (alternatively known as induced-charge electrokinetic phenomena (Squires & Quake, 2005), also discussed further in Chang and Yeo (2010)).

The simplest case of AC electroosmotic flow occurs due to capacitive charging over symmetric coplanar electrodes; it is also possible that AC electroosmotic flows can be generated due to Faradaic charging (Lastochkin, Zhou, Wang, Ben, & Chang, 2004; Ng, Lam, & Rodríguez, 2009), although we will refrain from discussing this mechanism here. In one half of the AC cycle, ions in the bulk are driven by the field toward electrodes of opposite polarity to form a double layer whose total charge balances that on the electrodes. In the next half cycle, the electrode polarity reverses and so does that of the double layer on each electrode. In both cases, however, an outward tangential Maxwell force arises, which does not reverse in direction upon reversal of the field. This, therefore, gives rise to a net nonzero time-average Maxwell stress and hence an electroosmotic slip to result in a pair of recirculating vortices with length scales comparable to the electrode dimension. This symmetric vortex pair, however, cancels, and hence no net flow is produced. In order to create a net global flow, it is, therefore, necessary to break the vortex symmetry with the use of asymmetric electrodes or an asymmetric field (e.g., a traveling wave) (Ajdari, 2000; Brown, Smith, & Rennie, 2000; Ramos, González, Castellanos, Green, & Morgan, 2003); practical devices also include an upper surface to suppress the back flow associated with the larger vortex. In fact, the most efficient flow can, therefore, be produced with maximum asymmetry through an orthogonal (T) electrode design given the near singular field at the tip of the vertical section of the "T" (Lastochkin, Zhou, Wang, Ben, & Chang, 2004). First derived by González, Ramos, Green, Castellanos, and Morgan (2000), the time-averaged AC electroosmotic slip on the electrode can be shown to assume the form:

$$u_s = -\frac{\varepsilon_l}{4\mu}\nabla_s\left|\Phi \mp \frac{V_0}{2}\right|^2. \tag{3.10}$$

where Φ is the potential in the bulk immediately adjacent to the double layer and $|V_0|$ the RMS amplitude of the applied voltage signal; ∇_s is a surface gradient operator across each electrode. It is then apparent from this, together with a charge balance across the double layer,

$$\sigma \frac{\partial \varphi}{\partial n} = i\omega C \left(\Phi - \frac{V_0}{2} \right) \qquad (3.11)$$

(where ω is the applied AC frequency, C the total capacitance in the double layer, and n the coordinate normal to the electrode surface) that the slip velocity reaches a maximum at an optimum frequency ω_0 associated with the RC or double layer charging time (R being the electrolyte resistance) $D/\lambda_D d$, where d is the electrode separation. Away from this optimum frequency, the slip velocity decays monotonically to zero. At low frequencies $\omega \to 0$, the double layer is completely polarized and completely screens the field such that the electrode resembles a perfect insulator; consequently, the potential drop occurs mainly across the double layer. At high frequencies $\omega \to \infty$, there is insufficient time to charge the double layer, and hence the electrode resembles a constant potential surface (i.e., a perfect conductor), and the potential drop occurs mainly across the bulk (Chang & Yeo, 2010).

Squires and Bazant (2004) later extended the analysis of AC electroosmotic flows to allow for charging on ideally polarizable surfaces other than electrodes. In particular, they examined a conducting cylinder (e.g., a metal wire) immersed in an electrolyte, which when subjected to a uniform field, attracted the normal field lines, thus facilitating normal field penetration into the double layer and giving rise to an electroosmotic slip (Fig. 3.5). Again, the time-averaged slip velocity exhibits a maximum due to complete screening in the low frequency limit and incomplete charging in the high frequency limit. In any case, the resulting flow is quadrupolar as shown in Fig. 3.5c, wherein fluid is drawn along the field lines at the poles and ejected radially at the equator.

In addition to micropumping applications, the planar converging stagnation flow associated with the recirculating vortex pair in AC electroosmosis above symmetric coplanar electrodes has also been exploited for linear particle assembly (Ben & Chang, 2005). A similar system was later used to convect single DNA molecules in a bulk suspension and immobilize them onto the electrode surface for subsequent stretching (Lin, Tsai, Chi, & Chen, 2005). Long-range convective trapping of DNA has also been demonstrated using the T-electrode design—the horizontal section of the "T" being used to sweep particles in the bulk toward the vertical section of the "T" which then funnels the concentrated particles into a conical region (Du, Juang, Wu, & Wei, 2008). While such long-range convective mechanisms are not extremely effective at local trapping, since flow conservation renders a true stagnation point impossible, it is possible to combine the AC electroosmotic flow with short-range forces to provide enhanced particle localization. Dielectrophoresis (DEP) is one such short-range mechanism, which we shall discuss next.

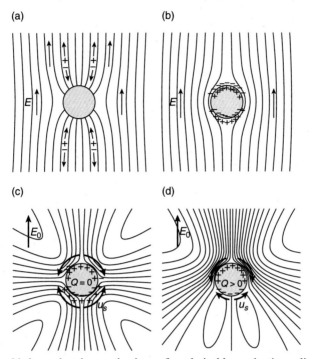

Figure 3.5 Double layer charging mechanisms of a polarizable conducting cylinder immersed in an electrolyte solution. Field lines (a) before and (b) after charging of the double layer. (c) Resulting electroosmotic flow streamlines, and (d) the corresponding streamlines obtained if the net charge on the cylinder surface is nonzero.
Reprinted with permission from Squires and Bazant (2004). Copyright 2004, American Physical Society.

3.2.5 Dielectrophoresis

Upon application of an electric field, a dielectric particle suspended in a dielectric medium acquires an interfacial charge due to the discontinuity in the permittivity across the phases. The interfacial polarization, however, is dependent on the orientation of the field due to the alignment of the individual dipoles within the particle and medium with the field, which can collectively be described by a single particle dipole that produces an effective dipole moment. For a spherical particle of radius a under an external AC field **E**, upon solving for the potential of the particle and the medium through an expansion in spherical harmonics, this takes the form (Chang & Yeo, 2010):

$$\mathbf{p} = 3\varepsilon_m f_{CM} V \mathbf{E}, \tag{3.12}$$

where

$$f_{CM} = \frac{\widetilde{\varepsilon}_p - \widetilde{\varepsilon}_m}{\widetilde{\varepsilon}_p + 2\widetilde{\varepsilon}_m} \otimes \quad (3.13)$$

is the Clausius–Mossotti factor that describes the polarizability of the particle. In the above, V is the particle volume, and

$$\widetilde{\varepsilon}_i = \varepsilon_i - i\frac{\sigma_i}{\omega} \quad (3.14)$$

is a complex permittivity in which the subscripts p and m denote particle and medium properties, respectively. When subject to an applied AC electric field with constant phase, this induced effective particle dipole then results in a time-averaged force on the particle, which reads (Green & Morgan, 1999):

$$\langle \mathbf{F} \rangle = \frac{1}{T}\int_0^T (\mathbf{p}\cdot\nabla)\widetilde{\mathbf{E}}\,dt = \pi\varepsilon_m a^3 \mathrm{Re}[f_{CM}]\nabla|\mathbf{E}|^2, \quad (3.15)$$

where T denotes the period of AC forcing.

We note that the force is short range, depending on the particle dimension cubed as well as the electric field gradient. This nonuniform field is necessary since the net interfacial charge on both ends of the particle are of opposite polarities but equal magnitudes; the force, therefore, cancels out in a uniform field since there is no effective dipole moment. The resulting particle motion that arises from this interaction between the nonuniform field with the induced dipole moment is, therefore, known as DEP.

The versatility of DEP manipulation arises from the reversal in the polarizability specified by the real part of the Clausius–Mossotti factor $\mathrm{Re}[f_{CM}]$ about a crossover frequency:

$$\omega_c = \frac{1}{2\pi}\sqrt{\frac{(\sigma_m - \sigma_p)(\sigma_m + 2\sigma_p)}{(\varepsilon_p - \varepsilon_m)(\varepsilon_p + \varepsilon_m)}}. \quad (3.16)$$

For frequencies at which $\mathrm{Re}[f_{CM}] > 0$, particles are, thus, drawn toward regions of high field intensity (positive DEP), whereas for frequencies at which $\mathrm{Re}[f_{CM}] < 0$, particles are drawn toward regions of low field intensity (negative DEP). The dependence of f_{CM} on the particle and medium conductivities and permittivities also allow the design of a DEP sorter that endows one particle species with a positive DEP force and another with a negative DEP force through judicious choice of a specific applied frequency (Gagnon & Chang, 2005). Multiple species, for example, can also be sorted by different DEP mobilities, which can be estimated from a balance between the DEP force in Eq. (3.15) and the Stokes drag on the particle:

$$v_{\text{DEP}} = \frac{\varepsilon_m a^2 \text{Re}[f_{\text{CM}}]}{6\mu}. \tag{3.17}$$

An integrated multiplex continuous flow microfluidic platform for filtering debris and for sorting and trapping of colloidal beads or pathogens at a rate of 100 particle/s is shown in Fig. 3.6 (Cheng, Chang, Hou, & Chang, 2007). While this sorting rate is still two orders of magnitude smaller than conventional flow cytometry, the technology offers the possibility for carrying out cell sorting and identification with costs and portability that are not afforded by laboratory-based cell sorters.

Consequently, DEP has emerged as a powerful tool for size-based discrimination for microfluidic detection and sorting. Numerous applications for DEP cell (blood cells, stem cells, neuronal cells, pathogens) sorting and characterization, pathogen (bacterial and viral) detection, and DNA, protein, and chromosomal manipulation are summarized in the excellent review by Pethig (2010). Given the emergence of bead-based assays to enhance detection, for example, in DNA hybridization and sequencing assays (Yeo et al., 2011), we anticipate DEP will play a major role in facilitating rapid and precise bead identification and sorting in microfluidic devices. Already, it has been shown that DNA concentration and the hybridized DNA

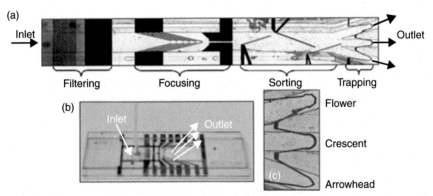

Figure 3.6 Bioparticle filtering, focusing, sorting, trapping, and detection using an integrated dielectrophoretic chip. (a) Image of the setup comprising different bioparticle manipulation stages. (b) Image showing the electrodes fabricated on two glass slides, giving rise to three-dimensional effects. (c) A top view of the three different trapping electrode configuration, comprising a flower—multiple curved electrode, crescent—a semicircle electrode, and an arrowhead—a pointed electrode.
Reprinted with permission from Cheng et al. (2007). Copyright 2007, American Institute of Physics.

conformation has a strong influence on the crossover frequency and the effective bead hydrodynamic radius (Gagnon, Senapati, Gordon, & Chang, 2009). This was exploited for trapping silica nanocolloids functionalized with oligonucleotides complementary to specific target DNA sequences for rapid microfluidic DNA identification in under 10 min. Beyond diagnostics and biosensing applications, DEP has also been used for isolating and positioning single cells in a similar manner to optical tweezers but with the advantage of design simplicity and significantly lower costs, primarily given that an expensive and complex laser is not required (Menachery, Graham, Messerli, Pethig, & Smith, 2011).

3.3 Acoustics

Despite its many advantages, electrokinetic actuation technology is hampered by the necessity for external ancillary equipment such as signal generators and amplifiers, which render complete miniaturization and integration with the microfluidic chip difficult. This is further compounded by the limitation of electrolyte solutions, which may be prohibitive in certain cases, and the requirement for high voltages in some other cases. An alternative mechanism that has demonstrated significant promise is the use of acoustic fields to drive microfluidic actuation, which has the ability to generate relatively large throughput and high pressures. While fairly low voltages are required, this is, however, compromised by the large sizes of the piezoelectric transducers often required to generate bulk ultrasonic manipulation that do not facilitate easy integration and miniaturization. Further, the large stresses that arise from the vibration, with frequencies typically of the order of 10−100 kHz and up to 1 MHz, and, in many cases, the accompanying cavitation that ensues, inflict considerable biomolecular and cellular damage.

These limitations, however, can be circumvented with a technology that has attracted considerable traction of late—the use of surface acoustic waves (SAWs) (Friend & Yeo, 2011; Yeo & Friend, 2009). Since the piezoelectric substrate required could comprise the microfluidic chip itself and as the interdigital transducer (IDT) electrodes required to generate the SAW can be integrated on the substrate, there is no need for the large transducers typically used in conventional ultrasonic microfluidics. Moreover, it has been shown that the ability to access high (MHz order and above) frequencies significantly limits the amount of molecular damage caused. One further advantage is the typically low powers (≤ 1 W) required to drive fluid and particle actuation with SAWs, even to the point of fluid atomization, thereby allowing the entire operation to be driven using a portable driver circuit powered by camera batteries, which, together with the chip-scale substrate (Fig. 3.7a), potentially allows for complete miniaturization and integration into a truly handheld and portable microfluidic device (Yeo & Friend, 2009). During the past years, acoustic particle

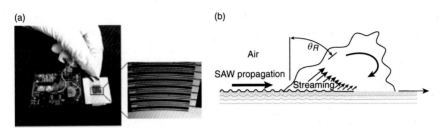

Figure 3.7 (a) A typical surface acoustic wave device comprising a piezoelectric substrate on which interdigital transducer electrodes are patterned (as shown in the enlarged inset) and a portable battery-operated electronic circuit and power supply. (b) Schematic depiction of the Eckart streaming generated when energy leaks into a drop at the Rayleigh angle θ_R when it is irradiated by SAWs propagating along the underlying substrate.

manipulation has been mainly used to focus, concentrate, and separate particles in various of one-phase microfluidic systems. Recently, acoustophoresis also has been implemented in two-phase systems to manipulate particles inside droplets (Fornell & Cushing, 2017; Park et al., 2017).

Here, we briefly discuss the basic principles underlying acoustic fluid and particle actuation, and review developments in the field to date, particularly focusing on the SAW technology.

3.3.1 Basic principles of acoustic fluid and particle manipulation

A sound wave is the result of pressure or velocity oscillations that propagate through a compressible medium and can be generated through bulk or surface vibration of solid materials. A convenient way to produce such vibration, especially at small scales in microfluidic systems, is with the use of oscillating electric fields by exploiting the electromechanical coupling afforded by piezoelectric transducers or substrates. There are primarily two broad strategies employed for acoustic particle and fluid actuation, which we describe next.

The first, generally known as *acoustophoresis,* exploits standing acoustic waves set up in a resonator configuration to spatially trap and move cells. The fundamental basis of the particle localization at pressure nodes/antinodes of the standing wave, and hence the ability to carry out particle separation arises from a competition between the dominant forces acting on the particle (assuming that sedimentation and buoyancy forces are negligible), namely, the primary acoustic radiation force,

$$F_a = -kE_a V_p \phi(\beta, \rho)\sin(2kx), \qquad (3.18)$$

assuming a one-dimensional planar standing wave, and the drag force,

$$F_d = -6\pi\mu u a \qquad (3.19)$$

acting on the particle of dimension a and volume V_p, in which x is the distance from a pressure node along the wave propagation axis. In the above, $k = 2\pi f/c_l$ is the wave number, with f denoting the applied frequency and c_l the sound speed in the fluid medium, $E_a = p_0^2\beta_l/4 = p_0^2/4K_l = p_0^2/4\rho_l c_l^2$ the acoustic energy density of the standing wave, with p_0 being the pressure amplitude of the standing wave, β_l the liquid compressibility, K_l the bulk modulus, ρ_l the liquid density, and

$$\phi = \frac{5\rho_p - 2\rho_l}{2\rho_p + \rho_l} - \frac{\beta_p}{\beta_l}, \qquad (3.20)$$

is an acoustic contrast factor in which ρ_p and β_p are the particle density and compressibility, respectively. Particles, therefore, aggregate at the pressure nodes for $\varphi > 0$ and at the antinodes for $\varphi < 0$.

The second exploits the fluid flow that results as the acoustic wave propagates through a fluid, known as *acoustic streaming* (Friend & Yeo, 2011). Different acoustic streaming phenomena are observed to occur over a variety of length scales imposed by the system geometry. In a thin boundary layer of fluid immediately adjacent to the vibrating surface with a characteristic thickness defined by the viscous penetration depth $(2\nu/\omega)^{1/2}$, strong viscous dissipation of the acoustic wave gives rise to flow known as *Schlichting streaming* (Schlichting, 1932), which is vortical in nature due to the no-slip condition at the oscillating solid boundary; ν is the kinematic viscosity, and ω the frequency. At the edge of the boundary layer (also known as the Stokes layer) over a length scale on the order of the sound wavelength in the liquid λ_L (which, in turn, is related to the excitation frequency), a steady irrotational drift flow, known as *Rayleigh streaming*, occurs as a consequence of the periodic recirculation in the boundary layer (Manor, Yeo, & Friend, 2012; Rayleigh, 1884). Over longer length scales $>>\lambda_L$, the viscous dissipation of the acoustic radiation due to absorption in the fluid, whose pressure and velocity fluctuations gives rise to a time-averaged particle displacement and hence steady momentum flux (i.e., Reynolds stress), which is nonzero despite the harmonic oscillation due to the nonlinear effects arising from viscous attenuation of the wave (Lighthill, 1978); the resultant flow being known as *Eckart streaming* (Eckart, 1948). It is not uncommon for a combination or all of the various streaming phenomena to exist together in a system, although one particular mechanism typically dominates, contingent on the system geometry. This is reflected in the flow phenomena observed, which can be remarkably distinct depending on the particular streaming mechanism that gives rise to them (Rezk, Manor, Friend, & Yeo, 2012).

3.3.2 Bulk ultrasonic vibration

The majority of the early work on acoustically driven microfluidic actuation was focused on the use of bulk ultrasonic transducers. These typically consisted of thin plates or membranes comprising a piezoelectric ceramic along which flexural waves (i.e., asymmetric Lamb waves) were generated, the plate/membrane thickness being a fraction of the wavelength of the flexural wave. For example, Moroney, White, and Howe (1991) and Meng, Nguyen, and White (2000) coated silicon nitride onto a ground plate, followed by the deposition of a thin zinc oxide layer and subsequently the aluminium interdigital electrodes. The bulk vibration that ensued then drove acoustic streaming, which due to the large attenuation length for the 1 MHz order employed, extended over a long range, typically a few centimetres from the membrane (Luginbuhl et al., 1997); as such, the device can also be used for mixing applications (Yaralioglu, Wygant, Marentis, & Khuri-Yakub, 2004). Nevertheless, these flexural wave pumps are not as efficient compared to the SAW fluid actuation which we discuss in the next section, with larger powers required, and one to two orders of magnitude lower in the velocity (typically up to 100 μm/s) that can be produced, even when focusing electrodes are employed (Meng et al., 2000).

In a similar manner, it is also possible to exploit substrate vibration to depin contact lines and to drive droplet motion in open microfluidic platforms. In the former, a contact line hysteresis condition for a drop subject to vibration was derived in which the depinning was dependent on the vibrational acceleration (Noblin, Buguin, & Brochard-Wyart, 2004); in other work, the drop could be shown to spread under 1 MHz order piston-like thickness mode vibration of the underlying substrate, which induced a boundary layer streaming flow that endowed an additional surface force at the contact line (Manor, Dentry, Friend, & Yeo, 2011). In the latter, a flexurally vibrating beam was employed by Alzuaga, Manceau, and Bastien (2005) on which different modes were excited in order to translate the drop between nodal locations.

Ultrasound-induced bubble oscillation can also be exploited to induce oscillatory flows, particularly useful for micromixing, or to facilitate nucleic acid transfection across cell membranes (i.e., sonoporation), even to the point of cell lysis (Ohl et al., 2006). In these cases, the bubbles are sonicated at resonance (typically kHz order) to induce a strong flow known as *cavitational microstreaming* that arises as the sound energy is dissipated due to the fluid viscosity in a boundary layer surrounding the bubble (Nyborg, 1958). Pumping flows of around several mm/s can be achieved, for example, with multiple bubbles housed in a cavity array and can be used to drive micromixing (Tovar & Lee 2009) or even cell sorting (Patel, Tovar, & Lee, 2012). More examples of the use of bubble oscillation in microfluidics can be found in the review by Hashmi, Yua, Reilly-Collette, Heiman, and Xu (2012). While relatively fast flows with reasonable throughput on the order of 100 μL/min and efficient mixing can be generated using bubble-based microfluidic actuators, difficulties associated with generating, trapping, and maintaining the stability of bubbles are a common problem that has yet to be adequately resolved, in addition to limitations arising from molecular/cell lysis due to cavitational damage that can be undesirable in bioapplications other than gene transfection.

Much more progress has been observed on the acoustophoretic front, on the other hand, in which ultrasonic standing waves are employed to focus particles onto nodal lines for cell sorting (Harris, Hill, Townsend, White, &, Beeby, 2005), colloidal filtering (Hawkes & Coakley, 2001) or particle switching (Manneberg et al., 2009) applications. Particles can also be separated based on size by exploiting the discrepancy in the size scaling between Eqs. (3.18) and (3.19) and hence the dependence of the particle migration time on the particle dimension (larger particles aggregate more quickly compared to smaller ones); such fractionation is more specifically known as free-flow acoustophoresis when conducted in a continuous flow system with the particles being driven orthogonally to the flow. Other design variations have also been investigated, for example flow splitting (Johnson & Feke, 1995) and frequency switching (Liu & Lim, 2011). Two vastly different particle species can also be separated given that the acoustic radiation force switches directions between positive and negative contrast factors in Eq. (3.20)—a property that was exploited for separating lipids from red blood cells (Petersson, Nilsson, Holm, Jönsson, & Laurell, 2004). The reader is referred to Laurell, Petersson, and Nilsson (2007) for a more detailed discussion on acoustophoresis and its applications.

3.3.3 Surface acoustic waves

Nanometre amplitude surface vibrations on a substrate in the form of Rayleigh waves offer an attractive and arguably superior alternative for microfluidic actuation compared to bulk ultrasound. The energy localization of these SAWs on the substrate and their efficient coupling into the fluid allows fluid actuation to be carried out with significantly lower dispersive losses, and hence the power requirement to drive comparable fluid actuation to that generated by bulk acoustics is significantly less, by one to two orders of magnitude, therefore offering the possibility for battery-powered operation, which, together with the chip-scale SAW device in Fig. 3.7a, enables attractive miniaturization possibilities (Yeo & Friend, 2009). Further, the low powers, together with the higher frequencies accessible with the SAWs, 10 MHz, and above, have been found to suppress shear or cavitation damage on molecules (Qi, Yeo, Friend, & Ho, 2010), thus making them attractive for bioapplications.

The SAW can be generated on a piezoelectric substrate by applying a sinusoidal electrical signal to IDT electrodes patterned on the substrate, whose finger width d - determines the frequency f of the SAW and hence its wavelength λ_{saw}, i.e., $f = c_s/4d = c_s/\lambda_{SAW}$. As illustrated in Fig. 3.7b, the coupling of acoustic energy into the fluid to drive Eckart streaming (Section 3.3.1) then arises from the diffraction of the SAW front in the presence of the fluid, which leads to leakage of the energy into the fluid at the Rayleigh angle, defined as the ratio between the sound speed of the Rayleigh wave on the substrate c_s to the speed of sound in the fluid c_l, i.e., $\theta_R = \sin^{-1}(c_s/c_l)$. In addition to the recirculation within the fluid, the acoustic radiation pressure also imparts a force at the interface that together with the momentum transfer to the interface due to Eckart streaming imparts a body force on the drop whose horizontal component causes it to translate in the direction of the SAW. Similarly, the elliptical retrograde motion of solid elements on the substrate as the SAW traverses underneath the drop also induces Schlichting and Rayleigh streaming, which has been shown to pull out a thin front-running wetting film in the opposite direction to that of the SAW propagation (Manor et al., 2012; Rezk et al., 2012). In the same way that ultrasonic standing waves and acoustic streaming can be exploited to drive microscale fluid actuation and particle manipulation, we provide a short discussion of the use of SAWs for this purpose and their associated applications. For a more detailed discussion on SAW microfluidics, see, for example, Friend and Yeo (2011).

3.3.3.1 SAW particle manipulation

Acoustophoretic manipulation can also be carried out using standing SAWs in a similar manner to bulk ultrasonic standing waves (Section 3.3.2). The standing wave in the SAW devices, however, arises when diffraction of the SAW from the substrate into the liquid (Fig. 3.7b) generates sound waves in the liquid bulk that reflects off the walls of the microchannel (often fabricated from polydimethylsiloxane (PDMS) and placed on top of the SAW substrate). Depending on the channel dimension and the sound wavelength in the fluid, the particles then aggregate along one or more pressure nodal (or antinodal) lines along the channel. Conventionally, the IDTs are placed perpendicular to the channel and hence flow direction (Shi, Mao, Ahmed, Colletti, & Huang, 2008) to achieve linear focusing and subsequent separation/sorting, for example, by size, compressibility, or density (Nam, Lim, Kim, Kang, & Shin, 2012). In addition, the IDTs can also be arranged orthogonally at two lateral sides of a square chamber to obtain two-dimensional patterning (Shi et al., 2009). A discussion on the use of these devices as "acoustic tweezers" for cell manipulation is given by Lin, Mao, and Huang (2012).

In addition, the nodal and hence particle positions can also be shifted along the axis of the standing wave by shifting the relative phase between the input IDT signal (Meng et al., 2011; Orloff et al., 2011). Particle alignment and sorting can also be carried out using IDTs placed at the ends of the channel such that the SAW propagates along the channel axis (Tan, Yeo, & Friend, 2009a). One advantage of this configuration is the ability to alter between fluid pumping and particle focusing simply by switching the frequency from the fundamental mode to a higher harmonic (Tan, Yeo, & Friend, 2010).

3.3.3.2 SAW fluid actuation and manipulation

SAW particle aggregation, trapping, patterning, and separation are typically carried out at low input powers, considerably below 1 W, where the SAW displacement amplitude and velocity are relatively small, on the order of 0.1 nm and 0.01 m/s, respectively, such that the streaming is weak in order to avoid dispersion of the particles. At these low powers, other particle patterning phenomena are also observed, for example, those that form on the nodes or antinodes of capillary waves induced on the free surface of drops vibrated by the SAW excitation (Li, Friend, & Yeo, 2008).

At moderate power levels (approximately up to 1 W), it is possible to dispense and transport drops (Renaudin, Tabourier, Zhang, Camart & Druon, 2006). For example, sessile drops can be translated on the substrate when the acoustic radiation pressure and acoustic streaming results are sufficient to impart momentum transfer to the interface to overcome the pinning of the contact line (Brunet, Baudoin, Matar, & Zoueshtiagh, 2010). This was shown for a variety of applications in open microfluidic systems such as polymerase chain reactions (Wixforth et al., 2004), bioparticle sampling, collection and concentration (Tan, Friend, & Yeo, 2007), scaffold cell seeding (Li, Friend, & Yeo, 2007a), and protein unfolding (Schneider et al., 2007). In addition, SAW droplet manipulation, such as mixing and particle concentration as well as sensing, has also been combined with electrowetting to enhance drop manipulation operations such as drop positioning and splitting (Li, Fu, Brodie, Alghane, & Walton, 2012).

At these powers, the SAW can also be used to drive strong convective flows both within the drop and in channels. For example, it is possible to break the planar symmetry of the SAW to drive azimuthal recirculation in a drop or a microfluidic chamber to generate a rapid microcentrifugation effect (Li, Friend & Yeo, 2007b; Shilton, Tan, Yeo, & Friend, 2008). This was used for example for inducing rapid and chaotic mixing (Shilton, Yeo, & Friend, 2011) (Fig. 3.8a), which can be used to enhance chemical

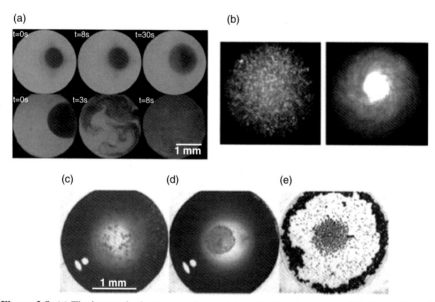

Figure 3.8 (a) The images in the top row show mixing of a dye due to pure diffusion without the action of the surface acoustic wave (SAW), whereas the images in the bottom row show effective mixing under chaotic flow conditions driven by the SAW with an input power of ∼1 W. (b) Concentration of particles in a 0.5 μL drop via drop rotation induced by acoustic radiation due to the SAW. (c)–(e) Separation of pollen and synthetic particles. (c) Prior to the application of the SAW, the pollen and synthetic particles were suspended homogeneously throughout the entire quiescent drop. (d) After 3 s of applying the SAW, the pollen particles appear to concentrate in the center of the drop and are hence separated from the synthetic particles, which tend to concentrate along the periphery of the drop. (e) The two species remain separated even after removal of the SAW and when the drop is fully evaporated after 1 min. After Shilton et al. (2011), (2008); Rogers et al. (2010).

and biochemical reactions (Kulkarni, Friend, Yeo, & Perlmutter, 2009, 2010), or for particle concentration/separation (Fig. 3.8b). It is also possible to sort two particle species based on size in this microcentrifugation flow by exploiting the discrepancy in the scaling between the acoustic radiation force and the drag force exerted on the particle (Eqs. 3.18 and 3.20): from a balance between these two forces, it is then possible to derive a frequency-dependent crossover particle size (which, in certain respects, is an analogue to the dielectrophoretic crossover frequency in Eq. (3.15)) below which the drag force dominates to drive smaller particles to the center of the drop and above which the acoustic force dominates to drive larger particles to the periphery (Fig. 3.8c) (Rogers, Friend, & Yeo, 2010). Finally, the drop rotation can also be used to spin 100 μm–10 mm thin SU-8 discs on which microfluidic channels, and chambers can be patterned, as a miniaturized counterpart to the Lab-on-a-CD (Madou et al., 2006) for centrifugal microfluidic operations; unlike the Lab-on-a-CD; however, the SAW miniaturized Lab-on-a-Disc (miniLOAD) platform does not require a laboratory bench-scale motor, as the SAW can be driven using a portable driver circuit (Fig. 3.7a), therefore constituting a completely handheld microfluidic platform (Fig. 3.9) (Glass, Shilton, Chan, Friend, & Yeo, 2012).

SAW streaming has been demonstrated for fluid actuation in PDMS channels placed atop the substrate (Masini et al., 2010), in channels ablated into the SAW substrate (Tan et al., 2009a), and even on paper (Rezk, Qi, Friend, Li, & Yeo, 2012b). In addition, it was also shown that the SAW can be used to deflect the interfaces of coflowing streams for directing emulsion droplets (Franke, Abate, Weitz, & Wixforth, 2009) and sorting cells (Franke, Braunmüller, Schmid, Wixforth, & Weitz, 2010). While the body of earlier work was carried out in open microchannels, which have severe limitations due to evaporation and possible contamination, recent work has focused on fluid actuation in a closed PDMS microchannel loop (Schmid, Wixforth, Weitz, & Franke, 2012) although the efficiency of the pump remained modest as a consequence of the strong absorption of the acoustic energy by the PDMS channel placed atop the SAW substrate. A way to circumvent this limitation was proposed by Langelier, Yeo, and Friend (2012), in which a glass superstrate housing the microchannel was directly bonded to the SAW substrate using UV epoxy; alternatively, an SU-8 glue layer can also be used (Johanssen et al., 2012). Importantly, it was shown that the SAW is retained at the interface between the substrate and superstrate. This is in contrast to previous uses of a superstrate, first proposed by Hodgson, Tan, Yeo, and Friend (2009), in which a fluid layer between the SAW substrate and the superstrate was employed to couple the acoustic energy into the latter, resulting in a Lamb wave on the superstrate. Nevertheless, it was shown that it is possible to achieve similar fluid actuation and particle manipulation on the superstrate through Lamb wave excitation, albeit at a cost of considerably lower efficiency. Regardless, the use of a superstrate remains attractive since the microfluidic operations can be carried out in conventional silicon-based materials, which are considerably cheaper, thus allowing the option of disposability. Bourquin, Reboud, Wilson, and Cooper (2010) later showed that it was possible to pattern periodic arrays of holes or posts in the

Actuation mechanisms for microfluidic biomedical devices 151

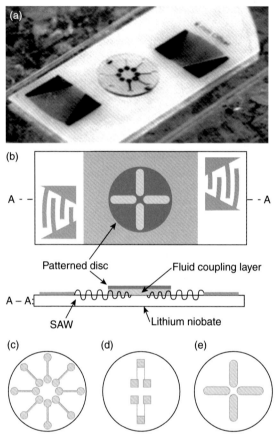

Figure 3.9 (a) Image and (b) schematic depiction of the miniLOAD platform comprising a 10 mm diameter SU-8 disc on which microchannels with a variety of designs ((c)–(e)) are fabricated to demonstrate capillary valving, micromixing, and particle concentration/separation on a miniaturized centrifugal platform. The disc rotation is driven by coupling an asymmetric pair of surface acoustic waves into the fluid underneath the disc.
Reprinted with permission from Glass et al. (2012). Copyright 2012, Wiley.

superstrate to form a phononic crystal lattice that acted as a bandgap to drive similar azimuthal recirculation to that discussed for a drop above, or to filter, scatter, reflect, or focus the Lamb wave. This was employed for the development of a biosensor platform for the concentration of beads labeled with antibodies onto surface sites for subsequent binding and fluorescent detection (Bourquin, Reboud, Wilson, Zhang, & Cooper, 2011).

At higher power, above 1 W, it is possible to drive sufficient interfacial deformation of a film or a drop to extrude fluid jets (Bhattacharjee, McDonnell, Prabhakar, Yeo, & Friend, 2011; Tan, Yeo, & Friend, 2009b) or to drive atomization (Qi, Yeo, & Friend, 2008). Given that a monodispersed distribution of 1–10 μm aerosol droplets can be formed in the latter without requiring nozzles or orifices, the latter is particularly useful for pulmonary drug delivery (Qi et al., 2009), especially the next generation of therapeutic agents such as DNA, peptides, and proteins, in a miniaturized portable platform for point-of-care therapeutics and personalized medicine. A significant advantage of the SAW pulmonary delivery platform over conventional nebulizers is the ability to preserve the viability of the drug, particularly shear-sensitive molecules such as DNA and peptides. In addition to drug delivery, the SAW atomization platform has been shown to be an efficient ionization source for microfluidic mass spectrometry interfacing (Heron, Wilson, Shaffer, Goodlett, & Cooper, 2010; Ho et al., 2011). The atomization of polymer solutions using the SAW is also a rapid technique for template-free polymer patterning for microarray applications (Alvarez, Friend, & Yeo, 2008a) as well as for synthesizing 100 nm dimension protein and polymer nanoparticles (Alvarez, Friend, & Yeo, 2008b; Friend, Yeo, Arifin, & Mechler, 2008) within which drugs can be encapsulated (Alvarez, Friend, & Yeo, 2009). This was more recently extended to synthesize nanocapsules of complementary polyelectrolyte layers for DNA encapsulation, as an example of tunable controlled release delivery (Qi et al., 2011).

3.4 Limitations and future trends

Microscale and nanoscale fluid actuation and particle manipulation comprises the underpinning technology which enables a revolutionary field that could potentially provide innovative solutions for chemical and biological applications by performing tasks much faster, cheaper, with considerably less reagent volume, and ideally more easily—tasks that include DNA amplification by polymerase chain reaction, chemical synthesis, proteomics, and point-of-care diagnostics, among others (Robinson & Dittrich, 2013). Yet, the primary limitation that besets this enabling technology is at present posing a severe bottleneck in the development of true integrated and miniaturized devices for these applications: the inability to scale down and incorporate compact and efficient fluid actuation and particle manipulation with the rest of the microfluidic operations on the chip device. While bench-scale capillary pumps and ancillary equipment such as amplifiers, signal generators, lasers, transducers, and motors are adequate in driving reasonably fast and efficient fluid actuation in a microfluidic chip for demonstrative purposes, such large and cumbersome components, and the difficulties of incorporating them on the chip, are impracticable when true portable functionality—the underlying motivation for adopting microfluidics in many applications—is desired.

Beyond miniaturization, another considerable challenge that has yet to be overcome is actuation efficiency. At present, the best fluidic actuation technologies that can be incorporated onto a chip, although not without their own challenges, are not comparable with their macroscopic counterparts in terms of efficiency. Electrokinetic and acoustic pumps, for example, have the ability to generate fast flow rates, but cannot match capillary pumps as far as the pressures that can be generated are concerned.

Particle and cell manipulation schemes have sorting efficiencies and throughputs that are well below those achievable with conventional fluorescent activated cell sorting (FACS) technology, often by over two to three orders of magnitude. Further, long-term reliability of microfluidic actuation technology has yet to be demonstrated. Another challenge that has yet to be widely addressed is chip automation and control—without which the device would be inoperable by an untrained user, thus defeating the goal of the "Lab on a Chip" for point-of-care use and rendering the device closer in concept to a "Chip-in-a-Lab."

With continued advances in the research and development in microscale fluid actuation, we nevertheless believe that these challenges can be overcome. It is our opinion, however, that the solution may not necessarily lie with a single technology, but rather by combining several complementary technologies such that the limitations of a particular technology may be overcome with the strengths of another. An example of such that has already been demonstrated is the combination of fast, long-range electroosmotic convection and precise, short-range trapping offered by DEP. We anticipate further technology combinations in the future, especially cross-platform technologies such as the integration of acoustofluidics and electrokinetics.

Nanoscale actuation is another exciting area in which we foresee further growth given the promise for nanofluidic platforms (Mukhopadhyay, 2006; Napoli, Eijkel, & Pennathur, 2010; Piruska, Gong, Sweedler, & Bohn, 2010), in particular for single molecule manipulation and sensing. Considerable work has been undertaken to date to elucidate mechanisms that govern nanoscale transport (Chang & Yossifon, 2009; Rauscher & Dietrich, 2008; Schoch, Han, & Renaud, 2008; Sparreboom, van den Berg, & Eijkel, 2009; Zhou, Perry, & Jacobson, 2011), and we anticipate their widespread translation into practical technology in the near future. Nanofluidic actuation, nevertheless, faces similar, if not more challenging, hurdles to those encountered by its microfluidic counterpart, most importantly in practical device integration, given the additional complication of dealing with the micro/nano interface.

References

Abi-Samra, K., Clime, L., Kong, L., Gorkin, R., III, Kim, T. H., Cho, Y. K., et al. (2011). Thermo-pneumatic pumping in centrifugal microfluidic. *Microfluidics and Nanofluidics, 11*, 643—652.

Ahmed, D., Mao, X., Juluri, B. K., & Huang, T. J. (2009a). A fast microfluidic mixer based on acoustically driven sidewall-trapped microbubble. *Microfluidics and Nanofluidics, 7*, 727—731.

Ahmed, D., Mao, X., Shi, J., Juluria, B. K., & Huang, T. J. (2009b). A millisecond micromixer via single-bubble-based acoustic streaming. *Lab on a Chip, 9*, 2738—2741.

Ajdari, A. (1995). Electro-osmosis on inhomogeneously charged surfaces. *Physical Review Letters, 75*, 755—758.

Ajdari, A. (2000). Pumping liquids using asymmetric electrode arrays. *Physical Review E - Statistical Physics, Plasmas, Fluids, and Related Interdisciplinary Topics, 61*, R45—R48.

Al-Halhoulia, A. T., Kilanib, M. I., & Büttgenb, S. (2010). Development of a novel electromagnetic pump for biomedical applications. *Sensors and Actuators, A: Physical, 162*, 172−176.

Alvarez, M., Friend, J. R., & Yeo, L. Y. (2008a). Surface vibration induced spatial ordering of periodic polymer patterns on a substrate. *Langmuir, 24*, 10629−10632.

Alvarez, M., Friend, J. R., & Yeo, L. Y. (2008b). Rapid generation of protein aerosols and nanoparticles via SAW atomisation. *Nanotechnology, 19*, 455103.

Alvarez, M., Friend, J. R., & Yeo, L. Y. (2009). Rapid production of protein loaded biodegradable microparticles using surface acoustic waves. *Biomicrofluidics, 3*, 014102.

Alzuaga, S., Manceau, J.-F., & Bastien, F. (2005). Motion of droplets on solid surface using acoustic radiation pressure. *Journal of Sound and Vibration, 282*, 151−162.

Bae, B., Han, J., Masel, R. I., & Shannon, M. A. (2007). A bidirectional electrostatic microvalve with microsecond switching performance. *Journal of Microelectromechanical Systems, 16*, 1461−1471.

Baroud, C. N., Vincent, M. R. S., & Delville, J.-P. (2007). An optical toolbox for total control of droplet microfluidics. *Lab on a Chip, 7*, 1029−1033.

Basu, A. S., & Gianchandani, Y. B. (2008). Virtual microfluidic traps, filters, channels and pumps using Marangoni flows. *Journal of Micromechanics and Microengineering, 18*, 115031.

Bau, H. H., Zhong, J., & Yi, M. (2001). A minute magneto hydro dynamic (MHD) mixer. *Sensors and Actuators B: Chemical, 79*, 205−213.

Benard, W. L., Kahn, H., Heuer, A. H., & Huff, M. A. (1998). Thin-film shape-memory alloy actuated micropumps. *Journal of Microelectromechanical Systems, 7*, 245−251.

Ben, Y., & Chang, H. C. (2005). Nonlinear electrokinetic devices. In M. Gad-el-Hak (Ed.), *The MEMS handbook*. Boca Raton: CRC Press.

Bhattacharjee, P. K., McDonnell, A. G., Prabhakar, R., Yeo, L. Y., & Friend, J. R. (2011). Extensional flow of low-viscosity fluids in capillary bridges formed by pulsed surface acoustic wave jetting. *New Journal of Physics, 13*, 023005.

Bourquin, Y., Reboud, J., Wilson, R., & Cooper, J. M. (2010). Tuneable surface acoustic waves for fluid and particle manipulations on disposable chips. *Lab on a Chip, 10*, 1898−1901.

Bourquin, Y., Reboud, J., Wilson, R., Zhang, Y., & Cooper, J. M. (2011). Integrated immunoassay using tuneable surface acoustic waves and lensfree detection. *Lab on a Chip, 11*, 2725−2730.

Brown, A. B. D., Smith, C. G., & Rennie, A. R. (2000). Pumping of water with ac electric fields applied to asymmetric pairs of microelectrodes. *Physical Review E - Statistical Physics, Plasmas, Fluids, and Related Interdisciplinary Topics, 63*, 016305.

Brunet, P., Baudoin, M., Matar, O. B., & Zoueshtiagh, F. (2010). Droplets displacement and oscillations induced by ultrasonic surface acoustic waves: A quantitative study. *Physical Review E - Statistical Physics, Plasmas, Fluids, and Related Interdisciplinary Topics, 81*, 036315.

Camp, J. P., & Capitano, A. T. (2005). Size-dependent mobile surface charge model of cell electrophoresis. *Biophysical Journal, 113*, 115−122.

Chang, H.-C., & Yeo, L. Y. (2010). *Electrokinetically driven microfluidics and nanofluidics*. New York: Cambridge University.

Chang, H.-C., & Yossifon, G. (2009). Understanding electrokinetics at the nanoscale: A perspective. *Biomicrofluidics, 3*, 012001.

Cheng, I.-F., Chang, H.-C., Hou, D., & Chang, H.-C. (2007). An integrated dielectrophoretic chip for continuous bioparticle filtering, focusing, sorting, trapping, and detecting. *Biomicrofluidics, 1*, 021503.

Chen, S. B., & Koch, D. L. (1996). Rheology of dilute suspensions of charged fibres. *Physics of Fluids, 8*, 2792−2807.

Chen, Z., Wang, P., & Chang, H.-C. (2005). An electro-osmotic micro-pump based on monolithic silica for micro-flow analyses and electro-sprays. *Analytical and Bioanalytical Chemistry, 382*, 817−824.

Chiou, P. Y., Ohta, A. T., & Wu, M. C. (2005). Massively parallel manipulation of single cells and microparticles using optical images. *Nature, 436*, 370−372.

Darhuber, A. A., & Troian, S. M. (2005). Principles of microfluidic actuation by modulation of surface stresses. *Annual Review of Fluid Mechanics, 37*, 425−455.

Debye, P., & Hückel, E. (1923). Zut Theorie der Electrolyte. II. Das Grenzgesetz für die elektrishe Leitfähigkeit. *Physikalische Zeitschrift, 24*, 305−325.

Delville, J. P., de Saint Vincent, M. R., Schroll, R. D., Chraibi, H., Issenmann, B., Wunenburger, R., et al. (2009). Laser microfluidics: Fluid actuation by light. *Journal of Optics, 11*, 034015.

Dholakia, K., MacDonald, M., & Spalding, G. (2002). Optical tweezers: The next generation. *Physics World, 15*, 31−35.

Dixit, S. S., Kim, H., Vasilyev, A., Eid, A., & Faris, G. W. (2010). Light driven formation and rupture of droplet bilayers. *Langmuir, 26*, 6193−6200.

Du, J.-R., Juang, Y.-J., Wu, J.-T., & Wei, H.-H. (2008). Long-range and superfast trapping of DNA molecules in an ac electrokinetic funnel. *Biomicrofluidics, 2*, 044103.

Eckart, C. (1948). Vortices and streams caused by sound waves. *Physical Review, 73*, 68−76.

Eijel, J. C. T., Dalton, C., Hayden, C. J., Burt, J. P. H., & Manz, A. (2003). A circular AC magnetohydrodynamic micropump for chromatographic applications. *Sensors and Actuators B: Chemical, 92*, 215−221.

Fainman, Y., Lee, L., Psaltis, D., & Yang, C. (2010). *Optofluidics: Fundamentals, devices, and applications*. New York: McGraw-Hill.

Footz, T., Somerville, M. J., Tomaszewski, R., Elyas, B., & Backhouse, C. J. (2004). Integration of combined heteroduplex/restriction fragment length polymorphism analysis on an electrophoresis microchip for the detection of hereditary haemochromatosis. *The Analyst, 129*, 25−31.

Fornell, A., Cushing, K., et al. (2017). Binary particle separation in droplet microfluidics using acoustophoresis. *Applied Physics Letters, 11*, 06412.

Franke, T., Abate, A. R., Weitz, D. A., & Wixforth, A. (2009). Surface acoustic wave (SAW) directed droplet flow in microfluidics for PDMS devices. *Lab on a Chip, 9*, 2625−2627.

Franke, T., Braunmüller, S., Schmid, L., Wixforth, A., & Weitz, D. A. (2010). Surface acoustic wave actuated cell sorting (SAWACS). *Lab on a Chip, 10*, 789−794.

Friend, J. R., & Yeo, L. Y. (2011). Microscale acoustofluidics: Microfluidics driven via acoustics and ultrasonics. *Reviews of Modern Physics, 83*, 647−704.

Friend, J. R., Yeo, L. Y., Arifin, D. R., & Mechler, A. (2008). Evaporative self-assembly assisted synthesis of polymer nanoparticles by surface acoustic wave atomization. *Nanotechnology, 19*, 145301.

Gagnon, Z., & Chang, H.-C. (2005). Aligning fast alternating current electroosmotic flow fields and characteristic frequencies with dielectrophoretic traps to achieve rapid bacteria detection. *Electrophoresis, 26*, 3725−3737.

Gagnon, Z., Senapati, S., Gordon, J., & Chang, H.-C. (2009). Dielectrophoretic detection and quantification of hybridized DNA molecules on nano-genetic particles. *Electrophoresis, 29*, 4808−4812.

Gervais, L., & Delamarche, E. (2009). Toward one-step point-of-care immunodiagnostics using capillary-driven microfluidics and PDMS substrates. *Lab on a Chip, 9*, 3330−3337.

Glass, N. R., Shilton, R. J., Chan, P. P. Y., Friend, J. R., & Yeo, L. Y. (2012). Miniaturized lab-on-a-disc (miniLOAD). *Small, 8*, 1881−1888.

González, A., Ramos, A., Green, N. G., Castellanos, A., & Morgan, H. (2000). Fluid flow induced by nonuniform ac electric fields in electrolytes on microelectrodes. II. A linear double-layer analysis. *Physical Review E - Statistical Physics, Plasmas, Fluids, and Related Interdisciplinary Topics, 61*, 4019−4028.

Gorkin, R., III, Clime, L., Madou, M., & Kido, H. (2010). Pneumatic pumping in centrifugal microfluidic platforms. *Microfluidics and Nanofluidics, 9*, 541−549.

Green, N. G., & Morgan, H. (1999). Dielectrophoresis of submicrometer latex spheres. 1. Experimental results. *The Journal of Physical Chemistry B, 103*, 41−50.

Grier, D. G. (1997). Optical tweezers in colloid and interface science. *Current Opinion in Colloid Interface Science, 2*, 264−270.

Grigoriev, R. O. (2005). Optical tweezers in colloid and interface science. *Physics of Fluids, 17*, 033601.

Grover, W. H., Ivester, R. H. C., Jensen, E. C., & Mathies, R. A. (2006). Development and multiplexed control of latching pneumatic valves using microfluidic logical structures. *Lab on a Chip, 6*, 623−631.

Harris, N. R., Hill, M., Townsend, R., White, N. M., & Beeby, S. P. (2005). Performance of a micro-engineered ultrasonic particle manipulator. *Sensors and Actuators B: Chemical, 111*, 481−486.

Hart, S. J., & Terray, A. V. (2003). Refractive-index-driven separation of colloidal polymer particles using optical chromatography. *Applied Physics Letters, 83*, 5316−5318.

Hart, S. J., Terray, A., Arnold, J., & Leski, T. A. (2007). Sample concentration using optical chromatography. *Optics Express, 15*, 2724−2731.

Hashmi, A., Yua, G., Reilly-Collette, M., Heiman, G., & Xu, J. (2012). Oscillating bubbles: A versatile tool for lab on a chip applications. *Lab on a Chip, 12*, 4216−4227. https://doi.org/10.1039/C2LC40424A

Hawkes, J. J., & Coakley, W. T. (2001). Force field particle filter, combining ultrasound standing waves and laminar flow. *Sensors and Actuators B: Chemical, 75*, 213−222.

Heron, S. R., Wilson, R., Shaffer, S. A., Goodlett, D. R., & Cooper, J. M. (2010). Surface acoustic wave nebulization of peptides as a microfluidic interface for mass spectrometry. *Analytical Chemistry, 82*, 3985−3989.

Herr, A. E., Molho, J. I., Santiago, J. G., Mungal, M. G., Kenny, T. W., & Garguilo, M. G. (2000). Electroosmotic capillary flow with nonuniform zeta potential. *Analytical Chemistry, 72*, 1053−1057.

Hodgson, R. P., Tan, M., Yeo, L. Y., & Friend, J. R. (2009). Transmitting high power RF acoustic radiation via fluid couplants into superstrates for microfluidics. *Applied Physics Letters, 94*, 024102.

Ho, J., Tan, M. K., Go, D., Yeo, L. Y., Friend, J. R., & Chang, H.-C. (2011). A paper-based microfluidic surface acoustic wave sample delivery and ionization source for rapid and sensitive ambient mass spectrometry. *Analytical Chemistry, 83*, 3260−3266.

Hunter, R. J. (1987). *Foundations of colloid science* (Vol. 1). Oxford: Oxford University.

Ichikawa, N., Hosokawa, K., & Maeda, R. (2004). Interface motion of capillary-driven flow in rectangular microchannel. *Journal of Colloid and Interface Science, 280*, 155−164.

Imasaka, T. (1998). Optical chromatography. A new tool for separation of particles, *Analusis 26*, 53−53. https://doi.org/10.1051/analusis:199826050053.

Jang, J., & Lee, S. S. (2000). Theoretical and experimental study of MHD (magnetohydrodynamic) micropump. *Sensors and Actuators, A: Physical, 80*, 84-85.

Jang, L. S., Li, Y. J., Lin, S. J., Hsu, Y. C., Yao, W. S., Tsai, M. C., et al. (2007). A stand-alone peristaltic micropump based on piezoelectric actuation. *Biomedical Microdevices, 9*, 185−194.

Jeong, O. K., & Yang, S. S. (2000). Fabrication and test of a thermopneumatic micropump with a corrugated p+ diaphragm. *Sensors and Actuators, A: Physical, 83*, 249−255.

Johansson, L., Enlund, J., Johansson, S., Katardjiev, I., Wiklund, M., & Yantchev, V. (2012). Surface acoustic wave-induced precise particle manipulation in a trapezoidal glass microfluidic channel. *Journal of Micromechanics and Microengineering, 22*, 025018.

Johnson, D. A., & Feke, D. L. (1995). Methodology for fractionating suspended particles using ultrasonic standing wave and divided flow fields. *Separations Technology, 5*, 251−258.

Kabata, A., Suzuki, H., Kishigami Y., & Haga, M. (2005). Micro system for injection of insulin and monitoring of glucose concentration. https://doi.org/10.1109/ICSENS.2005.1597663.

Kenyon, S. M., Meighan, M. M., & Haye, M. A. (2011). Recent developments in electrophoretic separations on microfluidic devices. *Electrophoresis, 32*, 482−493.

Khoo, M., & Liu, C., (2000). A novel micromachined magnetic membrane microfluidic pump. *Proceedings of the 22nd Annual EMBS International Conference,* July 23−28, Chiago, IL, pp. 2394−2397.

Kim, J.-H., Na, K.-H., Kang, C. J., & Kim, Y.-S. (2005). A disposable thermopneumatic-actuated micropump stacked with PDMS layers and ITO-coated glass. *Sensors and Actuators, A: Physical, 120*, 365−369.

Koch, M., Harris, N., Evans, A. G. R., White, N. M., & Brunnschweiler, A. (1998). A novel micromachined pump based on thick-film piezoelectric actuation. *Sensors and Actuators, A: Physical, 70*, 98−103.

Kulkarni, K. P., Friend, J. R., Yeo, L. Y., & Perlmutter, P. (2009). Surface acoustic waves as an energy source for drop scale synthetic chemistry. *Lab on a Chip, 9*, 754−755.

Kulkarni, K. P., Ramarathinam, S. H., Friend, J. R., Yeo, L. Y., Purcell, A. W., & Perlmutter, P. (2010). Rapid microscale in-gel processing and digestion of proteins using surface acoustic waves. *Lab on a Chip, 10*, 1518−1520.

Langelier, S. M., Yeo, L. Y., & Friend, J. R. (2012). UV epoxy bonding for enhanced SAW transmission and microscale acoustofluidic integration. *Lab on a Chip, 12*, 2970−2976.

Lastochkin, D., Zhou, R., Wang, P., Ben, Y., & Chang, H.-C. (2004). Electrokinetic micropump and micromixer design based on ac Faradaic polarisation. *Journal of Applied Physics, 96*, 1730−1733.

Laurell, T., Petersson, F., & Nilsson, A. (2007). Chip integrated strategies for acoustic separation and manipulation of cells and particles. *Chemical Society Reviews, 36*, 492−506.

Lazar, I. M., & Karger, B. L. (2002). Multiple open-channel electroosmotic pumping system for microfluidic sample handling. *Analytical Chemistry, 74*, 6259−6268.

Lemoff, A. V., & Lee, A. P. (2000). An AC magnetohydrodynamic micropump. *Sensors and Actuators B: Chemical, 63*, 178−185.

Li, H., Friend, J. R., & Yeo, L. Y. (2007a). A scaffold cell seeding method driven by surface acoustic waves. *Biomaterials, 28*, 4098−4104.

Li, H., Friend, J. R., & Yeo, L. Y. (2007b). Surface acoustic wave concentration of particle and bioparticle suspensions. *Biomedical Microdevices, 9*, 647–656.

Li, H., Friend, J. R., & Yeo, L. Y. (2008). Microfluidic colloidal island formation and erasure induced by surface acoustic wave radiation. *Physical Review Letters, 101*, 084502.

Li, Y., Fu, Y. Q., Brodie, S. D., Alghane, M., & Walton, A. J. (2012). Integrated microfluidics system using surface acoustic wave and electrowetting on dielectrics technology. *Biomicrofluidics, 6*, 012812.

Lighthill, J. (1978). Acoustic streaming. *Journal of Sound and Vibration, 61*, 391–418.

Lin, S. C., Mao, X., & Huang, T. J. (2012). Surface acoustic wave (SAW) acoustophoresis: Now and beyond. *Lab on a Chip, 12*, 2766–2770.

Lin, H., Storey, B. D., Oddy, M. H., Chen, C.-H., & Santiago, J. G. (2004). Instability of electrokinetic microchannel flows with conductivity gradients. *Physics of Fluids, 16*, 1922–1935.

Lin, H.-Y., Tsai, L.-C., Chi, P.-Y., & Chen, C.-D. (2005). Positioning of extended individual DNA molecules on electrodes by non-uniform AC electric fields. *Nanotechnology, 16*, 2738–2742.

Liu, Y., & Lim, K. M. (2011). Particle separation in microfluidics using a switching ultrasonic field. *Lab on a Chip, 11*, 3167–3173.

Luginbuhl, P., Collins, S. D., Racine, G., Gretillat, M. A., Rooij, N. F. D., Brooks, K. G., et al. (1997). Microfabricated lamb wave device based on PZT Sol–gel thin film for mechanical transport of solid particles and liquids. *Journal of Microelectromechanical Systems, 6*, 337–345.

Machauf, A., Nemirovsky, Y., & Dinnar, U. (2005). A membrane micropump electrostatically actuated across the working fluid. *Journal of Micromechanics and Microengineering, 15*, 2309–2316.

Madou, M., Zoval, J., Jia, G., Kido, H., Kim, J., & Kim, N. (2006). Lab on a CD. *Annual Review of Biomedical Engineering, 8*, 601–628.

Manneberg, O., Hagsäter, M. S., Svennebring, J., Hertz, H. M., Kutter, J. P., Bruus, H., et al. (2009). Spatial confinement of ultrasonic force fields in microfluidic channels. *Ultrasonics, 49*, 112–119.

Manor, O., Dentry, M., Friend, J. R., & Yeo, L. Y. (2011). Substrate dependent drop deformation and wetting under high frequency vibration. *Soft Matter, 7*, 7976–7979.

Manor, Yeo, L. Y., & Friend, J. R. (2012). The appearance of boundary layers and drift flows due to high-frequency surface waves. *Journal of Fluid Mechanics, 707*, 482–495.

Martinez, A. W., Phillips, S. T., & Whitesides, G. M. (2010). Diagnostics for the developing world: Microfluidic paper-based analytical devices. *Analytical Chemistry, 82*, 3–10.

Masini, L., Cecchini, M., Girardo, S., Cingolani, R., Pisignano, D., & Beltram, F. (2010). Surface-acoustic-wave counterflow micropumps for on-chip liquid motion control in two-dimensional microchannel arrays. *Lab on a Chip, 10*, 1997–2000.

Meagher, R. J., Won, J. I., McCormick, L. C., Nedelcu, S., Bertrand, M. M., Bertram, J. L., et al. (2005). End-labeled free-solution electrophoresis of DNA. *Electrophoresis, 26*, 331–350.

Menachery, A., Graham, D., Messerli, S. M., Pethig, R., & Smith, P. J. S. (2011). Dielectrophoretic tweezer for isolating and manipulating target cells. *IET Nanobiotechnology, 5*, 1–7.

Menachery, A., Graham, D., Messerli, S. M., Pethig, R., & Smith, P. J. S. (2011). Dielectrophoretic, tweezer for isolating and manipulating target cells. *IET Nanobiotechnology*.

Meng, L., Cai, F., Zhang, Z., Niu, L., Jin, Q., Yan, F., et al. (2011). Transportation of single cell and microbubbles by phase-shift introduced to standing leaky surface acoustic waves. *Biomicrofluidics, 5*, 044104.

Meng, A. H., Nguyen, N.-T., & White, R. M. (2000). Focused flow micropump using ultrasonic flexural plate waves. *Biomedical Microdevices, 2*, 169–174.

Minerick, A. R., Ostafin, A. E., & Chang, H.-C. (2002). Electrokinetic transport of red blood cells in microcapillaries. *Electrophoresis, 23*, 2165–2173.

Moroney, R. M., White, R. M., & Howe, R. T. (1991). Microtransport induced by ultrasonic Lamb waves. *Applied Physics Letters, 59*, 774–776.

Mugele, F., & Baret, J.-C. (2005). Electrowetting: From basics to applications. *Journal of Physics: Condensed Matter, 17*, R705–R774.

Mukhopadhyay, R. (2006). What does nanofluidics have to offer? *Analytical Chemistry, 78*, 7379–7382.

Nam, J., Lim, H., Kim, C., Kang, J. Y., & Shin, S. (2012). Density-dependent separation of encapsulated cells in a microfluidic channel by using a standing surface acoustic wave. *Biomicrofluidics, 6*, 024120.

Napoli, M., Eijkel, J. C., & Pennathur, S. (2010). Nanofluidic technology for biomolecule applications: A critical review. *Lab on a Chip, 10*, 957–985.

Natraj, V., & Chen, S. B. (2002). Primary electroviscous effect in a suspension of charged porous spheres. *Journal of Colloid and Interface Science, 251*, 200–207.

Neale, S. L., Macdonald, M. P., Dholakia, K., & Krauss, T. F. (2005). All-optical control of microfluidic components using form birefringence. *Nature Materials, 4*, 53–533.

Ng, W. Y., Lam, Y. C., & Rodríguez, I. (2009). Experimental verification of Faradaic charging in ac electrokinetics. *Biomicrofluidics, 3*, 022405.

Noblin, X., Buguin, A., & Brochard-Wyart, F. (2004). Vibrated sessile drops: Transition between pinned and mobile contact line oscillations. *European Physical Journal E, 14*, 395–404.

Nyborg, W. L. (1958). Acoustic streaming near a boundary. *Journal of the Acoustical Society of America, 30*, 329–339.

Ohl, C.-D., Arora, M., Ikink, R., Jong, N. D., Versluis, M., Delius, M., et al. (2006). Sonoporation from jetting cavitation bubbles. *Biophysical Journal, 91*, 4285–4295.

Orloff, N. D., Dennis, J. R., Cecchini, M., Schonbrun, E., Rocas, E., Wang, Y., et al. (2011). Manipulating particle trajectories with phase-control in surface acoustic wave microfluidics. *Biomicrofluidics, 5*, 044107.

Paegel, B. M., Emrich, C. A., Wedemayer, G. J., Scherer, J. R., & Mathies, R. A. (2002). High throughput DNA sequencing with a microfabricated 96-lane capillary array electrophoresis bioprocessor. *Proceedings of the National Academy of Sciences of the United States of America, 99*, 574–579.

Pan, Y.-J., Ren, C.-M., & Yang, R.-J. (2007). Electrokinetic flow focusing and valveless switching integrated with electrokinetic instability for mixing enhancement. *Journal of Micromechanics and Microengineering, 17*, 820–827.

Park, K., Park, J., Jung, J. H., et al. (2017). In-droplet microparticle separation using travelling surface acoustic wave. *Biomicrofluidics, 11*, 06412.

Patel, M. V., Tovar, A. R., & Lee, A. P. (2012). Lateral cavity acoustic transducer as an on-chip cell/particle microfluidic switch. *Lab on a Chip, 12*, 139–145.

Petersson, F., Nilsson, A., Holm, C., Jönsson, H., & Laurell, T. (2004). Separation of lipids from blood utilizing ultrasonic standing waves in microfluidic channels. *The Analyst, 129*, 938–943.

Pethig, R. (2010). Dielectrophoresis: Status of the theory, technology, and applications. *Biomicrofluidics, 4*, 022811.

Petsev, D. N. (2010). Transport in fluidic nanochannels. *Surfactant Science Series, 147*, 221−247.

Piruska, A., Gong, M., Sweedler, J. V., & Bohn, P. W. (2010). Nanofluidics in chemical analysis. *Chemical Society Reviews, 39*, 1060−1072.

Pol, F. C. M., Lintel, H. T. G., Elwenspoek, M., & Fluitman, J. H. J. (1990). A thermopneumatic micropump based on micro-engineering techniques. *Sensors and Actuators, A: Physical, 21*, 198−202.

Qiao, R., & Aluru, N. R. (2003). Ion concentrations and velocity profiles in nanochannel electroosmotic flows. *The Journal of Chemical Physics, 118*, 4692−4701.

Qi, A., Chan, P., Ho, J., Rajapaksa, A., Friend, J. R., & Yeo, L. Y. (2011). Template-free synthesis and encapsulation technique for layer-by-layer polymer nanocarrier fabrication. *ACS Nano, 5*, 9583−9591.

Qi, A., Friend, J. R., Yeo, L. Y., Morton, D. A., McIntosh, M. P., & Spiccia, L. (2009). Miniature inhalation therapy platform using surface acoustic wave microfluidic atomization. *Lab on a Chip, 9*, 2184−2193.

Qi, A., Yeo, L. Y., & Friend, J. R. (2008). Interfacial destabilization and atomization driven by surface acoustic waves. *Physics of Fluids, 20*, 074103.

Qi, A., Yeo, L. Y., Friend, J. R., & Ho, J. (2010). The extraction of liquid, protein molecules and yeast cells from paper through surface acoustic wave atomization. *Lab on a Chip, 10*, 470−476.

Ramos, A., González, A., Castellanos, A., Green, N. G., & Morgan, H. (2003). Pumping of liquids with ac voltages applied to asymmetric pairs of microelectrodes. *Physical Review E - Statistical Physics, Plasmas, Fluids, and Related Interdisciplinary Topics, 67*, 0563.

Ramos, & Morgan. (2016). AC electrokinetics of conducting microparticles: A review. *Current Opinion in Colloid & Interface Science, 24*, 79−90.

Rauscher, M., & Dietrich, S. (2008). Wetting phenomena in nanofluidics. *Annual Review of Materials Research, 38*, 143−172.

Rayleigh, L. (1884). On the circulation of air observed in Kundt's tubes and on some allied acoustical problems. *Philosophical Transactions of the Royal Society of London, 175*, 1−21.

Renaudin, A., Tabourier, P., Zhang, V., Camart, J. C., & Druon, C. (2006). SAW nanopump for handling droplets in view of biological applications. *Sensors and Actuators B: Chemical, 113*, 389−397.

Rezk, A. R., Manor, O., Friend, J. R., & Yeo, L. Y. (2012a). Acoustowetting: Film spreading, fingering instabilities and soliton-like wave propagation. *Nature Communications, 3*, 1167.

Rezk, A. R., Qi, A., Friend, J. R., Li, W. H., & Yeo, L. Y. (2012b). Uniform mixing in paper-based microfluidic systems using surface acoustic waves. *Lab on a Chip, 12*, 773−779.

Robinson, T., & Dittrich, P. S. (2013). Microfluidic technology for molecular diagnostics. *Advances in Biochemical Engineering, 133*, 89−114. https://doi.org/10.1007/10_2012_139

Rogers, P. R., Friend, J. R., & Yeo, L. Y. (2010). Exploitation of surface acoustic waves to drive size-dependent microparticle concentration within a droplet. *Lab on a Chip, 10*, 2979−2985.

Schabmueller, C. G. J., Koch, M., Mokhtari, M. E., Evans, A. G. R., Brunnschweiler, A., & Sehr, H. (2002). Self-aligning gas/liquid micropump. *Journal of Micromechanics and Microengineering, 12*, 420−424.

Schlichting, H. (1932). Calculation of even periodic barrier currents. *Physikalische Zeitschrift, 33*, 327−335.

Schmid, L., Wixforth, A., Weitz, D. A., & Franke, T. (2012). Novel surface acoustic wave (SAW)-driven closed PDMS flow chamber. *Microfluidics and Nanofluidics, 12*, 229−235.

Schneider, S. W., Nuschele, S., Wixforth, A., Gorzelanny, C., Alexander-Katz, A., Netz, R. R., et al. (2007). Shear-induced unfolding triggers adhesion of von Willebrand factor fibers. *Proceedings of the National Academy of Sciences of the United States of America, 104*, 7899−7903.

Schoch, R. B., Han, J., & Renaud, P. (2008). Transport phenomena in nanofluidics. *Reviews of Modern Physics, 80*, 839−883.

Shi, J., Ahmed, D., Mao, X., Lin, S. C. S., Lawit, A., & Huang, T. J. (2009). Acoustic tweezers: Patterning cells and microparticles using standing surface acoustic waves (SSAW). *Lab on a Chip, 9*, 2890−2895.

Shilton, R., Tan, M. K., Yeo, L. Y., & Friend, J. R. (2008). Particle concentration and mixing in microdrops driven by focused surface acoustic waves. *Journal of Applied Physics, 104*, 014910.

Shilton, R. J., Yeo, L. Y., & Friend, J. R. (2011). Quantification of surface acoustic wave induced chaotic mixing-flows in microfluidic wells. *Sensors and Actuators B: Chemical, 160*, 1565−1572.

Shi, J., Mao, X., Ahmed, D., Colletti, A., & Huang, T. J. (2008). Focusing microparticles in a microfluidic channel with standing surface acoustic waves (SSAW). *Lab on a Chip, 8*, 221−223.

Shubin, V. E., Hunter, R. J., & O'Brien, R. W. (1993). Electroacoustic and dielectric study of surface conduction. *Journal of Colloid and Interface Science, 159*, 174−183.

Sparreboom, W., van den Berg, A., & Eijkel, J. C. T. (2009). Principles and applications of nanofluidic transport. *Nature Nanotechnology, 4*, 713−720.

Squires, T. M., & Bazant, M. A. (2004). Induced-charge electro-osmosis. *Journal of Fluid Mechanics, 509*, 217−252.

Squires, T. M., & Quake, S. R. (2005). Microfluidics: Fluid physics at the nanoliter scale. *Reviews of Modern Physics, 77*, 977−1026.

Stern, O. (1924). The theory of electrical double layer. *Zeitschrift fuer Elektrochemie, 30*, 508−516.

Suzuki, H., & Yoneyama, R. (2002). A reversible electrochemical nanosyringe pump and some considerations to realize low power consumption. *Sensors and Actuators, A: Chemical, 86*, 242−250.

Szántai, E., & Guttman, A. (2006). Genotyping with microfluidic devices. *Electrophoresis, 27*, 4896−4903.

Takamura, Y., Onoda, H., Inokuchi, H., Adachi, S., Oki, A., & Horiike, Y. (2003). Low-voltage electroosmosis pump for stand-alone microfluidics devices. *Electrophoresis, 24*, 185−192.

Tan, M. K., Friend, J. R., & Yeo, L. Y. (2007). Microparticle collection and concentration via a miniature surface acoustic wave device. *Lab on a Chip, 7*, 618−625.

Tan, M. K., Yeo, L. Y., & Friend, J. R. (2009a). Rapid fluid flow and mixing induced in microchannels using surface acoustic waves. *Europhysics Letters, 87*, 47003.

Tan, M. K., Yeo, L. Y., & Friend, J. R. (2009b). Interfacial jetting phenomena induced by focused surface vibrations. *Physical Review Letters, 103*, 024501.

Tan, M. K., Yeo, L. Y., & Friend, J. R. (2010). Unique flow transitions and particle collection switching phenomena in a microchannel induced by surface acoustic waves. *Applied Physics Letters, 97*, 234106.

Tovar, A. R., & Lee, A. P. (2009). Lateral cavity acoustic transducer. *Lab on a Chip, 9*, 41−43.

Vyawahare, S., Sitaula, S., Martin, S., Adalianb, D., & Scherer, A. (2008). Electronic control of elastomeric microfluidic circuits with shape memory actuators. *Lab on a Chip, 8,* 1530−1535.

Wang, P., Chen, Z., & Chang, H.-C. (2006). A new electro-osmotic pump based on silica monoliths. *Sensors and Actuators B: Chemical, 113,* 500−509.

Wang, C., Jalikop, S. V., & Hilgenfeldt, S. (2012). Efficient manipulation of microparticles in bubble streaming flows. *Biomicrofluidics, 6,* 012801.

Wang, X., Wang, S., Gendhar, B., Cheng, C., Byun, C. K., Li, G., et al. (2009). Electroosmotic pumps for microflow analysis. *Trends in Analytical Chemistry, 28,* 64−74.

Wheeler, A. R. (2008). Putting electrowetting to work. *Science, 322,* 539−540.

Wixforth, A., Strobl, C., Gauer, C. H., Toegl, A., Scriba, J., & Guttenberg, Z. V. (2004). Acoustic manipulation of small droplets. *Analytical and Bioanalytical Chemistry, 379,* 982−991.

Wu, D., Qin, J., & Lin, B. (2008). Electrophoretic separations on microfluidic chips. *Journal of Chromatography A, 1184,* 542−559.

Xu, D., Wang, L., Ding, G., Zhou, Y., Yu, A., & Cai, B. (2001). Characteristics and fabrication of NiTi/Si diaphragm micropump. *Sensors and Actuators, A: Physical, 93,* 87−92.

Yaralioglu, G. G., Wygant, I. O., Marentis, T. C., & Khuri-Yakub, B. T. (2004). Ultrasonic mixing in microfluidic channels using integrated transducers. *Analytical Chemistry, 76,* 3694−3698.

Yeo, L. Y., & Chang, H.-C. (2005). Static and spontaneous electrowetting. *Modern Physics Letters B, 19,* 549−569.

Yeo, L. Y., Chang, H.-C., Chan, P. P. Y., & Friend, J. R. (2011). Microfluidic devices for bioapplications. *Small, 7,* 12−48.

Yeo, L. Y., & Friend, J. R. (2009). Ultrafast microfluidics using surface acoustic waves. *Biomicrofluidics, 3,* 012002.

Yin, Z., & Prosperetti, A. (2005). A microfluidic 'blinking bubble' pump. *Journal of Micromechanics and Microengineering, 15,* 643−651.

Yoshimi, Y., Shinoda, K., Mishima, M., Nakao, K., & Munekane, K. (2004). Development of an artificial synapse using an electrochemical micropump. *Journal of Artificial Organs, 7,* 210−215.

Zengerle, R., Richter A. et al. (1992) Conference: MicroElectroMechanical Systems, MEMS '92, Proceedings. An Investigation of Micro Structures, Sensors, Actuators, Machines and Robot. IEEE.

Zhou, Y., & Amirouche, F. (2011). An electromagnetically-actuated all-PDMS valveless micropump for drug delivery. *Micromachines, 2,* 345−355.

Zhou, K., Perry, J. M., & Jacobson, S. C. (2011). Transport and sensing in nanofluidic devices. *Annual Review of Analytical Chemistry, 4,* 321−341.

Droplet microfluidics for biomedical devices

Marie Hébert, Carolyn L. Ren
Mechanical and Mechatronics Engineering, University of Waterloo, Waterloo, Ontario, Canada

Reading questions

1. Why does droplet microfluidics work?
2. How can the necessary manipulations be achieved?
3. What do microfluidic devices contribute to biomedical applications?

4.1 Introduction—droplets in the wider context of microfluidics

The early development of microfluidic technologies aimed to take advantage of the smaller dimension to achieve short reaction times as well as to lower reagent consumption and cost (Manz, Graber, & Widmer, 1990). The early microfluidic devices initially included a single fluid phase and were presented as the precursors of micro total analysis systems (μTAS). The promise of achieving complex laboratory procedures on an integrated miniaturized device led to the advancement of microfluidics as a field. However, challenges encountered dissuaded researchers that single-phase microfluidic devices could indeed achieve the envisioned global impact of μTAS. Firstly, the parabolic flow profile led to significant sample dispersion. Secondly, mixing was mainly dictated by diffusion rather than convection, and thus, was prohibitively slow. Finally, the cross-contamination between samples in combination with the other two drawbacks spurred the community toward the development of droplet microfluidics.

The introduction of a second immiscible fluid within the system—the continuous phase—isolates the sample—the dispersed phase—in short segments aptly referred to as droplets. The main advantages of the smaller dimension (short reaction time, low reagent consumption, low cost) are preserved while the main issues associated with single-phase flow are avoided. Droplet microfluidics provides compartmentalization with the continuous phase confining each droplet; additionally, there is a strong potential for increased throughput while maintaining uniformity. The capabilities of droplet microfluidics led to the advancement of this new subfield within microfluidics. The studies can generally be categorized as either fundamentals-focused or application-focused. For the latter, one or multiple droplet manipulations are at the core of every application; manipulations include droplet generation, splitting, merging, mixing, incubation, and sorting.

Microfluidic Devices for Biomedical Applications. https://doi.org/10.1016/B978-0-12-819971-8.00001-9
Copyright © 2021 Elsevier Ltd. All rights reserved.

Droplet microfluidics has grown substantially within the microfluidic community because of its advantageous trade-off comparatively to single-phase microfluidics. The numerous application-focused studies range across variety of fields including but not limited to material synthesis (Hua, Du, Song, Sun, & He, 2019), single-cell analysis (Wen et al., 2016), water quality assessment (Lee, Thio, Park, & Bae, 2019), and drug discovery (Kulesa, Kehe, Hurtado, Tawde, & Blainey, 2018). Although some key disadvantages are addressed, other obstacles are introduced. Certain drawbacks of droplet microfluidics limit its adoption as an enabling technology by end-users outside of the developers' field. The barrier to entry of droplet microfluidics must provide a worthwhile trade-off to end-users; however, currently, the following challenges are typically deemed too important for end-users to adopt droplet microfluidics as a tool.

- Manufacturing tolerances challenge the microfluidic chip operation both for single-phase and droplet microfluidic devices.
- The microfluidic chip performance requires pristine wetting conditions.
- Device operation requires a thorough understanding of microfluidic principles to properly operate.
- Different users can obtain variable results because the repeatability is influenced by operational skills such as those related to surface treatment of microfluidic chips and priming of the chip with oil.
- The necessary peripheral equipment to the microfluidic chip itself (microscope, pressure pump, microfabrication facilities) is costly.
- The design process is iterative, and, thus, time- and resource-consuming due to manufacturing and operation uncertainties in addition to the coupled fluid dynamics. The integration of multiple droplet manipulations in series is especially challenging.
- Small changes such as droplet size require a reassessment of the design by knowledgeable users because the channels are coupled and the changes in droplet size, spacing, and frequency would influence the hydrodynamic resistance and, thus, other droplet manipulations accordingly.
- If required, the surfactant must match both the continuous and dispersed phases, and the associated dynamics add another layer of complexity to the experiments as well as an added cost.

Nevertheless, researchers within the droplet microfluidic field developed solutions and continue to innovate to circumvent these disadvantages. Droplet microfluidic technologies are promising and have high potential as enabling tools. A main area of interest is biomedical applications. This book chapter will summarize the key concepts of droplets microfluidics to understand not only its potential, but also its limitations. The main approaches to perform droplet manipulations are categorized according to their working principle as either passive or active methods. In order to assess the impact of droplet microfluidic within the biomedical application field, an overview of the different categories of applications is presented. The scope of this chapter is not meant to be comprehensive, but rather to give an introductory overview to the field of droplet microfluidics with a particular emphasis on biomedical applications. This chapter aims to address the following questions: Why does droplet microfluidics work? How can the necessary manipulations be achieved? What do microfluidic devices contribute to biomedical applications?

4.2 Fundamental principles of droplet microfluidics

Our working definition of *droplet microfluidics* refers specifically to devices with characteristic length about ~ 50−500 μm that require two immiscible liquid phases for operation. Some notable exclusions from this definition are digital microfluidic devices as well as liquid−gas flow. The fundamentals underlying the operation of droplet microfluidic devices will first be explored from the perspective of the physical principles. Then, the advantages and disadvantages previously introduced will be elaborated upon and justified in relation to the underlying fundamental principles.

4.2.1 Droplet flow in microchannels
4.2.1.1 Dimensionless numbers

The analysis of fluid flow is facilitated by dimensionless numbers; the combination of meaningful variables such that the obtained quantity is dimensionless provides information about the flow as summarized in Table 4.1. The small characteristic length associated with microchannels indicates that some forces are negligible compared to interfacial tension and viscous forces. The flow conditions are, thus, meaningfully

Table 4.1 Dimensionless number definition and relative importance (Kumacheva & Garstecki, 2011).

Dimensionless number	Qualitative description	Quantitative description[a]		Relative importance
Capillary	viscous / interfacial	$Ca = \frac{\mu U}{\gamma}$	$\propto 1^0$	1st (most important)
Reynolds	inertia / viscous	$Re = \frac{\rho U l}{\mu}$	$\propto 1^1$	2nd
Weber	inertia / interfacial	$We = \frac{\rho U^2 l}{\gamma}$	$\propto 1^1$	2nd
Bond	gravitational / interfacial	$Bo = \frac{l^2(\rho_1 - \rho_2)g}{\gamma}$	$\propto 1^2$	3rd
Grashoff	buoyancy / viscous	$Gr = \frac{l^3 \rho^2 \beta \Delta T}{\mu^2}$	$\propto 1^3$	4th (least important)

[a]where $\propto$ is the symbol for "proportional to," μ is dynamic viscosity [Pa.s], U is characteristic velocity [m/s], γ is interfacial tension [N/m], ρ is density [kg/m³], l is characteristic length [m], g is the gravitational acceleration [m/s²], β is coefficient of thermal expansion [1/K], ΔT is temperature difference [K].

characterized using the Capillary (Ca). The Reynolds (Re) number is used to characterize flow as laminar, turbulent, or somewhere in between in the transition regime. Although the Reynolds number depends on density, velocity, and viscosity, the characteristic length in the nominator signifies a laminar regime for microflow (Re $\ll$ 1). Other typical dimensionless numbers such as the Weber, Bond, and Grashoff numbers are insignificantly small due to their dependence on the characteristic length. The very small dimensionless numbers justify neglecting certain forces that are relatively much less impactful such as inertia and gravity.

The introduction of the second immiscible phase that transitioned single-phase microfluidics toward droplet microfluidics introduces the important physics of interfacial tension, and hence, the importance of the Capillary number in characterizing microflow conditions. The interfacial tension between the two fluids is primordial in maintaining their immiscibility but also plays an important role in the shape of the droplet. The flow rate is the variable used during experiments to modulate the Capillary number because the viscosity and interfacial tension are fixed by the choice of the two fluids.

4.2.1.2 Flow patterns

The flow profile of an enclosed single phase follows a parabolic profile. Although the shape is simple, the parabolic shape is the source of the undesirably increased sample dispersion. More thorough information is available from the literature about the dispersion phenomena referred to as "Taylor dispersion" (Beard, 2001). For droplets, the fluid flow involves two immiscible fluids. The flow patterns are much more complex than a parabola (Wong, Radke, & Morris, 1995a, 1995b). Nonetheless, high-level phenomena such as the thin film, the gutter region, and the vortices patterns are accessible without requiring to understand the complex equations.

Droplet flow is classified in different regimes: jetting, squeezing, and leaking (Korczyk et al., 2019). When in the squeezing regime, the droplet occupies most of the space in the cross-sectional direction; there is nonetheless a thin film isolating the droplet from the wall. The continuous phase fully surrounds the droplet on all sides because of its preferable wetting of the walls (this will be further discussed subsequently with surface wetting conditions). The complete isolation of the sample is an important advantage of droplet microfluidics.

Circular cross-section channels such as copper capillaries exhibit a uniform thin film around its perimeter. Oppositely, rectangular cross-sections—typically obtained when manufacturing devices using soft lithography or 3D printing techniques—exhibit a different profile around the droplet. The interface cannot conform closely to the cross-section shape due to the sharp corners. Consequently, the so-called gutter region in the corners is filled by the continuous phase (Baroud, Gallaire, & Dangla, 2010). The complex flow of the continuous phase with respect to the thin film and gutter region results in a mismatch between the velocity of the continuous phase and the velocity of the droplet. This mismatch is quantified by the slip factor and depends on different parameters such as the Capillary number, the droplet length-to-width ratio, and the viscosity contrast between the continuous and dispersed phases (Jakiela, Makulska, Korczyk, & Garstecki, 2011).

The ratio of viscosity between the dispersed and continuous phases affects the vortex patterns. In a straight microchannel, the flow pattern within and outside of the droplet follows a symmetric axis along the direction of travel (Baroud et al., 2010). Each half rotates within its droplet hemisphere. The convective mixing inside each vortex is rapid. However, the symmetry of the laminar flow pattern signifies that no convective mixing occurs across each half; diffusion governs the mixing between the two vortices and is correspondingly slower than desired. Various strategies will be explored in more detail in the manipulation section, but they primarily rely on breaking the symmetry to provide convective mixing between the two halves and to overcome diffusive mixing timescales.

4.2.1.3 Independent variables for experiments

Fundamental studies investigate changes in variables to better understand the flow, while for application studies, the tuning of these variables achieves the desired manipulations. Common variables that are adjusted are the flow rate ratio between different channels, viscosity contrast, and channel resistance. The flow rate ratio (generally ϕ) is adjusted while operating the microfluidic device and is primordial to generating the desired droplet size. The viscosity contrast affects the vortex patterns and correspondingly, the slip factor. Channel resistance can be used to decouple certain regions by decreasing the relative impact of the in and out motion of single droplets (Glawdel & Ren, 2012).

The choice of the two fluids is important for the experiments. The dispersed phase contains the sample, and hence, is specifically related to the study; an aqueous solution is typically used. For the continuous phase, a wide range of oils has been used for the numerous microfluidic studies with different trade-offs for each of them: silicone oil (5 cst, 10 cst, ..., 100 cst), mineral oil (light and heavy), FC-40, HFE-7500, and many more.

The flow conditions are commonly summarized using the Capillary number (the independent variable) while observing and quantifying changes in behavior (the targeted dependent variable).

4.2.1.4 Interfacial tension and surfactants

Surfactants are chemicals that modify the interfacial tension between the continuous and dispersed phases. The specialized chemical needs to match the chemistry of the continuous and dispersed phase to be effective.

The additional dynamics introduced by incorporating surfactant in the system can be challenging to understand and to adjust its concentration for the desired behavior (Baret, Kleinschmidt, El Harrak, & Griffiths, 2009; Wang, Lu, Xu, & Luo, 2009). However, the main two advantages of using a surfactant are long-term droplet stabilization and proper surface wetting; the cost and complexity are justified when the advantages are critical. By reducing the interfacial tension, the surfactant limits droplet merging that is especially important when incubating droplets for a long time in reservoirs for instance.

4.2.1.5 Surface wetting conditions

The stability of the operation of droplet microfluidic devices relies heavily on wetting conditions. The continuous phase must preferably wet the channel walls such that the dispersed phase is fully surrounded by the continuous phase. Correspondingly, the thin film and gutter region encloses and isolates each droplet containing the dispersed phase. Inadequate surface wetting conditions compromise the integrity of the droplet leading to potential cross-contamination through wall contact as well as the undesirable dynamics introduced within the flow when droplets adhere to the walls. The wetting conditions must also be maintained throughout the experiments.

The preferable wetting of the walls by the continuous phase is dictated by the three-way interfacial tension relationship between the continuous phase, the dispersed phase, and the solid substrate (Kumacheva & Garstecki, 2011). Considering aqueous droplets, the interfacial tension between the dispersed phase and the solid must be larger than between the solid and the continuous phase as well as between the dispersed and continuous phases.

Polydimethylsiloxane (PDMS) is a ubiquitous material used to fabricate microfluidic devices (Qin, Xia, & Whitesides, 2010). The surface properties—either hydrophobic or hydrophilic—are adjusted through the fabrication procedure (Choi, Lee, & Weitz, 2018; Hwang, Choi, & Lee, 2012). For example, after bonding using plasma treatment, quickly exposing the microchannels to water results in a hydrophilic chip. Oppositely, baking the chip for a long time will produce hydrophobic walls. However, the dual nature of surface properties of PDMS can be treacherous due to the potential instability of its surface properties.

Certain combinations of continuous and dispersed phases such as fluorocarbonated oil (FC-40) and aqueous samples require surfactant to sufficiently lower the interfacial tension such that FC-40 preferably wets the wall. As previously explained, surfactants introduce an added cost and complexity. But in the case of FC-40, the permeability to oxygen of the oil is crucial for studies involving cells. Thus, the trade-off is nevertheless advantageous.

4.2.2 Comparison and contrast of single-phase and droplet microfluidics

The fundamental principles of droplet flow in microchannels allow to better understand and elaborate upon the advantages and disadvantages of droplet microfluidics, more specifically compared to single-phase microfluidics.

The research at the early stages of microfluidics involved a single-phase, typically an aqueous solution to process. Although the advantages of the microfluidic devices proved to be significant enough to motivate the emergence of the field, the drawbacks eventually led to the onset of droplet microfluidics. Droplet microfluidic devices have potential as an enabling technology for numerous applications in a variety of fields such as biomedical assays, water treatment, material synthesis, and many more. New challenges are nevertheless introduced by the addition of the second fluid.

4.2.2.1 General advantages of microfluidic flow

Both single-phase and multiphase microfluidic devices provide key advantages that motivated the development of the technology at its early stage, and that continues to this day to stimulate further research in the now mature microfluidic field. The main advantages are low reagent consumption, short reaction time, and low cost.

By definition, microfluidics involves a characteristic length on the order of micrometers. Therefore, the volume consumed for each reaction is typically on the order of nanolitres (10^{-9} L) while pipettes can handle volumes on the order of microliters (10^{-6} L). Consequently, microfluidic devices innately consume less reagent per reaction. Moreover, the reaction time is shortened compared to larger volume (Zhao, He, Qiao, & Middelberg, 2011); the reactions at the microscale benefit from a much larger surface-to-volume ratio. The cost savings associated with microfluidic devices come from multiple sources. Saving reagent is particularly impactful financially when using high-cost chemicals involved in drug screening assays, for example. Shorter assays lead to cost savings as the objective is achieved faster. Finally, the apparatus, as well as the microfluidic chip itself, has a high potential for cost savings.

Furthermore, the small characteristic length is at the core of the fundamental principles of microflow that provide unique behavior. By controlling the flow appropriately, the application of microfluidic flow to many fields is possible.

4.2.2.2 Disadvantages of single-phase microfluidics

Although single-phase microfluidics provides low reagent consumption, short reaction time, and lower cost, obstacles related to the nature of single-phase flow slowed down the development of microfluidics as an enabling technology. The main drawbacks that affect single-phase flow are sample cross-contamination, dispersion, and slow mixing.

For single-phase flow, the fluid within the microfluidic device is in contact with the walls. A ubiquitous material used for devices is PDMS that is well known to be porous (Wang, Douville, Takayama, & ElSayed, 2012). Consequently, cross-contamination from wall contact can easily occur and is problematic. Dispersion issues arise from the parabolic flow profile of single-phase flow in microchannels. Taylor dispersion increases the diffusion of the solute sample through the buffer (Beard, 2001). This problem is significant for electrophoresis that targets specific separation peaks for subsequent analysis; the dispersion deteriorates the separation. The laminar nature of microflow is directly related to the small characteristic length. Although the micrometer scale provides key advantages, slow mixing is an important disadvantage when short reaction times are required. Reactions involving more than one reagent requires thorough mixing of the samples. The laminar nature of the flow limits convective mixing; rather, diffusive mixing dominates. Longer mixing delays limit the benefits from the shorter reaction time. Nevertheless, the laminar nature of single-phase flow can be positively used for hydrodynamic focusing for example.

4.2.2.3 Advantages of droplet microfluidics

The disadvantages associated with single-phase microfluidics drove the field toward droplet microfluidics. The aim was to retain the advantages of microfluidic flow while circumventing the disadvantages associated with single-phase flow. The introduction of another immiscible phase into the system in combination with the appropriate surface properties encapsulates the dispersed phase within the continuous phase. The continuous phase fully surrounds the droplets with a thin film separating the droplet from the wall. The compartmentalization avoids any potential of cross-contamination because the continuous phase is the only fluid in contact with the wall at all times while the samples are contained within the droplets.

Although convective mixing dominates within each half of the droplet (see the flow patterns subsection for further details), the symmetry of the vortex pattern is detrimental to the thorough mixing within the droplet. Strategies to break the symmetry of the vortices must be implemented to enhance mixing and take full advantage of the short reaction times.

Furthermore, the generation of droplets of uniform size at a high rate ensures uniformity and increased throughput. The samples are contained within the droplets and do not disperse.

4.2.2.4 Disadvantages of droplet microfluidics

Although droplet microfluidics provides key advantages that transformed and advanced the microfluidic field, the adoption of droplet technologies outside of the developers' field is limited. The end-users face barriers and challenges that are deemed too extensive to adopt microfluidics as a tool.

End-users require a thorough understanding of droplet microfluidics to operate properly the devices. The operation is further complicated by the manufacturing and operational uncertainties. These uncertainties lead to a lack of robustness between different users irrespective of their skill level. The operation process is challenging even after going through the time- and resource-consuming iterative design process. Moreover, the coupled dynamics makes the design of multiple droplet manipulations difficult. The design specificity is significant; thus, small changes such as droplet size typically requires further iterations of the design to adjust for the modifications. Furthermore, although microfluidic chips themselves are rather inexpensive, the apparatus required for microfabrication as well as operation such as the microscope and pressure pump is costly. Another costly aspect of droplet microfluidics experiments is the typical use of surfactant to lower interfacial tension. The development of surfactants requires the chemistry to match both the dispersed and continuous phases. Finally, the successful operation of the droplet microfluidic device relies on pristine surface wetting conditions (either hydrophobic or hydrophilic) that must remain stable throughout the duration of the experiment.

The trade-off with respect to macroscale equivalent experiments can nevertheless be beneficial, especially considering the advent of open-source apparatuses and the growing body of knowledge about droplets microfluidics. Nonetheless, more work is still required to develop accessible droplet microfluidic solutions capable of performing a series of droplet manipulations.

4.3 Droplet microfluidic approaches

All applications of droplet microfluidics are rooted in achieving different droplet manipulations, most commonly, starting with the generation of droplets containing the samples. There is a variety of methods to accomplish the droplet manipulations: droplet generation, splitting, merging, mixing, incubating, and sorting. An overview of various approaches using droplet microfluidics is herein presented. The content is not meant to be comprehensive; rather, the objective is to provide a brief survey of the literature to contextualize the biomedical applications. More thorough reviews are available in the literature for droplet manipulations (Yang, Xu, & Wang, 2010) and, more specifically, for passive droplet generation (Anna, 2016), for active droplet generation (Chong et al., 2016), and for both active and passive droplet generation (Zhu & Wang, 2017).

4.3.1 Passive microfluidics

Passive microfluidic devices rely on the predetermined channel geometry and the flow of the fluid to achieve the various droplet manipulations. The actuation—either pressure-driven or flow-driven—is devised to be constant after the initial setup phase. The device is designed for a range of operation, but the operator's judgment is required to compensate for operational and fabrication uncertainties. Thoughtful designs mitigate the effects of coupling dynamics for easier operation (Glawdel & Ren, 2012). Nonetheless, integrating multiple manipulations in series requires an in-depth understanding of microfluidic principles. The development of more robust passive devices typically requires time- and resource-intensive iterative design.

Passive microfluidic approaches nevertheless exhibit desirable advantages such as high throughput and uniformity. Numerous studies focus on individual manipulations that passive microfluidic devices can achieve, namely, droplet generation, splitting, merging, mixing, incubation, and sorting.

4.3.1.1 Generation

Droplet generation is essential to all droplet-based microfluidic devices because it is the first step to the other manipulations (Thorsen, Roberts, Arnold, & Quake, 2001). Passive generation of droplets generally falls into three categories of geometry: T-junction, coflow, or flow focusing. Additionally, droplets are formed in different regimes defined by the underlying physics of the generation process: jetting, squeezing, and the newly identified leaking regime (Korczyk et al., 2019). A vast literature covers the details of droplet generation (Anna, 2016; Zhu & Wang, 2017). Essentially, the channel geometry is used to force part of the continuous phase in between the isolated segments of the disperse phase which constitute the droplets.

Comparatively to other methods such as bulk emulsion, droplet generation in microdevices allows unprecedented control that enables the production of complex droplet architecture with multiple emulsions (Chong et al., 2015); the generation of such microstructures is leveraged particularly in biomedical applications.

The generation of droplets can also incorporate another layer of complexity when requiring the encapsulation of certain components. Commonly, single cells must be encapsulated. However, controlling the number of cells within each droplet is challenging. The encapsulation rate is limited in efficiency by the Poisson's distribution. The concentration of particle within the dispersed phase dictates the proportion of produced droplets containing 0, 1, 2, 3, etc. cells. The encapsulation of more than 1 cell is minimized by tuning the concentration. However, the trade-off is a low encapsulation efficiency due to the large majority of empty droplets produced (Collins, Neild, DeMello, Liu, & Ai, 2015).

The small volume of the droplet generated is a decisive advantage as previously discussed. However, the small size challenges the throughput in terms of mass per unit of time. The production of high-value components using microfluidics is widely achieved in laboratory settings (Nawar et al., 2020), but the transfer of the technology to the industry is limited partly due to the low throughput. The main approach to increase the throughput is parallelization (Yadavali, Jeong, Lee, & Issadore, 2018). Although passive devices require a constant input, manufacturing uncertainties in addition to coupling dynamics between the parallelized units can challenge the uniformity of the droplets produced.

4.3.1.2 Splitting

The splitting of droplets is very challenging to achieve robustly. Passive methods are further challenged by the limitations to flow and geometry; without additional forces, the device must geometrically disrupt the droplet interface to separate into two daughter droplets. Although certain studies successfully proved the concept (Link, Anna, Weitz, & Stone, 2004), certain applications such as washing require more than robustly achieving an even split; the daughter droplets might be required to respect a ratio, or solid particles should be contained within only one of the two daughter droplets.

4.3.1.3 Merging

The merging of droplets is desired when combining different samples on-chip. Various methods such as pillar arrays (Niu, Gulati, Edel, & deMello, 2008) and fluid viscosities

(Simone & Donk, 2019) demonstrate potential ways to achieve merging. Higher interfacial tension entails easier merging due to the lowered energy barrier. Conversely, if a surfactant is used, desirable merging is more challenging. Surfactant lowers the interfacial tension to prevent unintentional merging that is especially important when collecting many droplets in a reservoir for incubation, for example.

4.3.1.4 Mixing

Single-phase microfluidics mix samples slowly because of the laminar flow and dominating diffusive mixing. When droplets flow in the microchannels, vortices form within the two halves of the droplet; the axis of symmetry is along the direction of travel of the droplet. The sample quickly mixes within each half because of the convective mixing. However, the mixing between the two halves is dictated by the diffusion coefficient that limits the speed of mixing within the entire droplet.

A commonly used tactic to passively increase mixing speed is the serpentine channel. As the droplet follows the curvature, the vortices' symmetry is broken such that mixing is enhanced (Bringer, Gerdts, Song, Tice, & Ismagilov, 2004). The serpentine feature can easily be manufactured using soft lithography.

4.3.1.5 Incubation

Many applications require additional time for a reaction to complete. Although reaction times at the microfluidic scale are shorter compared to larger scales, special measures must nonetheless be implemented. The incubation of a vast number of droplets is generally applied for a uniform condition. Multiple empty droplets are expected when single encapsulation follows Poisson's distribution unless special measures are implemented (Collins et al., 2015). An appropriate surfactant is required to prevent undesirable merging in the incubation chamber. The chamber can take many forms such as an on-chip collection area or an external tubing in which droplets are stored.

Another tactic for incubation when encapsulation is not involved—and thus, the high number of empty droplets from the Poisson's distribution is avoided—is the trapping mechanism. Typically used for shorter times, on-chip trapping mechanisms immobilizes droplets to monitor their output (Chen & Ren, 2017). However, trapping droplet passively is challenging due to the dependence of the trap design on the droplet size, and the droplet size variations from operational and manufacturing uncertainties.

4.3.1.6 Sorting

The encapsulation of single cells in droplets is a good example for which sorting is pertinent. The empty droplets generated do not contribute information and would benefit from being sorted out as waste (Lim, Tran, & Abate, 2015). However, passive microfluidics changes are restricted to flow and geometry; therefore, sorting based on an external factor such as the presence of a cell within the droplet or fluorescent signal is not possible.

Nevertheless, inertial microfluidics spatially orders particles based on their size due to their different motion with the flow (Di Carlo, 2009). However, inertial microfluidics is generally applied to a single phase. Droplet microfluidics does benefit from particle ordering nevertheless to position cells in an ordered fashion before a junction, for instance (Lagus & Edd, 2013; Moon et al., 2018).

4.3.2 Active microfluidics

Similarly to passive microfluidics, active microfluidics relies on flow and geometry, but an additional and/or varying force is integrated within the system to provide more control. The additional control affects multiple or individual droplets.

4.3.2.1 Control of multiple droplets

Multiple droplets are affected by a single source of added and/or varying input through a layering approach to a passive device. For instance, the added control is used to tune the size of the generated droplets. The actuation and feedback are provided by different mechanisms. Visual feedback requires a fast algorithm for online monitoring of the droplet size (up to thousands per seconds), but oppositely to the complexity and robustness of the algorithm, the implementation does not require special additional hardware; the computer serves as the host for the controller that can communicate with the actuation method based on the feedback obtained visually through a camera (Crawford, Smith, & Whyte, 2017). Alternatively, an electric potential is used to tune the droplet size (He, Kim, Luo, Marquez, & Cheng, 2010). Different forces such as magnetic are implemented to tune the droplet generation process (Chong et al., 2016).

Another manipulation that benefits from the added control of multiple droplets is mixing. Passive mixing is achieved passively by breaking the vortices symmetry using a serpentine channel design. A faster mixing is accomplished using microwave heating by similarly breaking the vortices' symmetry (Boybay, Jiao, Glawdel, & Ren, 2013; Yesiloz, Boybay, & Ren, 2017).

4.3.2.2 Control of individual droplets

Individual droplets are controlled through a variety of ways; generating droplets on demand and sorting droplets are both closely intertwined with passive microfluidic designs. Generation on demand is performed using different approaches such as with surface acoustic waves (SAWs) (Collins, Alan, Helmerson, & Neild, 2013) and pressure (Churski, Nowacki, Korczyk, & Garstecki, 2013; Zhou & Yao, 2014). Similarly, active sorting typically uses the added control to divert droplets to the desired stream based on available feedback. The "push" is provided by voltage (Chung, Núñez, Cai, & Kurabayashi, 2017), SAW (Collins, Neild, & Ai, 2016; Franke, Abate, Weitz, & Wixforth, 2009), or laser (Won, Lee, & Song, 2017) to name a few. However, these techniques typically are linked to a passive network, and the active component is limited to one manipulation.

More versatile platforms perform various manipulations on droplets and provide advantageous additional control. The added control decouples the different manipulations such that they are independently performed. Garstecki's group developed such a platform that uses solenoid valves to control the flow (Churski, Korczyk, & Garstecki, 2010; Churski et al., 2012; Jakiela, Kaminski, Cybulski, Weibel, & Garstecki, 2013; Postek, Kaminski, & Garstecki, 2017). Although generation, merging, and splitting are performed, the robustness is limited due to the lack of automation. Moreover, the fixed pressure that the solenoid valves turn on and off must be properly tuned. A platform developed in Prof. Ren's group uses visual feedback to adjust the applied pressure. The calculations are based on the physical properties of the system that are entered by the user (Wong & Ren, 2016). Furthermore, robustness is improved through the implementation of a semiautomated algorithm to perform individual manipulations automatically based on quantitative parameters provided by the user (Hébert, Courtney, & Ren, 2019).

Although the recent advances in the development of active droplet control platforms are promising, much work remains to be done for the usage of microfluidic tools by end-users. A modular active platform is envisioned to mitigate the barrier to the adoption of microfluidics as a tool by end-users. The knowledge barrier in addition to the ease of operation is lowered by automation that only requires high-level information from the user such as the microchip geometry and the manipulation parameters. The significance of such an active droplet control platform would greatly increase the impact of microfluidics as a field through novel applications by end-users in various fields.

4.4 Biomedical applications

Since its beginnings, droplet microfluidic devices have been used in applications ranging across of variety of fields; the vast array of applications demonstrates the potential of droplet microfluidics as an enabling technology. The scope of this section will be limited to biomedical applications to maintain the thematic focus, but droplet microfluidics is applied to many more fields. Once again, the studies herein presented are not meant to be comprehensive, but rather, to provide an overview of what droplet microfluidics can contribute to biomedical applications. Review articles cover in more detail certain areas of biomedical applications (Feng et al., 2019; Li et al., 2018; Luo, Su, Zhang, & Raston, 2019). Biomedical applications rely on the microfluidic principles presented above, and as illustrated in Fig. 4.1, multiple areas of applications exist.

The applications of droplet microfluidics are grouped into three categories: biomaterials, isolated element screening, and bioreactors. The focus of each application is generally either to produce a high-value-added material or to collect information. Although biomaterials applications could fit in either the production-focused or

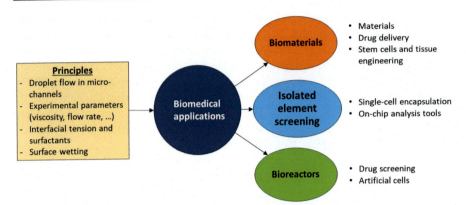

Figure 4.1 Schematic representation of the principles underlying microfluidic devices for biomedical applications in many categories of applications.

information-focused category, the selected studies are generally production rather than information-focused. Screening and bioreactor applications provide information as the end product. Review articles specific to each application usually compare and contrast different methods to achieve the particular application whereas this chapter focuses on providing compelling evidence on how droplet microfluidics is an enabling tool within the context of biomedical applications.

A clear working definition of biomedical applications is established to shape the scope of the works herein included. Biomedical applications are at the intersection of biology and medicine principles, and engineering problem-solving techniques; the overarching goal of these devices is to assist in the diagnostic and therapy of diseases through the comprehension, modification, and control of biological systems (Paras & Kanaris, 2019).

4.4.1 Biomaterials

The physics of droplets at the microscale enables not only the high-throughput of uniform simple beads but also the production of complex structures such as multiple emulsions and Janus particles. However, one main drawback is the yield of microfluidic devices that is generally too low for industrial or clinical applications, even with parallelization efforts. A clinical trial for a stem cell study requires $\sim 10^7$ to 10^{10} cells per patient (Choe, Park, Park, & Lee, 2018). The production of biomaterials using droplet microfluidics benefits from the compartmentalization, possible complex architecture, and uniformity, but the low output is prohibitive to translating the technology to industrial or clinical use.

Concerning the information-focused biomaterial studies, droplet microfluidics enables exploring a vast parameter space for biomaterial synthesis to optimize the process (Li & Ismagilov, 2010); the result of this type of application is the information about the set of parameters to achieve the specified outcome. Although applications such as protein crystallization are nevertheless an important area because of its contribution to the study of protein structures (Maeki, Yamaguchi, Tokeshi, & Miyazaki, 2016), the production of simple and complex structures will be the focus. The materials typically used for biomedical applications will first be covered before the two main application areas: drug delivery and tissue engineering. Fig. 4.2 visually regroups the three main subcategories of applications.

4.4.1.1 Materials

The material selection for any biomedical application is important. Various review articles cover the extensive array of materials involved for biomedical applications in more detail (Jo & Lee, 2019; Li et al., 2018; Luo et al., 2019).

Biopolymers are advantageous because of their biocompatibility, biodegradability, low antigenicity, and high bioactivity. The different biopolymers can generally be classified into three main categories: polysaccharides (e.g., alginate (Ling, Wu, Neish, & Champion, 2019; Utech et al., 2015), chitosan (Jiang et al., 2011; Mu et al., 2019), agarose (Zamora-Mora, Velasco, Hernández, Mijangos, & Kumacheva, 2014; Zhang, Zhang, Liu, Li, Zhu, & Yang, 2011)), proteins (Pepe, Podesva, & Simone, 2017; Yamada et al., 2015), and microbial polymers (Amoyav & Benny, 2019; Ekanem, Zhang, & Vladisavljević, 2017; Jeyhani, Gnyawali, Abbasi, Hwang, & Tsai, 2019). A wide range of properties such as chemical composition, porosity, stiffness, and cell adhesion is possible, but independently tailoring for a specific application is challenging (Velasco, Tumarkin, & Kumacheva, 2012).

In addition to the material itself, the method of formation of the particles is important (Alkayyali, Cameron, Haltli, Kerr, & Ahmadi, 2019). The common procedures are polymerization (Jeong et al., 2005; Liu et al., 2016), thermal (Comunian, Abbaspourrad, Favaro-Trindade, & Weitz, 2014), and ionic cross-linking (Tan & Takeuchi, 2007). More complex methods can circumvent the disadvantages of the simpler ones such as the damage caused to the compounds from the short UV radiation or increased temperature, for instance. Certain materials such as polylactic acid (PLA) exhibit desirable biocompatibility properties, but require solvent evaporation or diffusion (Bchellaoui, Hayat, Mami, Dorbez-Sridi, & El Abed, 2017; Hussain et al., 2019; Watanabe, Ono, & Kimura, 2011; Xu et al., 2009). More complex architectures such as Janus particles also require a complex formation process, namely, dewetting (Choi, Weitz, & Lee, 2013; Haase & Brujic, 2014; Shi & Weitz, 2017).

Separately, materials other than polymers are also involved in biomedical applications. Quantum dots (QDs) are 5–150 nm in diameter nanoparticles made of semiconductors that are used for biomedical applications. Droplet microfluidics serves both for the synthesis of various QDs (Bandulasena, Vladisavljević, & Benyahia, 2019; Dai, Yang, Hamon, & Kong, 2015; Edel, Fortt, deMello, & deMello, 2002; Kašpar, Koyuncu, Pittermannová, Ulbrich, & Tokárová, 2019) and the use of the nanoparticles for biomedical applications (Hu et al., 2014; Ji et al., 2011; Lan et al., 2016; Nguyen, Chen, Sedighi, Krull, & Ren, 2018; Park, Lee, Um, & Park, 2016; Seo, Gorelikov, Williams, & Matsuura, 2010). Environmental and health concerns about the traditional

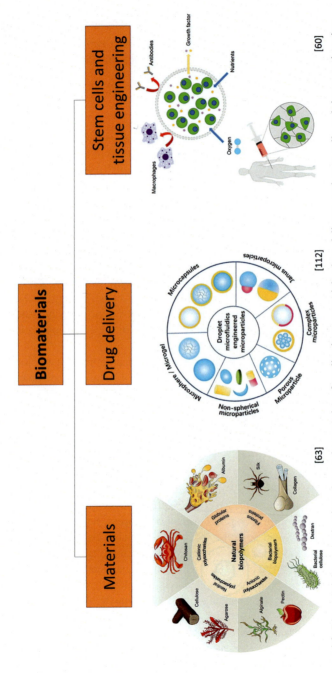

Figure 4.2 Biomaterials separation into three subcategories of applications: materials, drug delivery, and stem cells and tissue engineering. Reproduced from Jo and Lee (2019), Li et al., (2018), Choe et al., (2018) with permission from The Royal Society of Chemistry.

heavy metals used for QDs prompted a switch toward carbon dots (CDs) and fluorescent polymers instead (Li et al., 2014; Luo et al., 2018; Omidi, Hashemi, & Tayebi, 2019; Park & Park, 2018; Qu, Wang, Ren, & Qu, 2013). CDs exhibit similar luminescent properties—resistant to photobleaching—but are biocompatible as well (Gómez-de Pedro et al., 2014).

4.4.1.2 Drug delivery

The uniformity of the particles synthesized using microfluidic devices yields better releasing profiles and are made of a variety of materials such as polylactic-co-glycolic acid (PLGA) (Chiesa, Dorati, Modena, Conti, & Genta, 2018; Guo et al., 2018a, 2018b), polyethylene glycol (PEG) (Deveza et al., 2015), proteins (Shimanovich et al., 2015), and others (Wang et al., 2018). PLGA is particularly promising because of its Food and Drug Administration (FDA) approval for human use (Makadia & Siegel, 2011). However, challenges have hindered the widespread use of encapsulated nanoparticles due to concerns about biodistribution and toxicity (Bobo, Robinson, Islam, Thurecht, & Corrie, 2016).

The chemical and physical properties of the material govern the drug release dynamics. The important factors are molecular weight, mixed microparticles, crystalline degree, drug distribution, porosity, and particle size distribution (Chong et al., 2015). The most significant variable is the particle size. Smaller particles have larger surface-to-volume ratios that lead to fast release. The particle size must also be appropriate for the target area (Wang et al., 2004); small particles ($\sim$ 1–5 μm) can target cells to deliver DNA vaccines for instance; delivering drugs to the capillaries require particles about 10–20 μm. However, microfluidic devices typically produce larger monodisperse particles; particles 10–250 μm in size are suitable for oral intake and subcutaneous or intramuscular injections (Li et al., 2018).

In addition to spheres, more complex microstructures and properties bonify the control of the releasing profile such as with core—shell structures (Shum, Kim, & Weitz, 2008) and with stimuli-responsive microgels (Gu et al., 2018; Herranz-Blanco et al., 2014; Liu et al., 2011; Maher et al., 2017; Shah, Kim, Agresti, Weitz, & Chu, 2008). Janus particles feature two halves with different properties and are used for drug delivery purposes (Nisisako, Ando, & Hatsuzawa, 2012; Sun et al., 2019). Two drugs are coencapsulated and codelivered (Sundararajan, Wang, Rosen, Procopio, & Rosenberg, 2018; Xie, She, Wang, Sharma, & Smith, 2012). Alternatively, the inclusion of a marker instead of a second drug allows to track the particle location (Wu, Ross, Hong, & Lee, 2010).

4.4.1.3 Stem cells and tissue engineering

Tissue engineering aims to develop biocompatible and biodegradable scaffolds for cells. The scaffold provides support and stimulation for the cells to attach, migrate, proliferate, and differentiate. The physical characteristics of the scaffold have a complex impact on the application depending on: porosity, size, shape, spatial distribution, diameter, degree of fiber alignment, surface roughness, elasticity, mechanical strength (Hutmacher, 2000), and 3D geometry (Luo et al., 2019). The encapsulation process is exempt from the strict 1 cell per droplet requiring typical for information-focused applications; instead, multiple cells are encapsulated for proliferation within the scaffold (Sakai et al., 2011). Although stem cell therapy exhibits great potential, the death of the cells from the lack of proper support once injected leads to a lack of therapeutic in vivo effects. The versatility of the properties of hydrogel provides the support required for the encapsulated stem cells to provide the desired therapeutic effects.

The scaffold takes many shapes. The size of the spheres can be actively tuned (Costantini et al., 2018). Automation and control can also allow to interface between the passive microdevice and the world efficiently such that high throughput is maintained (Langer & Joensson, 2019). Alternatively to spheres, different shapes such as core−shell structures are used (Guo et al., 2018a, 2018b; Wang, Zhao, Tian, Ma, & Wang, 2015; Wang et al., 2019).

The 3D geometry of the cell structures creates a better model of a liver (Chen et al., 2016) or of a tumor (Agarwal et al., 2017; Jang, Koh, Lee, Cheong, & Kim, 2017), for example. The cell-laden particles can also be injected (Cha et al., 2014; Griffin, Weaver, Scumpia, Di Carlo, & Segura, 2015) such as for stem cell therapy (Feng et al., 2019; Guo et al., 2018a, 2018b; Li, Truong, Thissen, Frith, & Forsythe, 2017; Siltanen et al., 2016; Zhao et al., 2016).

Choe et al. (2018) provide valuable insight particularly about the challenges and future direction of stem cell microencapsulation in hydrogel. The selected microparticle production method can adversely affect cell viability. More specifically, photopolymerization produces radial initiators; the photoinitiator concentration and UV intensity are significant factors that can limit cell viability (Khademhosseini et al., 2006; Xia, Jiang, Debroy, Li, & Oakey, 2017). Moreover, the use of droplet microfluidics, and thus, the introduction of an oil phase can cause damage when the cell lipid membrane contacts the oil. Finally, typical stem cell therapy involves $\sim 10^7$ to 10^{10} cells per patient; consequently, high throughput is required to produce enough stem-cell-laden microparticles.

4.4.1.4 General perspective on droplet microfluidics and biomaterials

Droplet microfluidics technologies provide desirable characteristics for the production of biomaterials. Multiple fluids are injected to constitute complex structures. The encapsulation and isolation of the droplet content ensure the proper production of the biomaterials. The different solidification approaches can minimally impact the fragile content of the droplets such as bioactive proteins and live cells. The production-focused applications require a high throughput that is suitable for passive methods and control of multiple droplets only. More work is nonetheless required to increase throughput for large-scale manufacturing through parallelization (Jeong, Yelleswarapu, Yadavali, Issadore, & Lee, 2015; Romanowsky, Abate, Rotem, Holtze, & Weitz, 2012; Yadavali et al., 2018).

Moreover, further developments of the technologies are envisioned to increase the impact; useful capabilities to develop include but are not limited to: automated system to control the characteristics of the material that is produced, real-time and just-in-time processing, detection of leakage and blockage in the system, and online monitoring of a desired phenomenon such as nucleic growth. Furthermore, high-value-added biomaterials have a high-impact potential for a smaller amount, and thus, should be the focus of further applications.

4.4.2 Isolated element screening

The small size involved in droplet microfluidics is leveraged to encapsulate single species to be analyzed while preserving a strong signal by avoiding considerable dilution. Encapsulation of single elements allows perceiving the heterogeneity of the population, even if the target elements represent a low proportion of the large population. The lack of dilution, and thus, the large signal-to-noise ratio is suitable to complete the analysis process of the single elements on-chip. Such systems are coming closer to the envisioned μTAS. The applications are categorized into two subcategories as shown in Fig. 4.3: single-cell encapsulation and on-chip analysis tools.

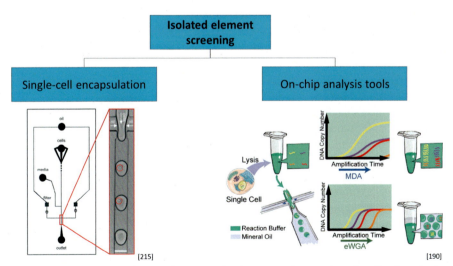

Figure 4.3 Isolated element screening separation into two subcategories of application: single-cell encapsulation and on-chip analysis tools.
From Shembekar et al., (2016), Fu et al., (2015).

4.4.2.1 Single-cell encapsulation

The passive encapsulation of single cells in droplets is a random process that is generally limited by the Poisson distribution (Collins et al., 2015); in order to ensure that very few droplets contain more than 1 cell, the sample is diluted such that most droplets are empty, but the occupied droplets contain only 1 cell. Certain methods developed both actively and passively increase the single-encapsulation efficiency (Abate, Chen, Agresti, & Weitz, 2009; Chung et al., 2017; Liu, Li, Wang, Piper, & Jiang, 2020; Schoendube, Wright, Zengerle, & Koltay, 2015). Active methods are typically at a disadvantage due to their significantly lower throughput; some applications require the analysis of large heterogeneous populations of cells ($O(10^5-10^6)$) (Mazutis et al., 2013)). Briefly, the challenge is to increase cell encapsulation efficiency without compromising throughput, monodispersity, and reproducibility. The following studies focus on large heterogeneous populations of cells to separate into droplets, and then, to perform the analysis off-chip, typically polymerase chain reaction (PCR) (Chung, Kurabayashi, & Cai, 2019; Klein et al., 2015; Lu et al., 2017; Zheng et al., 2017); the on-chip processing of single cells will be subsequently discussed. The small partitions enable the high-sensitivity process although it is performed off-chip (Kaushik, Hsieh, & Wang, 2018; Thibault et al., 2019).

'Droplet microfluidics supports a variety of materials for droplet formation. The properties such as stiffness are important for encapsulating living cells (Lee et al., 2017; Ma, Neubauer, Thiele, Fery, & Huck, 2014). Moreover, the control on the shape enabled by droplet microfluidics allows the production of spheres and of disk-shaped microgels. The disks easily maintain the same orientation which is desirable for long-term analysis without concerns about rotations and changes in planes (Liu et al., 2012). Another issue with encapsulated cells in microgels that is mediated through microfluidic tools is the cell egress. Centering the cell enables the growth to remain within the gel (Kamperman, Henke, Visser, Karperien, & Leijten, 2017; Lienemann et al., 2017).

The encapsulation allows the probing of gene expression at the single-cell level (Geng, Novak, & Mathies, 2013; Novak et al., 2011). Barcoding the droplets with unique identifiers enables the tracking of each individually encapsulated cell (Klein et al., 2015; Macosko et al., 2015). For example, immunoassays are important tools that provide useful information for drug discovery and that can be performed at the single-cell resolution through encapsulation in microgel (Akbari & Pirbodaghi, 2014; Shembekar, Hu, Eustace, & Merten, 2018). The single-cell encapsulation is streamlined as a commercial apparatus: *Cyto-mine* by *Sphere Fluidics*. The apparatus achieves basic encapsulation that is limited by Poisson's distribution. Nonetheless, the integrated workflow including the encapsulation, assay, sorting, and dispensing is well-suited for antibody discovery and cell line development. The commercial product streamlines the relatively basic single-cell encapsulation process but at the expense of flexibility and low cost. Whether the trade-off is worthwhile or not depends on the end-users usage.

Proteins initially are higher in quantity than DNA within the cells, but the lack of straightforward amplification techniques prohibits their analysis through traditional methods (Zare & Kim, 2010). Single-cell encapsulation limits the dilution and provides tools to analyze both the physical and chemical properties of the proteins which provide insight into how the cell works.

Bacteria are encapsulated in droplets for growth and analysis (Håti et al., 2016; Cui et al., 2018). Oppositely to other cells, the proliferation of bacteria provides a strong fluorescent signal (Duarte, Barbier, & Schaerli, 2017). Moreover, the encapsulation of multiple elements within a droplet creates a controlled environment to study bacteria cohabitation and cell−cell interactions (Terekhov et al., 2017; Zhang et al., 2018). Furthermore, antimicrobial susceptibility testing is performed using droplet-based microfluidic tools (Kaushik et al., 2017; Sabhachandani et al., 2017).

Multicellular organisms such as *C. elegans* are also encapsulated to provide a controlled environment for further analysis (Aubry & Lu, 2017; Clausell-Tormos et al., 2008; Wen, Yu, Zhu, Jiang, & Qin, 2015; Yan et al., 2016; Ying et al., 2012).

Generally, the small volume of droplet microfluidics allows analyzing secretion and uptake of trace biomolecules. Droplets that are too large have unfavorable signal-to-noise ratios; diffusion of nutrients through a too large droplet is too slow to properly support the encapsulated living cell. Moreover, aqueous droplets contained in an oil continuous phase can prevent the necessary nutrients such as oxygen from reaching the cell; encapsulating the water droplets in an aqueous phase to form water−oil−water emulsions is beneficial both for nutrient availability and subsequent aqueous phase−based analytical tools (Zhang et al., 2013). Certain oil phases such as FC-40 and HFE-7500 are sufficiently permeable to oxygen to sustain the cells within appropriately sized droplets. However, the required surfactant can introduce troublesome dynamics such as preventing the addition of reagents to the droplets in addition to the desired dynamics, more specifically, and the proper wetting conditions, and the lower interfacial tension that decreases undesirable droplet merging (Abate, Hung, Mary, Agresti, & Weitz, 2010). Furthermore, certain surfactants are prohibitively expensive. Most importantly, the surfactant should not be toxic to cells (Velasco, Tumarkin, & Kumacheva, 2012).

4.4.2.2 On-chip analysis tools

The previous subsection about single cell focused more particularly on the encapsulation process and the variety of potential downstream applications, but the analysis procedure could be performed off-chip. In contrast, the following subsection will focus on on-chip analysis methods such as PCR, multiple displacement amplification (MDA), and loop-mediated amplification (LAMP).

Similarly to the encapsulation of single cells, the small partitions encapsulate single target DNA for subsequent amplification with high sensitivity. The partitioning increases the signal-to-noise ratio of the rare elements to analyze. Moreover, the small volume involved drastically reduces the amount of reagent required comparatively to an equivalent well-plate procedure. The sensitivity and accuracy of the analysis are limited by the false-positive and false-negative rates of the assay such that the number of partitions cannot be arbitrarily increased to improve sensitivity. For droplet-based PCR (ddPCR), the sample application to detection of foodborne pathogens is shown to be more sensitive than comparable conventional methods (Jang et al., 2017).

The unprecedented sensitivity and ability to analyze heterogeneous populations make droplet-based PCR particularly impactful for cancer research (Hajji et al., 2020; Li et al., 2019; Ma et al., 2016). Moreover, the low count of circulating tumor cells (CTCs) within a sample challenges traditional analysis approaches; microfluidic devices can provide the required throughput and sensitivity to identify the CTCs (Bithi & Vanapalli, 2017; Chiu et al., 2015; Ribeiro-Samy et al., 2019; Watanabe et al., 2018). Alternatively to PCR, single-cell studies within the context of cancer research are performed using surface-enhanced Raman scattering (SERS) (Cong et al., 2019; Gao, Cheng, deMello, & Choo, 2016). *Mission Bio* offers commercial products to characterize both genotype and phenotype cells using their *Tapestri* platform; their platform is especially impactful for the analysis of tumor biology. The platform enables cell barcoding and most importantly, multiomics solutions at the single-cell resolution. However, the trade-off with the commercial product is whether its capabilitiesjustifies its cost.

An alternative to PCR for whole-genome amplification is MDA. Similarly, the small volume of the droplets limits the dilution while performing accurate and uniform sequencing of minute amounts of DNA (Fu et al., 2015; Hammond, Homa, Andersson-Svahn, Ettema, & Joensson, 2016; Hosokawa, Nishikawa, Kogawa, & Takeyama, 2017; Kim et al., 2017; Nishikawa et al., 2015; Novak et al., 2011; Rhee, Light, Meagher, & Singh, 2016; Sidore, Lan, Lim, & Abate, 2015; Spits et al., 2006; Zhang et al., 2018).

The combination of aptamers and microfluidics has tremendous potential for diagnostics and biosensing (Fraser et al., 2019). Microfluidics is useful for the production of not only aptamers (Autour, Westhof, & Ryckelynck, 2016; Autour, Bouhedda, Cubi, & Ryckelynck, 2019; Lee et al., 2018) but also their inclusion with other elements such as cells for analysis (Abatemarco et al., 2017; Giuffrida, Cigliana, & Spoto, 2018; Li, Wang, Feng, Tong, & Tang, 2014; Qiu et al., 2017; Zhang, Ye, Yang, & Xu, 2019).

Digital LAMP provides an analysis tool for nucleic acids that takes advantage of the high throughput, and of the small droplet volume allowing increased partitioning. The on-chip integration has been achieved for use in laboratory settings with conventional microfluidic peripheral apparatus (Azizi, Zaferani, Cheong, & Abbaspourrad, 2019; Chung et al., 2019; Ma, Luo, Chang, & Lee, 2018; Rane, Chen, Zec, & Wang, 2015; Schuler et al., 2016; Wan et al., 2017) as well as with point-of-care platforms that are portable (Lin, Huang, Urmann, Xie, & Hoffmann, 2019; Wan et al., 2019; Zhu et al., 2012).

The relatively standardized procedure for the nucleic acid quantification enables the development of automated commercial products. For example, *RainDance* and *QX ONE Droplet Digital PCR* (ddPCR) by *Bio-Rad* is capable of high throughput multiplexed and integrated ddPCR as an off-the-shelf system. Similarly, *Agilent* offers a real-time PCR (qPCR) system under their *AriaMx* products. *Fluidigm* proposes nucleic acid analysis platform under their *Access Array* product line.

4.4.2.3 General perspective on droplet microfluidics and isolated element analysis

The encapsulation of single elements such as cells, multicellular organisms, and DNA templates leverage the isolation capabilities of droplets microfluidics to create controlled environments. The separation of the elements allows the study of heterogeneous populations by considering each individual component separately. Moreover, the high throughput capabilities of droplet microfluidics enable the analysis of large populations with rare target elements that would other not be detected due to a poor signal-to-noise ratio. The sensitivity is, thus, increased by separating the elements and considering them individually.

Although the assays are information-focused rather than production-focused, the high throughput is nonetheless required due to the large populations to analyze ($O(10^5-10^6)$). Consequently, passive methods or active methods allowing the control over multiple droplets are better suited to the high throughput requirement. Nevertheless, the encapsulation process is random in nature, and the Poisson distribution dictates a majority of empty droplets to limit the encapsulation to a single unit per droplet. Some studies attempt to circumvent the Poisson distribution, but it is challenging to do so without compromising throughput, monodispersity, and reproducibility.

4.4.3 Bioreactors

The effective compartmentalization of the droplets surrounded by the continuous is leveraged to perform many reactions that provide information as the output. The small volume involved for each reaction spares precious and expensive samples. Moreover, reactions complete faster than for comparable assays at a larger scale. The main usage of droplets as bioreactors is for drug screening; building artificial cells from the ground up is another usage that is much more novel but promising nonetheless. The two subcategories are illustrated in Fig. 4.4.

4.4.3.1 Drug screening

The intersection of droplet microfluidics and pharmacology is fruitful not only for drug *delivery* as previously covered in the biomaterials section but also for drug *screening*. While the focus of delivery is the production of high-value-added particles as vehicles to administer the drugs, screening aims to develop the drugs themselves. The reagents involved in drug screening are often expensive. Consequently, the smaller volume translates to significant cost savings. Moreover, the reaction can complete in a shorter

186 Microfluidic Devices for Biomedical Applications

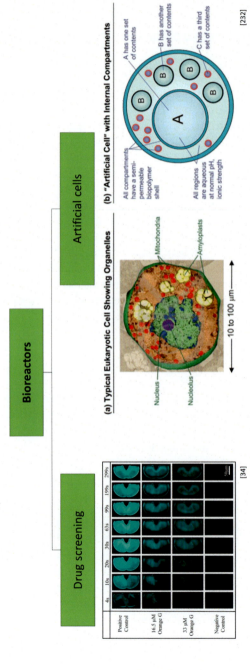

Figure 4.4 Bioreactors separation into two subcategories of applications: drug screening and artificial cells. From Chen et al., (2017), Lu et al., (2017).

timeframe (from hours to minutes (Pennemann, Watts, Haswell, Hessel, & Löwe, 2004)) while providing the same information. A more thorough categorization of the intersection of drug screening with microfluidics is found in pertinent review articles (Shembekar, Chaipan, Utharala, & Merten, 2016; Zhai, Yi, Jia, Mak, & Martins, 2019).

The potential contribution of droplet microfluidics to the field of drug discovery has been recognized since the early 2000s (Dittrich & Manz, 2006). A drug screening assay requires the formation of two droplets; one droplet contains the target molecules to study with the marker, and the other droplet contains the drug (or inhibitor) as well as the triggering agent. Merging the two droplets starts the reaction that is monitored with the marker's fluorescent intensity. The reaction completes over minutes; thus, the droplets must be trapped such that the data are collected. Changing the content and the concentration of the components allow running positive and negative controls as well as to investigate the impact of the drug concentration. A single microfluidic chip is shown to achieve such assay both with passive methods (Chen & Ren, 2017; Courtney et al., 2016; Mao et al., 2015; Miller et al., 2012) and active methods (Hébert et al., 2019; Kuo et al., 2019). Furthermore, the effects on *E. coli* of a combination of compounds forming a complex multidimensional response space are also efficiently investigated using droplets (Cao, Goldhan, Martin, & Köhler, 2013; Scanlon, Dostal, & Griswold, 2014).

The potential use of droplet microfluidics for drug screening moreover intersects with other application areas involving cells. The effect of chemotherapy drugs on single and clustered tumor cells is investigated (Bithi & Vanapalli, 2017; Wong et al., 2017). The 3D environment supported by microgels enables both the study of drugs on single and grouped cells as well as their long-term culture (Du et al., 2018; Sabhachandani et al., 2016; Sart, Tomasi, Amselem, & Baroud, 2017; Sun et al., 2018; Wang & Wang, 2014).

4.4.3.2 Artificial cells

Artificial cells aim to model biological systems at the cell-level analogously to organs-on-a-chip for organs. Organs-on-a-chip aim to construct and study models of organs, but the required expertise falls outside of *droplet* microfluidics. The intricate architecture involved in building artificial cells from the ground up is conceptually more complex than microparticles due to the importance of the interaction between the different components rather than their isolation. A more detailed review covers more extensively the topic of artificial cells (Majumder, Wubshet, & Liu, 2019), and a perspective article puts into context the progression of this application within the microfluidic community (Friddin, Elani, Trantidou, & Ces, 2019).

Cells can be built using only aqueous solutions (Douliez, Perro, & Béven, 2019; Lu, Oh, Terrell, Bentley, & Raghavan, 2017), but the introduction of another phase to build liposomes and polymersomes enhance their stability. The cell membrane is an important component that the structure of liposomes allows to study through the formation of giant unilamellar vesicles (GUVs) (Arriaga et al., 2014; Paterson, Reboud, Wilson, Tassieri, & Cooper, 2014; Stein, Spindler, Bonakdar, Wang, & Sandoghdar, 2017) with various membrane proteins (Deshpande, Caspi, Meijering, & Dekker, 2016; Ho, Lee, Durand, Majumder, & Liu, 2017) to study reactions across the membrane (Elani, Law, & Ces, 2014; Elani, Casadevall i Solvas, Edel, Law, & Ces, 2016; Schlicht & Zagnoni, 2015). Polymersomes are promising due to their better stability facilitating the study of the cell behavior, but studies are comparatively more limited (Bayoumi, Bayley, Maglia, & Sapra, 2017; Kubilis, Abdulkarim, Eissa, & Cameron, 2016; Martino et al., 2012; Mason et al., 2019). Focused review articles provide more detailed information about the use of droplet microfluidic to mimic cells (Armada-Moreira, Taipaleenmäki, Itel, Zhang, & Städler, 2016; Martino & deMello, 2016; Trantidou et al., 2017; Spoelstra, Deshpande, & Dekker, 2018). Generally, the characteristics required for the high-impact artificial cells are enhanced stability, better functionality, and environment interactivity that can be achieved by a promising recent study (Liu, Guo, & Liang, 2019).

4.4.3.3 General perspective on droplet microfluidics and bioreactors

The information-focused bioreactor applications leverage many advantages of droplets microfluidics. The small volume involved in each reaction saves reagent, and thus, also money. Shorter reaction times complete the assays faster. The lower throughput required—especially comparatively to high-throughput applications such as heterogeneous cell population analysis—means that both active and passive methods are promising. The trade-off of throughput for control involved in active methods is envisioned to be impactful to build complex artificial cells from the ground up.

4.5 Conclusion—perspective on the future of biomedical applications using droplet microfluidics

The field of droplet microfluidics exhibits a rich and expansive literature that investigates its fundamental principles as well as demonstrates its tremendous potential as an enabling technology, more specifically, for impactful biomedical applications.

Fundamentally, the physics of droplet microfluidics involves most importantly the viscous forces and interfacial tension between the continuous and dispersed phase as quantified by the Capillary number. The small characteristic length means the flow is laminar. The main advantages of droplet microfluidics are low reagent consumption, low cost, short reaction time, compartmentalization, high throughput, and uniformity. The physical behavior of droplets is leveraged through either passive or active methods. Passive methods rely on the flow and channel geometry to achieve droplet generation, splitting, merging, mixing, and incubation. Separately, active methods involve a varying and/or additional force to better control one or multiple droplets. The different droplet microfluidic manipulation methods are implemented for a variety of biomedical applications with one main target, either production or information. Biomaterials generally focus on producing high-value-added simple or complex materials for drug delivery and tissue engineering. Single-element screenings provide a highly sensitive analysis of cells, bacteria, or DNA such that the heterogeneity of the population is perceptible. Bioreactors perform reactions at a small scale, for example, to efficiently screen drugs or to mimic living cells. The involvement to a different degree of each of the subcategories (biomaterials, encapsulation, bioreactors) within each study highlights the complexity of the applications. For example, a drug screening assay can involve the encapsulation of single tumor cells in a hydrogel for culturing and assessment of the response to different drugs.

In spite of the vast research using droplet microfluidics fundamentals for biomedical studies, much work remains to be done to fully achieve the potential of droplet microfluidics as an enabling tool providing novel and advantageous capabilities to end-users in biomedical fields. The impact of droplet microfluidics would be most influential when the end-users can easily use it as a tool within their application. The numerous applications are nonetheless promising and lead to the development of new microfluidic technologies. However, the variety of applications entails a wide range of requirements. The variation in requirements implies that the selected application must be the driver for the development of the technological innovations, and not vice versa. The platform development should concentrate on one application and its specific requirements. Furthermore, the achievement of droplet microfluidic as an enabling technology requires ease of use without in-depth knowledge. Therefore, impactful developments can fall outside of the typical academic standpoint. For example, *Dolomite*'s connector is key in their success because of its ability to enable modularity.

The targeted application and the fulfilled requirements by the microfluidic platform need to engage numerous people to enlarge its impact. Innovations within the academic sphere equates to scientific publications and patent acquisition. The recent push toward collaboration with the end-users during the development in academia typically led to the creation of spin-off companies. However, the effort required to develop a tool enabling chemists and biologists to leverage droplet microfluidics is problematically large. Thus, currently, the translation from academic projects to viable commercial products is weak. The commercial systems offer researchers a trade-off: cost and flexibility must be sacrificed for ease of use and reliability. The latter can be challenging to achieve by the innovative droplet microfluidic platforms. Nevertheless, ease of use and reliability are primordial to the success of a commercial product and should not be underestimated. The adoption by end-users is envisioned to be greatly improved by the development of a modular active droplet control platform that requires only high-level information (Zhong et al., 2020).

References

Abate, A. R., Chen, C.-H., Agresti, J. J., & Weitz, D. A. (2009). Beating poisson encapsulation statistics using close-packed ordering. *Lab on a Chip, 9*, 2628−2631.

Abate, A. R., Hung, T., Mary, P., Agresti, J. J., & Weitz, D. A. (2010). High-throughput injection with microfluidics using picoinjectors. *Proceedings of the National Academy of Sciences of the United States of America, 107*, 19163−19166.

Abatemarco, J., Sarhan, M. F., Wagner, J. M., Lin, J.-L., Liu, L., Hassouneh, W., et al. (2017). RNA-aptamers-in-droplets (RAPID) high-throughput screening for secretory phenotypes. *Nature Communications, 8*, 1−9.

Agarwal, P., Wang, H., Sun, M., Xu, J., Zhao, S., Liu, Z., et al. (2017). Microfluidics enabled bottom-up engineering of 3D vascularized tumor for drug discovery. *ACS Nano, 11*, 6691−6702.

Akbari, S., & Pirbodaghi, T. (2014). A droplet-based heterogeneous immunoassay for screening single cells secreting antigen-specific antibodies. *Lab on a Chip, 14*, 3275−3280.

Alkayyali, T., Cameron, T., Haltli, B., Kerr, R. G., & Ahmadi, A. (2019). Microfluidic and cross-linking methods for encapsulation of living cells and bacteria-A review. *Analytica Chimica Acta, 1053*, 1−21.

Amoyav, B., & Benny, O. (2019). Microfluidic based fabrication and characterization of highly porous polymeric microspheres. *Polymers, 11*, 419.

Anna, S. L. (2016). Droplets and bubbles in microfluidic devices. *Annual Review of Fluid Mechanics, 48*, 285−309.

Armada-Moreira, A., Taipaleenmäki, E., Itel, F., Zhang, Y., & Städler, B. (2016). Droplet-microfluidics towards the assembly of advanced building blocks in cell mimicry. *Nanoscale, 8*, 19510−19522.

Arriaga, L. R., Datta, S. S., Kim, S.-H., Amstad, E., Kodger, T. E., Monroy, F., et al. (2014). Ultrathin shell double emulsion templated giant unilamellar lipid vesicles with controlled microdomain formation. *Small, 10*, 950−956.

Aubry, G., & Lu, H. (2017). Droplet array for screening acute behaviour response to chemicals in Caenorhabditis elegans. *Lab on a Chip, 17*, 4303−4311.

Autour, A., Bouhedda, F., Cubi, R., & Ryckelynck, M. (2019). Optimization of fluorogenic RNA-based biosensors using droplet-based microfluidic ultrahigh-throughput screening. *Methods, 161*, 46−53.

Autour, A., Westhof, E., & Ryckelynck, M. (2016). iSpinach: a fluorogenic RNA aptamer optimized for in vitro applications. *Nucleic Acids Research, 44*, 2491−2500.

Azizi, M., Zaferani, M., Cheong, S. H., & Abbaspourrad, A. (2019). Pathogenic bacteria detection using RNA-based loop-mediated isothermal-amplification-assisted nucleic acid amplification via droplet microfluidics. *ACS Sensors, 4*, 841−848.

Bandulasena, M. V., Vladisavljević, G. T., & Benyahia, B. (2019). Droplet-based microfluidic method for robust preparation of gold nanoparticles in axisymmetric flow focusing device. *Chemical Engineering Science, 195*, 657−664.

Baret, J.-C., Kleinschmidt, F., El Harrak, A., & Griffiths, A. D. (2009). Kinetic aspects of emulsion stabilization by surfactants: A microfluidic analysis. *Langmuir, 25*, 6088−6093.

Baroud, C. N., Gallaire, F., & Dangla, R. (2010). Dynamics of microfluidic droplets. *Lab on a Chip, 10*, 2032−2045.

Bayoumi, M., Bayley, H., Maglia, G., & Sapra, K. T. (2017). Multi-compartment encapsulation of communicating droplets and droplet networks in hydrogel as a model for artificial cells. *Scientific Reports, 7*, 45167.

Bchellaoui, N., Hayat, Z., Mami, M., Dorbez-Sridi, R., & El Abed, A. I. (2017). Microfluidic-assisted formation of highly monodisperse and mesoporous silica soft microcapsules. *Scientific Reports, 7*, 16326.

Beard, D. A. (2001). Taylor dispersion of a solute in a microfluidic channel. *Journal of Applied Physics, 89*, 4667−4669.

Bithi, S. S., & Vanapalli, S. A. (2017). Microfluidic cell isolation technology for drug testing of single tumor cells and their clusters. *Scientific Reports, 7*, 41707.

Bobo, D., Robinson, K. J., Islam, J., Thurecht, K. J., & Corrie, S. R. (2016). Nanoparticle-based medicines: A review of FDA-approved materials and clinical trials to date. *Pharmaceutical Research, 33*, 2373−2387.

Boybay, M. S., Jiao, A., Glawdel, T., & Ren, C. L. (2013). Microwave sensing and heating of individual droplets in microfluidic devices. *Lab on a Chip, 13*, 3840−3846.

Bringer, M. R., Gerdts, C. J., Song, H., Tice, J. D., & Ismagilov, R. F. (2004). Microfluidic systems for chemical kinetics that rely on chaotic mixing in droplets. *Philosophical Transactions of the Royal Society of London, Series A: Mathematical, Physical and Engineering Sciences, 362*, 1087−1104.

Cao, J., Goldhan, J., Martin, K., & Köhler, J. M. (2013). Investigation of mixture toxicity of widely used drugs caffeine and ampicillin in the presence of an ACE inhibitor on bacterial growth using droplet-based microfluidic technique. *Green Processing and Synthesis, 2*, 591−601.

Cha, C., Oh, J., Kim, K., Qiu, Y., Joh, M., Shin, S. R., et al. (2014). Microfluidics-assisted fabrication of gelatin-silica core–shell microgels for injectable tissue constructs. *Biomacromolecules, 15*, 283−290.

Chen, X., & Ren, C. L. (2017). A microfluidic chip integrated with droplet generation, pairing, trapping, merging, mixing and releasing. *RSC Advances, 7*, 16738−16750.

Chen, Q., Utech, S., Chen, D., Prodanovic, R., Lin, J.-M., & Weitz, D. A. (2016). Controlled assembly of heterotypic cells in a core–shell scaffold: Organ in a droplet. *Lab on a Chip, 16*, 1346−1349.

Chiesa, E., Dorati, R., Modena, T., Conti, B., & Genta, I. (2018). Multivariate analysis for the optimization of microfluidics-assisted nanoprecipitation method intended for the loading of small hydrophilic drugs into PLGA nanoparticles. *International Journal of Pharmaceutics, 536*, 165−177.

Chiu, T.-K., Lei, K.-F., Hsieh, C.-H., Hsiao, H.-B., Wang, H.-M., & Wu, M.-H. (2015). Development of a microfluidic-based optical sensing device for label-free detection of circulating tumor cells (CTCs) through their lactic acid metabolism. *Sensors, 15*, 6789−6806.

Choe, G., Park, J., Park, H., & Lee, J. Y. (2018). Hydrogel biomaterials for stem cell microencapsulation. *Polymers, 10*, 997.

Choi, C.-H., Lee, H., & Weitz, D. A. (2018). Rapid patterning of PDMS microfluidic device wettability using syringe-vacuum-induced segmented flow in nonplanar geometry. *ACS Applied Materials and Interfaces, 10*, 3170−3174.

Choi, C.-H., Weitz, D. A., & Lee, C.-S. (2013). One step formation of controllable complex emulsions: From functional particles to simultaneous encapsulation of hydrophilic and hydrophobic agents into desired position. *Advanced Materials, 25*, 2536−2541.

Chong, D., Liu, X., Ma, H., Huang, G., Han, Y. L., Cui, X., et al. (2015). Advances in fabricating double-emulsion droplets and their biomedical applications. *Microfluidics and Nanofluidics, 19*, 1071–1090.

Chong, Z. Z., Tan, S. H., Gañán-Calvo, A. M., Tor, S. B., Loh, N. H., & Nguyen, N.-T. (2016). Active droplet generation in microfluidics. *Lab on a Chip, 16*, 35–58.

Chung, M. T., Kurabayashi, K., & Cai, D. (2019). Single-cell RT-LAMP mRNA detection by integrated droplet sorting and merging. *Lab on a Chip, 19*, 2425–2434.

Chung, M. T., Núñez, D., Cai, D., & Kurabayashi, K. (2017). Deterministic droplet-based co-encapsulation and pairing of microparticles via active sorting and downstream merging. *Lab on a Chip, 17*, 3664–3671.

Churski, K., Kaminski, T. S., Jakiela, S., Kamysz, W., Baranska-Rybak, W., Weibel, D. B., et al. (2012). Rapid screening of antibiotic toxicity in an automated microdroplet system. *Lab on a Chip, 12*, 1629–1637.

Churski, K., Korczyk, P., & Garstecki, P. (2010). High-throughput automated droplet microfluidic system for screening of reaction conditions. *Lab on a Chip, 10*, 816–818.

Churski, K., Nowacki, M., Korczyk, P. M., & Garstecki, P. (2013). Simple modular systems for generation of droplets on demand. *Lab on a Chip, 13*, 3689–3697.

Clausell-Tormos, J., Lieber, D., Baret, J.-C., El-Harrak, A., Miller, O. J., Frenz, L., et al. (2008). Droplet-based microfluidic platforms for the encapsulation and screening of mammalian cells and multicellular organisms. *Chemistry and Biology, 15*, 427–437.

Collins, D. J., Alan, T., Helmerson, K., & Neild, A. (2013). Surface acoustic waves for on-demand production of picoliter droplets and particle encapsulation. *Lab on a Chip, 13*, 3225–3231.

Collins, D. J., Neild, A., & Ai, Y. (2016). Highly focused high-frequency travelling surface acoustic waves (SAW) for rapid single-particle sorting. *Lab on a Chip, 16*, 471–479.

Collins, D. J., Neild, A., DeMello, A., Liu, A.-Q., & Ai, Y. (2015). The Poisson distribution and beyond: Methods for microfluidic droplet production and single cell encapsulation. *Lab on a Chip, 15*, 3439–3459.

Comunian, T. A., Abbaspourrad, A., Favaro-Trindade, C. S., & Weitz, D. A. (2014). Fabrication of solid lipid microcapsules containing ascorbic acid using a microfluidic technique. *Food Chemistry, 152*, 271–275.

Cong, L., Liang, L., Cao, F., Sun, D., Yue, J., Xu, W., et al. (2019). Distinguishing cancer cell lines at a single living cell level via detection of sialic acid by dual-channel plasmonic imaging and by using a SERS-microfluidic droplet platform. *Microchimica Acta, 186*, 367.

Costantini, M., Guzowski, J., Żuk, P. J., Mozetic, P., De Panfilis, S., Jaroszewicz, J., et al. (2018). Electric field assisted microfluidic platform for generation of tailorable porous microbeads as cell carriers for tissue engineering. *Advanced Functional Materials, 28*, 1800874.

Courtney, M., Chen, X., Chan, S., Mohamed, T., Rao, P. P. N., & Ren, C. L. (2016). Droplet microfluidic system with on-demand trapping and releasing of droplet for drug screening applications. *Analytical Chemistry, 89*, 910–915.

Crawford, D. F., Smith, C. A., & Whyte, G. (2017). Image-based closed-loop feedback for highly mono-dispersed microdroplet production. *Scientific Reports, 7*, 1–9.

Cui, X., Ren, L., Shan, Y., Wang, X., Yang, Z., Li, C., et al. (2018). Smartphone-based rapid quantification of viable bacteria by single-cell microdroplet turbidity imaging. *Analyst, 143*, 3309–3316.

Dai, J., Yang, X., Hamon, M., & Kong, L. (2015). Particle size controlled synthesis of CdS nanoparticles on a microfluidic chip. *Chemical Engineering Journal, 280*, 385−390.

Deshpande, S., Caspi, Y., Meijering, A. E. C., & Dekker, C. (2016). Octanol-assisted liposome assembly on chip. *Nature Communications, 7*, 10447.

Deveza, L., Ashoken, J., Castaneda, G., Tong, X., Keeney, M., Han, L.-H., et al. (2015). Microfluidic synthesis of biodegradable polyethylene-glycol microspheres for controlled delivery of proteins and DNA nanoparticles. *ACS Biomaterials Science and Engineering, 1*, 157−165.

Di Carlo, D. (2009). Inertial microfluidics. *Lab on a Chip, 9*, 3038−3046.

Dittrich, P. S., & Manz, A. (2006). Lab-on-a-chip: Microfluidics in drug discovery. *Nature Reviews Drug Discovery, 5*, 210.

Duarte, J. M., Barbier, I., & Schaerli, Y. (2017). Bacterial microcolonies in gel beads for high-throughput screening of libraries in synthetic biology. *ACS Synthetic Biology, 6*, 1988−1995.

Douliez, J.-P., Perro, A., & Béven, l. (2019). Stabilization of all-in-water emulsions to form capsules as artificial cells. *ChemBioChem, 20*(20), 2546−2552.

Du, X., Li, W., Du, G., Cho, H., Yu, M., Fang, Q., et al. (2018). Droplet array-based 3D coculture system for high-throughput tumor angiogenesis assay. *Analytical Chemistry, 90*, 3253−3261.

Edel, J. B., Fortt, R., deMello, J. C., & deMello, A. J. (2002). Microfluidic routes to the controlled production of nanoparticles. *Chemical Communications*, 1136−1137.

Ekanem, E. E., Zhang, Z., & Vladisavljević, G. T. (2017). Facile microfluidic production of composite polymer core-shell microcapsules and crescent-shaped microparticles. *Journal of Colloid and Interface Science, 498*, 387−394.

Elani, Y., Casadevall i Solvas, X., Edel, J. B., Law, R. V., & Ces, O. (2016). Microfluidic generation of encapsulated droplet interface bilayer networks (multisomes) and their use as cell-like reactors. *Chemical Communications, 52*, 5961−5964.

Elani, Y., Law, R. V., & Ces, O. (2014). Vesicle-based artificial cells as chemical microreactors with spatially segregated reaction pathways. *Nature Communications, 5*, 5305.

Feng, Q., Li, Q., Wen, H., Chen, J., Liang, M., Huang, H., et al. (2019). Injection and self-assembly of bioinspired stem cell-laden gelatin/hyaluronic acid hybrid microgels promote cartilage repair in vivo. *Advanced Functional Materials, 29*, 1906690.

Feng, H., Zheng, T., Li, M., Wu, J., Ji, H., Zhang, J., et al. (2019). Droplet-based microfluidics systems in biomedical applications. *Electrophoresis, 40*, 1580−1590.

Franke, T., Abate, A. R., Weitz, D. A., & Wixforth, A. (2009). Surface acoustic wave (SAW) directed droplet flow in microfluidics for PDMS devices. *Lab on a Chip, 9*, 2625−2627.

Fraser, L. A., Cheung, Y.-W., Kinghorn, A. B., Guo, W., Shiu, S. C.-C., Jinata, C., et al. (2019). Microfluidic technology for nucleic acid aptamer evolution and application. *Advanced Biosystems, 3*, 1900012.

Friddin, M. S., Elani, Y., Trantidou, T., & Ces, O. (2019). New directions for artificial cells using prototyped biosystems. *Analytical Chemistry, 91*, 4921−4928.

Fu, Y., Li, C., Lu, S., Zhou, W., Tang, F., Xie, X. S., et al. (2015). Uniform and accurate single-cell sequencing based on emulsion whole-genome amplification. *Proceedings of the National Academy of Sciences of the United States of America, 112*, 11923−11928.

Gao, R., Cheng, Z., deMello, A. J., & Choo, J. (2016). Wash-free magnetic immunoassay of the PSA cancer marker using SERS and droplet microfluidics. *Lab on a Chip, 16*, 1022−1029.

Geng, T., Novak, R., & Mathies, R. A. (2013). Single-cell forensic short tandem repeat typing within microfluidic droplets. *Analytical Chemistry, 86*, 703−712.

Giuffrida, M. C., Cigliana, G., & Spoto, G. (2018). Ultrasensitive detection of lysozyme in droplet-based microfluidic devices. *Biosensors and Bioelectronics, 104*, 8−14.

Glawdel, T., & Ren, C. L. (2012). Global network design for robust operation of microfluidic droplet generators with pressure-driven flow. *Microfluidics and Nanofluidics, 13*, 469−480.

Gómez-de Pedro, S., Salinas-Castillo, A., Ariza-Avidad, M., Lapresta-Fernández, A., Sánchez-González, C., Martínez-Cisneros, C. S., et al. (2014). Microsystem-assisted synthesis of carbon dots with fluorescent and colorimetric properties for pH detection. *Nanoscale, 6*, 6018−6024.

Griffin, D. R., Weaver, W. M., Scumpia, P. O., Di Carlo, D., & Segura, T. (2015). Accelerated wound healing by injectable microporous gel scaffolds assembled from annealed building blocks. *Nature Materials, 14*, 737−744.

Gu, X., Liu, Y., Chen, G., Wang, H., Shao, C., Chen, Z., et al. (2018). Mesoporous colloidal photonic crystal particles for intelligent drug delivery. *ACS Applied Materials and Interfaces, 10*, 33936−33944.

Guo, S., Kang, G., Phan, D. T., Hsu, M. N., Por, Y. C., & Chen, C. H. (2018a). Polymerization-Induced phase separation formation of structured hydrogel particles via microfluidics for scar therapeutics. *Scientific Reports, 8*, 1−10.

Guo, S., Kang, G., Phan, D. T., Hsu, M. N., Por, Y. C., & Chen, C. H. (2018b). Polymerization-Induced phase separation formation of structured hydrogel particles via microfluidics for scar therapeutics. *Scientific Reports, 8*, 2245.

Haase, M. F., & Brujic, J. (2014). Tailoring of high-order multiple emulsions by the liquid–liquid phase separation of ternary mixtures. *Angewandte Chemie International Edition, 53*, 11793−11797.

Hajji, I., Serra, M., Geremie, L., Ferrante, I., Renault, R., Viovy, J.-L., et al. (2020). Droplet microfluidic platform for fast and continuous-flow RT-qPCR analysis devoted to cancer diagnosis application. *Sensors and Actuators B: Chemical, 303*, 127171.

Hammond, M., Homa, F., Andersson-Svahn, H., Ettema, T. J. G., & Joensson, H. N. (2016). Picodroplet partitioned whole genome amplification of low biomass samples preserves genomic diversity for metagenomic analysis. *Microbiome, 4*, 52.

Håti, A. G., Arnfinnsdottir, N. B., Østevold, C., Sletmoen, M., Etienne, G., Amstad, E., et al. (2016). Microarrays for the study of compartmentalized microorganisms in alginate microbeads and (W/O/W) double emulsions. *RSC Advances, 6*, 114830−114842.

Hébert, M., Courtney, M., & Ren, C. L. (2019). Semi-automated on-demand control of individual droplets with a sample application to a drug screening assay. *Lab on a Chip, 19*, 1490−1501.

He, P., Kim, H., Luo, D., Marquez, M., & Cheng, Z. (2010). Low-frequency ac electro-flow-focusing microfluidic emulsification. *Applied Physics Letters, 96*, 174103.

Herranz-Blanco, B., Arriaga, L. R., Mäkilä, E., Correia, A., Shrestha, N., Mirza, S., et al. (2014). Microfluidic assembly of multistage porous silicon–lipid vesicles for controlled drug release. *Lab on a Chip, 14*, 1083−1086.

Ho, K. K. Y., Lee, J. W., Durand, G., Majumder, S., & Liu, A. P. (2017). Protein aggregation with poly (vinyl) alcohol surfactant reduces double emulsion-encapsulated mammalian cell-free expression. *PLoS One, 12*, e0174689.

Hosokawa, M., Nishikawa, Y., Kogawa, M., & Takeyama, H. (2017). Massively parallel whole genome amplification for single-cell sequencing using droplet microfluidics. *Scientific Reports, 7*, 5199.

Hua, M., Du, Y., Song, J., Sun, M., & He, X. (2019). Surfactant-free fabrication of pNIPAAm microgels in microfluidic devices. *Journal of Materials Research, 34*, 206−213.

Hussain, M., Xie, J., Wang, K., Wang, H., Tan, Z., Liu, Q., et al. (2019). Biodegradable polymer microparticles with tunable shapes and surface textures for enhancement of dendritic cell maturation. *ACS Applied Materials and Interfaces, 11*, 42734−42743.

Hutmacher, D. W. (2000). Scaffolds in tissue engineering bone and cartilage. *Biomaterials, 21*, 2529−2543.

Hu, S., Zeng, S., Zhang, B., Yang, C., Song, P., Danny, T. J. H., et al. (2014). Preparation of biofunctionalized quantum dots using microfluidic chips for bioimaging. *Analyst, 139*, 4681−4690.

Hwang, S., Choi, C.-H., & Lee, C.-S. (2012). Regioselective surface modification of PDMS microfluidic device for the generation of monodisperse double emulsions. *Macromolecular Research, 20*, 422−428.

Jakiela, S., Kaminski, T. S., Cybulski, O., Weibel, D. B., & Garstecki, P. (2013). Bacterial growth and adaptation in microdroplet chemostats. *Angewandte Chemie International Edition, 52*, 8908−8911.

Jakiela, S., Makulska, S., Korczyk, P. M., & Garstecki, P. (2011). Speed of flow of individual droplets in microfluidic channels as a function of the capillary number, volume of droplets and contrast of viscosities. *Lab on a Chip, 11*, 3603−3608.

Jang, M., Jeong, S. W., Bae, N. H., Song, Y., Lee, T. J., Lee, M. K., et al. (2017). Droplet-based digital PCR system for detection of single-cell level of foodborne pathogens. *BioChip Journal, 11*, 329−337.

Jang, M., Koh, I., Lee, S. J., Cheong, J.-H., & Kim, P. (2017). Droplet-based microtumor model to assess cell-ECM interactions and drug resistance of gastric cancer cells. *Scientific Reports, 7*, 1−10.

Jeong, W. J., Kim, J. Y., Choo, J., Lee, E. K., Han, C. S., Beebe, D. J., et al. (2005). Continuous fabrication of biocatalyst immobilized microparticles using photopolymerization and immiscible liquids in microfluidic systems. *Langmuir, 21*, 3738−3741.

Jeong, H.-H., Yelleswarapu, V. R., Yadavali, S., Issadore, D., & Lee, D. (2015). Kilo-scale droplet generation in three-dimensional monolithic elastomer device (3D MED). *Lab on a Chip, 15*, 4387−4392.

Jeyhani, M., Gnyawali, V., Abbasi, N., Hwang, D. K., & Tsai, S. S. H. (2019). Microneedle-assisted microfluidic flow focusing for versatile and high throughput water-in-water droplet generation. *Journal of Colloid and Interface Science, 53*, 382−389.

Jiang, K., Xue, C., Arya, C., Shao, C., George, E. O., DeVoe, D. L., et al. (2011). A new approach to in-situ "micromanufacturing": Microfluidic fabrication of magnetic and fluorescent chains using chitosan microparticles as building blocks. *Small, 7*, 2470−2476.

Ji, X.-H., Cheng, W., Guo, F., Liu, W., Guo, S.-S., He, Z.-K., et al. (2011). On-demand preparation of quantum dot-encoded microparticles using a droplet microfluidic system. *Lab on a Chip, 11*, 2561−2568.

Jo, Y. K., & Lee, D. (2019). Biopolymer microparticles prepared by microfluidics for biomedical applications. *Small*, 1903736.

Kamperman, T., Henke, S., Visser, C. W., Karperien, M., & Leijten, J. (2017). Centering single cells in microgels via delayed crosslinking supports long-term 3D culture by preventing cell escape. *Small, 13*, 1603711.

Kašpar, O., Koyuncu, A. H., Pittermannová, A., Ulbrich, P., & Tokárová, V. (2019). Governing factors for preparation of silver nanoparticles using droplet-based microfluidic device. *Biomedical Microdevices, 21*, 88.

Kaushik, A. M., Hsieh, K., Chen, L., Shin, D. J., Liao, J. C., & Wang, T.-H. (2017). Accelerating bacterial growth detection and antimicrobial susceptibility assessment in integrated picoliter droplet platform. *Biosensors and Bioelectronics, 97*, 260−266.

Kaushik, A. M., Hsieh, K., & Wang, T.-H. (2018). Droplet microfluidics for high-sensitivity and high-throughput detection and screening of disease biomarkers. *Wiley Interdisciplinary Reviews: Nanomedicine and Nanobiotechnology, 10*, e1522.

Khademhosseini, A., Eng, G., Yeh, J., Fukuda, J., Blumling, J., III, Langer, R., et al. (2006). Micromolding of photocrosslinkable hyaluronic acid for cell encapsulation and entrapment. *Journal of Biomedical Materials Research Part A, 79*, 522−532.

Kim, S. C., Premasekharan, G., Clark, I. C., Gemeda, H. B., Paris, P. L., & Abate, A. R. (2017). Measurement of copy number variation in single cancer cells using rapid-emulsification digital droplet MDA. *Microsystems and Nanoengineering, 3*, 17018.

Klein, A. M., Mazutis, L., Akartuna, I., Tallapragada, N., Veres, A., Li, V., et al. (2015). Droplet barcoding for single-cell transcriptomics applied to embryonic stem cells. *Cell, 161*, 1187−1201.

Korczyk, P. M., Van Steijn, V., Blonski, S., Zaremba, D., Beattie, D. A., & Garstecki, P. (2019). Accounting for corner flow unifies the understanding of droplet formation in microfluidic channels. *Nature Communications, 10*, 1−9.

Kubilis, A., Abdulkarim, A., Eissa, A. M., & Cameron, N. R. (2016). Giant polymersome protocells dock with virus particle mimics via multivalent glycan-lectin interactions. *Scientific Reports, 6*, 32414.

Kulesa, A., Kehe, J., Hurtado, J. E., Tawde, P., & Blainey, P. C. (2018). Combinatorial drug discovery in nanoliter droplets. *Proceedings of the National Academy of Sciences of the United States of America, 115*, 6685−6690.

Kumacheva, E., & Garstecki, P. (2011). *Microfluidic reactors for polymer particles*. John Wiley & Sons.

Kuo, C.-T., Wang, J.-Y., Lu, S.-R., Lai, Y.-S., Chang, H.-H., Hsieh, J.-T., et al. (2019). A nanodroplet cell processing platform facilitating drug synergy evaluations for anti-cancer treatments. *Scientific Reports, 9*, 1−9.

Lagus, T. P., & Edd, J. F. (2013). High-throughput co-encapsulation of self-ordered cell trains: Cell pair interactions in microdroplets. *RSC Advances, 3*, 20512−20522.

Lan, J., Chen, J., Li, N., Ji, X., Yu, M., & He, Z. (2016). Microfluidic generation of magnetic-fluorescent Janus microparticles for biomolecular detection. *Talanta, 151*, 126−131.

Langer, K., & Joensson, H. N. (2019). *Rapid production and recovery of cell spheroids by automated droplet microfluidics.* SLAS TECHNOLOGY: Translating Life Sciences Innovation. p. 2472630319877376.

Lee, K., Hong, J., Roh, H. J., Kim, S. H., Lee, H., Lee, S. K., et al. (2017). Dual ionic crosslinked interpenetrating network of alginate-cellulose beads with enhanced mechanical properties for biocompatible encapsulation. *Cellulose, 24*, 4963−4979.

Lee, S. H., Lee, H. W., Kwon, H. G., Lee, J. H., Kim, Y.-H., Jeong, O. C., et al. (2018). A droplet-based microfluidic approach and microsphere-PCR amplification for single-stranded DNA amplicons. *Journal of Visualized Experiments*, e57703.

Lee, S., Thio, S. K., Park, S.-Y., & Bae, S. (2019). An automated 3D-printed smartphone platform integrated with optoelectrowetting (OEW) microfluidic chip for on-site monitoring of viable algae in water. *Harmful Algae, 88*, 101638.

Lienemann, P. S., Rossow, T., Mao, A. S., Vallmajo-Martin, Q., Ehrbar, M., & Mooney, D. J. (2017). Single cell-laden protease-sensitive microniches for long-term culture in 3D. *Lab on a Chip, 17*, 727−737.

Li, S., Hu, K., Cao, W., Sun, Y., Sheng, W., Li, F., et al. (2014). pH-responsive biocompatible fluorescent polymer nanoparticles based on phenylboronic acid for intracellular imaging and drug delivery. *Nanoscale, 6*, 13701−13709.

Li, L., & Ismagilov, R. F. (2010). Protein crystallization using microfluidic technologies based on valves, droplets, and SlipChip. *Annual Review of Biophysics, 39*, 139−158.

Li, L., Lu, M., Fan, Y., Shui, L., Xie, S., Sheng, R., et al. (2019). High-throughput and ultrasensitive single-cell profiling of multiple microRNAs and identification of human cancer. *Chemical Communications, 55*, 10404−10407.

Lim, S. W., Tran, T. M., & Abate, A. R. (2015). PCR-activated cell sorting for cultivation-free enrichment and sequencing of rare microbes. *PLoS One, 10*.

Ling, K., Wu, H., Neish, A. S., & Champion, J. A. (2019). Alginate/chitosan microparticles for gastric passage and intestinal release of therapeutic protein nanoparticles. *Journal of Controlled Release, 295*, 174−186.

Lin, X., Huang, X., Urmann, K., Xie, X., & Hoffmann, M. R. (2019). Digital loop-mediated isothermal amplification on a commercial membrane. *ACS Sensors, 4*, 242−249.

Link, D. R., Anna, S. L., Weitz, D. A., & Stone, H. A. (2004). Geometrically mediated breakup of drops in microfluidic devices. *Physical Review Letters, 92*, 054503.

Li, F., Truong, V. X., Thissen, H., Frith, J. E., & Forsythe, J. S. (2017). Microfluidic encapsulation of human mesenchymal stem cells for articular cartilage tissue regeneration. *ACS Applied Materials and Interfaces, 9*, 8589−8601.

Liu, K., Deng, Y., Zhang, N., Li, S., Ding, H., Guo, F., et al. (2012). Generation of disk-like hydrogel beads for cell encapsulation and manipulation using a droplet-based microfluidic device. *Microfluidics and Nanofluidics, 13*, 761−767.

Liu, J., Guo, Z., & Liang, K. (2019). Biocatalytic metal-organic framework-based artificial cells. *Advanced Functional Materials, 29*, 1905321.

Liu, H., Li, M., Wang, Y., Piper, J., & Jiang, L. (2020). Improving single-cell encapsulation efficiency and reliability through neutral buoyancy of suspension. *Micromachines, 11*, 94.

Liu, H., Qian, X., Wu, Z., Yang, R., Sun, S., & Ma, H. (2016). Microfluidic synthesis of QD-encoded PEGDA microspheres for suspension assay. *Journal of Materials Chemistry B, 4*, 482−488.

Liu, L., Yang, J.-P., Ju, X.-J., Xie, R., Liu, Y.-M., Wang, W., et al. (2011). Monodisperse core-shell chitosan microcapsules for pH-responsive burst release of hydrophobic drugs. *Soft Matter, 7*, 4821−4827.

Li, L., Wang, Q., Feng, J., Tong, L., & Tang, B. (2014). Highly sensitive and homogeneous detection of membrane protein on a single living cell by aptamer and nicking enzyme assisted signal amplification based on microfluidic droplets. *Analytical Chemistry, 86*, 5101−5107.

Li, W., Zhang, L., Ge, X., Xu, B., Zhang, W., Qu, L., et al. (2018). Microfluidic fabrication of microparticles for biomedical applications. *Chemical Society Reviews, 47*, 5646−5683.

Lu, H., Caen, O., Vrignon, J., Zonta, E., El Harrak, Z., Nizard, P., et al. (2017). High throughput single cell counting in droplet-based microfluidics. *Scientific Reports, 7*, 1366.

Lu, A. X., Oh, H., Terrell, J. L., Bentley, W. E., & Raghavan, S. R. (2017). A new design for an artificial cell: Polymer microcapsules with addressable inner compartments that can harbor biomolecules, colloids or microbial species. *Chemical Science, 8*, 6893–6903.

Luo, X., Al-Antaki, A. H. M., Pye, S., Meech, R., Zhang, W., & Raston, C. L. (2018). High-shear-imparted tunable fluorescence in polyethylenimines. *ChemPhotoChem, 2*, 343–348.

Luo, X., Su, P., Zhang, W., & Raston, C. L. (2019). Microfluidic devices in fabricating nano or micromaterials for biomedical applications. *Advanced Materials Technologies, 4*, 1900488.

Macosko, E. Z., Basu, A., Satija, R., Nemesh, J., Shekhar, K., Goldman, M., et al. (2015). Highly parallel genome-wide expression profiling of individual cells using nanoliter droplets. *Cell, 161*, 1202–1214.

Maeki, M., Yamaguchi, H., Tokeshi, M., & Miyazaki, M. (2016). Microfluidic approaches for protein crystal structure analysis. *Analytical Sciences, 32*, 3–9.

Maher, S., Santos, A., Kumeria, T., Kaur, G., Lambert, M., Forward, P., et al. (2017). Multifunctional microspherical magnetic and pH responsive carriers for combination anticancer therapy engineered by droplet-based microfluidics. *Journal of Materials Chemistry B, 5*, 4097–4109.

Majumder, S., Wubshet, N., & Liu, A. P. (2019). Encapsulation of complex solutions using droplet microfluidics towards the synthesis of artificial cells. *Journal of Micromechanics and Microengineering, 29*, 083001.

Makadia, H. K., & Siegel, S. J. (2011). Poly lactic-co-glycolic acid (PLGA) as biodegradable controlled drug delivery carrier. *Polymers, 3*, 1377–1397.

Ma, Y., Luk, A., Young, F. P., Lynch, D., Chua, W., Balakrishnar, B., et al. (2016). Droplet digital PCR based androgen receptor variant 7 (AR-V7) detection from prostate cancer patient blood biopsies. *International Journal of Molecular Sciences, 17*, 1264.

Ma, Y.-D., Luo, K., Chang, W.-H., & Lee, G.-B. (2018). A microfluidic chip capable of generating and trapping emulsion droplets for digital loop-mediated isothermal amplification analysis. *Lab on a Chip, 18*, 296–303.

Ma, Y., Neubauer, M. P., Thiele, J., Fery, A., & Huck, W. T. S. (2014). Artificial microniches for probing mesenchymal stem cell fate in 3D. *Biomaterials Science, 2*, 1661–1671.

Manz, A., Graber, N., & Widmer, H. M. (1990). Miniaturized total chemical analysis systems: A novel concept for chemical sensing. *Sensors and Actuators B: Chemical, 1*, 244–248.

Mao, Z., Guo, F., Xie, Y., Zhao, Y., Lapsley, M. I., Wang, L., et al. (2015). Label-free measurements of reaction kinetics using a droplet-based optofluidic device. *Journal of Laboratory Automation, 20*, 17–24.

Martino, C., & deMello, A. J. (2016). Droplet-based microfluidics for artificial cell generation: A brief review. *Interface Focus, 6*, 20160011.

Martino, C., Kim, S.-H., Horsfall, L., Abbaspourrad, A., Rosser, S. J., Cooper, J., et al. (2012). Protein expression, aggregation, and triggered release from polymersomes as artificial cell-like structures. *Angewandte Chemie International Edition, 51*, 6416–6420.

Mason, A. F., Yewdall, N. A., Welzen, P. L. W., Shao, J., Stevendaal, M., Hest, J. C. M., et al. (2019). Mimicking cellular compartmentalization in a hierarchical protocell through spontaneous spatial organization. *ACS Central Science, 5*, 1360–1365.

Mazutis, L., Gilbert, J., Ung, W. L., Weitz, D. A., Griffiths, A. D., & Heyman, J. A. (2013). Single-cell analysis and sorting using droplet-based microfluidics. *Nature Protocols, 8*, 870.

Miller, O. J., El Harrak, A., Mangeat, T., Baret, J.-C., Frenz, L., El Debs, B., et al. (2012). High-resolution dose–response screening using droplet-based microfluidics. *Proceedings of the National Academy of Sciences of the United States of America, 109*, 378−383.

Moon, H.-S., Je, K., Min, J.-W., Park, D., Han, K.-Y., Shin, S.-H., et al. (2018). Inertial-ordering-assisted droplet microfluidics for high-throughput single-cell RNA-sequencing. *Lab on a Chip, 18*, 775−784.

Mu, X.-T., Ju, X.-J., Zhang, L., Huang, X.-B., Faraj, Y., Liu, Z., et al. (2019). Chitosan microcapsule membranes with nanoscale thickness for controlled release of drugs. *Journal of Membrane Science, 590*, 117275.

Nawar, S., Stolaroff, J. K., Ye, C., Wu, H., Xin, F., Weitz, D. A., et al. (2020). Parallelizable microfluidic dropmakers with multilayer geometry for the generation of double emulsions. *Lab on a Chip, 20*, 147−154.

Nguyen, T. H., Chen, X., Sedighi, A., Krull, U. J., & Ren, C. L. (2018). A droplet-based microfluidic platform for rapid immobilization of quantum dots on individual magnetic microbeads. *Microfluidics and Nanofluidics, 22*, 63.

Nishikawa, Y., Hosokawa, M., Maruyama, T., Yamagishi, K., Mori, T., & Takeyama, H. (2015). Monodisperse picoliter droplets for low-bias and contamination-free reactions in single-cell whole genome amplification. *PLoS One, 10*, e0138733.

Nisisako, T., Ando, T., & Hatsuzawa, T. (2012). High-volume production of single and compound emulsions in a microfluidic parallelization arrangement coupled with coaxial annular world-to-chip interfaces. *Lab on a Chip, 12*, 3426−3435.

Niu, X., Gulati, S., Edel, J. B., & deMello, A. J. (2008). Pillar-induced droplet merging in microfluidic circuits. *Lab on a Chip, 8*, 1837−1841.

Novak, R., Zeng, Y., Shuga, J., Venugopalan, G., Fletcher, D. A., Smith, M. T., et al. (2011). Single-cell multiplex gene detection and sequencing with microfluidically generated agarose emulsions. *Angewandte Chemie International Edition, 50*, 390−395.

Omidi, M., Hashemi, M., & Tayebi, L. (2019). Microfluidic synthesis of PLGA/carbon quantum dot microspheres for vascular endothelial growth factor delivery. *RSC Advances, 9*, 33246−33256.

Paras, S. V., & Kanaris, A. G. (2019). *Experimental and numerical studies in biomedical engineering*. Multidisciplinary Digital Publishing Institute.

Park, Y.-H., Lee, D.-H., Um, E., & Park, J.-K. (2016). On-chip generation of monodisperse giant unilamellar lipid vesicles containing quantum dots. *Electrophoresis, 37*, 1353−1358.

Park, H.-I., & Park, S.-Y. (2018). Smart fluorescent hydrogel glucose biosensing microdroplets with dual-mode fluorescence quenching and size reduction. *ACS Applied Materials and Interfaces, 10*, 30172−30179.

Paterson, D. J., Reboud, J., Wilson, R., Tassieri, M., & Cooper, J. M. (2014). Integrating microfluidic generation, handling and analysis of biomimetic giant unilamellar vesicles. *Lab on a Chip, 14*, 1806−1810.

Pennemann, H., Watts, P., Haswell, S. J., Hessel, V., & Löwe, H. (2004). Benchmarking of microreactor applications. *Organic Process Research and Development, 8*, 422−439.

Pepe, A., Podesva, P., & Simone, G. (2017). Tunable uptake/release mechanism of protein microgel particles in biomimicking environment. *Scientific Reports, 7*, 6014.

Postek, W., Kaminski, T. S., & Garstecki, P. (2017). A precise and accurate microfluidic droplet dilutor. *Analyst, 142*, 2901−2911.

Qin, D., Xia, Y., & Whitesides, G. M. (2010). Soft lithography for micro-and nanoscale patterning. *Nature Protocols, 5*, 491.

Qiu, L., Wimmers, F., Weiden, J., Heus, H. A., Tel, J., & Figdor, C. G. (2017). A membrane-anchored aptamer sensor for probing IFNγ secretion by single cells. *Chemical Communications, 53*, 8066–8069.

Qu, K., Wang, J., Ren, J., & Qu, X. (2013). Carbon dots prepared by hydrothermal treatment of dopamine as an effective fluorescent sensing platform for the label-free detection of iron (III) ions and dopamine. *Chemistry–A European Journal, 19*, 7243–7249.

Rane, T. D., Chen, L., Zec, H. C., & Wang, T.-H. (2015). Microfluidic continuous flow digital loop-mediated isothermal amplification (LAMP). *Lab on a Chip, 15*, 776–782.

Rhee, M., Light, Y. K., Meagher, R. J., & Singh, A. K. (2016). Digital droplet multiple displacement amplification (ddMDA) for whole genome sequencing of limited DNA samples. *PLoS One, 11*, e0153699.

Ribeiro-Samy, S., Oliveira, M. I., Pereira-Veiga, T., Muinelo-Romay, L., Carvalho, S., Gaspar, J., et al. (2019). Fast and efficient microfluidic cell filter for isolation of circulating tumor cells from unprocessed whole blood of colorectal cancer patients. *Scientific Reports, 9*, 1–12.

Romanowsky, M. B., Abate, A. R., Rotem, A., Holtze, C., & Weitz, D. A. (2012). High throughput production of single core double emulsions in a parallelized microfluidic device. *Lab on a Chip, 12*, 802–807.

Sabhachandani, P., Motwani, V., Cohen, N., Sarkar, S., Torchilin, V., & Konry, T. (2016). Generation and functional assessment of 3D multicellular spheroids in droplet based microfluidics platform. *Lab on a Chip, 16*, 497–505.

Sabhachandani, P., Sarkar, S., Zucchi, P. C., Whitfield, B. A., Kirby, J. E., Hirsch, E. B., et al. (2017). Integrated microfluidic platform for rapid antimicrobial susceptibility testing and bacterial growth analysis using bead-based biosensor via fluorescence imaging. *Microchimica Acta, 184*, 4619–4628.

Sakai, S., Ito, S., Inagaki, H., Hirose, K., Matsuyama, T., Taya, M., et al. (2011). Cell-enclosing gelatin-based microcapsule production for tissue engineering using a microfluidic flow-focusing system. *Biomicrofluidics, 5*, 013402.

Sart, S., Tomasi, R. F.-X., Amselem, G., & Baroud, C. N. (2017). Multiscale cytometry and regulation of 3D cell cultures on a chip. *Nature Communications, 8*, 469.

Scanlon, T. C., Dostal, S. M., & Griswold, K. E. (2014). A high-throughput screen for antibiotic drug discovery. *Biotechnology and Bioengineering, 111*, 232–243.

Schlicht, B., & Zagnoni, M. (2015). Droplet-interface-bilayer assays in microfluidic passive networks. *Scientific Reports, 5*, 9951.

Schoendube, J., Wright, D., Zengerle, R., & Koltay, P. (2015). Single-cell printing based on impedance detection. *Biomicrofluidics, 9*, 014117.

Schuler, F., Siber, C., Hin, S., Wadle, S., Paust, N., Zengerle, R., et al. (2016). Digital droplet LAMP as a microfluidic app on standard laboratory devices. *Analytical Methods, 8*, 2750–2755.

Seo, M., Gorelikov, I., Williams, R., & Matsuura, N. (2010). Microfluidic assembly of monodisperse, nanoparticle-incorporated perfluorocarbon microbubbles for medical imaging and therapy. *Langmuir, 26*, 13855–13860.

Shah, R. K., Kim, J.-W., Agresti, J. J., Weitz, D. A., & Chu, L.-Y. (2008). Fabrication of monodisperse thermosensitive microgels and gel capsules in microfluidic devices. *Soft Matter, 4*, 2303–2309.

Shembekar, N., Chaipan, C., Utharala, R., & Merten, C. A. (2016). Droplet-based microfluidics in drug discovery, transcriptomics and high-throughput molecular genetics. *Lab on a Chip, 16*, 1314−1331.

Shembekar, N., Hu, H., Eustace, D., & Merten, C. A. (2018). Single-cell droplet microfluidic screening for antibodies specifically binding to target cells. *Cell Reports, 22*, 2206−2215.

Shimanovich, U., Efimov, I., Mason, T. O., Flagmeier, P., Buell, A. K., Gedanken, A., et al. (2015). Protein microgels from amyloid fibril networks. *ACS Nano, 9*, 43−51.

Shi, W., & Weitz, D. A. (2017). Polymer phase separation in a microcapsule shell. *Macromolecules, 50*, 7681−7686.

Shum, H. C., Kim, J.-W., & Weitz, D. A. (2008). Microfluidic fabrication of monodisperse biocompatible and biodegradable polymersomes with controlled permeability. *Journal of the American Chemical Society, 130*, 9543−9549.

Sidore, A. M., Lan, F., Lim, S. W., & Abate, A. R. (2015). Enhanced sequencing coverage with digital droplet multiple displacement amplification. *Nucleic Acids Research, 44*, e66.

Siltanen, C., Yaghoobi, M., Haque, A., You, J., Lowen, J., Soleimani, M., et al. (2016). Microfluidic fabrication of bioactive microgels for rapid formation and enhanced differentiation of stem cell spheroids. *Acta Biomaterialia, 34*, 125−132.

Simone, G., & Donk, O. (2019). On demand coalescence in microchannel: Viscosity matters. *Chemical Engineering Science, 208*, 115173.

Spits, C., Le Caignec, C., De Rycke, M., Van Haute, L., Van Steirteghem, A., Liebaers, I., et al. (2006). Whole-genome multiple displacement amplification from single cells. *Nature Protocols, 1*, 1965.

Spoelstra, W. K., Deshpande, S., & Dekker, C. (2018). Tailoring the appearance: What will synthetic cells look like? *Current Opinion in Biotechnology, 51*, 47−56.

Stein, H., Spindler, S., Bonakdar, N., Wang, C., & Sandoghdar, V. (2017). Production of isolated giant unilamellar vesicles under high salt concentrations. *Frontiers in Physiology, 8*, 63.

Sundararajan, P., Wang, J., Rosen, L. A., Procopio, A., & Rosenberg, K. (2018). Engineering polymeric Janus particles for drug delivery using microfluidic solvent dissolution approach. *Chemical Engineering Science, 178*, 199−210.

Sun, X.-T., Guo, R., Wang, D.-N., Wei, Y.-Y., Yang, C.-G., & Xu, Z.-R. (2019). Microfluidic preparation of polymer-lipid Janus microparticles with staged drug release property. *Journal of Colloid and Interface Science, 553*, 631−638.

Sun, Q., Tan, S. H., Chen, Q., Ran, R., Hui, Y., Chen, D., et al. (2018). Microfluidic formation of coculture tumor spheroids with stromal cells as a novel 3D tumor model for drug testing. *ACS Biomaterials Science and Engineering, 4*, 4425−4433.

Tan, W.-H., & Takeuchi, S. (2007). Monodisperse alginate hydrogel microbeads for cell encapsulation. *Advanced Materials, 19*, 2696−2701.

Terekhov, S. S., Smirnov, I. V., Stepanova, A. V., Bobik, T. V., Mokrushina, Y. A., Ponomarenko, N. A., et al. (2017). Microfluidic droplet platform for ultrahigh-throughput single-cell screening of biodiversity. *Proceedings of the National Academy of Sciences of the United States of America, 114*, 2550−2555.

Thibault, D., Jensen, P. A., Wood, S., Qabar, C., Clark, S., Shainheit, M. G., et al. (2019). Droplet Tn-Seq combines microfluidics with Tn-Seq for identifying complex single-cell phenotypes. *Nature Communications, 10*, 1−13.

Thorsen, T., Roberts, R. W., Arnold, F. H., & Quake, S. R. (2001). Dynamic pattern formation in a vesicle-generating microfluidic device. *Physical Review Letters, 86*, 4163.

Trantidou, T., Friddin, M., Elani, Y., Brooks, N. J., Law, R. V., Seddon, J. M., et al. (2017). Engineering compartmentalized biomimetic micro-and nanocontainers. *ACS Nano, 11*, 6549−6565.

Utech, S., Prodanovic, R., Mao, A. S., Ostafe, R., Mooney, D. J., & Weitz, D. A. (2015). Microfluidic generation of monodisperse, structurally homogeneous alginate microgels for cell encapsulation and 3D cell culture. *Advanced Healthcare Materials, 4*, 1628−1633.

Velasco, D., Tumarkin, E., & Kumacheva, E. (2012). Microfluidic encapsulation of cells in polymer microgels. *Small, 8*, 1633−1642.

Wan, L., Chen, T., Gao, J., Dong, C., Wong, A. H.-H., Jia, Y., et al. (2017). A digital microfluidic system for loop-mediated isothermal amplification and sequence specific pathogen detection. *Scientific Reports, 7*, 1−11.

Wan, L., Gao, J., Chen, T., Dong, C., Li, H., Wen, Y.-Z., et al. (2019). LampPort: A handheld digital microfluidic device for loop-mediated isothermal amplification (LAMP). *Biomedical Microdevices, 21*(9).

Wang, J. D., Douville, N. J., Takayama, S., & ElSayed, M. (2012). Quantitative analysis of molecular absorption into PDMS microfluidic channels. *Annals of Biomedical Engineering, 40*, 1862−1873.

Wang, C., Ge, Q., Ting, D., Nguyen, D., Shen, H.-R., Chen, J., et al. (2004). Molecularly engineered poly (ortho ester) microspheres for enhanced delivery of DNA vaccines. *Nature Materials, 3*, 190−196.

Wang, H., Liu, H., Liu, H., Su, W., Chen, W., & Qin, J. (2019). One-step generation of core-shell gelatin methacrylate (GelMA) microgels using a droplet microfluidic system. *Advanced Materials Technologies, 4*, 1800632.

Wang, K., Lu, Y. C., Xu, J. H., & Luo, G. S. (2009). Determination of dynamic interfacial tension and its effect on droplet formation in the T-shaped microdispersion process. *Langmuir, 25*, 2153−2158.

Wang, Y., Shang, L., Chen, G., Shao, C., Liu, Y., Lu, P., et al. (2018). Pollen-inspired microparticles with strong adhesion for drug delivery. *Applied Materials Today, 13*, 303−309.

Wang, Y., & Wang, J. (2014). Mixed hydrogel bead-based tumor spheroid formation and anticancer drug testing. *Analyst, 139*, 2449−2458.

Wang, Y., Zhao, L., Tian, C., Ma, C., & Wang, J. (2015). Geometrically controlled preparation of various cell aggregates by droplet-based microfluidics. *Analytical Methods, 7*, 10040−10051.

Watanabe, M., Kenmotsu, H., Ko, R., Wakuda, K., Ono, A., Imai, H., et al. (2018). Isolation and molecular analysis of circulating tumor cells from lung cancer patients using a microfluidic chip type cell sorter. *Cancer Science, 109*, 2539−2548.

Watanabe, T., Ono, T., & Kimura, Y. (2011). Continuous fabrication of monodisperse polylactide microspheres by droplet-to-particle technology using microfluidic emulsification and emulsion–solvent diffusion. *Soft Matter, 7*, 9894−9897.

Wen, H., Yu, Y., Zhu, G., Jiang, L., & Qin, J. (2015). A droplet microchip with substance exchange capability for the developmental study of C. elegans. *Lab on a Chip, 15*, 1905−1911.

Wen, N., Zhao, Z., Fan, B., Chen, D., Men, D., Wang, J., et al. (2016). Development of droplet microfluidics enabling high-throughput single-cell analysis. *Molecules, 21*, 881.

Wong, A. H.-H., Li, H., Jia, Y., Mak, P.-I., Silva Martins, R. P., Liu, Y., et al. (2017). Drug screening of cancer cell lines and human primary tumors using droplet microfluidics. *Scientific Reports, 7*, 9109.
Wong, H., Radke, C. J., & Morris, S. (1995a). The motion of long bubbles in polygonal capillaries. Part 1. Thin films. *Journal of Fluid Mechanics, 292*, 71−94.
Wong, H., Radke, C. J., & Morris, S. (1995b). The motion of long bubbles in polygonal capillaries. Part 2. Drag, fluid pressure and fluid flow. *Journal of Fluid Mechanics, 292*, 95−110.
Wong, D., & Ren, C. L. (2016). Microfluidic droplet trapping, splitting and merging with feedback controls and state space modelling. *Lab on a Chip, 16*, 3317−3329.
Won, J., Lee, W., & Song, S. (2017). Estimation of the thermocapillary force and its applications to precise droplet control on a microfluidic chip. *Scientific Reports, 7*, 1−9.
Wu, L. Y., Ross, B. M., Hong, S., & Lee, L. P. (2010). Bioinspired nanocorals with decoupled cellular targeting and sensing functionality. *Small, 6*, 503−507.
Xia, B., Jiang, Z., Debroy, D., Li, D., & Oakey, J. (2017). Cytocompatible cell encapsulation via hydrogel photopolymerization in microfluidic emulsion droplets. *Biomicrofluidics, 11*, 044102.
Xie, H., She, Z.-G., Wang, S., Sharma, G., & Smith, J. W. (2012). One-step fabrication of polymeric Janus nanoparticles for drug delivery. *Langmuir, 28*, 4459−4463.
Xu, Q., Hashimoto, M., Dang, T. T., Hoare, T., Kohane, D. S., Whitesides, G. M., et al. (2009). Preparation of monodisperse biodegradable polymer microparticles using a microfluidic flow-focusing device for controlled drug delivery. *Small, 5*, 1575−1581.
Yadavali, S., Jeong, H.-H., Lee, D., & Issadore, D. (2018). Silicon and glass very large scale microfluidic droplet integration for terascale generation of polymer microparticles. *Nature Communications, 9*, 1222.
Yamada, M., Hori, A., Sugaya, S., Yajima, Y., Utoh, R., Yamato, M., et al. (2015). Cell-sized condensed collagen microparticles for preparing microengineered composite spheroids of primary hepatocytes. *Lab on a Chip, 15*, 3941−3951.
Yan, Y., Boey, D., Ng, L. T., Gruber, J., Bettiol, A., Thakor, N. V., et al. (2016). Continuous-flow C. elegans fluorescence expression analysis with real-time image processing through microfluidics. *Biosensors and Bioelectronics, 77*, 428−434.
Yang, C.-G., Xu, Z.-R., & Wang, J.-H. (2010). Manipulation of droplets in microfluidic systems. *TrAC Trends in Analytical Chemistry, 29*, 141−157.
Yesiloz, G., Boybay, M. S., & Ren, C. L. (2017). Effective thermo-capillary mixing in droplet microfluidics integrated with a microwave heater. *Analytical Chemistry, 89*, 1978−1984.
Ying, D., Zhang, K., Li, N., Ai, X., Liang, Q., Wang, Y., et al. (2012). A droplet-based microfluidic device for long-term culture and longitudinal observation of Caenorhabditis elegans. *BioChip Journal, 6*, 197−205.
Zamora-Mora, V., Velasco, D., Hernández, R., Mijangos, C., & Kumacheva, E. (2014). Chitosan/agarose hydrogels: Cooperative properties and microfluidic preparation. *Carbohydrate Polymers, 111*, 348−355.
Zare, R. N., & Kim, S. (2010). Microfluidic platforms for single-cell analysis. *Annual Review of Biomedical Engineering, 12*, 187−201.
Zhai, J., Yi, S., Jia, Y., Mak, P.-I., & Martins, R. P. (2019). Cell-based drug screening on microfluidics. *TrAC Trends in Analytical Chemistry, 117*, 231−241.

Zhang, L., Chen, K., Zhang, H., Pang, B., Choi, C.-H., Mao, A. S., et al. (2018). Microfluidic templated multicompartment microgels for 3D encapsulation and pairing of single cells. *Small, 14*, 1702955.

Zhang, Y., Ho, Y.-P., Chiu, Y.-L., Chan, H. F., Chlebina, B., Schuhmann, T., et al. (2013). A programmable microenvironment for cellular studies via microfluidics-generated double emulsions. *Biomaterials, 34*, 4564−4572.

Zhang, Y., Ye, W., Yang, C., & Xu, Z. (2019). Simultaneous quantitative detection of multiple tumor markers in microfluidic nanoliter-volume droplets. *Talanta, 205*, 120096.

Zhang, W. Y., Zhang, W., Liu, Z., Li, C., Zhu, Z., & Yang, C. J. (2011). Highly parallel single-molecule amplification approach based on agarose droplet polymerase chain reaction for efficient and cost-effective aptamer selection. *Analytical Chemistry, 84*, 350−355.

Zhao, C.-X., He, L., Qiao, S. Z., & Middelberg, A. P. J. (2011). Nanoparticle synthesis in microreactors. *Chemical Engineering Science, 66*, 1463−1479.

Zhao, X., Liu, S., Yildirimer, L., Zhao, H., Ding, R., Wang, H., et al. (2016). Injectable stem cell-laden photocrosslinkable microspheres fabricated using microfluidics for rapid generation of osteogenic tissue constructs. *Advanced Functional Materials, 26*, 2809−2819.

Zheng, G. X. Y., Terry, J. M., Belgrader, P., Ryvkin, P., Bent, Z. W., Wilson, R., et al. (2017). Massively parallel digital transcriptional profiling of single cells. *Nature Communications, 8*, 14049.

Zhong, J., Riordon, J., Wu, T., Edwards, H., Wheeler, A. R., Pardee, K., et al. (2020). When robotics met fluidics. *Lab on a Chip, 20*(4), 709−716.

Zhou, H., & Yao, S. (2014). A facile on-demand droplet microfluidic system for lab-on-a-chip applications. *Microfluidics and Nanofluidics, 16*, 667−675.

Zhu, Q., Gao, Y., Yu, B., Ren, H., Qiu, L., Han, S., et al. (2012). Self-priming compartmentalization digital LAMP for point-of-care. *Lab on a Chip, 12*, 4755−4763.

Zhu, P., & Wang, L. (2017). Passive and active droplet generation with microfluidics: A review. *Lab on a Chip, 17*, 34−75.

Controlled drug delivery using microdevices

Ning Gao[1], XiuJun (James) Li[2]
[1]RD&E Dispensing Systems Engineering, Sensor Technology, Ecolab, Naperville, IL, United States; [2]Department of Chemistry and Biochemistry, University of Texas at El Paso, El Paso, TX, United States

Guided reading questions:

1. What working principles are used in the microreservoir-based and the micro/nanofluidic-based drug delivery systems?
2. How different types of drug delivery devices are fabricated?

5.1 Introduction

Drug delivery is the method or process of administering pharmaceutical compounds to achieve a therapeutic effect on disease treatment. Conventional dosage means, such as oral delivery and injection, are the predominant routes for drug administration. The main drawbacks of these types of dosages are nonlocal treatment and toxic to healthy tissues (Sharma et al., 2006). Effective drug delivery plays a critical role in disease treatment. With the development of advanced manufacturing and materials science, a variety of drug delivery devices have been created for controlled drug delivery. The distinct drug delivery devices that allow precise, local, and controlled dosing with lower toxicity have tremendous potential to address unmet medical needs. The approach of drug release has shown a significant impact on therapeutic efficacy. Ideally, it should maintain drug levels within a therapeutic window to avoid potential health hazards, maximize therapeutic efficiency, and provide a well-controlled drug dose. A drug when is used above the therapeutic window will be toxic, and below the therapeutic window will lose efficacy.

Conventional drug-delivery systems generally have a high initial level of the drug after the first administration, followed by a sharp decrease in blood concentration (Fig. 5.1(a)), in many cases resulting in a lower therapeutic efficacy and severe side effects. Controlled drug delivery aims to inject drugs at desired rates and time, thus enhancing the therapeutic efficacy and minimizing the toxicity. Fig. 5.1(b) shows two profiles of the most common time-depended release, sustained and pulsatile release. A sustained release can offer a constant drug concentration within the therapeutic window. However, a pulsatile release provides a continuous burst drug delivery. Based on compounds or therapeutic needs, drug delivery in different strategies can

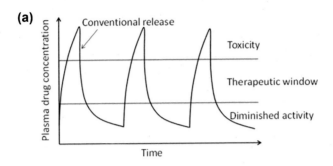

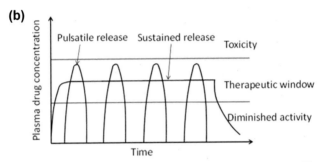

Figure 5.1 Profile of conventional, sustained, and pulsatile drug release. (a) Plasma concentration versus time curve for conventional drug administration. (b) Plasma concentration versus time curve for pulsatile and sustained drug release.

improve the treatment efficiency. Most of the disease treatments require sustained drug delivery at a constant rate over long periods. For certain drugs, such as insulin and hormones, the drug release should mimic the body's natural pulsatile.

In recent years, with several remarkable features, microfluidics has been utilized to address the above issues for more efficient therapy (Li, 2016; Riahi et al., 2015; Sanjay et al., 2018). For example, microfluidic systems are capable of: (1) precisely handling and manipulating the drug in nanoliter volumes, (2) a localized/tunable drug release to minimize side effects on healthy tissues, (3) integrating with sensing function for responsive drug administration, and (4) reducing degradation of drugs with a short lifetime or high risk of cytotoxicity. Over the years, a variety of microfluidic drug delivery systems have been created by different methods and materials, typically including polymer and silicon-based microneedles, microreservoirs, and microfluidic systems. Controlled drug delivery on these devices can be triggered by different stimuli and different microfluidic systems. Here, to avoid duplication with other chapters dedicated to microneedles, we will just focus on the microreservoir and micro/nanofluidic devices.

5.2 Microreservoir-based drug delivery systems

5.2.1 Working principle

The microreservoir-based drug delivery system typically consists of reservoirs containing drugs, controlled release systems, biodegradable polymers, or metallic layers as membranes. Individual or multiple drugs can be sealed in a single or multiple reservoirs, isolating them from the environment. Generally, the metallic or polymer layer covering the reservoir is opened or degraded on demand to expose their contents to the body. The covers or reservoirs are triggered by different mechanisms, such as temperature/thermal (Elman, Masi, Cima, & Langer, 2010; Prescott et al., 2006), light (Timko et al., 2014), ultrasound (Husseini & Pitt, 2008), and magnetic (Pirmoradi, Jackson, Burt, & Chiao, 2011) and electric fields (Fine et al., 2011; John Santini Jr, Cima, & Langer, 1999) to release the drug.

5.2.2 Microreservoir fabrication

Microreservoirs are usually fabricated with silicon and polymers. A microelectromechanical system (MEMS) process—deposition, lithography, patterning, and etching—enables to produce a desired configuration of features on the microsized devices, such as reservoirs, valves, and membranes to trigger systems. Silicon-based microreservoirs are commonly created by MEMS manufacturing techniques, such as bulk micromachining and surface micromachining. Fig. 5.2a is a schematic of a typical fabrication process of bulk micromachining (Ziaie, Baldi, Lei, Gu, & Siegel, 2004). It starts with anisotropic silicon etch using an oxide mask (Fig. 5.2a (i, ii)), and then followed by oxide deposition through conformal plasma-enhanced chemical vapor deposition (Fig. 5.2a (iii)). Subsequently, an anisotropic oxide etch is used to remove the oxide at the bottom of the trenches leaving the sidewall oxide intact (Fig. 5.2a (iv)). In the end, isotropic silicon etch (SF_6) is performed which results in undercut and finalization of the silicon structures (Fig. 5.2a (v)). Surface micromachining usually includes three steps: (1) construct a sacrificially patterned layer on the top of a silicon substrate, (2) deposit the structural material, and (3) remove the sacrificial layer for the desired microstructures. See Chapter 1 for more details of microfabrication.

For polymer-based devices, photolithography, replica molding, and surface machining are three major fabrication techniques (Hand & Gärtner, 2008). Among these three techniques, photolithograph allows constructing devices with thin membranes. SU-8 and poly(methyl methacrylate) (PMMA) are two popular polymers used in the fabrication process. Using SU-8 as an example, the photolithography fabrication process is illustrated in Fig. 5.2b (Truong and Nguyen, 2004). Two techniques, molding or embossing, can be utilized to construct polymeric structures. Here, for the molding technique, a master mold is generally created with a hard material, like silicon wafer, through a standard MEMS fabrication process. A prepolymer is deposited in the mold and solidified after surface treatment to reduce the adhesion of the mold to the

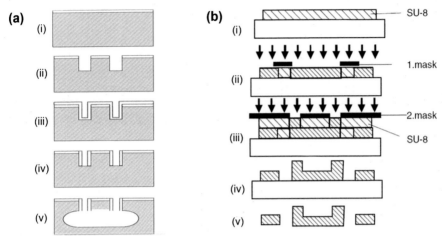

Figure 5.2 Microfabrication of microreservoir-based devices (a) Cross-section of bulk micromachining process include (i) wafer with oxide layer, (ii) anisotropic oxide etch,
(iii) deposition, (iv) anisotropic oxide etch, and (v) undercut. (b) Schematic of the photolithographic steps with an SU-8 photoresist. (i) Spin-coating SU-8 photoresist on silicon. (ii) SU-8 was exposed to UV light using the first mask. (iii) The second mask was used for the second exposure. (iv) The two SU-8 layers were hard baked and developed using propylene glycol methyl ether (PGMEA). (v) The SU-8 discs were released in 30% KOH solution.
(a) Copyright permission from Elsevier (Ziaie et al., 2004). (b) Copyright permission from IOP Science (Truong & Nguyen, 2004).

polymeric materials. The polymeric structure is then removed. The advantage of molding is that the mold can be repeatedly used to create microsize structures. Surface machining capable of creating a small size structure is another important technique to build polymeric structures on the top of a silicon substrate. However, due to the increased surface nonplanarity with the additional layer, there are limitations when creating a multilayer structure. To date, the polymer-based device has attracted more attention due to a better mechanical match with tissues.

5.2.3 Applications
5.2.3.1 Silicon-based devices

Microreservoir-based devices have been developed over the years (Staples, 2010). Silicon-based microreservoirs typically have an array of cavities with metallic walls. The top and bottom basis can be sealed by metallic or polymeric layers. Drugs are released from microreservoirs when the sealed layer is opened. Fig. 5.3(a) is an example of the multipulse drug delivery system which was fabricated on a silicon substrate using electrochemical dissolution to control the drug release (John Santini Jr et al., 1999). Gold membranes with excellent biocompatible properties as anodes

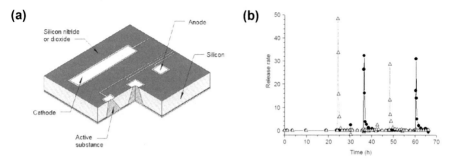

Figure 5.3 (a) A prototype microchip for controlled release showing the shape of a single reservoir. (b) Pulsatile release of multiple substances from a single microchip device. Copyright permission from Nature publishing group (John Santini Jr et al., 1999).

are on top of the reservoirs, protecting drug exposure before the trigger. Gold anodes were dissolved in the presence of chloride ions when anodic voltage was applied to the membrane. The drug, 20 nL each reservoir, was released after the application of a voltage for several seconds. This profile of drug release presented a burst drug delivery. Fig. 5.3(b) shows the drug release profile of a prototype device filled with two model chemicals. The results demonstrated that the activation of each reservoir was capable of individual control with a separate circuit. Varying amounts of drugs in solid, liquid, or gel could be released into solution in a pulsatile manner, a continuous manner, or a combination of both. In addition, the applied potential of the device was just 1.04 V versus saturated calomel electrode (SCE) with low power consumption.

More recently, Microchips Inc. created a controlled pulsatile release of the polypeptide leuprolide from microchip implants over 6 months in dogs (Prescott et al., 2006). In this design, each microchip contains an array of discrete 300 nL reservoirs from which dose delivery can be individually controlled by telemetry (Fig. 5.4). The filled and titanium hermetically sealed chip was electrically connected to wireless communication hardware, power supply, and circuit boards of the implant (Fig. 5.4(c)). The implant was remotely programmed to open selected reservoirs, initiating drug released. The profile of the maximum drug concentration (C_{max}) in Fig. 5.4(d) showed release kinetics of the drug over a period of 25 weeks.

As a traditional technique, electrothermal induction has also been applied in controlled drug delivery (Elman et al., 2010). In this work, an electrothermally induced single reservoir was sealed by a silicon nitride membrane. A gold strip deposited on the silicon nitride membrane served as a fuse to control the drug release. Activation caused the thermal shock of the suspended membrane allowing the drugs inside of the reservoir to diffuse out into the target region. Engineering the size and thickness of fuses can vary the flux of the multiplex reservoirs and provide the release rate on demand. This work explored a fuse activation mechanism that operates controlled release via an electrothermal approach. Because the fuse for opening membranes is geometrically laid out on the weakest point of the membranes, it has low energy consumption.

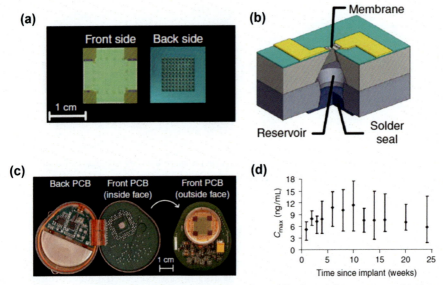

Figure 5.4 Images of the microchip reservoirs and implantable drug delivery system. (a) Front and back of the 100-reservoir microchip. (b) Representation of a single reservoir. (c) Electronic components on the printed circuit board (PCB) in the device package. (d) Average C_{max} for each release event throughout the 6-month study.
Copyright permission from Nature publishing group (Prescott et al., 2006).

The energy consumption for the in-vitro release is approximately 134 μJ, which reduced four orders of magnitude over the previous devices made with a full gold membrane. The reported device can provide a sustained drug release for more than 200 hours.

5.2.3.2 Polymer-based device

Polymer devices, as low-cost drug delivery systems, have been successfully fabricated for the administration of biopharmaceuticals. For the polymer-based devices, the time of drug release can be controlled with the different biodegradable rates of the materials used, the molecular mass, the composition, and the thickness of the membranes. In the Fig. 5.5(a), a multipulse drug delivery device, with 1.2 cm in diameter and 480–560 μm thick, consists of 36 poly (L-lactic acid) reservoirs covered with poly (D, L-lactic-co-glycolic acid) (PLGA) membrane (Richards Grayson et al., 2003). This device allows drug release from reservoirs maintained over a period of months. Fig. 5.5(b) shows the percentage of initial loading released from the representative device, in which both heparin and dextran were loaded into reservoirs sealed with different molecular weight PLGA. The in vivo study of the devices exhibited a pulsatile release that was analogous to that observed in other in-vitro studies.

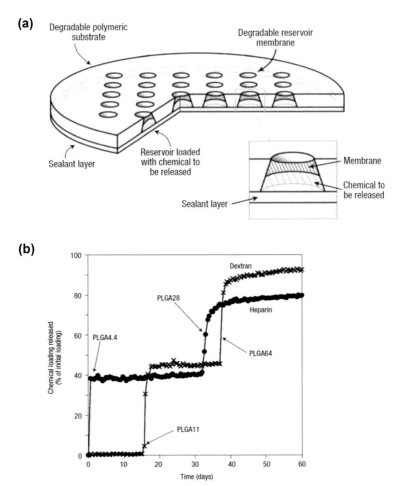

Figure 5.5 (a) Diagram of a polymeric microchip device. The main body of the device is composed of a reservoir-containing substrate that is fabricated from a degradable polymer. Truncated conical reservoirs in the substrate are loaded with the chemical to be released and sealed with polymeric degradable reservoir membranes on one end and a sealant layer (polyester tape) on the opposite end. Inset, close-up of a reservoir, reservoir membrane, sealant layer, and chemical to be released. (b) Cumulative percentage of initial loading released from microchip device in vitro. Release results are shown for a representative device that was loaded with both 14C-dextran (*crosses*) and 3H-heparin (*circles*).
Copyright permission from Nature publishing group (Richards Grayson et al., 2003).

Different from the above approach, a magnetically controlled device capable of on-demand release of an antiproliferative drug, docetaxel (DTX), was reported by Pirmoradi et al. (2011). The device consists of a drug-loaded reservoir (Ø 6 × ~550 mm) that was sealed by an elastic magnetic polydimethylsiloxane (PDMS) membrane. The reservoir was created with molding PDMS on SU-8 pattern through standard photolithography. When applying for a magnetic field, the magnetic PDMS membrane deformed, causing the discharge of the drug solution from the device. Controlled DTX with a sustained leakage release at a rate of 171 ± 16.7 ng per actuation interval was achieved for 35 days. In the cell viability experiment, cell viability in HUVEC and PC3 cells decreased to 24% and 58% after one actuation and to 21% and 34% after 10 actuations, respectively. This device made with biocompatible PDMS presents a promising prospect on in vivo implantation.

In other reports (Ainslie et al., 2010; Chirra & Desai, 2012), the researchers built the PMMA microdevices using photolithography and reactive-ion etching (Fig. 5.6). The different individual model drugs were loaded in each reservoir on the device. The use of different hydrogel systems in each reservoir showed an independent rate-controlled release of the respective drugs over the same release period. In addition, the PMMA surface was functionalized with lectin to improve bioadhesion of the device and epithelium, enhancing drug retention time. Fig. 5.6(a) is the fabrication process of both single drug and multidrug loaded devices.

The reservoir can also be triggered by light. The near-infrared (NIR) radiation with minimal absorbance by skin and tissue and deeper penetration in tissue has a great potential for safe in vivo drug delivery. Timko et al. (2014) proposed a NIR-triggered device that enables on-demand control of the timing and dose of drug released. As shown in Fig. 5.7, while in the presence of NIR, hollow Au nanoshells produced heat to the reservoir, resulting in the drug release from thermosensitive nanogels. Based on the need, this tunable device performed sustained and pulse drug release for at least 3 hours and 10 cycles, respectively. Further in vivo studies demonstrated reproducible dosing controlled by the intensity and timing of irradiation and showed a mild inflammatory response over a 2-week period. In addition, in 2012, for the first time, an implantable reservoir-based microchip was reported in human testing (Farra et al., 2012). In the clinical trial, the devices were implanted in eight osteoporotic postmenopausal women for 4 months and wirelessly programmed to release doses once daily to treat osteoporosis for up to 20 days. Currently, scientists have put more efforts on implantable and programming device for controlled drug delivery.

5.3 Micro/nanofluidics-based drug delivery systems

5.3.1 Working principle

Micro/nanofluidics is the science of manipulating, controlling, and studying fluids at the micro/nanodimensions. This unique characteristic allows micro/nanofluidic devices as controllable platforms to precisely perform drug delivery. In general, reservoirs, channels, pumps, and valves are primary components of micro/nanofluidic devices for precise drug delivery by implanted or transdermal techniques. Drugs stored in reservoirs are precisely moved to desired locations by control parts such as

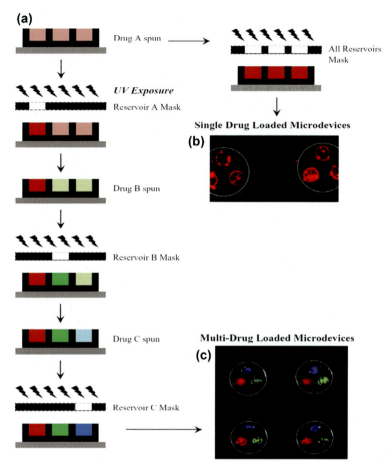

Figure 5.6 (a) Schematic process overview for fabricating single or multidrug loaded microdevices using photolithography. (b) A fluorescent micrograph showing the presence of a single model drug (Texas red-BSA) loaded in all three reservoirs of the same microdevice. (c) A fluorescent micrograph composite of a multidrug (Texas red-BSA; red, FITC-BSA; green, DNP-BSA; blue) loaded microdevice as individual drug in separate reservoirs. The *white circle* highlights the microdevice area.
Copyright permission from John Wiley and Sons Inc. (Chirra & Desai, 2012).

micropumps and valves. One advantage of a micro-/nanochannel-based drug delivery system is that it can provide a stable drug concentration in bodies. Compared to a device that directly exposes the whole reservoirs to the environment, the device with a long channel, especially for a long and narrow channel, can minimize the drug degradation. It is very valuable for delivering a sensitive, unstable, and easy-contaminated drug. In the beginning, the rate of drug delivery was mostly manipulated with flow diffusion (Garcia, Kirkham, Hatch, Hawkins, & Yager, 2004; Lee et al., 2012; Su & Lin, 2004). More control systems were reported recently, such as systems using

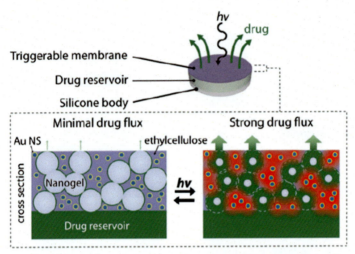

Figure 5.7 Schematic of proposed device (Upper) and membrane cross-section (Lower). Copyright permission from Proc Natl Acad Sci U S A (Timko et al., 2014).

electrokinetic force (Ainslie et al., 2010; Fine et al., 2010, 2011; Grattoni et al., 2009), pressure injection (Kleinstreuer, Li, & Koo, 2008; Metz, Bertsch, Bertrand, & Renaud, 2004), pH tunable nanofluidic diode (Ali, Ramirez, Mafé, Neumann, & Ensinger, 2009), and pumps (Kim et al., 2014; Kim, Kim, & Lee, 2016; Uguz et al., 2017). Mostly, micro- and nanochannel-based devices provide a sustained drug release.

5.3.2 Fabrication of micro/nanofluidic drug delivery systems

Microfluidic-based devices for drug delivery are mostly constructed with polymers. Similar to microreservoir-based devices, microfluidic devices are usually fabricated by standard photolithography, etching, deposition, and molding techniques.

Regarding nanofluidic devices, due to their tiny dimensions, fabrication of nanochannels needs to be done in a cleanroom to minimize the contamination of particles. Standard semiconductor processing techniques are utilized to construct nanofluidic devices. In general four highly effective and reproducible methods are used: (1) bulk nanomachining, (2) surface nanomachining, (3) buried channel technology, and (4) nanoimprint lithography (NIL) (Perry & Kandlikar, 2006).

In a bulk nanomachining process (Fig. 5.8), the wafer is lithographically patterned and the oxide mask is etched with an HF solution. After silicon is anisotropically etched with a developer solution, the oxide mask is stripped and bonded to a borofloat glass wafer. For surface nanomachining, the fabrication of nanofluidic devices is similar to that used in microreservoir devices. Buried channel technology is one approach to fabricate nanofluidic devices, especially to reservoir-based nanofluidic devices. An detailed fabrication process is shown in Fig. 5.9 (left) (Fintshenko & van den Berg, 1998). The process can be implemented in several stages: deep reactive ion etch to form a trench, trench coating with protective material, etch coating at bottom of the

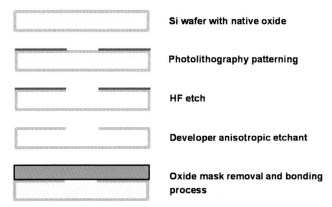

Figure 5.8 A fabrication process for bulk nanomachining with wafer bonding.

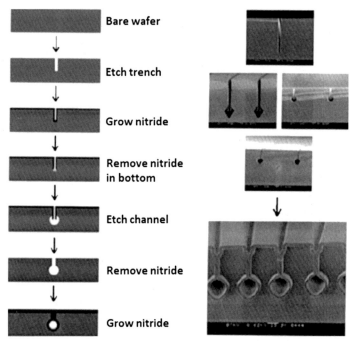

Figure 5.9 Process sequence (left) and SEM micrographs (right) of buried channels. Copyright permission from Elsevier. (Fintshenko & van den Berg, 1998).

trench, second isotropic etch to round out the bottom, strip coating and channel closing by trench filling. On the right of Fig. 5.9 is scanning electron microscope (SEM) images of the device.

Additionally, NIL with a two-step process is an alternative fabrication method (Perry & Kandlikar, 2006). The first process is the imprint step, which duplicates the nanostructures on the mold in the polymer. The polymer is heated to become a viscous liquid which allows for it to deform into the shape of the mold. The second step is the pattern transfer where an etching anisotropic process, such as RIE, is used to remove the residual polymer in the compressed area. PMMA with a small thermal expansion and pressure shrinkage coefficient is a common polymer used in NIL.

5.3.3 Applications

Before the 2000s, the applications of microfluidic and nanofluidic devices were concentrated on diagnosis, microchemical reactors, protein and DNA separation, and cellular analysis. In recent decades, more efforts have been devoted to developing micro/nanofluidic drug delivery and disease therapy. Here, a few drug delivery systems of micro/nanofluidics will be introduced as examples of tremendous applications.

One of the simplest approaches of microfluidic drug delivery devices is a diffusion release. In one example, the microchip was fabricated with PMMA, including one or more microwells and microchannels to serve as drug reservoirs and drug diffusion barriers, respectively (Lee et al., 2012).With the length of channel increasing, the onset time and duration of drug release increased and the device exhibited a sustained drug release. This microchip embedded with multiple sets of microwells, and microchannels of different lengths can be designed to enable sustained drug release for controlled and prolonged periods of time. When the matrix was exposed to flowing liquid, the reagent was dissolved, resulting in the controlled release of the reagent from the cavity (Garcia et al., 2004; Lee et al., 2012; Su & Lin, 2004). Although the fabrication of diffusion delivery devices is simple, in some cases it has limitations of performing precise drug delivery.

Fig. 5.10(a) shows a polymer-based implantable device with embedded microelectrodes and microfluidic channels (Metz et al., 2004). This implanted device allows simultaneous selective chemical delivery/probing and performs multichannel recording/stimulation of bioelectric activity. The drug delivery was performed in fluidic microchannels with pressure injection techniques. The device enables the monitoring of chemical and electrical information exchange among cells and combined for the first time simultaneous electric and fluidic interfacing to tissue with a flexible microimplant.

Nanodrugs can sometimes be combined with microfluidics for controlled drug delivery. As shown in Fig. 5.10(b) (Kleinstreuer et al., 2008), the plenum chamber as a reservoir provides the nutrient supply and/or purging fluid. The microchannels can alter the incoming fluid by adjusting the individual inlet pressure. Nanodrugs are supplied by setting the supply pressure of the nanodrug solution higher than that of the fluid supply side. An appropriate wall heat flux beneath the microchannels ensures that the delivery of a drug-fluid mixture to the living cells occurs at an optimal temperature. Controlled dosages of nanodrugs allow simultaneous testing of living cells and stimuli responses. Such microsystems, featuring controlled transport processes for

Controlled drug delivery using microdevices 217

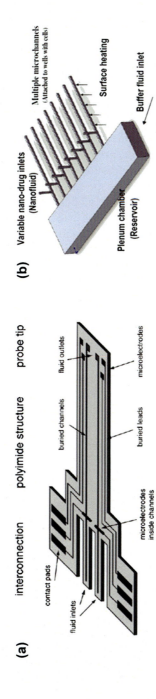

Figure 5.10 (a) An illustration of implantable, flexible polyimide probe with microelectrodes and microfluidic channels. (b) Nanomedicine delivery system with eight microchannels.
(a) Copyright permission from Elsevier (Metz et al., 2004). (b) Copyright permission from Elsevier (Kleinstreuer et al., 2008).

optimal nanodrug delivery, are important in laboratory testing of predecessors of implantable smart devices which could offer closed-loop sensing for interpretation and automatic nanodrug dispensation.

An electrokinetic actuator is another approach to control drug release. In one study (Fine et al., 2011), an implantable and mechanically robust nanofluidic membrane was manufactured with precise silicon nanofabrication techniques. Two integrated platinum electrodes at the inlet and outlet played the roles in reversing the nanoflow by applying opposite voltages as well as controlling the rate of nanoflow. An electrokinetically actuated nanofluidic membrane provided a sustained drug release at a low applied voltage. The delivery performance of the nanochannel membrane was measured and monitored with a fluorescence microscope during a period of 33 days. This nanofluidic membrane can achieve rhythmic delivery by electrokinetic actuator and control the range of release rates by the mechanical dimension of the fluidic network, the voltage, and the electrophoretic mobility of the molecules.

Moreover, integrating different techniques with microfluidics can offer more functions to improve drug administration. For example, a proposed device that combines functional materials, the porous supraparticle functioning as a reservoir to store drug, with a PDMS microfluidic channel provides a sustained drug release (Rastogi, Velikov, & Velev, 2010). A stable rate of drug release was achieved by controlling porosity, size, and chemical properties of particles and drugs. Microfluidics can also be integrated with the needle structure for controlled drug release (Bodhale, Nisar, & Afzulpurkar, 2010; Kim & Lee, 2007). On a nanoneedle drug release device, microfluidic channels as interconnectors and reservoirs provided fluidic interconnection of external devices and drug storage room (Kim & Lee, 2007). A microfluidic interconnector assembly was designed and fabricated using SU-8 and conventionally machined PMMA in a way that it had a male interconnectorwhich directly fitted into the fluidic reservoir of the microneedle array at one end, and the other male interconnector which provideed fluidic interconnection to external devices at the other end. In a different report, microfluidics is integrated with convection-enhanced drug delivery (CED), a promising therapeutic method to treat brain diseases (Fig. 5.11) (Neeves, Lo, Foley, Saltzman, & Olbricht, 2006). By increasing the rate of infusion at positive pressure, CED can enhance the drug penetration distance and overcome limitations of traditional treatment for brain tumors caused by the larger tumor size and the difficulty of delivering drugs into their dense tissue. Compared to the CED using needles and cannulas delivering drugs, this integrated microfluidic system offered several advantages, including small size to minimized tissue damage, low backflow, the rigid tip to penetrate deep into the tissue, and the fluidic outlet located away from the penetrating edge to avoid occlusion of the channel. To improve the precision of drug dose, different types of micropumps (e.g., ion pump, reciprocating micropump, and thermoresponsive leaf-inspired micropump) have also been developed and incorporated into the microfluidic/microreservoir drug delivery devices (Kim et al., 2014, 2016; Uguz et al., 2017).

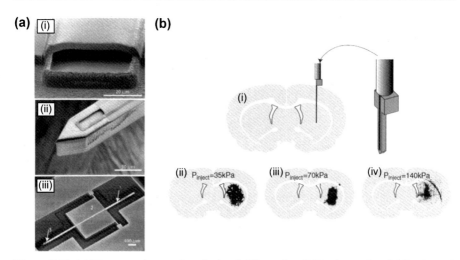

Figure 5.11 (a) Electron micrographs of microfluidic probe. (i) Parylene microfluidic channel with dimension of 50 × 10 μm. (ii) Pointed tip of insertable portion of probe. (iii) Entire probe with protrusion for fluidic connection (1), base for handling (2), and tissue penetrating insert (3). (b) Injecting pressure dependence of the dye distribution. (i) The microfluidic probe with attached fluid reservoir was inserted 3 mm laterally from bregma to a depth of 5 mm into the caudate nucleus (Top). (ii–iv) An overlay of the processed data on a cartoon of the insertion site illustrates the pressure dependence of the dye distribution at injection pressure of 35, 70, and 140 kPa.
Copyright permission from Elsevier (Neeves et al., 2006).

Another new rapidly growing field for the microfluidic platform is the application for neurological disorders and diseases. Due to the brain–blood barrier, traditional drug delivery is not able to penetrate enough doses without severe systemic cytotoxic effects for the therapy. The implantable and on-demand drug release device has opened up new opportunities for neurological disease therapy (Jeong et al., 2015; Lee et al., 2015; Minev et al., 2015). For example, an integrated neural probe includes an electrode array to record individual neuron signals and microchannels to localized deliver a small volume of drugs (<1 μL) to mice brain for chemical simulation (Lee et al., 2015). In the past few years, the flexible multifunctional platform that offers a better mechanical match with neural tissue and is capable of studying the complexity of the brain has attracted much attention from neuroscientists. In one design, a soft implant consists of a transparent silicone substrate, stretchable gold interconnects, soft electrodes, and drug injection microchannels (Minev et al., 2015). This implant incorporated high-resolution neural recording with localized electrical and chemical modulation, alleviating neurological deficits in freely moving rats for a long period of time. Compared to the stiff implant, the neural tissue showed significantly less neuroinflammatory responses to this soft implant. Besides, electrical performance of the device remains stable after applying a 20% strain over one million cycles. The second example is an optofluidic neural probe that has wireless capabilities for programmed drug delivery and photostimulation in freely moving animals (Jeong et al., 2015).

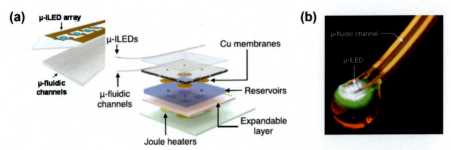

Figure 5.12 Wireless optofluidic neural probe for programmable pharmacology and optogenetics. (a) Exploded view schematic diagram that illustrates an array of m-ILEDs (left top) mounted on top of a soft microfluidic system that includes four separate microfluidic channels (left bottom), each connected to a set of fluid reservoirs that include copper membranes as hermetic seals, expandable composite materials as mechanical transducers, and microscale Joule heating elements as actuators. (b) Optofluidic neural probe during simultaneous drug delivery and photostimulation.
Copyright permission from Cell (Jeong et al., 2015).

Fig. 5.12a is a schematic of the device that combines ultrathin, soft, thermal-triggered microfluidic drug delivery with inorganic light-emitting diode (m-ILED) arrays. In this design, each of four microchannels connects to a separated reservoir capable of multiple drug delivery, and the cellular-scale ILEDs offer a high spatial photostimulation. Fig. 5.12b is an optical image of the device.

5.4 Future trends and challenges

Innovations in microreservoir and microfluidic drug delivery systems based on new materials, mechanical concepts, and advanced manufacturing lead to attractive personalized disease therapy. Except for providing well-controlled drug release, highly efficient treatment for diseases, and low toxicity for healthy tissues, the ideal drug delivery system should also include a monitored feedback to manage the drug release in real time, or even in response to a therapeutic marker of patients. The first closed-loop feedback control of drug levels in living animals is reported in 2017 (Mage et al., 2017). To date, developing low-cost drug delivery devices with a combination of biosensors and drug infusing networks remains challenging, such as the long-term stability of the sensor, biocompatible of the devices, and ability to treat chronic diseases, etc. Furthermore, a number of materials have been developed that exhibit sensitivity to light, ultrasound, or electrical and magnetic fields to remotely trigger drug delivery. Developing tunable materials that can switch on/off drug release will provide more options for closed-loop feedback devices. The new materials that can physically and mechanically match with tissues and have a high degradation rate, especially for those materials that can be used to create flexible micro-even nano-size structures through

MEMS/NEMS (nanoelectromechanical system), are essential for the implanted device. In addition, long-term drug delivery is critical for chronic disease treatment. However, the current implantable devices are often small and lack of ability to load enough drugs for long-term treatment. A novel refilling system is also required for the implantable devices to reload drugs. Though commercialization of microreservoir drug delivery is around 4 decades later than reservoir (larger size) drug delivery, several commercial products (e.g. Selution SLR (MedAlliance), Nitro Disc (G.D. Searle Pharmaceuticals), and MicroCHIPS) are already on the market or near to complete the clinical trials. For microfluidic drug delivery, with an expectation of incorporating multiple functions and components into a single device, commercialization is still in the early stage. As a multidisciplinary field, microfluidic-based drug delivery requires a more advanced integration of drug delivery, biosensors, electronics, manufacturing, automation, and data analysis to foster drug administration and personalized therapy.

References

Ainslie, K. M., Lowe, R. D., Beaudette, T. T., Petty, L., Bachelder, E. M., & Desai, T. A. (2010). Microfabricated devices for enhanced bioadhesive drug delivery: Attachment to and small-molecule release through a cell monolayer under flow. *Small, 6*(3), 355−360.

Ali, M., Ramirez, P., Mafé, S., Neumann, R., & Ensinger, W. (2009). A pH-tunable nanofluidic diode with a broad range of rectifying properties. *ACS Nano, 3*(3), 603−608.

Bodhale, D. W., Nisar, A., & Afzulpurkar, N. (2010). Structural and microfluidic analysis of hollow side-open polymeric microneedles for transdermal drug delivery applications. *Microfluidics and Nanofluidics, 8*, 373−392.

Chirra, H. D., & Desai, T. A. (2012). Multi-reservoir bioadhesive microdevices for independent rate-controlled delivery of multiple drugs. *Small*, 201201367.

Elman, N. M., Masi, B. C., Cima, M. J., & Langer, R. (2010). Electro-thermally induced structural failure actuator (ETISFA) for implantable controlled drug delivery devices based on Micro-Electro-Mechanical-Systems. *Lab on a Chip, 10*(20), 2796−2804.

Farra, R., Sheppard, N. F., Jr., McCabe, L., Neer, R. M., Anderson, J. M., Santini, J. T., Jr., et al. (2012). First-in-human testing of a wirelessly controlled drug delivery microchip. *Science Translational Medicine, 4*(122), 122ra21.

Fine, D., Grattoni, A., Hosali, S., Ziemys, A., De Rosa, E., Gill, J., et al. (2010). A robust nanofluidic membrane with tunable zero-order release for implantable dose specific drug delivery. *Lab on a Chip, 10*(22), 3074−3083.

Fine, D., Grattoni, A., Zabre, E., Hussein, F., Ferrari, M., & Liu, X. (2011). A low-voltage electrokinetic nanochannel drug delivery system. *Lab on a Chip, 11*(15), 2526−2534.

Fintshenko, Y., & van den Berg, A. (1998). Silicon microtechnology and microstructures in separation science. *Journal of Chromtography A, 819*, 3−12.

Garcia, E., Kirkham, J. R., Hatch, A. V., Hawkins, K. R., & Yager, P. (2004). Controlled microfluidic reconstitution of functional protein from an anhydrous storage depot. *Lab on a Chip, 4*(1), 78−82.

Grattoni, A., De Rosa, E., Ferrati, S., Wang, Z., Gianesini, A., Liu, X., et al. (2009). Analysis of a nanochanneled membrane structure through convective gas flow. *Journal of Micromechanics and Microengineering, 19*, 115018.

Hand, B., & Gärtner, C. (2008). Polymer microfabrication technologies for microfluidic systems. *Analytical and Bioanalytical Chemistry, 390*, 89−111.

Husseini, G. A., & Pitt, W. G. (2008). Micelles and nanoparticles for ultrasonic drug and gene delivery. *Advanced Drug Delivery Reviews, 60*(10), 1137−1152.

Jeong, J. W., McCall, J. G., Shin, G., Zhang, Y., Al-Hasani, R., Kim, M., et al. (2015). Wireless optofluidic systems for programmable in vivo pharmacology and optogenetics. *Cell, 162*(3), 662−674.

Santini, J. T., Jr., Cima, M. J., & Langer, R. (1999). A controlled-release microchip. *Nature, 397*(6717), 335−338.

Kim, E. S., Gustenhoven, E., Mescher, M. J., Pararas, E. E., Smith, K. A., Spencer, A. J., et al. (2014). A microfluidic reciprocating intracochlear drug delivery system with reservoir and active dose control. *Lab on a Chip, 14*(4), 710−721.

Kim, H., Kim, K., & Lee, S. J. (2016). Compact and thermosensitive nature-inspired micropump. *Scientific Reports, 6*, 36085.

Kim, K., & Lee, J. B. (2007). High aspect ratio tapered hollow metallic microneedle arrays with microfluidic interconnector. *Microsystem Technologies, 13*, 231−235.

Kleinstreuer, C., Li, J., & Koo, J. (2008). Microfluidics of nano-drug delivery. *International Journal of Heat and Mass Transfer, 51*, 5590−5597.

Lee, S. H., Park, M., Park, C. G., Lee, J. E., Prausnitz, M. R., & Choy, Y. B. (2012). Microchip for sustained drug delivery by diffusion through microchannels. *AAPS PharmSciTech, 13*(1), 211−217.

Lee, H. J., Son, Y., Kim, J., Lee, C. J., Yoon, E. S., & Cho, I. J. (2015). A multichannel neural probe with embedded microfluidic channels for simultaneous in vivo neural recording and drug delivery. *Lab on a Chip, 15*(6), 1590−1597.

Li, X. (2016). Thematic issue: Special issue for current pharmaceutical biotechnology miniaturized platforms & methods for pharmaceutical studies. *Current Pharmaceutical Biotechnology, 17*, 753−754.

Mage, P. L., Ferguson, B. S., Maliniak, D., Ploense, K. L., Kippin, T. E., & Soh, H. T. (2017). Closed-loop control of circulating drug levels in live animals. *Nature Biomedical Engineering, 1*, 0070.

Metz, S., Bertsch, A., Bertrand, D., & Renaud, P. (2004). Flexible polyimide probes with microelectrodes and embedded microfluidic channels for simultaneous drug delivery and multi-channel monitoring of bioelectric activity. *Biosensors and Bioelectronics, 19*(10), 1309−1318.

Minev, I. R., Musienko, P., Hirsch, A., Barraud, Q., Wenger, N., Moraud, E. M., et al. (2015). Electronic dura mater for long-term multimodal neural interfaces. *Science, 347*(6218), 159−163.

Neeves, K. B., Lo, C. T., Foley, C. P., Saltzman, W. M., & Olbricht, W. L. (2006). Fabrication and characterization of microfluidic probes for convection enhanced drug delivery. *Journal of Controlled Release, 111*(3), 252−262.

Perry, J. L., & Kandlikar, S. G. (2006). Review of fabrication of nanochannels for single phase liquid flow. *Microfluidics and Nanofluidics, 2*, 185−193.

Pirmoradi, F. N., Jackson, J. K., Burt, H. M., & Chiao, M. (2011). On-demand controlled release of docetaxel from a battery-less MEMS drug delivery device. *Lab on a Chip, 11*(16), 2744−2752.
Prescott, J. H., Lipka, S., Baldwin, S., Sheppard, N. F., Jr., Maloney, J. M., Coppeta, J., et al. (2006). Chronic programmed polypeptide delivery from an implanted multireservoir microchip device. *Nature Biotechnology, 24*(4), 437−438.
Rastogi, V., Velikov, K. P., & Velev, O. D. (2010). Microfluidic characterization of sustained solute release from porous supraparticles. *Physical Chemistry Chemical Physics, 12*(38), 11975−11983.
Riahi, R., Tamayol, A., Shaegh, S. A. M., Ghaemmaghami, A., Dokmeci, M. R., & Khademshosseini, A. (2015). Microfluidics for advanced drug delivery systems. *Current Opinion in Chemical Engineering, 7*, 101−112.
Richards Grayson, A. C., Choi, I. S., Tyler, B. M., Wang, P. P., Brem, H., Cima, M. J., et al. (2003). Multi-pulse drug delivery from a resorbable polymeric microchip device. *Nature Materials, 2*(11), 767−772.
Sanjay, S. T., Zhou, W., Dou, M., Tavakoli, H., Ma, L., Xu, F., et al. (2018). Recent advances of controlled drug delivery using microfluidic platforms. *Advanced Drug Delivery Reviews, 128*, 3−28.
Sharma, S., Nijdam, A. J., Sinha, P. M., Walczak, R. J., Liu, X., Cheng, M. M., et al. (2006). Controlled-release microchips. *Expert Opinion on Drug Delivery, 3*(3), 379−394.
Staples, M. (2010). Microchips and controlled- release drug reservoirs. *Wiley Interdisciplinary Reviews. Nanomedicine and Nanobiotechnology, 2*(4), 400−417.
Su, Y., & Lin, L. (2004). A water-powered micro drug delivery system. *Journal of Microelectromechanical System, 13*, 175−182.
Timko, B. P., Arruebo, M., Shankarappa, S. A., McAlvin, J. B., Okonkwo, O. S., Mizrahi, B., et al. (2014). Near-infrared-actuated devices for remotely controlled drug delivery. *Proceedings of the National Academy of Sciences of the United States of America, 111*(4), 1349−1354.
Truong, T. Q., & Nguyen, N. T. (2004). A polymeric piezoelectric micropump based on lamination technology. *Journal of Micromechanics and Microengineering, 14*, 632−638.
Uguz, I., Proctor, C. M., Curto, V. F., Pappa, A. M., Donahue, M. J., Ferro, M., et al. (2017). Microfluidic ion pump for in vivo drug delivery. *Advanced Materials*, 1701217.
Ziaie, B., Baldi, A., Lei, M., Gu, Y., & Siegel, R. A. (2004). Hard and soft micromachining for BioMEMS review of techniques and examples of applications in microfluidics and drug delivery. *Advanced Drug Delivery Reviews, 56*(2), 145−172.

Microneedles for drug delivery and monitoring

Emma McAlister, Melissa Kirkby, Ryan F. Donnelly
School of Pharmacy, Queen's University Belfast, Belfast, United Kingdom

Guided reading questions

1. How can the design of microneedle arrays be manipulated to maximise drug delivery?
2. What are the challenges associated with translation of microneedle arrays from benchtop to bedside?

6.1 Introduction

Microneedle (MN) arrays consist of multiple microprojections assembled on one side of a supporting base, ranging in height from 25 to 900 μm. MN arrays are minimally invasive devices that are applied to the skin surface and pierce the epidermis, creating temporary microscopic aqueous channels through which drug molecules can diffuse into the microcirculation. MN arrays enhance transdermal drug delivery by mechanically disrupting the stratum corneum (SC), bypassing this skin barrier altogether. This technology was first conceptualized in 1976 (Gerstel & Place, 1976), but it was not until 1998 when MN arrays became the subject of considerable research. Indeed, advancements in microfabrication technology enabled their manufacture and allowed for their practical realisation in 1998. Since then, this technology has been extensively investigated.

MN arrays have demonstrated great promise as a drug delivery platform. MN arrays combine the patient-friendly benefits of a transdermal patch with the potential delivery capabilities of a hypodermic injection. The unique attribute of MN arrays is that they penetrate the resilient skin barrier sufficiently to enable access to the skin's rich microcirculation, yet are short and narrow enough to avoid stimulation with nerve fibers or puncture blood vessels that primarily reside in the dermal layer. A painless application is, thus, considered the principal benefit of MN arrays with reports in the literature from those intimately involved in the scientific development of MN arrays supporting this (Birchall, Clemo, Anstey, & John, 2011; Donnelly, McCrudden et al., 2014; Gill, Denson, Burris, & Prausnitz, 2008). Compared to the hypodermic needle, there are additional advantages of MN arrays. Skin trauma is minimized, and bleeding is avoided after insertion. No reports on the development of skin infections exist with significantly less microbial penetration with MN arrays than the hypodermic needle (Donnelly, Marrow, McCarron et al., 2009). Needle phobia from the hypodermic needle is removed, which is experienced by many people and which can ultimately reduce adherence. In addition, needle-stick injuries and the issues surrounding sharps waste disposal are removed. Furthermore, in the literature, it has been documented that MN arrays can be reproducibly inserted into the skin by patients (self-application), without additional applicator devices (Donnelly, McCrudden et al., 2014; Vicente-Pérez et al., 2016).

6.2 Microneedle design parameters and structure

MN arrays are fabricated using a wide variety of fabrication techniques. Despite more recent novel fabrication techniques increasing in complexity, the majority of the techniques encompass microelectromechanical systems (MEMS). This technology was traditionally used in producing microprocessors but subsequently it has been applied effectively in the manufacture of a variety of microscale devices, such as MN arrays. There are three basic techniques in MEMS technology on which the fabrication processes of MN arrays are based on. These are lithography (patterning), deposition, and etching (wet or dry) (Larrañeta & Singh, 2018). These three techniques are applied depending on the choice of material used in the fabrication of MN arrays.

6.2.1 Microneedle geometry

The shape and geometry of MN is critical during design and fabrication. The needles must be capable of inserting into skin without breaking, and the needles should be of suitable length, width, and shape to avoid nerve contact (McAllister et al., 2003; Park, Allen, & Prausnitz, 2005; Yung et al., 2012). The elastic properties of human skin can prevent MNs from penetrating by twisting around the needles during MN application, particularly in the case of blunt and short MNs (McAllister et al., 2003). Metals are typically strong enough, whereas polymers must be selected in order to ensure they have sufficient mechanical strength. Typical MN geometries vary from 25 to 2500 µm in length, 50 to 250 µm in base width, and 1 to 25 µm in tip diameter (McAllister et al., 2003; Yung et al., 2012).

Based on the fabrication process, the MNs are classified as in-plane MNs, out-of-plane MNs, or a combination as seen in Fig. 6.1. Considering the in-plane designs (Fig. 6.1(a)), the MNs are parallel to the machined surface of the substrate (e.g., Si wafer). The major advantage of in-plane MNs is easily and accurately controlled production of MNs with various lengths during fabrication process. In out-of-plane designs (Fig. 6.1(b)), the MNs are perpendicular to the fabrication surface of Si wafer and are easier to produce in arrays than in-plane (Ashraf, Tayyaba, & Afzulpurkar, 2011).

MNs can be classified on the basis of overall shape and tip, ranging from cylindrical, rectangular, pyramidal, conical, octagonal to quadrangular, with different needle lengths and widths. The tip shape of MNs is important for skin penetration because

Microneedles for drug delivery and monitoring

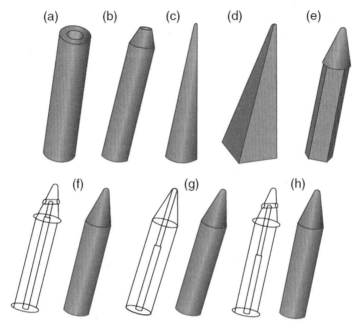

Figure 6.1 Shapes of MN: (a) Cylindrical; (b) Tapered tip; (c) Canonical; (d) Square base; (e) Pentagonal-based canonical tip; (f) Side-open single lumen; (g) Double lumen; (h) Side-open double lumen.
Adapted from Ashraf et al. (2011).

sharper MNs have a higher potential for penetrating the skin, but larger tip diameters require higher insertion forces, which may lead to bending or breaking of the needles in the skin (Arora, Prausnitz, & Mitragotri, 2008; Banga, 2009; Teo, Shearwood, Ng, Lu, & Moochhala, 2006). In addition, the shape of the tips of hollow MNs is essential for the flow rate; the flow from a blunt-tip MN is lower than a bevel-tip MN because a blunt-tip MN compacts the skin and, thus, has higher risk of clogging (Bodhale, Asim, Ae, & Afzulpurkar, 2010; Luttge et al., 2007). To overcome this problem, it should have very sharp tip, with the bore of the MN off-centered or on the side of the MN. Increasing the number of bores in hollow MNs will increase the flow rate; nevertheless, this results in decreased MN strength and a reduction in sharpness (Stoeber & Liepmann, 2002). Fig. 6.1 summarizes the multiple geometries of MN available.

6.2.2 Microneedle materials

MN arrays have been fabricated from a range of materials. In the literature, it has been demonstrated that MN arrays have been mainly fabricated from silicon, metal, and polymers (including carbohydrates) with other materials used such as ceramic (Bystrova & Luttge, 2011; Ita, 2018) and glass (Wang, Cornwell, Hill, & Prausnitz, 2006). The first MN arrays developed for drug delivery were fabricated from silicon, using the processes of photolithography and deep reactive ion etching (Henry, McAllister, Allen, & Prausnitz, 1998). Since then, silicon MN arrays have continued to be commonly prepared by modifications of the etching process, either wet (solution) or dry (water vapor). Although the manufacture of silicon MN arrays offers the potential for mass production of MN arrays, it is expensive, highly specialized, and includes complex multistep processes. Regarding patient safety, silicon is an untested biomaterial; thus, it is reasonable to suggest that this would lead to concerns regarding silicon debris in the skin (McAllister et al., 2003). As a result, there has been some movement away from the use of silicon MN arrays with other materials more commonly investigated.

An alternative material is metal as metals have been in medical use for decades e.g., hypodermic needles and implants. Classic examples of metals used for the fabrication of MN arrays include stainless steel (Martanto et al., 2004) and titanium (Liu, Yan, Yang, Jiang, & Yang, 2013), but other metals such as palladium, palladium-cobalt alloys nickel and gold have also been used. Approaches such as laser cutting (stainless steel), photochemical etching (titanium), and electroplating with subsequent etching (nickel) have been investigated for the fabrication of metal MN arrays (Donnelly, Garland et al., 2010). Metals have been found to be equally effective in skin penetration compared with silicon MN arrays but are less expensive to fabricate and hence are more advantageous. A further advantage of using metals such as stainless steel and titanium is that they are well characterized and already approved for medical applications. This may reduce the number of hurdles when trying to attain regulatory approval for an MN product. As metals, stainless steel, and titanium are commonly used within the medical field, limitations of this material are sparse. However, there are concerns surrounding the immune-inflammatory response of soft tissue around stainless steel and titanium implants. Also, it has been documented that caution should be used when employing nickel as a material for fabricating MN arrays due to the potential adverse allergic reactions and is known to be carcinogenic (Larrañeta, Lutton, Woolfson, & Donnelly, 2016).

Polymer MN arrays are most commonly fabricated by micromoulding, moving away from the typical MEMS processes employed in the fabrication of silicon and metal MN arrays. Micromoulding-based fabrication involves replication of master structures by means of molds (Donnelly, Singh, Morrow, & Woolfson, 2012). In simple terms, a master mold is manufactured which is otherwise known as the male master mold. These male master molds have been produced using different materials such as silicon and metal. This male master mold is then used to create the reciprocal master mold, namely the female master mold from which polymer MN arrays are fabricated from. It is reported that the most commonly used material for producing female master molds is polydimethylsiloxane (PDMS) or silicone elastomer. The popularity of this material is attributed to its flexibility, durability, low cost, and the accurate reproducibility of female master molds (Larrañeta & Singh, 2018; Park et al., 2007). It is important to note that lithography is often employed in the production of the male master mold that is used for the inverse female master mold based on silicone elastomer (Park et al., 2007). For the fabrication of polymer MN arrays, a polymer blend (with or without drug) is casted into female master molds made from silicone elastomer. Additional use of centrifugal force or vacuum is required during the filling of the material into the mold cavities and drying state (Yang et al., 2012). In the literature, a number of research groups have investigated carbohydrates as potential MN array materials. Examples of carbohydrate MN arrays include maltose (Miyano et al., 2005) and galactose (Donnelly, Marrow, Singh et al., 2009). However, Donnelly, Marrow, Singh et al. (2009) showed that due to high processing temperatures involved during the fabrication of carbohydrate MN arrays, substantial losses of the model drug molecules investigated (5-aminolevulinic acid) and bovine serum albumin (BSA) occurred. Also, galactose MN arrays were found to be unstable at ambient relative humidities (43% and 85%) and, thus, very difficult to work with. On the other hand, various polymer materials have been efficiently fabricated into MN arrays. Examples include poly(vinylpyrrolidone) (PVP) (Sullivan, Murthy, & Prausnitz, 2008), poly(vinyl alcohol) (PVA) (Nguyen et al., 2018), poly(lactic-co-glycolic) acid (PLGA) (Naves et al., 2017), carboxymethyl cellulose (CMC) (Lee, Choi, Felner, & Prausnitz, 2011), and the copolymer methyl vinyl ether and maleic acid (PMVE/MA) (Gantrez S-97) (Quinn, Bonham, Hughes, & Donnelly, 2015). A number of advantages are associated with the use of polymer MN arrays. In comparison to silicon MN arrays as previously described, a wide range of polymers are biocompatible and have long-standing safety records when used in drug delivery systems (Larrañeta et al., 2016). The use of biocompatible polymers will also effectively reduce the number of regulatory hurdles required for approval, compared with that required for nonapproved materials, such as silicon. In addition to their biocompatibility, a wide variety of polymers are biodegradable. The use of water-soluble and biodegradable polymers eliminates the risk of leaving biohazardous sharp waste in the skin as well as guarantees safe MN array disposal. In addition, the low cost of polymer materials and their less complex fabrication process *via* micromolding allows for mass production. Thus, through its unique properties, importantly the biocompatibility and biodegradability, which have been a concern with silicon and metal MN arrays, polymer MN arrays are gaining huge importance (Larrañeta & Singh, 2018).

A recognized disadvantage with the male master mold made from silicon or metal is the limitation of the MN array height and spacing (Donnelly, Singh, Morrow et al., 2012). In 2011, Donnelly's research group combined micromolding with laser micromachining to overcome the limitation with male master molds made from silicon and metal and offer greater flexibility for polymer MN arrays (Donnelly et al., 2011). In this novel laser-based fabrication method, a pulsed laser beam is used to create 3D structures on the micrometer scale into transparent silicone sheets, of dimensions warranted and programmed by a standard computer aided design file. These laser-engineered silicone sheets were subsequently attached to silicone elastomer female master molds. In this case, the silicone elastomer molds were prepared using custom-made aluminum holders, containing a teflon stub and laser-engineered silicone sheets. The fabrication of polymer MN arrays using silicone laser-engineered MN array molds described by Donnelly's research group is summarised and schematically presented in Fig. 6.2.

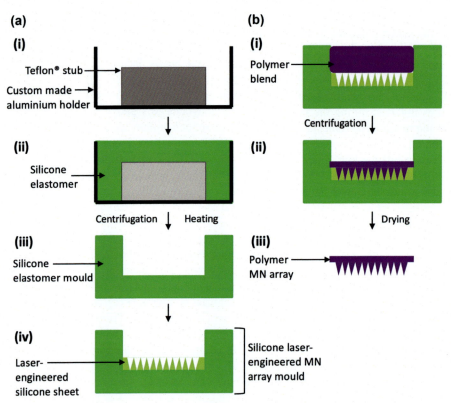

Figure 6.2 Schematic representation of the steps involved in the fabrication of polymer microneedle (MN) arrays. Firstly, (a) shows the production of silicone molds using laser-engineered silicone sheets. In this case, (i) a Teflon stub is attached to a custom-made aluminum holder. (ii) Silicone elastomer is poured into the custom-made aluminum holder and centrifuged. (iii) After curing overnight, the silicone elastomer mold is carefully removed from the custom-made aluminum holder. (iv) A laser-engineered silicone sheet is glued to the bottom of the silicone elastomer mold. Secondly, (b) shows the fabrication of polymer MN arrays from the silicone laser-engineered MN array molds. In this case, (i) polymer blend is transferred to the silicone laser-engineered MN array mold. (ii) The MN array mold is centrifuged. (iii) After drying, the polymer MN array is removed from the MN array mold. Produced using information from Donnelly et al. (2011).

6.3 Drug delivery strategies using microneedle arrays

MN arrays have been fabricated in a number of different designs. Drug delivery across the skin with the aid of MN arrays can be achieved *via* five main strategies. These are solid, coated, dissolving, hollow, and hydrogel-forming as illustrated in Fig. 6.3. The first strategy is *via* the use of solid MN arrays or also termed the "poke with patch" approach (Fig. 6.3(a)). Solid MN arrays require a two-step application process. Initially, a solid MN array is applied to the skin, puncturing the SC to create micropores. The MN array is then removed and a conventional drug formulation is placed over the site of MN array insertion, typically in the form of a transdermal patch,

Microneedles for drug delivery and monitoring 231

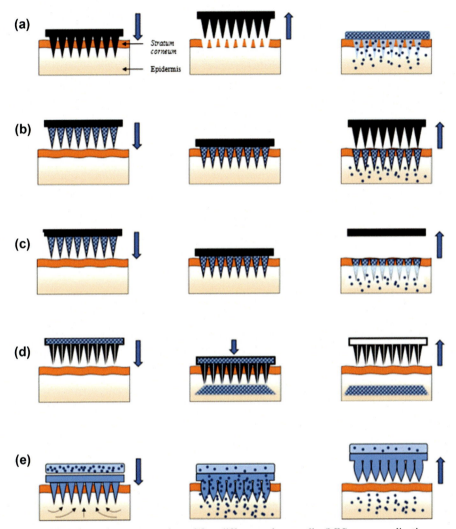

Figure 6.3 Schematic representation of five different microneedle (MN) array application strategies to facilitate drug delivery transdermally. (a) Solid MN arrays for increasing the permeability of a drug formulation by creating microholes across the skin pretreatment followed by the application of a conventional drug formulation; (b) Coated MN arrays for deposition and dissolution of a drug-containing layer into the skin; (c) Dissolving MN arrays for delivery of incorporated drug into the skin; (d) Hollow MN arrays for insertion into the skin and infusion of drug molecules *via* the central lumen of the MN array and (e) Hydrogel-forming MN arrays that take up skin ISF, inducing diffusion of the drug from a drug-containing reservoir through the swollen microprojections.
Adapted from Larrañeta et al. (2016).

gel, or solution. The creation of micropores in the skin increases skin permeability, and movement of drug molecules through these microchannels occurs *via* passive diffusion. Coated MN arrays or the "coat and poke" approach relies on coating the microprojections of the MN array with the drug formulation and subsequent insertion of the coated MN array into the skin (Fig. 6.3(b)). Drug deposition occurs through the dissolution of the coating after being applied to the skin. Dissolving MN arrays or the "poke and release" approach function by incorporating the drug molecules within the structure of the MN array (Fig. 6.3(c)). Following insertion into the skin and upon contact with the skin interstitial fluid (ISF), dissolution of the MN array and subsequent drug delivery occurs. Hollow MN arrays or the "poke and flow" approach allows delivery of drug molecules *via* the injection of a fluid drug formulation through the central lumen of the hollow MN arrays into the skin (Fig. 6.3(d)). Hydrogel-forming or swellable MN arrays are the most recent drug delivery strategy, fist described by Donnelly, Singh, Garland et al. (2012) (Fig. 6.3(e)). Following insertion into the skin, these MN arrays rapidly imbibe skin ISF and swell. As a result, continuous, unblockable hydrogel conduits are formed. In this drug delivery strategy, the drug molecule is not within the hydrogel-forming MN array but in a separate drug-containing reservoir. The moisture from the swellable hydrogel-forming MN array comes into contact with the attached drug-containing reservoir, and this causes the drug-containing reservoir to dissolve/disintegrate. This subsequently triggers diffusion of the drug molecule from the attached drug-containing reservoir through the hydrogel matrix. Thus, the numerous drug delivery strategies described reflect the extensive nature of research in this field. With each particular drug delivery strategy, associated technical challenges will also be discussed.

6.3.1 Solid microneedle arrays

Solid MN arrays (Fig. 6.4(a)) have been fabricated from silicon, metal, and polymer. Solid MN arrays were the first reported MN array strategy, and they were fabricated from silicon (Henry et al., 1998). Described by Henry et al. (1998), the first drug molecule delivered *via* silicon solid MN arrays was that of the low molecular weight model drug molecule, calcein. In this study, a four-fold increase in the permeability of calcein across human skin *in vitro* was demonstrated. Following this success, scientific research continued to explore the drug delivery capabilities of solid MN arrays made from silicon and metal. In 2003, McAllister et al. (2003) reported the successful delivery of different compounds, including BSA and insulin using metal solid MN arrays. Furthermore, Martanto et al. (2004) described the pretreatment with metal solid MN arrays, followed by application of a topical insulin solution, which resulted in the lowering of blood glucose levels in diabetic rats. The delivery of macromolecules transdermally, previously considered to be extremely challenging, such as insulin was, therefore, established as being possible. In the literature, solid MN arrays have also been used to deliver low molecular weight drug molecules, such as galantamine (Wei-Ze et al., 2010). Solid MN arrays, in the form of MN roller devices, have also been used for the delivery of drug molecules transdermally. In one example, Stahl, Wohlert, and Kietzmann (2012) showed the increased permeation of Non-steroidal

Microneedles for drug delivery and monitoring 233

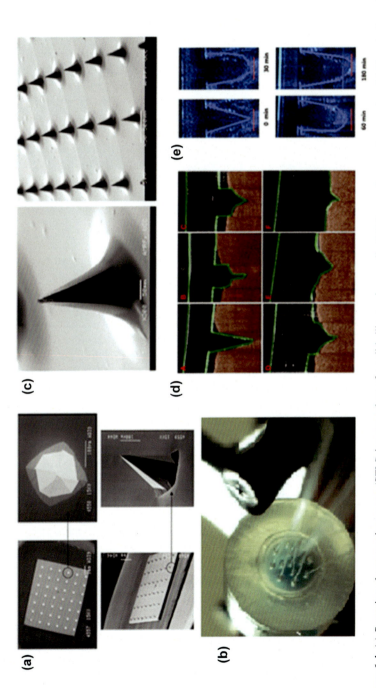

Figure 6.4 (a) Scanning electron microscope (SEM) images taken of a solid silicon microneedle (MN) array from various angles. (b) Flow testing of hollow MNs at 12 mL/min using blue dextran dye. (c) SEM image of a carboxymethyl cellulose (CMC) film coated single silicon MN and a CMC film coated MN array. (d) False color images of the *in vitro* dissolution profile of dissolving microneedles in porcine skin over a 3-hour period, as assessed by optical coherence tomography (A = time 0; B = time 15 min, C = time 30 min, D = 60 min, E = 120 min, F = 180 min). (*Scale bar* represents length of 300 μm). (e) False color images of the *in vitro* swelling profile of hydrogel-forming MN arrays in excised neonatal porcine skin recorded over a 3 h period, as assessed by optical coherence tomography (*Scale bar* represents 300 mm in each case).
(a) Reproduced from Donnelly, Singh et al. (2009), (b) Reproduced from (Farias et al., 2018), (c) Reproduced from McGrath et al. (2011) with permission, (d) Reproduced with permission from Donnelly, Singh, and Woolfson (2010), (e) Reproduced from Donnelly, Moffatt et al. (2014).

anti-inflammatories (NSAIDs), diclofenac, ibuprofen, ketoprofen, and paracetamol using a pretreatment step with an MN roller compared to untreated skin. The first study in humans using solid MN arrays as a drug delivery strategy was conducted using naltrexone as a model drug (Wermeling et al., 2008). This study successfully demonstrated the feasibility of using MN arrays to enhance transdermal delivery of hydrophilic drug molecules. The main technical challenge of this drug delivery strategy is the need for a two-step application, which is considered impractical for patient use. With this, silicon and metal are not necessarily the most appropriate choices of materials. There are concerns that such nonbiodegradable materials may present safety issues when inserted into the skin. Example of safety issues include silicone-related granulomas and reports of solid MN array tips remaining in the skin after removal of solid MN arrays (Henry et al., 1998; Millard & Maisels, 1966). Other drug delivery strategies using MN arrays have, therefore, now become more prevalent.

6.3.2 Coated microneedle arrays

Coated MN arrays are typically prepared from silicon or metal, but coated polymeric MN arrays have been investigated in a bid to move away from using less biocompatible materials (Quinn & Donnelly, 2018). Coated MN arrays have been employed for the delivery of a number of different drug molecules and peptides. Examples include salmon calcitonin (Tas et al., 2012), desmopressin (Cormier et al., 2004), parathyroid hormone (Daddona, Matriano, Mandema, & Maa, 2011), bleomycin (Lee, Ryu, Roh, & Park, 2017), and lidocaine (Baek, Shin, & Kim, 2017). While this drug delivery strategy offers a more efficient route of transdermal drug delivery than that described for skin pretreatment with solid MN arrays, a technical challenge of this drug delivery strategy is the amount of drug formulation that can be coated (and indeed, uniformly dispersed) over the surface of the MN array itself. Owing to the small size of the needles, the loading capacity of such an array is small. With dosing limited to typically microgram (μm) quantities, coated MN arrays are more restricted to high potency drug molecules (Quinn & Donnelly, 2018).

6.3.3 Dissolving microneedle arrays

Dissolving MN arrays (Fig. 6.4(d)) have been fabricated primarily from polymers with a considerable push in recent years toward developing dissolving MN arrays using biocompatible FDA(Food and Drug Administration)-approved materials. For the fabrication of dissolving MN arrays, materials include synthetic, natural, and copolymers. Examples of synthetic polymers include PVA (Donnelly et al., 2011), PVP (González-Vázquez et al., 2017), poly(lactic acid) PLA (Park, Allen, & Prausnitz, 2006), and PLGA (Naves et al., 2017). Natural polymers include CMC (Park & Kim, 2017) and the copolymer, Gantrez S-97 (Pamornpathomkul et al., 2018; Quinn et al., 2015). Given that the majority of polymers are water-soluble, dissolving MN arrays are particularly amenable to drugs with a more hydrophilic character (Quinn & Donnelly, 2018). Despite this, dissolving MN arrays have been used to deliver a range of molecules, from hydrophilic, low molecular weight drugs molecules to larger biopharmaceutical molecules, demonstrating the ability of such a platform to enhance transdermal delivery. Examples of hydrophilic, low molecular weight drug molecules include caffeine (Garland, Caffarel-Salvador, Migalska, Woolfson, & Donnelly, 2012), lidocaine (Garland et al., 2012), theophylline (Caffarel-Salvador, Brady et al., 2015), and acyclovir (Pamornpathomkul et al., 2018). On the other hand, examples of large biopharmaceuticals include insulin (Migalska et al., 2011), heparin (Gomaa et al., 2012; Ito et al., 2008), erythropoietin (Ito et al., 2007), and human growth hormone (Lee et al., 2011). Delivery of antibiotics using dissolving MN arrays has been investigated, but the number of antibiotics is sparse. In one study, González-Vázquez et al. (2017) investigated the transdermal delivery of gentamicin, a hydrophilic, low molecular weight aminoglycoside. Approximately, 75% of the total gentamicin was delivered across the skin *in vitro* after 24 h. In *in vivo* experimentation, therapeutically relevant doses of the antibiotic were delivered to rats, highlighting the potential for exploitation of this delivery route and promising technology for gentamicin administration (González-Vázquez et al., 2017). As dissolving MN arrays dissolve upon application and insertion into ISF, this drug delivery strategy is essentially self-disabling, meaning that not only is the reinsertion of dissolving MN arrays into another patient impossible, the risk of needle-stick injuries to healthcare professional (HCP) who may be involved in administration is none (Quinn & Donnelly, 2018). Another advantage related to this is that there is no need for safe disposal as there is no sharp waste remaining with dissolving MN arrays. However, one technical challenge is the inability of this platform to deliver therapeutically relevant concentrations of low potency drug molecules, due to reduced functionality of the MN array associated with high drug loading (Quinn, Kearney, Courtenay, McCrudden, & Donnelly, 2014). Indeed, many drug molecules require several hundred milligrams in order to achieve therapeutic plasma concentrations in humans. However, this technical challenge has since been demonstrated that therapeutically relevant concentrations of the low potency drug molecule, ibuprofen sodium was successfully delivered in rats (McCrudden et al., 2014). The deposition of polymer in the skin may be another concern with this drug delivery strategy. However, this is likely of little concern for medication that is used for occasional use, such as antibiotics compared with medications that require long-term MN array usage (Quinn & Donnelly, 2018).

6.3.4 Hollow microneedle arrays

Hollow MN arrays (Fig. 6.4(b)) have been fabricated mainly from silicon and metal (Brazzle, Papautsky, & Bruno Frazier, 2000; Griss & Stemme, 2003). In addition, glass hollow MN arrays have also been manufactured (Wang et al., 2006). Most studies regarding hollow MN arrays have focused on fabrication aspects, including design and characterization studies. As a result, less attention has been given to their actual efficiency in delivering drug molecules across the skin. To date, insulin has been the most extensively delivered molecule using hollow MN arrays (Davis, Martanto, Allen, & Prausnitz, 2005; Wang et al., 2006). For example, a human study using hollow MN arrays was performed to assess the effect of hollow MN arrays on insulin delivery in Type 1 diabetic adults (Gupta, Felner, & Prausnitz, 2009). A reduction in glucose levels occurred, thus proving the feasibility of using hollow MN arrays for the minimally invasive transdermal delivery of insulin. Hollow MN arrays enable continuous delivery of molecules across the skin through the central lumen of the hollow MN array either by passive diffusion or electrically driven flow of a liquid formulation. In comparison to solid or coated MN arrays, which are capable of delivering small quantities of drug molecules or peptides, this drug delivery strategy is considered to allow for infusion of larger amounts of drug molecules (Tuan-Mahmood et al., 2013). However, the successful use of hollow MN arrays can be hindered by potential clogging of the needle bore with tissue upon insertion, reducing the potential for drug delivery. There are also a number of technical challenges associated with this drug delivery strategy. In comparison to solid or coated MN arrays, hollow MN arrays present a complex design, with an inherently more challenging manufacturing process, in order to prepare needles with an appropriate bore for drug infusion. Hollow MN arrays require the incorporation of a drug reservoir, which contains the liquid to be delivered. In comparison to solid MN arrays, hollow MN arrays are inherently weaker in terms of mechanical strength and are, therefore, at a greater risk of breakage. This is owing to their complex design. Furthermore, insertion of hollow MN arrays into the skin could be more difficult because the bore opening for drug infusion reduces the overall sharpness of the needle.

6.3.5 Hydrogel-forming microneedle arrays

Hydrogel-forming MN arrays (Fig. 6.4(e)), a relatively new concept, have been fabricated from polymers which are crosslinked to form the hydrogel matrix. Described by Donnelly, Singh, Garland et al. (2012), the first hydrogel-forming MN array was fabricated from poly methyl vinyl ether and maleic anhydride (PMVE/MAH) (Gantrez AN-139), crosslinked with the polymer poly(ethylene glycol) (PEG). In the same research group, PMVE/MA (Gantrez S-97), crosslinked with PEG has also been used to fabricate hydrogel-forming MN arrays (Donnelly, Moffatt et al., 2014). Hydrogel-forming MN arrays have been shown to deliver various drug molecules and biopharmaceuticals of varying molecular weight. Examples of low molecular weight drug molecules include ibuprofen sodium (Donnelly, Moffatt et al., 2014), caffeine (Caffarel-Salvador, Tuan-Mahmood et al., 2015), donepezil (Kearney, Caffarel-Salvador, Fallows, McCarthy, & Donnelly, 2016), and metformin (Migdadi et al., 2018). On the other hand, examples of high molecular weight molecules include insulin (Donnelly, Singh, Garland et al., 2012), BSA (Donnelly, Singh, Garland et al., 2012), ovalbumin (Donnelly, Moffatt et al., 2014), and bevacizumab (Courtenay, McCrudden, McAvoy, McCarthy, & Donnelly, 2018). Regarding antibiotics, in the first report describing hydrogel-forming MN arrays, Donnelly, Singh, Garland et al. (2012) investigated the transdermal delivery of the low potency, low molecular weight, hydrophilic drug molecule, metronidazole. Approximately, 30% of the total amount of metronidazole was delivered across the skin *in vitro* after 24 h. In *in vivo* experimentation, metronidazole was found to rapidly appear in plasma and maintained at relatively constant levels over the 48 h study period (Donnelly, Singh, Garland et al., 2012). Developed in response to the challenges of the previously described drug-delivery strategies, this unique MN array design has its own advantages. Rather than transdermal drug delivery primarily controlled by the barrier properties of the SC, the control is now in the crosslink density of the hydrogel system. By altering the polymer crosslink density, the swelling rate of the hydrogel system can be controlled, thus conferring the ability to govern the drug release rate. This implies that the drug delivery can be tailored, on a case-by-case basis, to meet the requirements of different drug molecules, thus confirming the versatility of this novel MN array design. Hydrogel-forming MN arrays are also removed from the skin completely intact. Therefore, no measureable polymer residue is left behind. Hydrogel-forming MN arrays soften by the uptake of ISF, thus preventing reinsertion of the MN array. This reduces the risk of infection transmission that may arise from needle reuse. As the drug is prepared in a separate drug-containing reservoir, the loading capacity is not linked to MN array itself, removing any limitations on dosing. This is particularly useful for high dose drug molecules. Due to these advantages, this novel technology has the potential to increase the range of drug molecules that can be delivered transdermally.

6.4 Other microneedle array applications

6.4.1 Microneedle-mediated vaccine delivery

Vaccines are conventionally administered *via* the subcutaneous or intramuscular (IM) route of administration. The skin is an attractive vaccination target due to its rich immune cell population, specifically antigen presenting cells that generate adaptive immune responses (McCrudden, Courtenay, & Donnelly, 2018). The use of MN arrays for the facilitated delivery of vaccines has, thus, become an area of great interest and promise. It has been suggested by Al-Zahrani et al. (2012) that MN-mediated vaccination may provide a dose-sparing effect compared to IM vaccination. Vaccines are temperature sensitive biological products, requiring refrigeration. The thermostability of MN array vaccines eliminates cold-chain requirements, thus reducing costs and potentially improving distribution (Marshall, Sahm, & Moore, 2016). This would be particularly advantageous in low resource settings as this would combat the frequently encountered issue of supply shortage as stock piling could be permitted. In addition, MN array vaccines offer a simple and minimally invasive technique for reliable vaccination, which may be self-administered, with no sharp disposal waste. Self-administration with MN array vaccines could further improve vaccine coverage in low resource settings where there are shortages of medical personnel.

The two main MN array types for MN-mediated vaccine delivery discussed and researched at length in the literature are coated and dissolving MN arrays, with the influenza virus vaccine a popular vaccine target (Marshall et al., 2016). Coated MN arrays have shown success with regard to simulating an appropriate immune response following vaccine application. In one study, Kommareddy et al. (2013) found that coating influenza antigen onto solid MN arrays was comparable to IM vaccination. Conducted in guinea pigs, this study moved beyond initial mouse model studies.

Dissolving MN arrays show most promise with respect to potential future commercialization, due to mainly their self-disabling nature, thereby preventing reuse. In the first study investigating dissolving MN arrays for vaccination, Sullivan et al. (2010) introduced dissolving MN arrays for influenza vaccination using a simple patch-based system. MN array vaccination generated humoral and cellular immune responses in mice and provided complete protection against lethal challenge. Compared to conventional IM vaccination, MN vaccination also resulted in more efficient lung clearance. *The Lancet* published the results of the first-in-man Phase I study on dissolving MN arrays containing the influenza vaccine (Rouphael et al., 2017). In this study, results were comparable between dissolving MN arrays containing influenza vaccine and IM vaccination. Indeed, humoral immune responses were generated in participants, whether administered by HCPs or self-administered. Administration of the dissolving MN arrays was well tolerated, with the dissolving MN arrays preferred by participants over IM administration. Thus, MN vaccines could increase influenza vaccination rates and improve present vaccination coverage.

6.4.2 Microneedle-mediated skin appearance improvement and delivery of cosmeceuticals

Aging is a biological process and facial scarring, as a result of acne or a burn, can be a distressing phenomenon encountered by many people. Skin appearance has traditionally been improved *via* ablative methodologies such as chemical peels, collagen injections, and dermabrasion, all of which aim to destruct the epidermis (McAlister, McCrudden, & Donnelly, 2018). However, in ablative methodologies such as these, undesired postoperative changes in the skin can occur, resulting in lengthened healing times and in some cases, adverse side effects such as the development of dyschromias. In contrast, microneedling (a nonablative method), with needles of appropriate height, would negate the risks of negative side effects often seen with invasive ablative approaches.

Cosmetic MN devices have been designed and developed with the distinct function of disrupting the barrier properties of the SC to enable skin rejuvenation and improved skin appearance (McCrudden et al., 2015). The concept of skin microneedling technology in dermatology was pioneered in 1995 (Orentreich & Orentreich, 1995), and the principle of this technique was to induce collagen synthesis. Currently, there are a wide variety of commercially available MN devices used in cosmetic applications. The original concept design that is used for microneedling is known commercially as the Dermaroller, and the efficacy of this treatment alone has been investigated (Alam et al., 2014; Aust, Fernandes, Kolokythas, Kaplan, & Vogt, 2008; Fabbrocini, Fardella, Monfrecola, Proietti, & Innocenzi, 2009). In one study, Alam et al. (2014) conducted a split-face, placebo-controlled clinical trial, including 20 participants with acne scars on both sides of their face, randomized to receive either microneedling with topical anesthetic or topical anesthetic alone (control) to either side of the face. Three microneedling treatments were performed at 2 week intervals. Two dermatologists, blinded to the intervention, graded digital photographs of the participants' acne scars with the quantitative Goodman and Baron grading system. At 6 months posttreatment, using the grading system, there was a significant improvement in the appearance of acne scars compared with the control group (Alam et al., 2014).

The future commercial and clinical success of MN devices, not just cosmetic MN devices, will undoubtedly depend not only upon their ability to fulfill a designated function but also on their acceptability by both patient and HCPs. User perception studies are actively being conducted, with participants' having a "strongly positive" perception of MN arrays (Donnelly, McCrudden et al., 2014). Potentially detrimental to the impact of such studies, however, are reports, such as that published in the *Daily Mail* newspaper in 2009, which stated that the Dermaroller, specifically resembled an " … instrument of medieval torture … " despite the article concluding that the Dermaroller resulted in improved skin appearance (Mail Online, 2009). Media reports, such as this, reinforce the importance of clear message dissemination to the general public about the benefits of MN devices so that their reputation may not be harmed unnecessarily.

An area in the cosmeceutical industry that has garnered much interest is the exploitation of MN technologies in facilitating the delivery of cosmeceuticals (McAlister et al., 2018). In one study, two antiwrinkle compounds of different hydrophilicities, namely ascorbic acid and retinyl retinoate were incorporated into dissolving hyaluronic acid–based MN arrays, separately, for evaluation in combating wrinkles, on 24 women for 12 weeks (Kim, Yang, Kim, Jung, & Jung, 2014). Patients were randomly allocated to either the ascorbic acid or the retinyl retinoate group. All subjects applied dissolving hyaluronic acid–based MN arrays to the "crow's feet" area of the face twice daily, and these were left in place for 6 h. Improved skin appearance in terms of reduction in roughness and diminished wrinkle appearance resulted (Kim et al., 2014). Although test conditions are obviously not ideal for cosmetic purposes, this study serves as a promising indication of proof of concept for the delivery of antiaging compounds using MN technology.

6.5 Microneedle-mediated patient monitoring and diagnosis

Therapeutic patient monitoring represents a useful tool for clinicians in optimizing patient therapy and diagnosing illness (Donnelly, Mooney et al., 2014). Monitoring in this case relates to the determination of plasma concentration of drug molecules or endogenous markers during treatment or diagnosis. Plasma levels of these drug molecules or endogenous markers are conventionally measured from a blood sample, obtained using the traditional hypodermic needle and syringe. With the well-known drawbacks of hypodermic needles, MN arrays offer the potential to overcome these limitations. Hypodermic needles are associated with increased risk of needle stick injuries and crosscontamination, such as 37.6% of Hepatitis B infections, 39% of Hepatitis C infections, and 4.4% HIV/AIDS infections among world healthcare workers (Rapiti, Prüss-Üstün, & Hutin, 2005). In addition to the health implications, needlestick injuries also represent a significant economic burden, with one study estimating an annual cost of £500,000 per National Health Service (NHS) trust (Ball & Pike,

2009). Premature neonates, in particular, can exhibit blood volumes as low as 80 mL/kg, making blood sampling to any degree far from ideal and frequent sampling increasing the risk of anemia (Koren, 1997). From the patient's perspective, minimally invasive sampling offers less discomfort and could offer significant benefits for those with needle phobia and low sample volumes.

Minimally invasive monitoring methods include the use of reverse iontophoresis (Bouissou, Sylvestre, Guy, & Delgado-Charro, 2009; Ching, Chou, Sun, Huang, & Shieh, 2011; Ebah et al., 2012; Leboulanger, Aubry, Bondolfi, Guy, & Delgado-Charro, 2004), reverse iontophoresis combined with electroporation (Lee et al., 2010), low frequency ultrasound (Paliwal, Ogura, & Mitragotri, 2010), capillary microdialysis (Kim et al., 2008; Nielsen et al., 2009), and by pore creation using a near infrared laser (Venugopal et al., 2008). ISF monitoring is common practice and an alternative technique to blood extraction (Jian et al., 2007; Sun et al., 2010; Takshing Ching, Sun, Huang, Shieh, & Chen, 2010; Wang, Cornwell, & Prausnitz, 2005).

In one study, Li, Lee, Lee, and Jung (2013) described the fabrication and use of metallic hollow MN arrays, capable of extracting 20 µL of blood from the tail of a mouse. It must be noted, however, that the MN arrays were 1800 µm in height, exceeding the height of conventionally used MN arrays for drug delivery as previously described. Nonetheless, the authors of this study claimed that these MN arrays allow blood extraction with low risk of pain inducement (Li et al., 2013). Although a less invasive approach than the hypodermic needle, these MN arrays share the risks associated with crosscontamination, infection, and would require sharps waste disposal.

An alternative approach to blood extraction has recently been developed to collect ISF from the skin using MN arrays instead of blood extraction. ISF represents a good medium for analyte monitoring as concentrations in the ISF often accurately reflect concentrations in the blood (Larrañeta et al., 2016). Thus, MN arrays offer the possibility of a pain and blood free patient monitoring and diagnosis system. A number of publications document the use of MN arrays focusing on glucose monitoring. In one study, Wang et al. (2005) investigated the use of glass hollow MN arrays, in combination with vacuum pressure, to extract ISF from hairless rats and humans for glucose monitoring. Results showed that the concentrations of glucose in ISF correlated well with blood glucose levels (Wang et al., 2005). Hydrogel-forming MN arrays provide a unique mechanism to obtain ISF. In a publication by Caffarel-Salvador, Brady et al. (2015), the Donnelly Research Group first described the use of hydrogel-forming MN arrays to extract ISF from human volunteers for glucose monitoring. While the concentrations of glucose in ISF did not correlate directly with blood glucose levels, this study provides preliminary evidence and promise for the use of hydrogel-forming MN arrays in patient monitoring and diagnosis.

6.5.1 Fluid flow

Irrespective of the fluid to be accessed, technical challenges related to MN-mediated patient monitoring and diagnosis is adequate force to drive fluid flow and adequate fluid volume collected for subsequent analysis. In some cases, flow rates between 1 and 100 µL/h have been quoted as necessary (Gardeniers et al., 2003). Regarding adequate fluid volume collection, many designs rely on passive extraction alone, depending solely on capillary action to generate fluid flow. One such design proposed uses a bimask process to achieve sharp tips, a cylindrical body, and side ports to minimize blockage of the hollow MN, and is suggested for use in either drug delivery or microbiological sampling (Zhang & Jullien, 2003). The authors recommend this design as it is easily fabricated to provide a high needle density and it offers a low flow resistance and good structural strength. In a paper that follows, they describe this design further and investigate performance (Zhang & Jullien, 2005). The needles, fabricated using silicon dioxide, were capable of human skin penetration without breakage, but passive liquid extraction was only demonstrated on a potato. Another early study, describing a system amenable to both ISF and whole blood, used a hollow MN array with integrated fluidic microchannels, fabricated using silicon and glass, and conducted preliminary tests on the ear lobe of one human volunteer (Mukerjee, Collins, Isseroff, & Smith, 2004). The authors outline three needle tip designs including a "volcano-like design," a "microhypodermic" design, and a "snake-fang" design. A common issue with hollow designs is the potential for blockage, and the first two listed here exhibited this issue. The third, "snake-fang," design was reported as superior since it was found to be less susceptible to this difficulty, with the bore here placed 25 µm off-center. The fluid capture from the ear lobe by capillary action was described, but penetration testing conducted on the first knuckle of the thumb concluded that a 1.5 ± 0.25 N force was required for penetration. The risk of glass becoming embedded within the skin represented a major drawback with this design. Other work has focused more on the theoretical considerations behind fluid flow, driven by capillary action, in hollow MNs and the development of models and calculations to aid in the determination of optimal MN design for optimum fluid flow. Work by one group developed a theoretical fluid model to enable interpretation of microfluidic properties of Newtonian fluids within silicon MN and concluded a faster fluid filling when the length—width ratio of the microchannel was $\sqrt{2} + 1$ (Liu et al., 2006).

The employment of MN arrays with a high needle density has been suggested as a possible means to enable sufficient rates of flow, with the use of out-of-plane arrays recommended as most appropriate for achieving such specifications (Gardeniers et al., 2003). In contrasting with this, others discuss the need for more active extraction methods to ensure adequate fluid collection rather than reliance of capillary force alone. The use of vacuum force to assist with fluid withdrawal has been described (Tsuchiya, Jinnin, Yamamoto, Uetsuji, & Nakamachi, 2010), as well as more novel approaches such as exploitation of the phase transition of a gel to power sample extraction. The latter approach was first documented in the literature using poly (N-isopropylacrylamide) integration within a microsystem intended for glucose sensing (Kobayashi & Suzuki, 2001). The volume change exhibited by the gel in response to a variation in temperature was utilized in this study to power a micropump for fluid extraction, with the ultimate aim of achieving spontaneous sampling in response to the temperature of human skin. While successful sampling of a glucose solution was achieved through a 50 µm diameter MN using this concept, flow was only unidirectional and in response to temperature shifts between 30 and 40°C and, thus, not relevant for human body temperature. Work to instigate sampling at more relevant temperatures (30–37°C) was subsequently carried out (Suzuki, Tokuda, & Kobayashi, 2002). The improved design incorporated a silicon membrane to enable repeated gel use as a result of its elastic force. By shifting the system between hot plates maintained at 30 and 37°C, volume changes were found to occur within less than 1 min and 90% response time of the sensor reported to range between 30 and 40 s. This modified system could also successfully achieve bidirectional flow; however, the use of nonideal materials, such as silicon, for MN fabrication is again declared a challenge by the authors. Further work by this group then explored the possibility of continuous monitoring adopting this approach. Adjustment of pH, in addition to temperature, to induce the volume change was used. This study also explored the use of an enzyme-loaded gel to extend the time for volume reduction even further (Suzuki, Tokuda, Miyagishi, Yoshida, & Honda, 2004). Using this combined approach of pH and temperature-induced changes, the time for sampling was prolonged, while the use of the enzyme-loaded gel provided an opportunity for further adjustment. The work also demonstrated continuous glucose sampling using an external glucose sample solution.

6.5.2 Differential strategies for fluid extraction

While much work in the area of MN-mediated monitoring has focused on the development of hollow MNs for fluid collection, alternative approaches have also been explored. One group suggested a novel array to remove the use of conventional holes altogether, instead developing MNs with quadrupled grooves for blood storage following capillary force extraction (Khumpuang, Kawaguchi, & Sugiyama, 2004). This interesting suggestion used a biocompatible material, polymethacrylate (PMMA), for MN fabrication by a novel technique, plain pattern to cross section. Penetration of this array into chicken meat was confirmed using a liquid with similar viscosity to blood (aniline blue); however, they failed to successfully demonstrate fluid flow along the grooves with this approach.

Another approach described used a combination design based on both hollow and solid silicon MN for ISF extraction (Mukerjee, Issseroff, Collins, & Smith, 2003). This strategy used hollow MNs for fluid flow in the center only and designed with a beveled tip to impede pore blockage. The incorporation of an outer border of solid needles functioned to stretch the skin to facilitate successful penetration. Human skin penetration of this device was demonstrated using an *in vivo* confocal microscope, with some MN tip breakage identified. Such events are clearly not ideal, particularly when dealing with materials with poor biocompatibility. Application to the human ear lobe resulted in flow through the 80 μm wide channels, which was assumed to be ISF.

A two-stage approach to sample extraction has also been explored, using solid MN for skin pretreatment with subsequent fluid extraction, using vacuum force (Wang et al., 2005). This study used glass MNs for ISF extraction for subsequent glucose analysis, with insertion achieved using a vibration technique and involved both animal (rats) and human subjects. The vacuum was applied for 2–10 min and 5–10 min on rats and humans, respectively. In human volunteers, volumes of 1–10 μL were extracted from a 1 cm−2 area with 7–10 MN-created conduits. The vacuum procedure was reported to cause erythema in human subjects, but the overall procedure was defined as relatively painless. ISF glucose measurements obtained using this design were found proportional to that of the blood. However, the need for a calibration factor using blood was an obvious flaw for this system. Importantly, these authors showed detection of rapidly changing blood glucose levels without any associated time lag using this technique; an issue previously alluded to for other minimally invasive monitoring work (Potts, Tamada, & Tierney, 2002; Sieg, Guy, & Delgado-Charro, 2004). In work that followed, this group attempted to examine the accuracy of electrochemical monitors for glucose measurement by comparison with a gas chromatography—mass spectrometry method for the different matrices, blood, and ISF, with the conclusion that use of ISF results in a bias which must be accounted for (Vesper, Wang, Archibold, Prausnitz, & Myers, 2006).

Sato et al. (2011) adopted a similar approach by using polycarbonate MN arrays (305 MN arrays per 50 mm^2 area), with a length of 300 µm. In contrast to the vacuum approach outlined by Wang et al. (2005), a reservoir was used for ISF collection by passive diffusion and osmotic pressure only, allowing for sodium to be used as an internal standard. Two reservoir designs were proposed; the first was a plastic chamber containing 1.2% KCL solution, the second a hydrogel patch consisting of polyvinyl alcohol with 2% KCL solvent and adhesive tape. Interstitial glucose measurements were found to be in close correlation with blood measurements, but this was based only on data from healthy volunteers, thus exhibiting minimal glucose fluctuations, rather than for a more representative diabetic population. Furthermore, a recent patent has also outlined the possible use of this two-stage approach for extraction in a design which claims flexibility to, not only blood and ISF collection, but also other bodily fluids, including saliva, tears, lymph, and urine, for analytical evaluation (Brancazio, 2012). Again, the designs outlined here incorporated vacuums or chambers to ensure pressures lower than atmospheric to facilitate fluid flow rather than placing sole reliance on passive mechanisms.

6.5.3 Integrated designs

The development of integrated systems that negate the formal extraction of fluid and instead rely on the use of integrated sensors has also been explored. Analyte detection for MN-mediated monitoring can, therefore, be on-site, with the incorporation of integrated sensors, as well as off-site, using fluid extracted for subsequent analysis. In the case of the former, sensor development and optimization have been critical aspects of design progressions to date toward a complete, optimized, integrated system. One system to allow easy integration with a PDMS biochip involved the first single-crystal-silicon MN array fabricated in the plane of the substrate (Paik et al., 2003). The extraction fluid of interest in this design was blood, using MNs with lengths around 2 mm and microchannel diameters around 20 µm. Fluid flow *in vitro* and *in vivo*, with successful penetration into the tail vein of a mouse, was demonstrated. In a paper that followed, penetration was tested using agarose gel, chicken breast, rat-tail vein, and rabbit ear, and fluid flow confirmed using agarose gel and chicken breast (Paik et al., 2004). The authors outline potential optimisation of the design, highlighting the need to balance sharpness with mechanical strength and propose a tip taper angle of 30°C to be superior, producing a 6.28 N buckling load enabling penetration without breakage. However, the actual functioning of the integrated biochip was not addressed.

A group in the Netherlands proposed a combination of anisotropic wet etching and the BOSCH-DIRE process to produce an out-of-plane silicon hollow MN array, with flow channels positioned off-center to avoid blockage (Gardeniers et al., 2003). Subsequent works have also adopted this strategy in an attempt to avert this issue (Bodhale et al., 2010; Luttge et al., 2007). The triangular-tipped MNs produced had height of only 350 μm and maximum channel width of 70 μm. As already discussed, such heights seem insufficient for successful blood withdrawal, thus possibly indicating the fabrication approach as unfit for purpose. The diagnostic capabilities of the device were, therefore, examined using blood collected with a 1.8 mm lancet. Compatibility of the array with a capillary electrophoresis chip was demonstrated using 30 μL of the collected blood, but inaccuracies compared to expected blood concentrations were evident. In work that followed, water was used to fill the volume between the chip and the sampler, resulting in the successful demonstration of potassium, sodium, magnesium, and lithium measurement (Vrouwe & Luttge, 2005). However, this again was based only on a model for the MN system, composed of CE chip and sample collector, and failed to demonstrate actual MN blood extraction. The same group later suggested the use of SU-8 as a material for hollow MN fabrication, improving biocompatibility, and outlined novel fabrication methods to produce this polymeric MN patch, achieving needle heights ≥500 μm (Luttge et al., 2007). They suggest that this device enables blood collection for analysis off-site, as well as again describing integration with a CE chip. Only preliminary results were presented to show the capabilities of the device in blood diagnostics, proving the device suitable for sample transfer, such as to a CE chip, so facilitating the analysis of inorganic ions in blood.

Another integrated system for sampling and glucose sensing was suggested, using in-plane silicon hollow MN and gold microelectrodes (Liu, Wang, Tang, Feng, & Zhou, 2005). Here, a unique approach was taken to glucose sensing, using electrochemical detection as well as a novel technique for enzyme immobilisation, relying on capillary force to immobilise the enzymes on the microelectrode surface. The sensor showed good linearity for glucose in the concentration range 0−500 mg/dL when tested using standard solutions. Enzyme immobilisation was also a key component in the system described by Goud et al. (2007), consisting of a novel biosensor integrated with microfluidic channels and MNs fabricated using OrmocerR, an organically modified ceramic material for glucose monitoring (Goud et al., 2007). This design, unlike that proposed by (Liu et al., 2005), offered the advantage of MNs fabricated using a material described as biologically inert and nontoxic, i.e., OrmocerR. The biosensor used here incorporates electrodes, developed from carbon nanotubes and glassy carbon, alongside the enzyme, glucose oxidase, encapsulated within a zirconia/Nafi on matrix to offer improved sensitivity and specificity. This system displayed prompt glucose detection, using standard glucose solutions, signifying its potential value in glucose monitoring applications. In both instances, however, extensive evaluation of the integrated functioning of the entire system failed to be conducted.

The exploitation of enzyme-mediated bioluminescent reactions for detection has also been outlined as part of an autonomous MN system. This system consisted of an MN array with an associated reaction chamber and photodetector (Chandrasekaran, Brazzle, & Frazier, 2003). With this approach, metabolite concentrations were determined by coupling reactions with other enzyme-linked reactions that emitted light. Light emitted could then be subsequently measured. In this study, the production of adenosine triphosphate (ATP) during glucose consumption was exploited, since the enzyme-catalyzed process of luciferin oxidation uses ATP and results in bioluminescence. Subsequent measurement of light intensity was, thus, related to glucose concentration. The use of ATP in many biochemical reactions broadens the potential applications of this design. The hollow metal MNs integrated within the system demonstrated successful fluid flow (1000−4000 μL/h) without leakage, with a 1500 μm shaft length and 4.1 mm lumen length. The novel photo detection approach was illustrated as feasible with the sensor characterized within the range relevant to glucose detection (2.0−7.0 mM of ATP). However, the performance of this device was limited by a decreased light intensity.

A different integrated design focused on arrays composed of gold-coated silicon with a hetero-bifunctional PEG coated to its surface for protein biomarker capture (Corrie et al., 2010). The surface modifications were designed to enable selective detection of anti-FluVax®-immunoglobulin G (AF-IgG), which was tested using a 10% mouse serum. Application to mouse ear skin in this study illustrated the device to be capable of selective biomarker capture, and the ease of removal for subsequent analysis. As with many of the designs suggested, various modifications are essential prior to optimal human targeting, such as ensuring an adequate penetration depth and biocompatibility considerations, to name but a few.

A similar approach has also been outlined for hydrogen peroxide and lactate detection using an array of hollow MNs with integrated carbon-paste electrodes (Windmiller, Valdés-Ramírez et al., 2011). In this case, a biocompatible polymer was used to produce MNs with a height of 1500 μm and a vertical central bore of 425 μm. *In vitro* studies performed indicated the selectivity and sensitivity of this sensor, which demonstrated stability over the time period (2 h). This group have also proposed a different design to remove the need for fluid extraction for glutamate oxidase and glucose detection, with a view toward their continuous monitoring (Windmiller, Zhou et al., 2011). This design incorporates both hollow and solid MNs, using the same polymer during fabrication, to form a single array with multiple microcavities, in which the detection enzymes, glutamate oxidase, and glucose oxidase, are entrapped within a thin film of poly(o-phenylenediamine) (PPD) to minimize interference. High sensitivity and fast detection within clinically relevant ranges was shown for this biosensor using both a buffer matrix and human serum. A different paper also focuses on the use of an integrated design incorporating solid MNs, which themselves act as the sensor surface for glucose and lactate detection (Trzebinski et al., 2012). These were developed using SU-8 coated with gold and then an enzyme layer, before being surrounded in a protective epoxy-PU membrane. Stability of this device was claimed for the 48 h period. Again, glucose detection within the clinically relevant ranges was demonstrated for this device, and the concurrent detection of both glucose and lactate are suggested as a possibility.

With an aim of cost reduction, other researchers have proposed a microvalve for fluid extraction, which is intended for integration within an MN array and biosensing system (Moreno, Aracil, & Quero, 2008; Moreno, Aracil, & Quero, 2009). By removing the standard high energy need for valve operation, and through use of low cost polymers, which are easily fabricated, a cost reduction for this approach was intended. The valve design employs two chambers with varied pressures separated by an SU-8 wall and undergoes both thermal and mechanical activation. A gold wire, bonded to a copper line on a PCB substrate, crosses the wall and functions to collapse the wall *via* thermal destruction upon current flow. Different pressures between the chambers will also facilitate this destruction. Miniaturization of this system has yet to be demonstrated, however, as well as the actual sensing functionalities for biomedical monitoring purposes.

With biosensors clearly at the forefront of monitoring using an MN array—based approach, consideration has also been given to prolonging sensor lifetime. The destruction that proteins can impart on enzyme-based sensors has been addressed with suggestions made to exclude large molecular weight compounds, and, thus, prolong enzyme-based biosensor lifetime. One approach in an attempt to achieve this aim involved the integration of a dialysis membrane within the monitoring device (Zahn, Trebotich, & Liepmann, 2000). Two designs based on silicon MN for ISF extraction were suggested. First, the use of a diffusion membrane of layered polysilicon either side of a thin thermally grown oxide of approximately 10—50 μm with etch holes was described. The second design was based on a permeable polysilicon. It is concluded within this work that the latter design should offer superiority, in terms of mass transfer rates as well as filtration capabilities. In work that follows, this group go further with this concept in the design of an MN-based glucose monitoring system, with the addition of an integrated glucose sensor (Zimmermann, Fienbork, Stoeber, Flounders, & Liepmann, 2003). In this design, ISF flows through the out-of-plane MN (200 μm length) before passing through a porous polysilicon dialysis membrane, thus excluding larger proteins before coming into contact with the sensor for detection. This in-device glucose sensor had a suggested optimum flow rate of 25 μL/min, and response linearity was illustrated for glucose concentrations in the region of 0—160 mg/dL. While the capabilities for ISF sampling and glucose sensing with the integrated device are demonstrated, the use of only 8 MNs proved insufficient for a significant sensor response, relying on capillary action and evaporation alone for fluid extraction. An increased array density was, however, proposed as a solution. Work with this design is further explained within a later paper; however, results remain preliminary and are largely based upon models and estimations (Zahn, Trebotich, & Liepmann, 2005).

A recently published patent also cites the prevention of protein entry into the collection chamber as a crucial element of sensor design (Mischler & Werner, 2012), suggesting the incorporation of a filter membrane which prevents entry of molecules greater than 10 TDa, such as that previously outlined (Zahn et al., 2005). The invention functions to continuously monitor analytes in ISF using optical detection methods, negating the need for reagents and relying on the correlation between analyte concentration and absorbed radiation. A miniaturised system is described consisting of an array of hollow MNs that enable fluid flow to a chamber. The chamber has a window allowing radiation entry and transmission. A diamond coating is a suggestion to further minimize protein disruption by preventing protein attachment to the window surface. A detector on the other side of the window enables radiation detection and is coupled to a unit functioning to quantify analyte concentrations. Possible analytes outlined by the authors include glucose, cholesterol, creatinine, urea, and triglycerides. Importantly, this integrated design's on-site approach to sample analysis also eliminates the need for additional regents to be used for analyte quantification. The inventors here also suggest a watch-type design for this device, with needles attached to the portion of the watch face in contact with the arm, with the face displaying the calculated concentration. Such considerations regarding ease of use and convenience for the user are critical for the advancement of these alternative strategies from novel ideas into useful and applicable approaches to patient monitoring.

The amalgamation of drug delivery, alongside the processes of blood extraction, filtration, and insertion, has also been described for a device targeted for patients with renal disease (Tayyaba, Ashraf, & Afzulpurkar, 2011). The electronic components of this system include a microcontroller, which controls transport according to pressure, as determined by the flow sensors. Blood extraction with this system is achieved using 1700 μm polyglycolic-acid (PGA) MN with a double-radius structure, creating a pressure difference to prevent clogging. Following extraction, blood enters a heparin-containing mixing chamber before passing through the filtration membrane to remove molecules such as urea and vancomycin, with high molecular weight molecules. One such molecule, beta-2 microglobulin (β 2m), requires filtration, however, necessitating the inclusion of a β 2m absorbent material to ensure its removal. The dual lumens were constructed to have lengths of 800 and 900 μm with corresponding diameters of 60 and 100 μm. The authors highlight viscosity as an important determinant of flow rate and, based on a 5 × 5 array, flow rates for acetone, water, and blood for the system were defined at 1182, 971, and 845 μL/min, respectively. While the proposed system is outlined in terms of fabrication and theoretically analysed, progress toward the demonstration of the integrated system's actual functionality is needed. Furthermore, the advantage of using biocompatible PGA for MNs within the blood extraction component of this device seems degraded by the use of silicon for MNs within the drug delivery element of the design (Tayyaba et al., 2011).

6.6 Clinical translation and commercialisation of microneedle products

The transdermal delivery market has traditionally been limited to around 20 drugs. This small number is attributed to the strict physicochemical parameters which a drug must have (e.g., low molecular weight, lipophilic, high potency (Naik, Kalia, & Guy, 2000)) in order to be suitable for transdermal delivery. However, MNs have been shown to deliver drugs which previously were not considered as viable for delivery *via* the transdermal route (McCrudden et al., 2014). This, combined with the increasing prevalence of chronic diseases, which require long-term, convenient, and effective treatment, has driven the growth in the transdermal market, which is now predicted to grow by $1.79 billion between 2019 and 2023 (Technavio, 2019).

Despite the large volume of research in this field, to date, there are only two marketed MN products. The first MN product is BD (Becton Dickinson) Soluvia, a prefilled, ready-to-use microinjection system, developed by BD and launched in 2009 (Dickinson, 2009). It consists of a single 1.5 mm silicon hollow needle, with a 0.1 mL injected volume (Dickinson, 2009). The second MN product is MicronJet600, developed by Nanopass Technologies Ltd. and launched in 2010 (NanoPass Technologies Ltd, 2018). It is composed of four silicon hollow needles, each 0.6 mm in height, which is fixed to a plastic adaptor that could be mounted on a standard syringe. It is within reason to suggest that these MN products, in essence, reflect the nature of miniature hypodermic needles rather than the drug delivery strategies of MN arrays previously described. However, silicon is not biodegradable, and implanted silicon is prone to biofouling (Chow et al., 2001; Voskerician et al., 2003). Furthermore, many researchers and research groups have shifted their focus to the use of FDA-approved polymer materials given that inappropriate disposal of silicon or metal MNs remains a concern (Bernadete Riemma Pierre & Cristina Rossetti, 2014). Thus, the future development of commercial MN-based products must ensure that biocompatibility is high and the bioburden is low, demonstrated clearly by the more recent developments of dissolving MNs and hydrogel-forming MNs (Donnelly, Singh, Garland et al., 2012; Donnelly, Singh, Morrow et al., 2012; Migalska et al., 2011). Such designs are able to remove many disadvantages associated with previous MN designs, such as the two-step process associated with solid MNs and the potential for needle stick injuries by using self-disabling MNs. However, the clinical application of MNs does not solely rely on the production of a device which is able to effectively delivery a drug transdermally at therapeutic concentrations; the acceptance of patients, prescribers, and the regulatory authorities must also be considered.

Though patients are likely to accept MNs on the basis of reduced pain, blood, and needle stick injuries, and increased acceptability by patients with needle phobia (Birchall et al., 2011; Mooney, McElnay, & Donnelly, 2014), it must be demonstrated that patients can effectively apply the MN array themselves, particularly in elderly groups, where chronic conditions are more commonplace and patients may struggle with consistent array application (Quinn, Hughes, & Donnelly, 2018). Additionally, it is likely that regulatory authorities would require assurance than the MNs have been inserted correctly in order for the device to be formally approved. Previous studies have shown that patients can successfully apply MNs to their own skin following instruction provided by pharmacist counseling in conjunction with a patient information leaflet (Donnelly, McCrudden et al., 2014; Donnelly, Moffatt et al., 2014; Donnelly, Mooney et al., 2014). Furthermore, a "dosing indicator" has been developed to assure patients that application was successful (Vicente-Pérez et al., 2016) alongside appropriate instructions made available to the patient (Donnelly, McCrudden et al., 2014; Donnelly, Moffatt et al., 2014; Donnelly, Mooney et al., 2014; Norman et al., 2014).

Patient safety is also a legitimate concern, particularly when considering long-term use of MNs for treatment of chronic conditions. Compared to a traditional hypodermic needle, skin penetration using MNs results in a significantly lower microbial penetration (Donnelly, Morrow, McCarron et al., 2009; Donnelly, Morrow, Singh et al., 2009; Wei-Ze et al., 2010). In addition, hydrogel-forming MNs have exhibited antimicrobial properties (Donnelly et al., 2013). It is also statistically unlikely that MNs will ever pierce the same place twice due to their small size (Donnelly, 2018), which may be further assured by rotating the application side at regular intervals. Yes, these studies do not consider the implications of repeated use of MNs. Though studies involving dissolving MNs largely have mainly adopted the use of FDA-approved polymers, the long-term effects of repeated polymer deposition into the skin has yet to be studied in great detail. *In vivo* studies revealed that repeat application of both dissolving (once daily for 5 weeks) and hydrogel-forming (twice daily for 3 weeks) MNs did not alter skin appearance or barrier function and caused no measurable disturbance of serum biomarkers of infection, inflammation, or immunity (Vicente-Perez et al., 2017). Repeat application of hydrogel-forming MNs over a 5 day period did not lead to prolonged skin reactions or disruption in barrier function, and the concentration of systemic inflammation biomarkers were all found to be within the normal range (Al-Kasasbeh et al., 2020). These studies are promising; however, regulatory authorities may request ongoing studies on a drug-by-drug basis to be sure that the MN array used as a transdermal delivery device may be considered "safe."

One of the greatest concerns moving forward is whether MNs will be accepted as a drug delivery system, consumer product, or medical device. If MNs are to be considered closer to a traditional hypodermic injection than a transdermal patch, regulatory authorities are likely to request that the device is rendered sterile prior to use. Aseptic manufacture will be expensive and will present practical challenges if large-scale manufacturing is required (Kirkby, Hutton, & Donnelly, 2020). If this is the case, then any manufacturer wishing to develop MN products will need to make a substantial initial capital investment, which may be off-putting without the guarantee of substantial investment return. However, MNs as a medical device, rather than a drug product, could be CE marked and, therefore, may be accompanied with less regulatory requirements including the need for sterility. This could mean that pharmaceutical companies may be willing to invest in the device, offsetting the initial upfront costs by achieving rapid market commercialization. As a result, the infrastructure would be in place for the manufacture of drug containing MNs in the future (Kirkby et al., 2020).

For drug containing MNs, standardized tests for MNs will likely be required, in the same vein as those provided by the British Pharmacopoeia for oral dosage forms. In addition to those tests already discussed (assuring sterility, reliability of application, deposition of MN material into skin), MNs must show uniformity of content, either form the system as a whole, or potentially of individual needles, depending on the overall array design. Assurances regarding immunological safety will also be required. Furthermore, packaging must be secure, particularly from water ingress for dissolving and hydrogel-forming MNs. Patients must also be able to remove the MN from the packaging without accidental piercing of the skin prior to intended application (Donnelly, 2018). QC tests that are likely to be performed on MNs during the manufacturing process include dissolution, disintegration, friability, uniformity of dosage, stability, water content where appropriate, microbial limits, sterility (if required by the manufacturer), particulate matter, antimicrobial preservative content, extractables, functionality of delivery system, and osmolarity (Lutton et al., 2015). Further unanswered questions include the appropriate model membrane to test for sufficient MN insertion during manufacture, and whether repeated delivery of protein, peptide, and antibody based therapies could result in an immune response from the host given the large number of immune cells present in the skin (Huang, 2007; Lambert & Laurent, 2008).

Despite the ongoing questions surrounding commercialisation of MNs, the US FDA has published draft guidance on "microneedling" for cosmetic applications, and PATH have released a fact sheet illustrating their 4-year initiative for accelerating the development of MNs for drug and vaccine delivery (PATH, 2019; US Food and Drug Administration, 2017). Thus, the interest in MNs for these applications remains in place.

6.7 Conclusion

The use of MNs for drug and vaccine delivery and for diagnostic applications has been clearly demonstrated. The technology has proven adaptable for the delivery of a wide range of therapies, some of which was previously thought impossible for delivery *via* the transdermal route and thus, if pharmaceutical companies can view MNs as commercially viable, it is likely that we will see an MN-based device on the market within the coming years. The potential benefits to both the patient and the healthcare sector are evident, though the translation of MNs from benchtop to bedside will only become a reality through focused collaboration between academia, industry, HCPs, and patients. To this end, Zosano Pharma have developed a zolmitriptan-based intracutaneous MN system for the treatment of migraine headaches. This MN device successfully produced a therapeutic effect in clinical studies, and as result, is expected to receive FDA approval in 2021.

References

Al-Kasasbeh, R., Brady, A. J., Courtenay, A. J., Larrañeta, E., McCrudden, M. T. C., O'Kane, D., et al. (2020). Evaluation of the clinical impact of repeat application of hydrogel-forming microneedle array patches. *Drug Delivery and Translational Research, 10*, 690−705.

Al-Zahrani, S., Zaric, M., McCrudden, C. M., Scott, C., Kissenpfennig, A., & Donnelly, R. F. (2012). Microneedle-mediated vaccine delivery: Harnessing cutaneous immunobiology to improve efficacy. *Expert Opinion on Drug Delivery, 9*(5), 541−550.

Alam, M., Han, S., Pongprutthipan, M., Disphanurat, W., Kakar, R., Nodzenski, M., et al. (2014). Efficacy of a needling device for the treatment of acne scars: A randomized clinical trial. *JAMA Dermatology, 150*(8), 844−849.

Arora, A., Prausnitz, M. R., & Mitragotri, S. (2008). Micro-scale devices for transdermal drug delivery. *International Journal of Pharmaceutics, 364*(2), 227−236.

Ashraf, M. W., Tayyaba, S., & Afzulpurkar, N. (2011). Micro electromechanical systems (MEMS) based microfluidic devices for biomedical applications. *International Journal of Molecular Sciences, 12*(6), 3648−3704.

Aust, M. C., Fernandes, D., Kolokythas, P., Kaplan, H. M., & Vogt, P. M. (2008). Percutaneous collagen induction therapy: An alternative treatment for scars, wrinkles, and skin laxity. *Plastic and Reconstructive Surgery, 121*, 1421−1429.

Baek, S. H., Shin, J. H., & Kim, Y. C. (2017). Drug-coated microneedles for rapid and painless local anesthesia. *Biomedical Microdevices, 19*(1), 1−11.

Ball, J., & Pike, G. (2009). *Needlestick injury in 2008, Royal College of Nursing, result from a survey of RCN members*. Collaboration of Employment Research Royal College of Nursing. http://www.rcn.org.uk/_data/assets/pdf_file/0019/203374/003_304.pdf. (Accessed 15 March 2020).

Banga, A. K. (2009). Microporation applications for enhancing drug delivery. *Expert Opinion on Drug Delivery, 6*(4), 343−354.

Bernadete Riemma Pierre, M., & Cristina Rossetti, F. (2014). Microneedle-based drug delivery systems for transdermal route. *Current Drug Targets, 15*(3), 281−291.

Birchall, J. C., Clemo, R., Anstey, A., & John, D. N. (2011). Microneedles in clinical practice−an exploratory study into the opinions of healthcare professionals and the public. *Pharmaceutical Research, 28*(1), 95−106.

Bodhale, D. W., Asim, A. E., Ae, N., & Afzulpurkar, N. (2010). Structural and microfluidic analysis of hollow side-open polymeric microneedles for transdermal drug delivery applications. *Microfluidics and Nanofluidics, 8*, 373−392.

Bouissou, C. C., Sylvestre, J. P., Guy, R. H., & Delgado-Charro, M. B. (2009). Reverse iontophoresis of amino acids: Identification and separation of stratum corneum and subdermal sources in vitro. *Pharmaceutical Research, 26*(12), 2630−2638.

Brancazio, D. (2012). *Systems and interfaces for blood sampling*. US8808202B2.

Brazzle, J. D., Papautsky, I., & Bruno Frazier, A. (2000). Hollow metallic micromachined needle arrays. *Biomedical Microdevices, 2*(3), 197−205.

Bystrova, S., & Luttge, R. (2011). Micromolding for ceramic microneedle arrays. *Microelectronic Engineering, 88*(8), 1681−1684.

Caffarel-Salvador, E., Brady, A. J., Eltayib, E., Meng, T., Alonso-Vicente, A., Gonzalez-Vazquez, P., et al. (2015). Hydrogel-forming microneedle arrays allow detection of drugs and glucose in vivo: Potential for use in diagnosis and therapeutic drug monitoring. *PLoS One, 10*(12), 1−21.

Caffarel-Salvador, E., Tuan-Mahmood, T. M., McElnay, J. C., McCarthy, H. O., Mooney, K., Woolfson, A. D., et al. (2015). Potential of hydrogel-forming and dissolving microneedles for use in paediatric populations. *International Journal of Pharmaceutics, 489*(1−2), 158−169.

Chandrasekaran, S., Brazzle, J. D., & Frazier, A. B. (2003). Surface micromachined metallic microneedles. *Journal of Microelectromechanical Systems, 12*(3), 281−288.

Ching, C. T. S., Chou, T. R., Sun, T. P., Huang, S. Y., & Shieh, H. L. (2011). Simultaneous, noninvasive, and transdermal extraction of urea and homocysteine by reverse iontophoresis. *International Journal of Nanomedicine, 6*, 417−423.

Chow, A. Y., Pardue, M. T., Chow, V. Y., Peyman, G. A., Liang, C., Perlman, J. I., et al. (2001). Implantation of silicon chip microphotodiode arrays into the cat subretinal space. *IEEE Transactions on Neural Systems and Rehabilitation Engineering, 9*(1), 86−95.

Cormier, M., Johnson, B., Ameri, M., Nyam, K., Libiran, L., Zhang, D. D., et al. (2004). Transdermal delivery of desmopressin using a coated microneedle array patch system. *Journal of Controlled Release, 97*(3), 503−511.

Corrie, S. R., Fernando, G. J. P., Crichton, M. L., Brunck, M. E. G., Anderson, C. D., & Kendall, M. A. F. (2010). Surface-modified microprojection arrays for intradermal biomarker capture, with low non-specific protein binding. *Lab on a Chip, 10*(20), 2655−2658.

Courtenay, A. J., McCrudden, M. T. C., McAvoy, K. J., McCarthy, H. O., & Donnelly, R. F. (2018). Microneedle-mediated transdermal delivery of bevacizumab. *Molecular Pharmaceutics, 15*(8), 3545−3556.

Daddona, P. E., Matriano, J. A., Mandema, J., & Maa, Y. F. (2011). Parathyroid hormone (1-34)-coated microneedle patch system: Clinical pharmacokinetics and pharmacodynamics for treatment of osteoporosis. *Pharmaceutical Research, 28*(1), 159−165.

Davis, S. P., Martanto, W., Allen, M. G., & Prausnitz, M. R. (2005). Hollow metal microneedles for insulin delivery to diabetic rats. *IEEE Transactions on Biomedical Engineering, 52*(5), 909−915.

Dickinson, B. (2009). *BD Soluvia^{TM} microinjection system used for first approved intradermal influenza vaccine in the European Union*. https://www.bd.com/contentmanager/b_article.asp?Item_ID=23817&ContentType_ID=1&BusinessCode=20001&d=&s=&dTitle=&dc=&dcTitle=. (Accessed 2 November 2019).

Donnelly, R. F. (2018). Clinical translation and industrial development of microneedle-based products. In R. F. Donnelly, & T. R. R. Singh (Eds.), *Microneedles for drug and vaccine delivery and patient monitoring* (pp. 307−322). Chichester: John Wiley and Sons.

Donnelly, R. F., Garland, M. J., Morrow, D. I. J. J., Migalska, K., Singh, T. R. R., Majithiya, R., et al. (2010). Optical coherence tomography is a valuable tool in the study of the effects of microneedle geometry on skin penetration characteristics and in-skin dissolution. *Journal of Controlled Release, 147*(3), 333−341.

Donnelly, R. F., Majithiya, R., Singh, T. R. R., Morrow, D. I. J., Garland, M. J., Demir, Y. K., et al. (2011). Design, optimization and characterisation of polymeric microneedle arrays prepared by a novel laser-based micromoulding technique. *Pharmaceutical Research, 28*(1), 41−57.

Donnelly, R. F., McCrudden, M. T. C., Alkilani, A. Z., Larrañeta, E., McAlister, E., Courtenay, A. J., et al. (2014). Hydrogel-forming microneedles prepared from 'super swelling' polymers combined with lyophilised wafers for transdermal drug delivery. *PLoS One, 9*(10), e111547.

Donnelly, R. F., Moffatt, K., Alkilani, A. Z., Vicente-Pérez, E. M., Barry, J., McCrudden, M. T. C. C., et al. (2014). Hydrogel-forming microneedle arrays can be effectively inserted in skin by self-application: A pilot study centred on pharmacist intervention and a patient information leaflet. *Pharmaceutical Research, 31*(8), 1989−1999.

Donnelly, R. F., Mooney, K., Caffarel-Salvador, E., Torrisi, B. M., Eltayib, E., & McElnay, J. C. (2014). Microneedle-mediated minimally invasive patient monitoring. *Therapeutic Drug Monitoring, 36*(1), 10−17.

Donnelly, R. F., Morrow, D. I. J., McCarron, P. A., David Woolfson, A., Morrissey, A., Juzenas, P., et al. (2009). Microneedle arrays permit enhanced intradermal delivery of a preformed photosensitizer. *Photochemistry and Photobiology, 85*(1), 195−204.

Donnelly, R. F., Morrow, D. I. J., Singh, T. R. R., Migalska, K., McCarron, P. A., O'Mahony, C., et al. (2009). Processing difficulties and instability of carbohydrate microneedle arrays. *Drug Development and Industrial Pharmacy, 35*(10), 1242−1254.

Donnelly, R. F., Singh, T. R. R., Alkilani, A. Z., McCrudden, M. T. C., O'Neill, S., O'Mahony, C., et al. (2013). Hydrogel-forming microneedle arrays exhibit antimicrobial properties: Potential for enhanced patient safety. *International Journal of Pharmaceutics, 451*(1−2), 76−91.

Donnelly, R. F., Singh, T. R. R., Garland, M. J., Migalska, K., Majithiya, R., McCrudden, C. M., et al. (2012). Hydrogel-forming microneedle arrays for enhanced transdermal drug delivery. *Advanced Functional Materials, 22*(23), 4879−4890.

Donnelly, R. F., Singh, T. R. R., Morrow, D. I. J., & Woolfson, D. A. (2012). *Microneedle-mediated transdermal and intradermal drug delivery* (1st ed., p. 280pp). Sussex: John Wiley & Sons.

Donnelly, R. F., Singh, T. R. R., Tunney, M. M., Morrow, D. I. J., McCarron, P. A., O'Mahony, C., et al. (2009). Microneedle arrays allow lower microbial penetration than hypodermic needles in vitro. *Pharmaceutical Research, 26*(11), 2513−2522.

Donnelly, R. F., Singh, T. R. R., & Woolfson, A. D. (2010). Microneedle-based drug delivery systems: Microfabrication, drug delivery, and safety. *Drug Delivery, 17*(4), 187−207.

Ebah, L. M., Read, I., Sayce, A., Morgan, J., Chaloner, C., Brenchley, P., et al. (2012). Reverse iontophoresis of urea in health and chronic kidney disease: A potential diagnostic and monitoring tool? *European Journal of Clinical Investigation, 42*(8), 840−847.

Fabbrocini, G., Fardella, N., Monfrecola, A., Proietti, I., & Innocenzi, D. (2009). Acne scarring treatment using skin needling. *Clinical and Experimental Dermatology, 34*, 874−879.

Farias, C., Lyman, R., Hemingway, C., Chau, H., Mahacek, A., Bouzos, E., & Mobed-Miremadi, M. (2018). Three-Dimensional (3D) Printed Microneedles for Micro-encapsulated Cell Extrusion. *Bioengineering, 5*(3), 59.

Gardeniers, H. J. G. E., Luttge, R., Berenschot, E. J. W., De Boer, M. J., Yeshurun, S. Y., Hefetz, M., et al. (2003). Silicon micromachined hollow microneedles for transdermal liquid transport. *Journal of Microelectromechanical Systems, 12*(6), 855−862.

Garland, M. J., Caffarel-Salvador, E., Migalska, K., Woolfson, A. D., & Donnelly, R. F. (2012). Dissolving polymeric microneedle arrays for electrically assisted transdermal drug delivery. *Journal of Controlled Release, 159*(1), 52−59.

Gerstel, M. S., & Place, V. A. (1976). *Drug delivery device.* US3964482A.

Gill, H. S., Denson, D. D., Burris, B. A., & Prausnitz, M. R. (2008). Effect of microneedle design on pain in human volunteers. *The Clinical Journal of Pain, 24*(7), 585−594.

Gomaa, Y. A., Garland, M. J., Mcinnes, F., El-khordagui, L. K., Wilson, C., & Donnelly, R. F. (2012). Laser engineered dissolving microneedles for active transdermal delivery for nadroparin calcium. *European Journal of Pharmaceutics and Biopharmaceutics, 82*(2), 299−307.

González-Vázquez, P., Larrañeta, E., McCrudden, M. T. C., Jarrahian, C., Rein-Weston, A., Quintanar-Solares, M., et al. (2017). Transdermal delivery of gentamicin using dissolving microneedle arrays for potential treatment of neonatal sepsis. *Journal of Controlled Release, 265*, 30−40.

Goud, J. D., Raj, P. M., Liu, J., Narayan, R., Iyer, M., & Tummala, R. (2007). Electrochemical biosensors and microfluidics in organic system-on-package technology. In *Proceedings - electronic components and technology conference* (pp. 1550−1555).

Griss, P., & Stemme, G. (2003). Side-opened out-of-plane microneedles for microfluidic transdermal liquid transfer. *Journal of Microelectromechanical Systems, 12*(3), 296−301.

Gupta, J., Felner, E. I., & Prausnitz, M. R. (2009). Minimally invasive insulin delivery in subjects with type 1 diabetes using hollow microneedles. *Diabetes Technology and Therapeutics, 11*(6), 329−337.

Henry, S., McAllister, D. V., Allen, M. G., & Prausnitz, M. R. (1998). Microfabricated microneedles: A novel approach to transdermal drug delivery. *Journal of Pharmaceutical Sciences, 87*(8), 922−925.

Huang, C. M. (2007). Topical vaccination: The skin as a unique portal to adaptive immune responses. *Seminars in Immunopathology, 29*(1), 71−80.

Ita, K. (2018). Ceramic microneedles and hollow microneedles for transdermal drug delivery: Two decades of research. *Journal of Drug Delivery Science and Technology, 44*, 314−322.

Ito, Y., Murakami, A., Maeda, T., Sugioka, N., & Takada, K. (2008). Evaluation of self-dissolving needles containing low molecular weight heparin (LMWH) in rats. *International Journal of Pharmaceutics, 349*(1−2), 124−129.

Ito, Y., Shiroyama, K., Yoshimitsu, J., Ohashi, Y., Sugioka, N., & Takada, K. (2007). Pharmacokinetic and pharmacodynamic studies following percutaneous absorption of erythropoietin micropiles to rats. *Journal of Controlled Release, 121*(3), 176−180.

Jian, L., Chunxiu, L., Hongmin, L., Liying, J., Qingde, Y., & Xinxia, C. (2007). Study of noninvasive sampling of subcutaneous glucose by reverse iontophoresis. In *Proceedings of the 2nd IEEE international conference on nano/micro engineered and molecular systems* (pp. 707−710). IEEE NEMS.

Kearney, M. C., Caffarel-Salvador, E., Fallows, S. J., McCarthy, H. O., & Donnelly, R. F. (2016). Microneedle-mediated delivery of donepezil: Potential for improved treatment options in Alzheimer's disease. *European Journal of Pharmaceutics and Biopharmaceutics, 103*, 43−50.

Khumpuang, S., Kawaguchi, G., & Sugiyama, S. (2004). Quadruplets-microneedle array for blood extraction. In *Proceedings of the nanotechnology conference and trade show, Boston, MA* (pp. 205−208).

Kim, A., Suecof, L. A., Sutherland, C. A., Gao, L., Kuti, J. L., & Nicolau, D. P. (2008). In vivo microdialysis study of the penetration of daptomycin into soft tissues in diabetic versus healthy volunteers. *Antimicrobial Agents and Chemotherapy, 52*(11), 3941−3946.

Kim, M., Yang, H., Kim, H., Jung, H., & Jung, H. (2014). Novel cosmetic patches for wrinkle improvement: Retinyl retinoate and ascorbic acid-loaded dissolving microneedles. *International Journal of Cosmetic Science, 36*(3), 207−212.

Kirkby, M., Hutton, A. R. J., & Donnelly, R. F. (2020). Microneedle mediated transdermal delivery of protein, peptide and antibody based therapeutics: Current status and future considerations. *Pharmaceutical Research, 36*(6), 117−135.

Kobayashi, K., & Suzuki, H. (2001). A sampling mechanism employing the phase transition of a gel and its application to a micro analysis system imitating a mosquito. *Sensors and Actuators B: Chemical, 80*(1), 1−8.

Kommareddy, S., Baudner, B. C., Bonificio, A., Gallorini, S., Palladino, G., Determan, A. S., et al. (2013). Influenza subunit vaccine coated microneedle patches elicit comparable immune responses to intramuscular injection in Guinea pigs. *Vaccine, 31*(34), 3435−3441.

Koren, G. (1997). Therapeutic drug monitoring principles in the neonate. *Clinical Chemistry, 43*(1), 222−227.

Lambert, P. H., & Laurent, P. E. (2008). Intradermal vaccine delivery: Will new delivery systems transform vaccine administration? *Vaccine, 26*(26), 3197−3208.

Larrañeta, E., Lutton, R. E. M., Woolfson, A. D., & Donnelly, R. F. (2016). Microneedle arrays as transdermal and intradermal drug delivery systems: Materials science, manufacture and commercial development. *Materials Science and Engineering R: Reports, 104*, 1−32.

Larrañeta, E., & Singh, T. R. R. (2018). Microneedle manufacturing and testing. In R. F. Donnelly, T. R. R. Singh, E. Larrañeta, & M. T. C. McCrudden (Eds.), *Microneedles for drug and vaccine delivery and patient monitoring* (pp. 21−70). Sussex: John Wiley & Sons.

Leboulanger, B., Aubry, J.-M., Bondolfi, G., Guy, R. H., & Delgado-Charro, M. B. (2004). Lithium monitoring by reverse iontophoresis in vivo. *Clinical Chemistry, 50*(11), 2091−2100.

Lee, C. K., Ching, C. T. S., Sun, T. P., Tsai, C. L., Huang, W., Huang, H. H., et al. (2010). Noninvasive and transdermal measurement of blood uric acid level in human by electroporation and reverse iontophoresis. *International Journal of Nanomedicine, 5*(1), 991−997.

Lee, J. W., Choi, S. O., Felner, E. I., & Prausnitz, M. R. (2011). Dissolving microneedle patch for transdermal delivery of human growth hormone. *Small, 7*(4), 531−539.

Lee, H. S., Ryu, H. R., Roh, J. Y., & Park, J. H. (2017). Bleomycin-coated microneedles for treatment of warts. *Pharmaceutical Research, 34*(1), 101−112.

Li, C. G., Lee, C. Y., Lee, K., & Jung, H. (2013). An optimized hollow microneedle for minimally invasive blood extraction. *Biomedical Microdevices, 15*(1), 17−25.

Liu, R., Wang, X., Feng, Y., Wang, G., Liu, J., & Ding, H. (2006). Theoretical analytical flow model in hollow microneedles for non-forced fluid extraction. In *Proceedings of 1st IEEE international conference on nano micro engineered and molecular systems* (pp. 1039−1042). 1st IEEE-NEMS.

Liu, R., Wang, X. H., Tang, F., Feng, Y. Y., & Zhou, Z. Y. (2005). An in-plane microneedles used for sampling and glucose analysis. In *Digest of technical papers - international conference on solid state sensors and actuators and microsystems, TRANSDUCERS '05* (pp. 1517−1520).

Liu, J.-Q., Yan, X.-X., Yang, B., Jiang, S.-D., & Yang, C.-S. (2013). Fabrication and testing of porous Ti microneedles for drug delivery. *Micro and Nano Letters, 8*(12), 906−908.

Luttge, R., Berenschot, E. J. W., de Boer, M. J., Altpeter, D. M., Vrouwe, E. X., van den Berg, A., et al. (2007). Integrated lithographic molding for microneedle-based devices. *Journal of Microelectromechanical Systems, 16*(4), 872−884.

Lutton, R. E. M. M., Moore, J., Larrañeta, E., Ligett, S., Woolfson, A. D., & Donnelly, R. F. (2015). Microneedle characterisation: The need for universal acceptance criteria and GMP specifications when moving towards commercialisation. *Drug Delivery and Translational Research, 5*(4), 313−331.

Mail Online. (2009). *It costs £250 and looks like an instrument of medieval torture - but can the Dermaroller make you look younger?*. https://www.dailymail.co.uk/femail/beauty/article-1226193/Can-Dermaroller-make-look-younger.html. (Accessed 25 November 2019).

Marshall, S., Sahm, L. J., & Moore, A. C. (2016). The success of microneedle-mediated vaccine delivery into skin. *Human Vaccines and Immunotherapeutics, 12*(11), 2975−2983.

Martanto, W., Davis, S. P., Holiday, N. R., Wang, J., Gill, H. S., & Prausnitz, M. R. (2004). Transdermal delivery of insulin using microneedles in vivo. *Pharmaceutical Research, 21*(6), 947−952.

McAlister, E., McCrudden, M. T. C., & Donnelly, R. F. (2018). Microneedles in improving skin appearance and enhanced delivery of cosmeceuticals. In R. F. Donnelly, T. R. R. Singh, E. Larrañeta, & M. T. C. McCrudden (Eds.), *Microneedles for drug and vaccine delivery and patient monitoring* (pp. 259−282). Sussex: John Wiley & Sons.

McAllister, D. V., Wang, P. M., Davis, S. P., Park, J.-H., Canatella, P. J., Allen, M. G., et al. (2003). Microfabricated needles for transdermal delivery of macromolecules and nanoparticles: Fabrication methods and transport studies. *Proceedings of the National Academy of Sciences of the United States of America, 100*(24), 13755−13760.

McCrudden, M. T. C., Alkilani, A. Z., McCrudden, C. M., McAlister, E., McCarthy, H. O., Woolfson, A. D., et al. (2014). Design and physicochemical characterisation of novel dissolving polymeric microneedle arrays for transdermal delivery of high dose, low molecular weight drugs. *Journal of Controlled Release, 180*(1), 71−80.

McCrudden, M. T. C., Courtenay, A. J., & Donnelly, R. F. (2018). Microneedle-mediated vaccine delivery. In R. F. Donnelly, T. R. R. Singh, E. Larrañeta, & M. T. C. McCrudden (Eds.), *Microneedles for drug and vaccine delivery and patient monitoring* (pp. 93−127). Sussex: John Wiley & Sons.

Mccrudden, M. T. C., McAlister, E., Courtenay, A. J., González-Vázquez, P., Raj Singh, T. R., & Donnelly, R. F. (2015). Microneedle applications in improving skin appearance. *Experimental Dermatology, 24*(8), 561−566.

McGrath, M. G., Vrdoljak, A., O'Mahony, C., Oliveira, J. C., Moore, A. C., & Crean, A. M. (2011). Determination of parameters for successful spray coating of silicon microneedle arrays. *International Journal of Pharmaceutics, 415*(1−2), 140−149.

Migalska, K., Morrow, D. I. J., Garland, M. J., Thakur, R., Woolfson, A. D., & Donnelly, R. F. (2011). Laser-engineered dissolving microneedle arrays for transdermal macromolecular drug delivery. *Pharmaceutical Research, 28*, 1919−1930.

Migdadi, E. M., Courtenay, A. J., Tekko, I. A., McCrudden, M. T. C., Kearney, M. C., McAlister, E., et al. (2018). Hydrogel-forming microneedles enhance transdermal delivery of metformin hydrochloride. *Journal of Controlled Release, 285*, 142−151.

Millard, D. R., & Maisels, D. O. (1966). Silicon granuloma of the skin and subcutaneous tissue. *American Journal of Surgery, 112*, 119−123.

Mischler, R., & Werner, G. (2012). *Microneedle arrays with ATR sensor.* US8160665B2.

Miyano, T., Tobinaga, Y., Kanno, T., Matsuzaki, Y., Takeda, H., Wakui, M., et al. (2005). Sugar micro needles as transdermic drug delivery system. *Biomedical Microdevices, 7*(3), 185−188.

Mooney, K., McElnay, J. C., & Donnelly, R. F. (2014). Children's views on microneedle use as an alternative to blood sampling for patient monitoring. *International Journal of Pharmacy Practice, 22*(5), 335−344.

Moreno, M., Aracil, C., & Quero, J. M. (2008). High-integrated micro valve for lab-on-chip biomedical applications. In *2008 IEEE-BIOCAS biomedical circuits and systems conference, BIOCAS 2008* (pp. 313−316).

Moreno, J. M., Aracil, C., & Quero, J. M. (2009). Low cost fluid microextractor for lab-on-chip. In *Proceedings of the 2009 Spanish conference on electron devices, CDE'09* (pp. 274−277).

Mukerjee, E. V., Collins, S. D., Isseroff, R. R., & Smith, R. L. (2004). Microneedle array for transdermal biological fluid extraction and in situ analysis. *Sensors and Actuators, A: Physical, 114*(2−3), 267−275.

Mukerjee, E. V., Issseroff, R. R., Collins, S. D., & Smith, R. L. (2003). Microneedle array with integrated microchannels for transdermal sample extraction and in situ analysis. In *Transducers 2003 - 12th international conference on solid-state sensors, actuators and microsystems, digest of technical papers* (pp. 1439−1441). Institute of Electrical and Electronics Engineers Inc.

Naik, A., Kalia, Y. N., & Guy, R. H. (2000). Transdermal drug delivery: Overcoming the skin's barrier function. *Pharmaceutical Science and Technology Today, 3*(9), 318−326.

NanoPass Technologies Ltd. (2018). *MicronJet600 advanced intradermal solution.* https://www.nanopass.com/product/. (Accessed 20 April 2019).

Naves, L., Dhand, C., Almeida, L., Rajamani, L., Ramakrishna, S., & Soares, G. (2017). Poly(lactic-co-glycolic) acid drug delivery systems through transdermal pathway: An overview. *Progress in Biomaterials, 6*(1−2), 1−11.

Nguyen, H. X., Bozorg, B. D., Kim, Y., Wieber, A., Birk, G., Lubda, D., & Banga, A. K. (2018). Poly (vinyl alcohol) microneedles: Fabrication, characterization, and application for transdermal drug delivery of doxorubicin. *European Journal of Pharmaceutics and Biopharmaceutics, 129*, 88−103.

Nielsen, J. K., Freckmann, G., Kapitza, C., Ocvirk, G., Koelker, K. H., Kamecke, U., et al. (2009). Glucose monitoring by microdialysis: Performance in a multicentre study. *Diabetic Medicine, 26*(7), 714−721.

Norman, J. J., Arya, J. M., McClain, M. A., Frew, P. M., Meltzer, M. I., & Prausnitz, M. R. (2014). Microneedle patches: Usability and acceptability for self-vaccination against influenza. *Vaccine, 32*(16), 1856−1862.

Orentreich, D. S., & Orentreich, N. (1995). Subcutaneous incisionless (subcision) surgery for the correction of depressed scars and wrinkles. *Dermatologic Surgery, 21*(6), 543−549.

Paik, S. J., Byun, S., Lim, J. M., Park, Y., Lee, A., Chung, S., et al. (2004). In-plane single-crystal-silicon microneedles for minimally invasive microfluid systems. *Sensors and Actuators, A: Physical, 114*(2−3), 276−284.

Paik, S. J., Lim, J. M., Jung, I., Park, Y., Byun, S., Chung, S., et al. (2003). A novel microneedle array integrated with a PDMS biochip for microfluid systems. In *Transducers 2003 - 12th international conference on solid-state sensors, actuators and microsystems, digest of technical papers* (pp. 1446−1449). Institute of Electrical and Electronics Engineers Inc.

Paliwal, S., Ogura, M., & Mitragotri, S. (2010). Rapid sampling of molecules via skin for diagnostic and forensic applications. *Pharmaceutical Research, 27*(7), 1255−1263.

Pamornpathomkul, B., Ngawhirunpat, T., Tekko, I. A., Vora, L., McCarthy, H. O., & Donnelly, R. F. (2018). Dissolving polymeric microneedle arrays for enhanced site-specific acyclovir delivery. *European Journal of Pharmaceutical Sciences, 121*, 200−209.

Park, J.-H., Allen, M. G., & Prausnitz, M. R. (2005). Biodegradable polymer microneedles: Fabrication, mechanics and transdermal drug delivery. *Journal of Controlled Release, 104*(1), 51−66.

Park, J.-H., Allen, M. G., & Prausnitz, M. R. (2006). Polymer microneedles for controlled-release drug delivery. *Pharmaceutical Research, 23*(5), 1008−1019.

Park, J. H., Choi, S. O., Kamath, R., Yoon, Y. K., Allen, M. G., & Prausnitz, M. R. (2007). Polymer particle-based micromolding to fabricate novel microstructures. *Biomedical Microdevices, 9*(2), 223−234.

Park, Y., & Kim, B. (2017). Skin permeability of compounds loaded within dissolving microneedles dependent on composition of sodium hyaluronate and carboxymethyl cellulose. *Korean Journal of Chemical Engineering, 34*(1), 133−138.

PATH. (2019). *The PATH center of Excellence for Microarray patch technology*. https://www.path.org/resources/path-center-excellence-microarray-patch-technology/. (Accessed 20 April 2020).

Potts, R. O., Tamada, J. A., & Tierney, M. J. (2002). Glucose monitoring by reverse iontophoresis. *Diabetes Metabolism Research and Reviews, 18*(Suppl. 1), S49−S53.

Quinn, H. L., Bonham, L., Hughes, C. M., & Donnelly, R. F. (2015). Design of a dissolving microneedle platform for transdermal delivery of a fixed-dose combination of cardiovascular drugs. *Journal of Pharmaceutical Sciences, 104*(10), 3490−3500.

Quinn, H. L., & Donnelly, R. F. (2018). Microneedle-mediated drug delivery. In R. F. Donnelly, T. R. R. Singh, E. Larrañeta, & M. T. C. McCrudden (Eds.), *Microneedles for drug and vaccine delivery and patient monitoring* (pp. 71−91). Sussex: John Wiley & Sons.

Quinn, H. L., Hughes, C. M., & Donnelly, R. F. (2018). In vivo and qualitative studies investigating the translational potential of microneedles for use in the older population. *Drug Delivery and Translational Research, 8*(2), 307−316.

Quinn, H. L., Kearney, M.-C., Courtenay, A. J., McCrudden, M. T., & Donnelly, R. F. (2014). The role of microneedles for drug and vaccine delivery. *Expert Opinion on Drug Delivery, 11*(11), 1769−1780.

Rapiti, E., Prüss-Üstün, A., & Hutin, Y. (2005). *Sharps injuries: Assessing the burden of disease from sharps injuries to health-care at national and local levels*. https://apps.who.int/iris/bitstream/handle/10665/43051/924159232X.pdf?sequence=1&isAllowed=y. (Accessed 11 April 2020).

Rouphael, N. G., Paine, M., Mosley, R., Henry, S., McAllister, D. V., Kalluri, H., et al. (2017). The safety, immunogenicity, and acceptability of inactivated influenza vaccine delivered by microneedle patch (TIV-MNP 2015): A randomised, partly blinded, placebo-controlled, phase 1 trial. *The Lancet, 390*, 649−658.

Sato, T., Okada, S., Hagino, K., Asakura, Y., Kikkawa, Y., Kojima, J., et al. (2011). Measurement of glucose area under the curve using minimally invasive interstitial fluid extraction technology: Evaluation of glucose monitoring concepts without blood sampling. *Diabetes Technology and Therapeutics, 13*(12), 1194−1200.

Sieg, A., Guy, R. H., & Delgado-Charro, M. B. (2004). Electroosmosis in transdermal iontophoresis: Implications for noninvasive and calibration-free glucose monitoring. *Biophysical Journal, 87*(5), 3344−3350.

Stahl, J., Wohlert, M., & Kietzmann, M. (2012). Microneedle pretreatment enhances the percutaneous permeation of hydrophilic compounds with high melting points. *BMC Pharmacology and Toxicology, 13*(5), 1−7.

Stoeber, B., & Liepmann, D. (2002). Design, fabrication and testing of a MEMS syringe. In *Proceedings of the solid-state sensor, actuator and microsystems workshop, Hilton Head, SC* (pp. 1−4).

Sullivan, S. P., Koutsonanos, D. G., del Pilar Martin, M., Lee, J. W., Zarnitsyn, V., Choi, S.-O., et al. (2010). Dissolving polymer microneedle patches for influenza vaccination. *Nature Medicine, 16*(8), 915−920.

Sullivan, S. P., Murthy, N., & Prausnitz, M. P. (2008). Minimally invasive protein delivery with rapidly dissolving polymer microneedles. *Advanced Materials, 20*(5), 933−938.

Sun, T.-P., Shieh, H.-L., Ching, C. T.-S., Yao, Y.-D., Huang, S.-H., Liu, C.-M., et al. (2010). Carbon nanotube composites for glucose biosensor incorporated with reverse iontophoresis function for noninvasive glucose monitoring. *International Journal of Nanomedicine, 5*, 343.

Suzuki, H., Tokuda, T., & Kobayashi, K. (2002). A disposable 'intelligent mosquito' with a reversible sampling mechanism using the volume-phase transition of a gel. In *Sensors and actuators, B: Chemical* (pp. 53−59).

Suzuki, H., Tokuda, T., Miyagishi, T., Yoshida, H., & Honda, N. (2004). A disposable on-line microsystem for continuous sampling and monitoring of glucose. *Sensors and Actuators B: Chemical, 97*(1), 90−97.

Tak-shing Ching, C., Sun, T., Huang, S., Shieh, H., & Chen, C. (2010). A mediated glucose biosensor incorporated with reverse iontophoresis function for noninvasive glucose monitoring. *Annals of Biomedical Engineering, 38*(4), 1548−1555.

Tas, C., Mansoor, S., Kalluri, H., Zarnitsyn, V. G., Choi, S.-O., Banga, A. K., & Prausnitz, M. P. (2012). Delivery of salmon calcitonin using a microneedle patch. *International Journal of Pharmaceutics, 423*(2), 257−263.

Tayyaba, S., Ashraf, M., & Afzulpurkar, N. (2011). *Blood filtration system for patients with kidney diseases*. IET Communications, Manuscript ID COM-2011 0176.

Technavio. (2019). *Transdermal drug delivery market*. https://www.technavio.com/report/transdermal-drug-delivery-market-industry-analysis?tnplus. (Accessed 1 April 2020).

Teo, A. L., Shearwood, C., Ng, K. C., Lu, J., & Moochhala, S. (2006). Transdermal microneedles for drug delivery applications. *Materials Science and Engineering: B, 132*(1−2), 151−154.

Trzebinski, J., Sharma, S., Radomska-Botelho Moniz, A., Michelakis, K., Zhang, Y., & Cass, A. E. G. (2012). Microfluidic device to investigate factors affecting performance in biosensors designed for transdermal applications. *Lab on a Chip, 12*(2), 348−352.

Tsuchiya, K., Jinnin, S., Yamamoto, H., Uetsuji, Y., & Nakamachi, E. (2010). Design and development of a biocompatible painless microneedle by the ion sputtering deposition method. *Precision Engineering, 34*(3), 461−466.

Tuan-Mahmood, T. M., McCrudden, M. T. C., Torrisi, B. M., McAlister, E., Garland, M. J., Singh, T. R. R., et al. (2013). Microneedles for intradermal and transdermal drug delivery. *European Journal of Pharmaceutical Sciences, 50*(5), 623−637.

US Food and Drug Administration. (2017). *Regulatory considerations for microneedling devices: Draft guidance for industry and food and drug administration staff*. https://www.fda.gov/regulatory-information/search-fda-guidance-documents/regulatory-considerations-microneedling-devices. (Accessed 14 April 2020).

Venugopal, M., Feuvrel, K. E., Mongin, D., Bambot, S., Faupel, M., Panangadan, A., et al. (2008). Clinical evaluation of a novel interstitial fluid sensor system for remote continuous alcohol monitoring. *IEEE Sensors Journal, 8*(1), 71−80.

Vesper, H. W., Wang, P. M., Archibold, E., Prausnitz, M. R., & Myers, G. L. (2006). Assessment of trueness of a glucose monitor using interstitial fluid and whole blood as specimen matrix. *Diabetes Technology and Therapeutics, 8*(1), 76−80.

Vicente-Perez, E. M., Larrañeta, E., McCrudden, M. T. C., Kissenpfennig, A., Hegarty, S., McCarthy, H. O., et al. (2017). Repeat application of microneedles does not alter skin appearance or barrier function and causes no measurable disturbance of serum biomarkers of infection, inflammation or immunity in mice in vivo. *European Journal of Pharmaceutics and Biopharmaceutics, 117*, 400−407.

Vicente-Pérez, E. M., Quinn, H. L., McAlister, E., O'Neill, S., Hanna, L.-A., Barry, J. G., et al. (2016). The use of a pressure-indicating sensor film to provide feedback upon hydrogel-forming microneedle array self-application in vivo. *Pharmaceutical Research, 33*(12), 1−10.

Voskerician, G., Shive, M. S., Shawgo, R. S., Von Recum, H., Anderson, J. M., Cima, M. J., et al. (2003). Biocompatibility and biofouling of MEMS drug delivery devices. *Biomaterials, 24*(11), 1959−1967.

Vrouwe, E., & Luttge, R. (2005). Sampling for point-of-care analysis of lithium in whole blood with chip based (special issue). *Royal Society of Chemistry, 269*, 503−505.

Wang, P. M., Cornwell, M., Hill, J., & Prausnitz, M. R. (2006). Precise microinjection into skin using hollow microneedles. *Journal of Investigative Dermatology, 126*(5), 1080−1087.

Wang, P. M., Cornwell, M., & Prausnitz, M. R. (2005). Minimally invasive extraction of dermal interstitial fluid for glucose monitoring using microneedles. *Diabetes Technology and Therapeutics, 7*(1), 131−141.

Wei-Ze, L., Mei-Rong, H., Jian-Ping, Z., Yong-Qiang, Z., Bao-Hua, H., Ting, L., et al. (2010). Super-short solid silicon microneedles for transdermal drug delivery applications. *International Journal of Pharmaceutics, 389*, 122−129.

Wermeling, D. P., Banks, S. L., Hudson, D. A., Gill, H. S., Gupta, J., Prausnitz, M. R., et al. (2008). Microneedles permit transdermal delivery of a skin-impermeant medication to humans. *Proceedings of the National Academy of Sciences, 105*(6), 2058−2063.

Windmiller, J. R., Valdés-Ramírez, G., Zhou, N., Zhou, M., Miller, P. R., Jin, C., et al. (2011). Bicomponent microneedle array biosensor for minimally-invasive glutamate monitoring. *Electroanalysis, 23*(10), 2302−2309.

Windmiller, J. R., Zhou, N., Chuang, M. C., Valdés-Ramírez, G., Santhosh, P., Miller, P. R., et al. (2011). Microneedle array-based carbon paste amperometric sensors and biosensors. *Analyst, 136*(9), 1846−1851.

Yang, S., Feng, Y., Zhang, L., Chen, N., Yuan, W., & Jin, T. (2012). A scalable fabrication process of polymer microneedles. *International Journal of Nanomedicine, 7*, 1415−1422.

Yung, K. L., Xu, Y., Kang, C., Liu, H., Tam, K. F., Ko, S. M., et al. (2012). Sharp tipped plastic hollow microneedle array by microinjection moulding. *Journal of Micromechanics and Microengineering, 22*(1), 015016.

Zahn, J. D., Trebotich, D., & Liepmann, D. (2000). Microfabricated microdialysis microneedles for continuous medical monitoring. In *1st annual international IEEE-EMBS special topic conference on microtechnologies in medicine and biology - proceedings* (pp. 375−380). Institute of Electrical and Electronics Engineers Inc.

Zahn, J. D., Trebotich, D., & Liepmann, D. (2005). Microdialysis microneedles for continuous medical monitoring. *Biomedical Microdevices, 7*(1), 59−69.

Zhang, P., & Jullien, G. A. (2003). Micromachined needles for microbiological sample and drug delivery system. In *Proceedings - international conference on MEMS, NANO and smart systems, ICMENS 2003* (pp. 247−250). Institute of Electrical and Electronics Engineers Inc.

Zhang, P., & Jullien, G. A. (2005). Microneedle arrays for drug delivery and fluid extraction. In *Proceedings - 2005 international conference on MEMS, NANO and smart systems* (pp. 392−395). ICMENS.

Zimmermann, S., Fienbork, D., Stoeber, B., Flounders, A. W., & Liepmann, D. (2003). A microneedle-based glucose monitor: Fabricated on a wafer-level using in-device enzyme immobilization. In *Transducers 2003 - 12th international conference on solid-state sensors, actuators and microsystems, digest of technical papers* (pp. 99−102). Institute of Electrical and Electronics Engineers Inc.

Microfluidic systems for drug discovery, pharmaceutical analysis, and diagnostic applications

Dawei Ding[1], Sol Park[2], Jaspreet Singh Kochhar[3,*], Sui Yung Chan[4], Pei Shi Ong[4], Won Gu Lee[5], Lifeng Kang[2]

[1]College of Pharmaceutical Sciences, Soochow University, Suzhou, Jiangsu, China; [2]School of Pharmacy, Faculty of Medicine and Health, University of Sydney, Sydney, NSW, Australia; [3]Procter & Gamble, Singapore, Republic of Singapore; [4]Department of Pharmacy, National University of Singapore, Singapore, Republic of Singapore; [5]Department of Mechanical Engineering, College of Engineering, Yongin, Gyeonggi, Republic of Korea

Guided reading questions:

1. What is microfluidics? What is the role of microfluidics in drug discovery? How are microfluidics used in pharmaceutical analysis? How can microfluidic devices be used for diagnostic applications?

7.1 Introduction

The ascension of the microfabrication technology at the turn of the century opened several avenues for the biomedical sector. Microscale chips, with micrometre dimension channels, can be used to manipulate fluid flow on micron or submicron scale. The spatial control offered by this technology, known as "microfluidics," has potential applications in handling, processing, and analysis of fluids (Whitesides, 2006). The miniaturized ambit of these devices requires lower sample volumes in nanolitres as opposed to conventional microplate assays which require hundreds of microliters, hence making them economical alternatives. The minute dimensions of the device offer shorter diffusion path lengths, allowing for precise control of fluid flow and faster analysis leading to specificity in the chemical microreactors. Design manipulation, easily achievable by conventional lithographical and novel nanotechnology techniques, provides versatility in mixing of fluids that can be controlled by external

---

* The author has contributed in his personal capacity and the work represented is in no way linked to his current organization.

physical forces such as magnetic and electric fields. These microdevices may either be integrated to the existing devices or be a comprehensive analytical system by itself. The miniaturization provided by these high throughput devices endows a small chip with large number of replicates on, which make massive parallelization possible, thereby increasing efficiency and further cutting down the cost (Lombardi & Dittrich, 2010). The fluid flow properties at microscale are very different from that at macroscale, and this can be exploited using microfluidic devices (Beebe, Mensing, & Walker, 2002). These advantages make them an ideal choice in disciplines spanning across molecular analysis, biodefense programs, and discovery and development of new drugs in pharmaceutical and biotechnological industries.

Initially, the concept of microfluidics was applied to the field of analytical chemistry. Lithographic patterning/etching, used to produce chemical sensors and chemical analytical techniques on glass/silicon substrates, provided proof of concept for their applicability (Harrison et al., 1993; Manz, Graber, & Widmer, 1990). Afterward, chemical and biological sensors that could thwart the threats due to bioterrorism and aid in biodefense sample testing (Liszewski, 2003) were developed. With the surge in the biotechnological methods, proteomics, genomics, and discovery of protein-based therapeutics, microfluidics offers brighter prospects in DNA sequencing and genotyping as well as protein separation and analysis (Chen, Roller, & Huang, 2010; Gomez, 2011). Microfluidic devices have also provided commendable opportunities for drug discovery and development process with their plausible benefits at each stage from target identification (Malmstadt, Nash, Purnell, & Schmidt, 2006) to lead identification/optimization (Jones et al., 2005) and further to preclinical studies (Matsui et al., 2006), clinical trials (Herr et al., 2007), formulation development (Alsenz and Kansy, 2007), and manufacturing stage (Szita et al., 2005). Additionally, these devices have been used for improved confinement of cells in three dimensional scaffolds, cell-based testing, and cell component analysis. The cellular and molecular interactions at a scale proportional to their dimensions (Whitesides, 2003) are much different from that observed at macroscale volumes. An interesting application has been in the field of tissue engineering whereby microfluidic platforms provide three dimensional scaffolds mimicking natural environment for growth and mutual interaction between cells (Li, Valadez, Zuo, & Nie, 2012; Yamada, Sugaya, Naganuma, & Seki, 2012). They have also been investigated for transdermal and pulmonary delivery of drugs (Ashraf, Tayyaba, & Afzulpurkar, 2011; Yeo, Friend, McIntosh, Meeusen, & Morton, 2010) as well as for personalized diagnostic kits (Yager et al., 2006).

In this chapter, we will present an overview of the microfluidic devices that have been researched for drug discovery and drug analysis. First, we discuss the role played by microfluidics in the current paradigm for drug discovery, in identifying druggable targets, progress achieved by high throughput screening, that allowed for thousands of molecules to be screened on a chip, followed by optimizing lead molecules and assessing their pharmacokinetic and pharmacodynamic properties in preclinical systems. Lastly, we discuss the application of microfluidic devices in chemical analysis.

7.2 Microfluidics for drug discovery

Discovering new therapeutics for a pathophysiological condition involves identifying a specific target (Kang, Chung, Langer, & Khademhosseini, 2008). With the help of computational biology and/or experimental methods, such targets can be identified. This is followed by validating the target by a series of complicated cell or animal-based experiments. Once validated, screening of drug libraries, produced by combinatorial chemistry, composed of millions (usually $>10^6$ compounds) of drug molecules to find a few lead molecules for clinical trials is carried out. This is aimed at getting the safest, most reliable, and efficacious pharmaceutical compound that is then filed as a new drug application for approval by regulatory agents like United States Food and Drug Administration (USFDA). The complex and lengthy procedure of discovering a suitable drug candidate is exemplified by the fact that it takes 10−15 years for a drug to reach from bench to bedside and has been estimated to cost approximately one billion USD (Wu, Huang, & Lee, 2010). The attrition rate from thousands of new chemical structures in the drug library to a few lead compounds and a single successful therapeutic agent is a result of the inefficient procedures used in the conventional/current drug discovery and development process.

Progress in use of microscale platforms aims to accelerate the process of drug discovery by efficient and expeditious design of therapeutics and provision of information on biological targets (Lal & Arnsdorf, 2010). High throughput microfluidic devices have shown considerable promise over the conventional methods which required long processing times and expensive equipment, hence delaying the whole drug discovery process. In the following sections, we describe the contribution of microfluidics in various segments of drug discovery.

7.2.1 Identification of druggable targets

The process of drug discovery begins with the identification of the function of a potential drug target and comprehending its role in the disease process. Discovering pharmacological activities was conventionally carried out by testing various substances in living organisms to observe the changes caused in a phenotype. However, toward the end of the 20th century, this process of phenotype-based target identification was largely replaced by a target-based approach. With progressive acquisition of knowledge in the field of molecular biology and improvement in isolation techniques, identification of complex systems that are responsible for a drug's pharmacological response has evolved to be the new approach in identification of drug targets and has reduced the use of living organisms and living tissues (Terstappen, Schlupen, Raggiaschi, & Gaviraghi, 2007).

Drug targets, which may be a cellular receptor, an ion channel, nucleic acids, DNA or RNA, enzymes, polysaccharide, and lipids, are usually chemically well-defined molecular structures capable of interacting with therapeutic drug moieties (Imming, Sinning, & Meyer, 2006). This interaction leads to downstream clinical effects.

The most common drug targets belong to the class of kinases, phosphatases, nuclear receptors, and G protein coupled receptors (Santos et al., 2017). Ion channels proteins represent another attractive target in drug discovery paradigm as they have been implicated in neurological, cardiovascular, and metabolic diseases as well as cancer and immunomodulation (Dunlop, Bowlby, Peri, Vasilyev, & Arias, 2008) (NATURE REVIEWS DRUG DISCOVERY 2019, 18, 339−357). Around 40% of targets in drug discovery belong to the class of ligand-gated ion channels (Yin et al., 2008). They act as the main targets for the currently available pharmaceutical agents as well as majority of those agents in the drug development phase and hence have been the focus of intense research resulting in dedicated conferences and numerous publications (Perrin, Fremaux, & Scheer, 2006; Talwar & Lynch, 2014; Zagnoni, 2012).

As most of these targets are a part of the cell membrane lipid bilayer structure, their functionality depends on the membrane integrity. The proteins may be denatured once dissociated from the membrane and hence are required to be integrated into the membrane throughout the analytical procedure (Suzuki, Tabata, Kato-Yamada, Noji, & Takeuchi, 2004). Target validation employing isolated membrane proteins and ion channels offers many technological challenges as reproducing these nanoscale systems is very complex (Sandison, Zagnoni, & Morgan, 2007). However, incorporating these drug targets in artificially synthesized lipid bilayer membranes and by specifically controlling the membrane architecture and surface characteristics, simulating the natural environment of a drug target, is envisaged as an option for target identification (Zagnoni, 2012).

Microfluidic technology has played a key role in the fabrication of bilayer lipid membranes (BLMs) (Mayer, Kriebel, Tosteson, & Whitesides, 2003). Micron-sized BLMs with integrated membrane proteins and ion channels are advantageous over macrosystems, providing economical and time-saving analysis platforms. These BLMs bear remarkable electric sealing and, hence, are amenable to recording of electrical signals across single membrane protein. On chip planar bilayer structures were first introduced in 2004 by Suzuki et al. (2004). They fabricated a bilayer membrane chip using a silicon wafer having flow channels on both sides that are connected to apertures (Fig. 7.1(a)). Lipid solution and buffer, injected alternatively, resulted in the formation of the lipid bilayer.

The proteins were incorporated in the bilayer using protein laden liposomes. Integrated microelectrodes could be used for determining the membrane potential and, thus, could serve as a tool for ligand binding studies. However, silicon-based devices suffer from many disadvantages including high dielectric loss of silicon leading to high electrical noise. Apart from that, the manufacture of silicon-based devices is time consuming, and the reproducibility of the BLMs is questionable. Other materials or substrates used for fabrication include epoxy photoresist (Cheng et al., 2001), glass (Fertig, Blick, & Behrends, 2002), and Teflon (Mayer et al., 2003), but the resultant BLMs were fragile and unstable.

Polymeric microfluidic devices have the potential to overcome these drawbacks, offering advantages of economy and ease of fabrication. Poly(methyl methacrylate) (PMMA) has been seen as viable alternative due to its good optical and dielectric properties, low glass transition temperature, ease of processing, and ability to bond

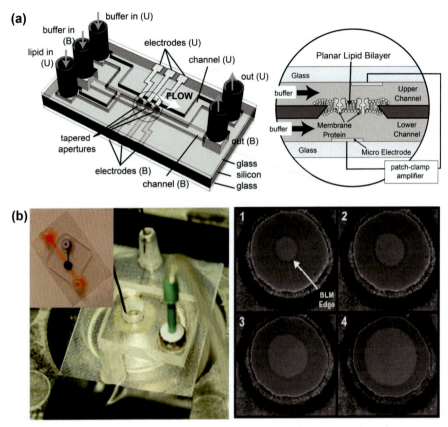

Figure 7.1 Formation of bilayer lipid membranes (BLMs) on microfluidic chips. (a) Conceptual diagram of a membrane fluid chip having fluid channels and apertures. Alternate flow of lipid and buffer solutions lead to formation of BLMs (Suzuki et al., 2004). (b) A microfluidic device with a channel extending out from a trench, where electrodes are inserted in both the upper well (containing lipid) and the lower channel (containing buffer). The bilayer is formed within an aperture upon exposure to air (left), the growth of which is monitored over 20 s (right). The setup was placed over a microscope to observe BLM formation (Sandison et al., 2007).

other materials unlike Teflon (Sandison et al., 2007). Suzuki et al. modified their previous silicon-based design, to make a PMMA-based device providing a tapered aperture for lipid flow and hence achieve a constant amount of lipid solution at the aperture. Further application of a static pressure to control film thickness yielded a more reproducible (90%) bilayer. With further optimization, embedding of four lipid bilayers on a single chip and gramicidin peptide, a monovalent cation channel, incorporated into the bilayer, was achieved (Suzuki, Tabata, Noji, & Takeuchi, 2006). One of the unique advantages of this microfluidic device is that it facilitates easy microscopic observation of the bilayer (Suzuki, Tabata, Noji, & Takeuchi, 2007). Sandison et al. created microfluidic channels on PMMA-coated glass substrates by using hot embossing and laser micromachining (Fig. 7.1(b)). PMMA surface was chemically treated to render it hydrophobic. Lower channel was filled with buffer, and lipid solution was applied to the upper well, which was later filled with the buffer. Lipid bilayers could be achieved by exposure of the top surface to air (Sandison et al., 2007).

Malmstadt et al. suggested that air required in triphasic PMMA-based BLMs can be problematic, and automation is limited as continuous operator vigilance is needed during device fabrication. Also, an annulus was formed around the membrane due to the solvent, limiting the miniaturization capability (Malmstadt et al., 2006). They developed a novel method based on hydrophobic properties of poly(dimethylsiloxane) (PDMS), used a microfluidic channel. A nonaqueous solution of the lipid was suspended in an aqueous flow stream through a microfluidic channel in PDMS. The hydrophobic solvent, partitions into PDMS, shrinking the lipid membranes together forming a bilayer (Fig. 7.2(a)). Ide and Ichikawa developed a microfluidic device based on successive stacking of a glass slide, plastic sheet, PDMS spacer, and agarose-coated coverslip (Fig. 7.2(b)). Lipid solution is first applied to plastic aperture and sucked by vacuum to form a thin layer over the coverslip. Electrolyte was then added to the well and aperture was moved toward the coverslip, compressing the spacer. Before applying a thin layer of lipid, excess electrolyte was removed. Another layer of electrolyte was applied over this, and excess lipid drained by the means of lateral diffusion, leaving behind central lipid bilayer. The area of the bilayer could be controlled by modulating the aperture movement (Ide & Ichikawa, 2005). This method offers the advantage of specific control of bilayer thickness due to application of vacuum and provision for aperture adjustment.

Kreier et al. developed a solvent free method for creating lipid bilayers, using giant unilamellar vesicles that were made to burst by suction through a micron-sized glass orifice. Ion channel proteins were integrated in the bilayer by incubation of giant unilamellar vesicles to obtain proteoliposomes in a simple and less time-consuming manner as opposed to the previous techniques. Typical gating phenomenon was observed by changes in pH and membrane voltage in the outer membrane protein OmpF obtained from *Escherichia coli* (Kreir, Farre, Beckler, George, & Fertig, 2008). Chip-based bilayers have been used for bacterial toxin binding studies. Using total internal reflection fluorescence microscopy, Cholera toxin B subunit and tetanus toxin C fragment could be detected as low as 100 pM (Moran-Mirabal et al., 2005). It was suggested that this method is adaptable for proteins and nucleic acids as well.

Recently, Schlicht reported a fully integrated microfluidic system to produce artificial lipid bilayers based on the miniaturization of droplet interface bilayer (DIB) techniques (Schlicht & Zagnoni, 2015). The microfluidic platform allowed the controlled positioning and storage of phospholipid-stabilized water-in-oil droplets, giving rise to the scalable and automated formation of DIB arrays which were able to mimic cell membrane processes. Based on the optimization of important parameters such as lipid concentration, immiscible phase flow velocities, and the device geometrical parameters, they were able to quantify diffusive transport of molecules and ions across on-chip DIBs by fluorescence-based assays. To further investigate the effect of inhibitors and promoters of ion channels in drug discovery, it would be beneficial to conduct a solution exchange of droplets to introduce membrane proteins.

Microfluidic systems for drug discovery, pharmaceutical analysis, and diagnostic applications 267

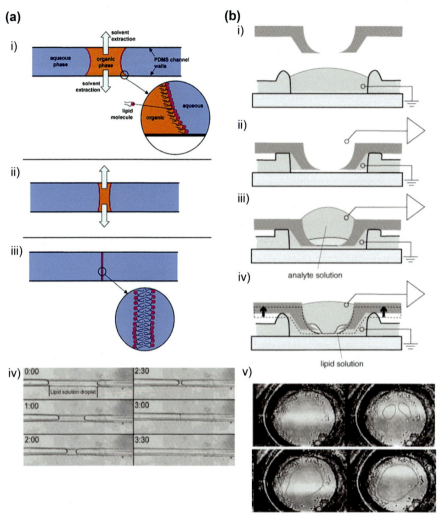

Figure 7.2 Formation of bilayer lipid membranes (BLMs). (a) By microfluidic solvent extraction, (i) droplet of organic solvent with dissolved lipid is formed in an aqueous stream of fluid. Lipids are organized on the hydrophobic—hydrophilic interface (inset). (ii) As solvent enters the poly(dimethyl siloxane) (PDMS), the two interfaces approach one another. (iii) Finally, only the lipid layers are left behind, forming a bilayer membrane. (iv) Images showing solvent extraction from a lipid solution droplet in a microfluidic channel, over a period (minutes: seconds), the BLM, although not visible in the last image, was formed and confirmed by electrical measurements (Malmstadt et al., 2006). (b) By microfluidic bilayer chamber method, (i) A drop of electrolyte was applied to the well of spacer. (ii) A plastic sheet was placed on the spacer and moved downward until the aperture hit the bottom. Then excess electrolyte was removed with a pipette. (iii) Small amount of lipid solution and a sample solution were added sequentially. Alternatively, lipid solution was sprayed through a fine pipette to the edge of the aperture with bubbling without removing the electrolyte in (ii). (iv) After formation of a thick membrane across the aperture, the plastic sheet was moved upwards. The membrane expanded, reached the agarose layer, and thinned to form a bilayer. (v) Successive bright-field images of BLM formation (Ide & Ichikawa, 2005).

To this end, Tsuji and coworkers designed a droplet contact method that allowed the solution exchange of droplets via microfluidic channels (Tsuji et al., 2013). The system allowed the injection of αHL blockers into a droplet and then washing them out. The injection flow rate and the exchange time were adjusted to control the concentration of blockers, which is of great importance since applying differing type of permeating ion, or applying modulators or drugs to the ion channels is often required in ion channel analysis. Moreover, the washing-out experiment demonstrated the binding behavior between ion channels and its ligands. Taken together, the solution exchangeable bilayer system is expected to be a powerful tool for the rapid analyses of ion channels. Similar multiplexed DIBs were prepared by using a mechanically operated linear PMMA chamber array (Barlow et al., 2016). The low cost, linear movable array chip allowed for the simultaneous formation and rapid and high throughput permeation analysis of sub-μL DIBs by the parallelization of DIBs.

These techniques to fabricate BLMs in vitro provide a good platform to identify ion channel proteins as drug targets. Also, once identified, these targets can then be used to screen new therapeutic agents and identify lead compounds for preclinical studies (Kongsuphol, Fang, & Ding, 2013). Syeda and coworkers designed 16-element "DIB-chips" for fast single potassium channel screenings (Syeda, Holden, Hwang, & Bayley, 2008), while Andersson et al. developed arrays of 14 BLMs for the screening of mechanosensitive ion channel (MscL) by forming an ionic reservoir between membrane and the gold electrodes (Andersson et al., 2008) (Fig. 7.3). They can also be used for determination of membrane properties under nonphysiological conditions and gain access to ion channels in intracellular membranes (Kreir et al., 2008).

Cellular receptors and the downstream signal transduction pathways are being increasingly recognized to play a critical role in drug action, and astounding progress has been made in characterizing their behavior. Signal transduction has also been enormously researched with many companies having dedicated programs for signal transduction-based drug discovery (Anonymous, 2000). Enzyme such as tyrosine kinase plays an important role in phosphorylating proteins, forming the essential links in signal transduction pathways (Wang et al., 2008). Wang et al. recently developed a novel microfluidic device combining the function of electroporation and flow cytometry to measure the translocation of fluorescently tagged tyrosine kinase to the cell membrane, at a single cell level. It was demonstrated that cells stimulated through antigen receptor retained more kinase than their nonstimulated counterparts. These results could have a marked impact in target-based drug discovery as kinases are frequently involved in common diseases such as cancer (Wang et al., 2008).

Analysis of protein molecules from a single cell has recently been envisaged as a potential tool to identify specific targets. Recently, single cell analysis has gained considerable attention in microfluidics-based drug discovery as these devices are able to perform manipulation, lysis, labeling, separation, and quantification of the protein contents in a single cell (Huang et al., 2007; Liu & Singh, 2013). Although, this technique is not amenable to live cell monitoring, it provides for simultaneous detection of multiple targets, endowing higher sensitivity in a high throughput capacity. Using single cell analysis chip, the number of β_2 adrenergic receptors was determined. The integrated microfluidic chip facilitated cell and chemical handling,

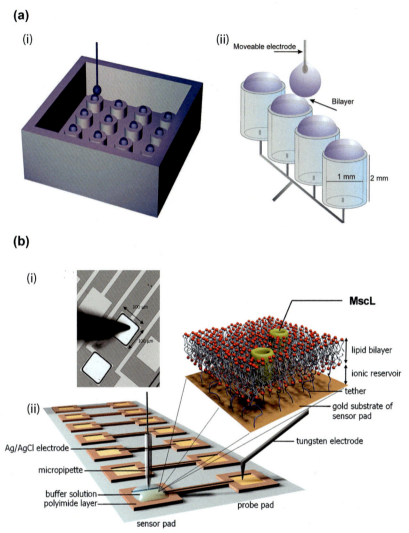

Figure 7.3 (a) Ion-channel screening chip. (i) Simplified schematic of the chip. Each well holds 1.5 µL of solution and presents a convex surface under the oil. A droplet containing the desired IVTT mixture is suspended from the moveable Ag/AgCl electrode, which is grounded. Ion channel blockers and a control (buffer only) are distributed in the wells, each of which contains a Ag/AgCl electrode connected to the working end of the patch clamp amplifier. A DIB is formed between the IVTT droplet and the control well to verify normal channel function. Subsequently, the DIB is separated and the droplet is moved to the next well, and so on. (ii) Detail showing the wiring of 4 of the 16 wells. (Syeda et al., 2008). (b) The engineered tethered bilayer membrane array. (i) Optical microscope image of the probe pad and the tungsten electrode. (ii) Graphical representation of the engineered tethered bilayer membrane array. The lower left corner shows the gold sensor pad covered by a tethered bilayer lipid membrane (tBLM) incorporating MscL ion channels. (Andersson et al., 2008).

cell lysis, electrophoretic separation, and detection of lysate using laser-induced fluorescence (LIF) (Gao, Yin, & Fang, 2004; Wu, Wheeler, & Zare, 2004). Separation of proteins and peptides has also been achieved on miniaturized electrophoretic cells (Schulze & Belder, 2012; Sikanen, Aura, Franssila, Kotiaho, & Kostiainen, 2012). Some of these techniques have been dealt with in greater detail in the subsequent section on analysis.

Understanding of interactions between receptors and their ligands provide insightful information on disease progression and exploration of such drug-receptor pairs provides us an opportunity to discover drugs selectively targeting a particular receptor (Goldberg, Lo, Abele, Macka, & Gomez, 2009). Modulation of physiological events such as cell differentiation and death, release of neurotransmitters and hormones is a result of activation/suppression of signal transduction pathways, which are often coupled to cellular receptors. This activation/suppression is in turn due to binding of specific ligands to these receptors. Much of the research work in discovering new receptor ligands has been focused on binding studies of low molecular weight molecules to macromolecular receptors, followed by screening of biochemical changes. However, it has been reported that lack of a biochemical event does not necessarily translate into lack of receptor activation. Other cellular components and events like second messengers, downstream processes, gene transcription, and change in receptor configuration shall be investigated. This, however, is not possible with the conventional assay procedures (Gurwitz & Haring, 2003). High throughput ligand binding assays provide a suitable alternative to perform multiple tasks on a small chip. Moreover, the discovery of many new "orphan" receptors, for which no ligands are currently known, offers a promising avenue for drug discovery.

Microfluidic devices are beneficial for ligand binding studies as they are able to reduce interaction times, enhance sensitivity and throughput (Kang et al., 2008), and aid in separation of complexed and uncomplexed molecules (Bange, Halsall, & Heineman, 2005). For these binding studies, receptor or ligand molecule can be immobilized on a PDMS substrate by adsorption (Makamba, Hsieh, Sung, & Chen, 2005) or covalent bonding (Sui et al., 2006) or by microcontact printing as achieved for solution hybridized oligonucleotides (Razumovitch, Meier, & Vebert, 2009). These binding interactions are usually quantified by the measurement of equilibrium dissociation constant (K_d) of the ligand—receptor complex.

Goldberg et al. demonstrated the interaction of glycopeptide antibiotics, teicoplanin, and vancomycin, immobilized on a PDMS microchannel with 5-carboxyfluorescein-d-Ala-d-Ala-d-Ala (5-FAM-(DA)$_3$). The K_d was reported to be similar to previously reported values as measured by commercial systems, even though it utilized a smaller amount of reagents (Goldberg et al., 2009). Centrifugal microfluidic platforms, which are disc-shaped microfluidic devices, have also been developed whereby the fluid flows by simple rotation of the disc. Interaction between phenothiazine antidepressants and calmodulin, attached to a green fluorescent protein, was studied. Drug binding affected the fluorescence properties and hence concentration of the drug bound to the protein receptor could be determined (Puckett et al., 2004). BLMs described earlier have been used extensively for ligand binding studies in the past two decades. Recently, phospholipid bilayers were patterned with bovine serum albumin by lithography. Following repeated cycles of patterning, ganglioside GM1 was coated along the microfluidic channels in different concentrations, and its interaction with varying concentrations of cholera toxin B was studied (Shi, Yang, & Cremer, 2008). Javanmard et al. demonstrated a novel method of coupling microfluidic device with shear force spectroscopy to study the interaction between protein molecules and DNA base pairs. The method could be used to measure the affinity of bond between the interacting molecules by measuring the drag force required to detach the ligand bound to the microfluidic channel when receptor attached on surface of microbeads is pressure driven through these channels (Javanmard, Babrzadeh, & Davis, 2010). Cheow and coworkers reported a protein−ligand binding assay based on a modified commercially available microfluidic platform, the Fluidigm Dynamic Array integrated fluidic circuit (IFC) which was originally designed for multiplexed nucleic acids analysis (Cheow et al., 2014). The analysis was streamlined and automated, where only a loading of 48 protein samples and 48 ligands by pipetting was needed before the benchtop instrument automatically combined the proteins and ligands, for instance chromatin binding proteins and various histone peptides in a pairwise way in 2304 independent chambers of 9 nL for fluorescence anisotropy imaging. The binding affinities turned out to be close to those achieved by a conventional microtiter plate platform which requires two orders of magnitude more reagents and more time. More recently, Glick et al. pioneered an in vitro tool for host−pathogen screening with protein arrays in order to understand important pathogenic processes (Glick et al., 2016) (Fig. 7.4). Around 2700 synthetic genes were arrayed and expressed as insoluble transmembrane proteins within a microfluidic platform using a cell-free protein expression system, and then screened against two important pathogenic proteins, the simian virus 40 (SV40) and hepatitis delta virus (HDV) to find new interactions. The effectiveness of using this microfluidic platform was demonstrated by performing a high-throughput screen of pathogen−membrane protein interactions, since specific interactions of interest were further validated by coimmunoprecipitation or protein−fragment complementation assay of luciferase activity.

7.2.2 Hit identification and lead optimization

After the identification of a druggable target, the next step in the drug discovery process is to identify a "hit" which involves phases of hit identification (HI), lead identification (LI), and leading to lead optimization (LO). A "hit" is a chemical or biological moiety that binds to a specific target which has been implicated in an ailment. Screening and optimization of millions of "hits" results in several "lead" compounds. This whole multiphase process, in which "leads" are optimized by an initial screening involving multiple "hits," is ascribed as a "hit-to-lead" process (Goodnow, 2006). Synthesizing and screening the right drug which can potentially be used and carried forward through a drug development program and enter a clinic starts from right identification of hits and leads. These steps are imperative and crucial since drug discovery is an expensive process (Katsuno et al., 2015). An error at this stage may lead to an expensive failure at a later stage.

Drug candidates may either be derived from combinatorial libraries or be of natural origin, and drug libraries have been estimated to be in the order of 10^{63}

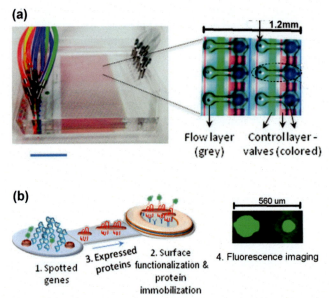

Figure 7.4 Membrane protein array generated by integrated microfluidic platform. (a) An integrated microfluidics platform (Left) was used for on-chip expression of membrane proteins, to serve as "baits" for protein interactions or modifications (29). The device consists of two polydimethylsiloxane (PDMS) layers, a flow layer with 64 × 64 unit cells array (gray), and a control layer with micromechanical valves (colored) that manipulate the flow of fluids in the experiment (Center). The sandwich valves (pink) separate neighboring unit cells; the neck valves (green) divide each unit cell into a DNA compartment and a reaction compartment. The button valves (blue) enable surface patterning to promote binding of proteins to an antibody surface. The button valves serve as mechanical traps of molecular interactions (MITOMI) and allow measurement at equilibrium concentration. MITOMI increases the sensitivity of the system, facilitating detection of weak and transient interactions (SI Appendix, Fig. S6). (b) Combining the microfluidic platform with microarray technology enables programming of the device with up to several thousand spotted genes (Right). Using assembly polymerase cycling assembly (PCR) (SI Appendix, Fig. S1), we added c-Myc (N-terminal) and His6 (C-terminal) tags to the open reading frame (ORFs), creating synthetic genes. On-chip in vitro protein expression, following the synthetic gene programming, combined with the corresponding antibody surface patterning, facilitates the self-assembly of an membrane protein array (MPA) using cell-free transcription and translation (TNT) (rabbit reticulocyte). The immobilized bait proteins are labeled with fluorescent antibodies and quantified by using a microarray scanner. Expressed proteins form a green circle below the button valve (Right) (Glick et al., 2016).

(Bohacek, McMartin, & Guida, 1996). Microfluidic chip−based combinatorial chemistry and high throughput screening together aim to result in a paradigm shift, leading to development of methods of sequential synthesis and testing of thousands of compounds in parallel (Knight, 2000; Li et al., 2018; MacConnell, Price, & Paegel, 2017).

7.2.2.1 Synthesis of drug libraries

Recognition of drug targets has kept pace with the fast progress in genomic and proteomic tools. Pharmaceutical companies on the other hand are facing challenges in generating drug compounds at fastest possible rate, in an inexpensive manner. Synthesis of drug libraries has been described as the biggest impediment in the drug discovery process (Jones et al., 2005). Improved methods in combinatorial chemistry have resulted in rapid synthesis of large number of chemical compounds and produced enormous drug libraries. This has been further accelerated by the improvement in the design of the microfluidic reactors. These microfluidic reactors can be classified into three types, based on the flow pattern, namely (i) flow thorough type, (ii) droplet or slug type, and (iii) batch type (Keng et al., 2012). The most common flow through type enables multiple reagents to be maintained at a temperature, which can be pressure driven through the channels. These reactors have been used greatly in extraction procedures as well as multiple chemical syntheses (Keng et al., 2012). Such application was firstly performed by Warrington and colleagues from GlaxoSmithKline (GSK) to synthesize a small set of pyrazoles using Knorr chemistry (Garcia-Egido, Spikmans, Wong, & Warrington, 2003). The semiautomated synthesis using this technique achieved a residence time in the microreactor of 210 s and ensured near quantitative conversion rates. In another example, an Automated Lead Optimization Equipment Platform, which could significantly reduce time gaps between the synthesis-assay-design cycles, was developed. Its software was equipped with an algorithm which could build predictive bioactivity models and prioritizing the selection of starting materials for subsequent compound generations (Pickett, Green, Hunt, Pardoe, & Hughes, 2011). More recently, Reutlinger et al. presented the optimization of the on-chip reaction and assembly of a combinatorial library of imidazopyridines through the Ugi chemistry (Reutlinger, Rodrigues, Schneider, & Schneider, 2014). The synthesis was conducted at a throughput of 0.3 s per compound with a total reaction volume of only 5 μL.

Parallel combinatorial synthesis in multiple microfluidic reactors has also been demonstrated utilizing continuous flow of reagents in microfluidic channels. A multiple microfluidic reactor assembly was fabricated to synthesize carbamates in a multistep procedure (Sahoo, Kralj, & Jensen, 2007). However, this method sacrifices the advantages of an integrated system for several reactions to be carried out on a single chip. Researchers then looked to fabricate a consolidated device with multiple layers of parallel chips. A multilayer glass chip was developed for a 2 × 2 series synthesis in parallel (Kikutani et al., 2002). Complexity and expense of fabrication of this multilayered device was a concern. Recently, Dexter and Parker exhibited parallel combinatorial synthesis of compounds on a single layered microfluidic chip (Fig. 7.5(a)). They fabricated a single layer PDMS chip for synthesizing a 2 × 2 series of amide formation products (Dexter & Parker, 2009).

However, the continuous flow reactors are not suitable for multistep reactions, especially involving sequential synthesis. A modified technique (batch microfluidics) in which specific microvalves control the delivery of reagents in batches has

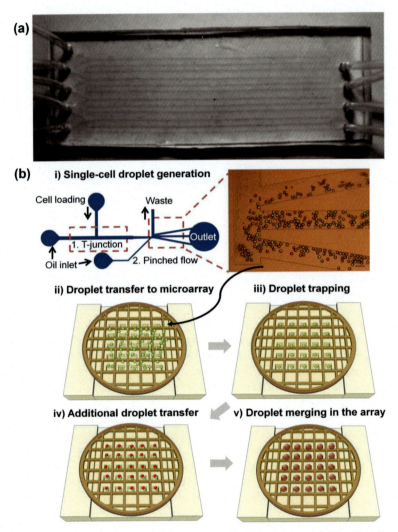

Figure 7.5 Different types of microfluidic reactors. (a) A continuous poly(dimethylsiloxane) (PDMS)-based microfluidic flow reactor for 2 × 2 parallel combinatorial synthesis. The tubing has been inserted at each inlet and outlet port (Dexter & Parker, 2009). (b) Schematic of a microdroplet manipulator, including functions for (i) droplet generation, (ii) transfer of droplets to a microwell array, (iii) migration of droplets into the wells, (iv) trapping of second droplets, and (v) oil change to induce droplet merging (Um, Rha, Choi, Lee, & Park, 2012).

been developed. These isolated batches can be delivered to the microfluidic reactor chamber at specific time points in a reaction cycle, exercising greater control over the reaction (Lee et al., 2005). A fluoride radiolabeled imaging probe, in nano/microgram scale, was synthesized in five sequential processes involving fluoride concentration, water evaporation, radiofluorination, solvent exchange, and hydrolytic deprotection.

A newer technology known as droplet microfluidics has recently come to the fore due to its merits such as consuming very little materials and reagents for large-scale studies, and a high degree of automation which facilitates high throughput screens (Shembekar, Chaipan, Utharala, & Merten, 2016). It is based on compartmentalization of each assay in a small droplet, usually in the range of 1 pL—10 nL which is 10^3-10^9 times smaller than the volume required by conventional systems, surrounded by an immiscible oil and can be manipulated and processed in a high throughput manner (Brouzes, 2012). Each of these droplets can act as a tiny microfluidic reactor, notably reducing the reagent volumes required. A mesh-grid design microwell array was fabricated by Um et al., which allows for continuous addition and trapping of picolitre single cell droplets in the microwells (Fig. 7.5(b)). Due to miniaturization, the device provides high throughput screening (HTS) of the droplets (Um et al., 2012), but multistep reactions using these devices are still a big challenge.

Besides the small molecular chemicals, the microchannel reactor was also employed in the synthesis of macromolecular therapeutics, such as DNA and proteins. Short synthetic oligonucleotides were joined under thermal cycling in a microfluidic PicoArray device to form DNA constructs up to 10 kb in an instant. The fabricated DNA construct was shown to express relevant proteins and may be used for cell free protein expression on a large scale (Zhou et al., 2004). Mei et al. developed a microfluidic array device for synthesis of chloramphenicol acetyltransferase and luciferase and reported the yield to be 13—22 times higher than that achieved in microcentrifuge tube, with a 5—10 times longer lasting protein expression. The device composed of an array of units that allowed for fabrication of different proteins, protein expression, and nutrient supply. The device is also capable of synthesis and analysis of proteins on a single chip, potentially eliminating the need to harvest proteins thereby reducing wastage and increasing process efficiency (Mei, Fredrickson, Simon, Khnouf, & Fan, 2007). A droplet-based microfluidic method was recently developed for on-chip protein synthesis. Production of a water-in-oil-in-water (W/O/W) emulsion was accomplished by formation of a water-in-oil emulsion on a PMMA chip, up first, followed by complete emulsion formation on a PDMS/glass microchip. Synthesis and expression of a green fluorescent protein from a DNA template was successfully demonstrated using a microfluidic platform (Wu et al., 2011). Recently, Timm reported a microfluidic-based cell-free system as a bioreactor for the production of a single dose of a therapeutic protein (Timm, Shankles, Foster, Doktycz, & Retterer, 2016). This new design integrated a long, serpentine channel bioreactor channel, and a nanofabricated membrane to allow exchange of materials between parallel "reactor" and "feeder" channels. The membrane was designed to facilitate the exchange of metabolites, energy, and inhibitory species between the two channels, and its surface could be modified to tune the exchange rate of small molecules, which enabled extended reaction times and higher yields than conventional tube—based batch synthesis.

Most of the devices developed use PDMS as the substrate materials due to its excellent optical properties as well as its mouldability. However, PDMS is incompatible with many organic solvents and adsorbs many hydrophobic compounds due to its surface properties. Keng et al. fabricated a microfluidic platform that is operated by electrowetting-on-dielectric (EWOD). The device was made from inorganic materials coated with perfluoro polymer and offers flexibility in use with organic and hydrophobic reagents (Keng et al., 2012). The device was shown to be suitable for diverse chemical reactions with minimal consumption of reagents, with suitability for multistep procedures requiring several solvent exchange rounds.

7.2.2.2 High throughput screening

Microfluidics-based devices have been put to efficient use to generate drug libraries which provide a powerful source that need to be screened to explore new drugs. To screen these large combinatorial libraries of compounds, pharmaceutical industry has looked at HTS methodologies in the past two decades. The conventional screening methods were able to screen 5000−20,000 compounds over a few years, resulting in inefficient screening of only 2%−20% of the compounds on the whole library. However, HTS or newly termed, ultrahigh throughput screening (uHTS) methodologies aim to screen 10,000−100,000 compounds over a period of 24 h, resulting in generation of 2−18 million screening results per year (Beggs, 2001). This logarithmic increase in screening capability has given a boost to the hit-to-lead discovery process.

Traditionally, high density microplates including 96, 384, 1536 and those with >1536 wells have been used extensively for HTS (Battersby & Trau, 2002; Brandish et al., 2006). However, liquid handling on a microliter scale in these microplates was found to be difficult due to their inability to be integrated with robotic liquid handling technologies as well as suitable detection platforms. Microfluidic platforms can further miniaturize the HTS platforms, lowering the assay volume required (Ding et al., 2015). Also, these platforms can be easily modeled for convenient liquid handling and integrated with analytical devices. Microfluidic HTS platforms for confining reagents have been studied in both serial and parallel configurations. Using serial method, compounds are screened in a successive manner with only one detector unit. However, in this approach, the throughput is largely dependent on flow rate and concentration of the sample as well as acquisition speed of the detector. In contrast, parallel screening offers faster analysis, segregating multiple samples into miniaturized compartments of a high-density microplate, and analyzed by a single detector (Ding et al., 2015). But parallel analysis is limited by the miniaturization capacity and hence the extent of parallelization (Thorsen, 2004). Nevertheless, both methods have been extensively used in microfluidic HTS. Generally, cell-based microfluidic HTS platforms include cell culture (El-Ali, Sorger, & Jensen, 2006; Wu, Huang, & Lee, 2010), introduction and transportation of samples (Melin & Quake, 2007; Stone, Stroock, & Ajdari, 2004), and characterization of cell viability (Barbulovic-Nad, Yang, Park, & Wheeler, 2008), with an effort to demonstrate the integration of these different components into a single microfluidic device. Among current microfluidic platforms for cell-based HTS, there are three major modes to manipulate microfluids: perfusion flow mode, droplet-based mode, and microarray mode (Du, Fang, & den Toonder, 2016), which will be elaborated in the following.

Microfluidic microwell arrays are a versatile tool for cell culture and high throughput experimentation through cell-based assays. They enable assays with many biological samples on a 2D solid substrate and are particularly important in drug screening. Nearly 50% of all drug discovery processes rely on cell-based assays (Fox et al., 2006). Seeding many cell types on a single chip offers the advantages of testing the effect on drugs on different cells types. It also offers the potential of testing many compounds on a single cell type in high throughput. A multiwall microelectrode array was fabricated using PDMS by conventional soft lithographic process. The array was then coated with a cell adhesive layer of poly-D-lysine followed by patterning a nonconducting agarose gel layer to isolate the individual neuronal microcircuits and record individual action potentials of drugs like bicuculline and N-methyl-D-aspartic acid (Kang, Lee, Lee, & Nam, 2009) (Fig. 7.6). Chen et al. developed a complementary microwell and microcolumn system for screening of drugs. They used microelectromechanical systems (MEMS) to first fabricate a microwell array on a glass substrate, to culture the cells. Employing a similar process, they fabricated complementary microcolumns that will carry the drugs to be topically applied onto the cells. The system was found to be suitable to deliver high throughput identification of epidermal growth factor receptor inhibitors (Chen, Huang, & Juang, 2011). An integrated multilayer microdevice incorporating a drug/medium concentration gradient generator, flow controlling microvalves, and microchambers for cell culture was recently fabricated by Liu et al. for testing the apoptosis behavior in a cisplatin resistant cancer cell line (Liu et al., 2012). A vertical perfusion mode was adopted in this device, as shear stress due to horizontal fluid flow can adversely impact the cells. Using the setup, sequential loading of cells, medium, drugs, and air was achieved in successive layers of the device.

The combination of two or more clinically available drugs, administered either simultaneously or sequentially, may enhance the therapeutic efficacy, as well as reduce the drug toxicity and resistance as a result of its multitarget treatment mechanisms. More importantly, drug combination is also considered as an effective way to increase the efficiency of drug discovery since most drug combinations are conducted using existing drugs which have passed the strict clinical and safety studies (Ashburn & Thor, 2004). Therefore, Ding et al. developed a low-cost, high-efficiency microfluidic print-to-screen (P2S) platform for high-throughput screening of anticancer drug combinations (Ding et al., 2015). The P2S platform utilized a microfluidic impact printer to generate large-scale combinatorial droplets containing multiple anticancer drugs, so-called combinatorial library in microarrays. Then, the hydrogel-based cell culture matrix was treated with the droplet arrays before stained and imaged for HI (Fig. 7.7). Compared with conventional techniques, the P2S platform completely automated the combinatorial library generation and significantly accelerated the screening process by performing thousands of cell-drug interaction analyses in parallel, which could facilitate the discovery cycle of potent drug combinations. Furthermore, taking advantage of the sequential operation droplet array (SODA) technique, Du and coworkers developed a drug combination screening platform with multisteps involving cell culture, medium changing, drug dosage and stimulation, and cell viability assay in an oil-covered nanolitre-scale droplet array system (Du et al., 2013). The drug consumption for each screening testing was substantially reduced to 5 ng—5 mg, considered as a significant reduction compared with conventional

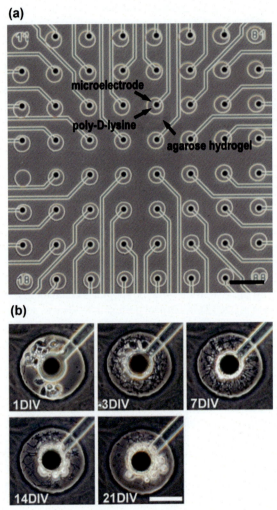

Figure 7.6 Microfluidic microarrays for cell-based high throughput screening. A multiwell microelectrode array, (a) phase contrast image of agarose microwells on a microelectrode array. Each microwell is composed of a microelectrode, poly-D-lysine coated surface, and agarose hydrogel wall, scale—200 μm. (b) The growth of neuronal conduits in microwells over a period of 3 weeks, scale—50 μm (DIV—days in vitro) (Kang et al., 2009).

drug screening systems. Despite a lot of progress in developing microscale arrays for cell culture, cell seeding in these arrays is a challenge. Kang et al. addressed this issue by developing a simple wiping method to seed cells in microwells. A coverslip was used to slowly wipe the cells suspended in the growth medium across the surface of the microwell array. Cell concentration, microwell geometry, and wiping speed controlled the cell seeding density (Kang, Hancock, Brigham, & Khademhosseini, 2010). They also developed an algorithm and software for automatic counting of cells

Microfluidic systems for drug discovery, pharmaceutical analysis, and diagnostic applications 279

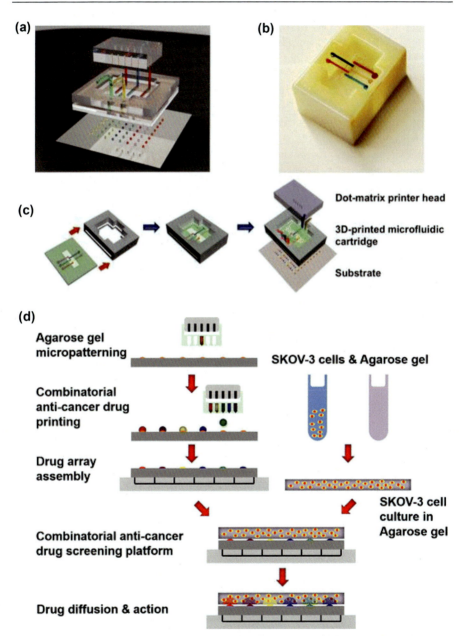

Figure 7.7 Microfluidic impact printing. (a) Illustration of the microfluidic impact printer, consisting of a dot matrix printer head, a traveling stage, and a microfluidic cartridge with a 3D printed adapter. (b) Microfluidic impact printer prototype. (c) Plug-and-play assembly of the microfluidic impact printer head (Ding et al., 2015).

in a microwell array. The software, named as Arraycount, detects the cell count from the fluorescent cell images in high throughput. The results were in close correlation between cell counts from the manual methods (Kachouie, Kang, & Khademhosseini, 2009).

Studying single cell characteristics offers the advantage over observing the behavior of a group of cells as single cell characteristics might be hugely different from the entire population of cells. Microwell arrays have been developed to confine single cells for observation of these cells and their progeny over a period. One of the first studies pertaining to single cell confinement in microwell arrays for drug screening was reported by Rettig and Folch (Rettig & Folch, 2005). PDMS microwells were fabricated by conventional soft lithography, and controlled seeding of single cells into microwells could be achieved by optimizing the geometry of the microwells. It was observed that microwells with an aspect ratio (diameter: depth) close to one had more than 85% wells with single cell occupancy for both adherent and non-adherent cells (Rettig & Folch, 2005). An interesting round bottom microwell array was recently developed by Liu et al. by creating PDMS microwell arrays by reverse molding using polystyrene microspheres melted on a glass substrate (Liu, Liu, Gao, Ding, & Lin, 2010) (Fig. 7.8). The size of these microwells could be tuned to 10–20 μm, which is difficult to achieve by conventional soft lithography. The PDMS microwells were then used to confine single cells by pouring excess of cell suspension over the microwells, which allowed the cells to settle in. The enzymatic activity of cells was studied by carrying out the carboxylesterase assay using calcein AM. Fluorescence intensities from single cells could be captured to reveal different kinetic behavior of entrapped cells, which was related to cell viability. Another novel way of constraining single cells in microwells was demonstrated by Wang, Shah, Phillips, Sims, and Allbritton (2012). The flexibility of PDMS was exploited by stretching the patterned PDMS array using a tube that delivered the cells onto the array. After loading, the tube was withdrawn and cells settled in the microwells, which were then amenable to further analytical treatments. They also demonstrated that cells within the microwells could be isolated by deforming the PDMS substrate using a microneedle (Wang et al., 2012). A further example was illustrated by Lew and coworkers who devised a plastic microwell array by using economical materials like shrink wrap film and tape. A carbon dioxide laser was used to cut holes in the tape which acts as a mask to etch wells in the shrink wrap by oxygen plasma (Lew, Nguyen, & Khine, 2011).

In a perfusion flow mode of drug screening, the microfluidic devices need a series of generic components for introducing reagents and samples, transferring fluids within a microchannel network, as well as combining and mixing reactants. By using the technique of reversible sealing of elastomeric PDMS, Ali et al. developed a double-layer device making use of a PDMS substrate layer with microwells and a PDMS cover layer with arrays of microchannels (Khademhosseini et al., 2005). Multiple cell types were seeded into microwells in the substrate layer through the microchannels of the first PDMS cover layer which was replaced with an orthogonally aligned second cover layer to deliver different fluids to the patterned cells for screening. Another method of on-chip drug screening relies on the controlled diffusive mixing of solutions in

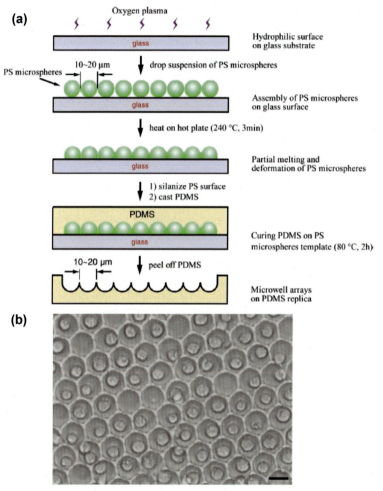

Figure 7.8 Fabrication of microwell assays. (a) Schematic illustration for the fabrication of PDMS microwell arrays. (b) Cell arrays on the microwells and single cell enzyme activity analysis. Micrograph of dense trapping of Ramos cells (Liu et al., 2010).

continuous laminar flow inside a network of microfluidic channels where drug concentration gradients were generated. Chung and coworkers reported a microfluidic device for high throughput capture and imaging of single cells by shear force in a continuous flow channel (Chung, Rivet, Kemp, & Lu, 2011). Coupled to gradient generators, this device was able to study heterogeneity in calcium oscillatory behavior in genetically identical cells and investigate kinetic cellular response to various chemicals. Due to the development of individual components, microfluidics also has potential in developing integrated automatic systems to perform cell culture, drug release, and cell activity detection together for drug discovery. Weltin et al. developed a microfluidic system for drug screening by real-time on-line monitoring of human cancer cell metabolism process (Weltin et al., 2014). The optically transparent multifunction microsystem comprised cell culture chambers and four chemo- and biosensors modules for the detection of pH, oxygen, lactate, and glucose, respectively. The drug screening application was demonstrated by monitoring the change and recovery effects of cellular metabolism induced by the addition of substances to the medium.

The droplet mode is the last type of microfluids manipulation in cell-based HTS which can perform a broad spectrum of experimental chemistry and biology screening. The typical droplet systems use water-in-oil emulsion droplets, where the continuous oil phase can prevent cross-contamination between reagents in neighboring droplets and minimize the nonspecific binding between the channel surface and reagents of dispersed phase. Another advantage of droplet system is that droplets can be split or merged to start or stop reactions or to conduct washing steps. Clausell-Tormos and coworkers first designed a droplet-based microfluidic platform where cells or multicellular organism could survive and proliferate for more than several days (Clausell-Tormos et al., 2008). This system offered a screening with a 1000-fold smaller volume and a 500 times higher throughput. Brouzes et al. reported a microfluidic droplet-based system for high throughput cytotoxicity screening of single cells (Brouzes et al., 2009). The cells were encapsulated in individual microdroplets and coalesced with optically coded droplets from a chemical library to identify drug composition and drug concentration in each droplet, before the coalesced droplets were merged with fluorescent dye droplets to stain the cells for the on-line fluorescence assay. Recently, Cao and coworkers developed a microfluidic droplet device for an assay of toxic effects on *Escherichia coli* via the generation of multidimensional concentrations of antibiotics (Cao et al., 2012). This device allowed more than 5000 distinct experiments with different combinations of antibiotic concentrations in a single experiment, making it suitable for the drug screening with the advantages of reduced experimental complexity and higher information density.

Multiplexed screening platforms have also been developed to screen multiple samples in one run. The ability to analyze multiple proteins, nucleic acids as well as small molecules reduces assay time, reagent volume, and cost. Multiplexed measurements provide the ability to increase the throughput without a simultaneous increase in the density of the microfluidic array. Multiplexing technology has been applied to two different types of microfluidic platforms: planar arrays and suspension (particle-based) arrays. For protein and DNA analysis, planar arrays have been used, whereby protein molecules have been patterned as microarrays onto substrates using lithography (MacBeath & Schreiber, 2000). Such systems offer application-specific advantages ranging from study of protein—protein interactions to establishing proteins as targets for small molecules and specific functions of enzymes. Suspension arrays on the other hand offer the advantages of studying the properties of compounds in solution, thereby providing ease of sample modification, higher throughput, and increased batch to batch uniformity (Nolan & Sklar, 2002).

A multiplexed system could be used to screen a compound against multiple kinases or study protein—protein interaction and detect changes in enzyme conformation (Xue, Wainright, Gangakhedkar, & Gibbons, 2001). In this report, four kinases were screened against a substrate. The reaction products/substrates could be separated by electrophoretic separation on a chip and analyzed. Multiplexed screening of picolitre-sized droplets that could be manipulated using an array of electrodes has also been reported. For example, caspase-3 activity, a marker of apoptosis which is an important tool in cancer drug discovery, was measured after human cervical adenocarcinoma HeLa cells were treated with different concentrations of staurosporine. The technique termed as digital microfluidics (DMF) was compared against conventional techniques involving 96-well plate. It resulted in a 33-fold reduction in sample volume together with a lower detection limit for caspase-3 analysis compared with conventional techniques. This can be attributed to the lack of delamination in apoptotic cells in the DMF platform that uses droplet manipulation system instead of pipetting or aspiration of liquids with conventional techniques (Bogojevic, Chamberlain, Barbulovic-Nad, & Wheeler, 2012).

Analyzing multiple samples by multiplexing, however, poses a challenge in sample recognition. Hence, it is necessary to have an encoding scheme integrated into the system to allow for rapid and precise analyte identification. Encoding schemes based on spectrometric (Han, Gao, Su, & Nie, 2001), graphical (Evans, Sewter, & Hill, 2003), electronic (Service, 1995), and physical techniques (Vaino & Janda, 2000) have been developed. An exhaustive review on various encoding techniques has been published by Braeckmans, De Smedt, Leblans, Pauwels, and Demeester (2002). Spectrometric techniques utilize specific wavelengths to analyze a compound. In contrast, graphical methods use certain optical elements that are chemically patterned onto the microarray. These techniques require much sophistication and are expensive and may require considerable amount of time for fabrication and integration.

Pregibon et al. recently developed a novel encoding scheme for multiplexed platforms (Pregibon, Toner, & Doyle, 2007). In this system, two poly(ethylene glycol) based monomer solutions, one being a fluorescent dye and another being an acrylate probe, were made to flow through microfluidic channels. The solutions during flow were exposed to ultraviolet light using conventional techniques of continuous flow lithography to develop a patterned particle (Pregibon et al., 2007). Morphological properties of the particles were determined by a photomask, inserted into a fluorescence microscope (Pregibon et al., 2007). A simple dot coding scheme was used on the photomask that could generate over two million particles, with each having a unique code. Although the particle size achieved in this method was larger than previous methods, the authors demonstrated that the sample volume required will be manageable, together with providing higher sensitivity and reproducibility. The system was able to detect DNA at concentrations as low as 10^{-18} mol, without signal amplification, proving it to be a completely integrated encoding device, with advantages of low cost, high efficiency with virtually unlimited number of codes possible, and all this achievable with the services of a simple fluorescence microscope.

Inkjet printing technology has been purported as a highly efficient screening alternative, providing efficiencies greater than 200,000 compounds per day, currently achievable with the microfluidic platforms described earlier. The technology offers capabilities to simultaneously deposit cells and drugs to be tested in a small picolitre volume. Postprocessing, the cell characteristics can be studied to evaluate the drug effects. Such a novel platform was developed by Rodríguez-Dévora, Zhang, Reyna, Shi and Xu (2012). They developed an inkjet printer—based method to pattern green fluorescent protein expressing *Escherichia coli* cells grown on a soy agar medium, on a coverslip. Live/Dead assay, used to assess bacterial cell viability, demonstrated high number of cell survival after imprinting. Fast screening utilizing low volumes to assess effect of three antibiotics patterned together with the bacterial cells could be carried out. This bioprinting approach was compared to the standard micropipetting approach and was found to yield similar results at much lower volumes (Rodríguez-Dévora et al., 2012).

These microfluidic platforms have significantly enhanced the profile of high throughput screening, leading to optimization of hits and leads, before the leads are put through preclinical testing for evaluation of their preliminary pharmacokinetic and toxicological properties.

7.2.3 Preclinical evaluation

Interaction with the molecular targets begins the journey of the drug in the human body. When a drug is administered, it must get absorbed across mucous membranes, followed by its distribution to its target site and metabolism to an inactive metabolite to get eliminated from the body. It should also be devoid of any toxic effects. These characteristics, known as Absorption, Distribution, Metabolism, Elimination, and Toxicology (ADMET) are essential factors in determining the path of the drug in the later stages of the drug discovery process. A fine balance between these pharmacokinetic characteristics is needed for the development of a drug from a chemical entity (Muster et al., 2008). Unsatisfactory ADMET profile accounts for attrition of 50%—60% drug candidates at the preclinical development stage (Smith, 2007), with lack of efficacy and undesirable toxicity being the major causes (Kramer, Sagartz, & Morris, 2007). It has been reported that the lack of efficacy accounts for 30% of failures of new drug entities and toxicity further accounts for another 30%. If these are detected at later stages in the drug development process, the overall cost of the program will be increased, as cost escalates with each stage (Kola & Landis, 2004). Therefore, pharmaceutical companies are nowadays adopting the *fail early; fail cheap* approach to identify the toxicological properties of drug compounds. This is done in lieu of savings if toxicological properties are identified at a much later stage or even after the launch of the product, necessitating an inevitable and highly expensive market recall. It has been reported that number of market recalls as a percentage of number of approvals in United States has reduced from 27.2% in 1980s to 5.2% in 2000s (Qureshi, Seoane-Vazquez, Rodriguez-Monguio, Stevenson, & Szeinbach, 2011). This has, in part, been the contribution of more novel and efficient toxicity screening platforms that have been developed in the past two decades. It also underlines the importance of proficient preclinical programs and the role played by them in drug development.

In vitro toxicological testing in cell models provides useful information about the drug candidates, much before the expensive animal experiments and first-in-human clinical trials are conducted. In vitro experiments have been long touted to replace animal testing, especially due to the ethical concerns surrounding animal experimentation (Wen, Zhang, & Yang, 2012). Moreover, in vitro toxicity in excised animal organs may not be extrapolated to correctly reflect human toxicities. On the other hand, in vivo preclinical testing in live animals requires large amount of compound under investigation, which is usually available in limited quantities and may be prohibitively expensive (Muster et al., 2008).

7.2.3.1 In vitro evaluation

Three dimensional (3D) cell culture mimics the natural environment of the cells, including cell—cell and cell—extracellular matrix interactions as opposed to planar two dimensional (2D) cultures that are used to maintain cells (Pampaloni, Reynaud, & Stelzer, 2007). An excellent collation of advantages of 3D cell culture over 2D format has been provided by Zhang and van Noort (2011). Also, these 3D cultures offer an ex vivo alternative to live animal testing and potentially reduce the cost of toxicity screening during drug development. Nonetheless, 3D cell cultures present a few shortcomings, especially with sample handling and imaging. Since these cultures are thicker than conventional "petri-dish" cultures, they are difficult to adapt to conventional microscopic techniques. Liquid handling in patterned microstructures requires sophisticated micro/nanolitre scale devices. However, the advantages of studying the cells in an environment outweigh the technological shortcomings, which, too, are being addressed simultaneously.

As hepatotoxicity has been the leading cause of failure at the clinical trial stages and postlaunch market withdrawals, many researchers have looked at developing in vitro cell-based hepatotoxicity assays. It is important to notice here that most of these agents went through preclinical animal testing and were assumed to be safe (Kaplowitz, 2005). Microfluidic 3D cell culture platforms aim to address this problem and have been designed to provide deeper insights into cell behavior, when exposed to cytotoxic agents. A multiwell 3D cell culture platform was designed using soft lithography to coculture primary hepatocytes with mouse 3T3-J2 fibroblasts. A PDMS stencil containing through holes in a 24-well format was first applied to a polystyrene plate, followed by application of collagen-I through the holes. After removal of the PDMS stencil and application of a 24 well PDMS blank, hepatocytes were cultured on the 24 wells, which attached to the collagen, surrounded by fibroblasts. The hepatocyte morphology was maintained in the wells for 4—6 weeks. Albumin and urea synthesis, measured as markers of protein synthesis and nitrogen metabolism and typically considered as a measure of liver function, was reported to be normal. On the other hand, pure cultures were reported to be morphologically unstable, and there was a loss of albumin and urea synthesis (Khetani & Bhatia, 2008).

Kane et al. designed a microfluidic 8 × 8 array, composed of PDMS. Each well in the array had two chambers, a primary chamber whose bottom was made of glass coated with collagen, for coculturing rat hepatocytes and 3T3-J2 fibroblasts. The collagen aided selective adhesion of hepatocytes. Continuous perfusion of medium and removal of waste products was achieved by microfluidic tubing connected to the chamber. The secondary chamber, which was separated from the primary chamber by a thin PDMS membrane, was linked to microfluidic channels supplying humidified air with 10% carbon dioxide at 37°C. They also reported similar results of increased albumin and urea production (Kane, Zinner, Yarmush, & Toner, 2006). Such microfluidic platforms have also been used to assess cardiotoxicity, neurotoxicity, embryotoxicity, and cytolysis, a summary of which has been provided in a review by Wen et al. (2012). These microfluidic devices, which can emulate an organ in vitro, are referred to as organ-on-a-chip devices.

Although the above listed cell-based assays provide information about a compound's therapeutic and toxic properties on the tissue under consideration, they do not tell anything about the effect on the whole body or interactions with other organs and related dose dynamics. As a drug in the body goes through the complex process of ADME, collectively called as pharmacokinetics (PK), with contribution from different organs, cell culture using cells-on-a-chip or organ-on-a-chip technology fails to capture these responses. Of late, scientists have developed miniaturized multicompartment cell culture platform better known as body-on-a-chip devices. These can promote tissue—tissue interactions by creation of environment and flow conditions scaled down to in vivo tissue sizes. They can also aid in studying interactions between organs in a high throughput manner, enabling the study of multiorgan metabolic and toxicity profiles of a compound. Microscale systems designed for physiologically based pharmacokinetic modeling (PBPK) having different compartments for different tissues can help to understand parameters such as tissue-to-blood perfusion, enzyme kinetics, liquid-to-cell ratio, and physiological stress on a particular tissue/organ (Esch, King, & Shuler, 2011).

Novel microfluidic systems called as microscale cell culture analog (μCCA) have been developed for multiorgan toxicity analysis. A multiorgan culture system termed as "Integrated discrete multiple organ culture" or "wells-within-a-well" system was designed by Li et al. Cells from different organs were cultured in small wells in their respective medium in a bigger well. They cultured primary cells from liver, kidney, lungs, central nervous system, blood vessels as well as human breast adenocarcinoma cancer cell line, MCF-7. For testing the toxicity of a model drug, the bigger wells were flushed with a medium containing the drug, tamoxifen. The effect of tamoxifen was evaluated, and its comparative toxicity toward various organs was also examined. Apart from this, the system offers another advantage in enabling the analysis of anticancer activity of a drug with respect to its effect on normal tissues. The authors did not delve upon multiorgan interactions; this, in principle, can be adapted for this purpose and its capabilities should be further investigated (Li, Bode, & Sakai, 2004).

In a model based on PBPK to emulate dynamics of human body, different compartments hosting different cell types were connected through microfluidic channels to mimic blood circulation. Four different cells were cultured on a μCCA, including hepatocytes (HepG2/C3A), bone marrow cells (MEG-01), uterine cancer cells (MES-SA), and a multidrug resistant (MDR) uterine cancer cell line (MES-SA/DX-5). In a combination drug therapy of chemotherapeutic doxorubicin, with MDR modulators cyclosporine and nicardipine, treated for 24 or 72 h, a selective toxicity toward MES-SA/DX-5 was observed, a synergy not observed in conventional 96-well plate assays. This device could, thus, be used in drug screening and selection of potential MDR modulators, as well as gather dose required and dose response

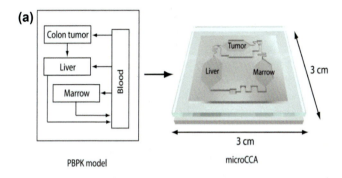

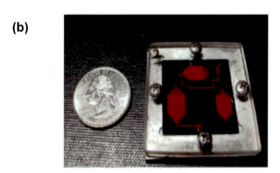

Figure 7.9 A mathematical PBPK model and a corresponding physical mCCA based on the human body. (a) A μCCA consists of liver, tumor, and marrow chambers, interconnected with channels mimicking the blood flow pattern in the human body. (b) An assembled μCCA with red dye for visualization of chambers and channels (Sung & Shuler, 2009).

curves for subsequent in vivo animal experiments or clinical trials (Tatosian & Shuler, 2009). 3D hydrogel cultures in μCCA format were developed by Sung and Shuler (Fig. 7.9). Three types of cells, hepatocytes (HepG3/C3A), myeloblasts (Kasumi-1), and colon cancer cells (HCT-116), were embedded in different chambers in 3D hydrogels, representing different organs. The cytotoxic effect of tegafur, a prodrug of active anticancer drug, 5-fluorouracil, commonly used in colon cancer was tested using this device. An interesting revelation as compared to conventional 96-well plate assay was that, although, the liver cells in μCCA showed metabolism of tegafur similar to 96 well plate, the metabolism lead to death of hepatocytes, an effect which was unnoticeable in well plate assays (Sung & Shuler, 2009). The literature is replete with tegafur toxicity data, particularly its hepatotoxicity (Maruyama, Hirayama, Abe, Tanaka, & Matsui, 1995). In such a scenario, development of microfluidic systems providing critical toxicity information in in vitro models bodes well for preclinical drug testing.

7.2.3.2 Ex vivo evaluation

Apart from in vitro microfluidic cell culture platforms, some researchers have also looked at ex vivo microfluidic platforms by isolating animal tissues, particularly liver, and culturing excised explants to analyze the toxicity of various compounds. It has been reported that precision cut liver slices fare better than hepatocytes alone with respect to metabolic activity (Graaf, Groothuis, & Olinga, 2007). Continuous perfusion of nutrient medium can further reduce the loss of metabolic activity and prolong protein expression in these slices. Microfluidic devices have been designed to continuously replenish the spent medium and remove waste material from these slices. van Midwoud et al. designed a PDMS-based "perifusion" device, with liver slices supported on polycarbonate membranes. The term "perifusion" was used instead of perfusion as the medium flowed around the slices. PDMS membranes were purposely kept thin to allow for efficient gaseous exchange. Comparable metabolic activity of 7-ethoxycoumarin to well plate based method was observed in this device (van Midwoud, Groothuis, Merema, & Verpoorte, 2010). Another PDMS based device was developed to analyze ethanol toxicity in liver explants. Using this device, concentrations as low as 20 mM produced a decrease in mitochondrial metabolic activity as well increased lactate dehydrogenase activity, a marker of cell death. These effects were observed in a concentration dependent manner, together with a decrease in albumin and urea synthesis (Hattersley, Greenman, & Haswell 2011). Such devices utilizing excised tissues represent clinically more relevant models to replace animal experimentation.

7.2.3.3 In vivo evaluation

Microfluidic platforms have also been used to assist in vivo animal experiments, for blood sampling, sample preparation, and analysis (Kang et al., 2008). An automatic blood collection microfluidic chip based on PDMS was developed by Wu et al. for withdrawal of blood from mice without the need of trained personnel. The device consisted of two layers, holding channels for blood inlet, outlet, heparin block, blood reservoir, and sample wells. A microfluidic device was used for processing blood samples from mice for determining hematotoxicity. In this device, a microcavity array was created by master molding PDMS structures to form a sieve-like structure that separates leukocytes from other blood cells (Fig. 7.10). Benzene toxicity was assessed by staining the leukocytes and counting them over a period of 2 weeks (Hosokawa et al., 2012). Microfluidic platforms have been designed to be integrated with novel analytical techniques such as matrix-assisted laser/desorption ionization—mass spectrometry (MALDI-MS), which can facilitate fast sample analysis with high precision and resolution of many metabolites in biological samples (Lee, Lee, Kim, & Kim, 2008; Xu, Little, & Murray, 2006).

These microfluidic systems have, thus, played a critical role in various stages of the drug development process. Beginning with the identification of targets, to synthesis of compounds for generation big compound libraries, to HTS and preclinical development, microfluidics has been effectively adapted to reduce the consumption of reagents and make the drug discovery process more efficient and cost effective. In the subsequent section, we will discuss about the application of microfluidics in analysis of chemical and biological drugs. We also discuss the role played by these devices in detection of diseases and routine diagnostic purposes, which may reduce the healthcare costs.

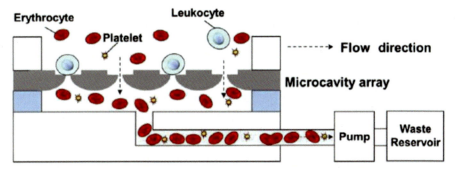

Figure 7.10 Microfluidic platforms for ex vivo experiments. For leukocyte counting and assessment of hematotoxicity. A microcavity array was created by PDMS to form a sieve-like structure that retained the leukocytes, while allowing other blood cells to pass through. The cells can then be separately analyzed for toxicity due to various drugs (Hosokawa et al., 2012).

7.3 Microfluidics for pharmaceutical analysis and diagnostic applications

Miniaturization of analytical tools has been propelled by the recent surge in the development and maturation of microfabrication techniques. The better control of physical processes and parameters at the micron scale has further fueled the interest in microscale analytical systems as new paradigms for pharmaceutical analysis. These systems are aimed at both reducing the sample volume and time of analysis, besides being amenable to integration with the other platforms and potential for high throughput. High parallelization made analysis of multiple compounds fast and easy (Lee et al., 2009). Moreover, design modification can provide integrated facilities for handling fluids, thermal and spatial control for targeting specific detection components to enhance selectivity (DeMello, 2006). Given that the mass fabrication of micronsized platforms now is possible via sophisticated instruments, the cost of production of these devices has come down, providing an opportunity to develop single use analytical device, and thereby reducing the possibility of cross-contamination (Lion, Reymond, Girault, & Rossier, 2004). In the following sections, we will discuss the application of microfluidic device in chemical/drug analysis followed by a brief description on microfluidic-based diagnostic applications.

7.3.1 Microfluidics for pharmaceutical analysis

Although there have been many mechanistic and experimental advancements in analysis of drugs, the basic analytical equipment and components have not changed much over the past few decades. Recently, with the application of microscale techniques adopted from the semiconductor industry, scientists are now poised for choices to carry out analytical assessments at an order 5–9 times lower than conventional counterparts (DeMello, 2006). Microscale analytical devices, also termed as micro total analytical systems (μTAS), comprise microchannel networks, which aim to replicate the analysis procedures on physically shrunk platforms, without compromising the analytical efficiency or sensitivity. Apart from this, µTAS can be designed to attain a high level of automation, thereby making multiplexed assays possible and providing a system that reduces manual errors and helps to increase the assay accuracy. In particular, these devices have been more popular in analysis of biological molecules like proteins and nucleic acids (Guo, Rotem, Heyman, & Weitz, 2012; Meagher & Thaitrong, 2012) and have been the subject of other chapters in this book. Here, we would limit our focus to discuss about the application of microfluidics in the analysis of drug entities in both pharmaceutical and biological samples.

Analysis of pharmaceutical compounds has been carried out using high performance liquid chromatography (HPLC) equipped with various detection modules including ultraviolet and fluorescence spectrophotometers as well as mass spectrometry, electrophoresis, potentiometry, colorimetry, radioisotopic assay, microbiological methods, enzymatic methods, surface plasmon resonance based biosensor assays, surface-enhanced Raman spectroscopy (SERS), conductivity, and chemiluminescence (CL) among many others. Microfluidic platforms, due to the flexibility in their design, are docile to integration with most of the above listed analytical methods. With the increasing demand for highly sensitive and miniscule working volume platforms, it is imperative that the chosen methods detect low amounts of the analyte. CL-based methods have been used for microfluidic detection of vitamin B_{12} and L-phenylalanine. It was reported to be a highly sensitive technique which was capable of detecting vitamin B_{12} as low as 5 pg/mL (Kumar, Chouhan, & Thakur, 2009). This testing stands on luminol oxidation by hydrogen peroxide in the presence of externals catalyst ions such as cobalt (II) and copper (II) and amino acid like L-phenylalanine under alkaline conditions. The resultant product is a blue compound (3-aminopthalate ion) that can be detected at a wavelength of 425 nm (Chen, Gao, He, & Cui, 2007; Wang et al., 2007).

Lok et al. developed a microfluidic chip to detect the concentration of vitamin B_{12} using a continuous flow microfluidic chip (Fig. 7.11). The device consisted of three layers which contained two passive mixing reaction chambers and a double spiral microchannel network as an optical detection unit. The first layer was located on top of the second one, where there were a mixing chamber and a clockwise spiral detection unit. The third layer had the other mixing chamber and an anticlockwise spiral detection module. The mixing chambers were designed in layers to counter the problem of mixing in the laminar flow. The spirally designed detection channels present a better CL signal to the optical detector as compared to a single loop unit. The microchip also had a chamber for acidification of vitamin B_{12}, as cobalt present in vitamin B_{12} complex is not released passively to catalyze the reaction. Using the device, up to 0.3 pg/mL of vitamin B_{12} could be detected (Lok, Abdul Muttalib, Lee, Kwok, & Nguyen, 2012). In another CL-based microfluidic chip based on the same principle of oxidation of luminol catalyzed by copper sulfate was used to detect L-phenylalanine, as the CL signal increased in the presence of L-phenylalanine in alkaline medium. PDMS was used to fabricate the device by soft lithography. The device was provided with four sample inlets and one outlet and was able to detect

Microfluidic systems for drug discovery, pharmaceutical analysis, and diagnostic applications   291

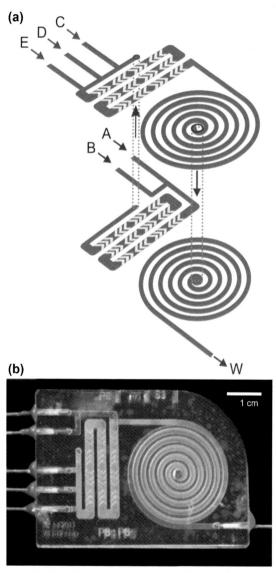

Figure 7.11 Lab-on-a-chip for determination of vitamin B12 concentration: (a) microchannel network (A to E are inlets; W is outlet to waste; arrows indicate the fluid flow); (b) Fabricated microchip. The chip measures 45 6 30 6 3 mm (Lok et al., 2012).

around 39 pg/mL of L-phenylalanine in commercial soft drinks as well as pharmaceutical injections (Kamruzzaman et al. 2012).

In contrast to CL, a larger number of microfluidic devices rely on the electrochemical detection of analytes for drug analysis. Won et al. developed a microfluidic device on glass slides for simultaneous detection of five sulphonamide drugs.

The device was provided with modules for preconcentration and electrokinetic (EK) separation of drugs using the field-amplified sample stacking (FASS) and field-amplified sample injection (FASI) techniques in two parallel channels (Shiddiky & Shim, 2007). Subsequent electrochemical detection of sulphonamides was carried out at the end of separation channel which consisted of a silver/silver chloride, platinum wire, and aluminum-gold nanoparticles modified carbon paste electrode. The device was able to detect femto-molar level concentration of sulphonamide drugs and provides an opportunity to simultaneously detect these drugs in clinical samples. Later, they further developed a highly sensitive and robust microfluidic device integrating the preconcentration, separation, and electrochemical detection for simultaneous analysis of multiple sulphonamide drugs (Won, Chandra, Hee, & Shim, 2013). The microfluidic device comprised both FASS and FASI channels for the preconcentration process and the EK separation for sulphonamides detection by chronoamperometry. In this study, they pioneered the simultaneous detection of preconcentrated sulphonamides in a microfluidic device. Thanks to the optimization of various experimental parameters affecting the analytical performances of the method, the detection limits of the analytes were brought down to approximately 1−2 fM. In addition, the reliability of the proposed method was confirmed by detecting the spiked concentrations of drugs in various meat samples. Wu et al. developed a micellar electrokinetic chromatography (MEKC) technique with the help of microchips for the detection of antibiotics (Wu et al., 2015). An on-line multiple-preconcentration device coupled FASS and reversed-field stacking (RFS) for the simultaneous analysis of three antibiotics including kanamycin, vancomycin, and gentamycin by microchip MEKC with LIF detection. This strategy allows the detection of antibiotics in river water samples, which could be successfully focused and well separated with high efficiency and sensitivity. In addition, Chong et al. also developed a portable microchip electrophoresis (MCE) coupled with on-chip contactless conductivity detection system for the detection of vancomycin in human plasma (Chong, Thang, Quirino, & See, 2017). To increase the sensitivity, a new online multistacking preconcentration technique based on field-enhanced sample injection (FESI) and micelle-to-solvent stacking (MSS) was designed and implemented in MCE-C^{4}D system combined with a commercially available double T-junction glass chip. The cationic analytes from the two sample reservoirs were injected under FESI conditions and subsequently focused by MSS within the sample-loading channel. They achieved a detection limit of vancomycin at 1.2 μg/mL, recoveries in spiked human plasma around 99.0%−99.2%, as well as intraday and interday repeatability relative standard deviation (RSDs) of 2.6% and 4.3%, respectively. Similarly, Rudasova et al. developed a novel MCE method for the rapid detection of N-acetylcysteine, a pharmaceutically active ingredient with isotachophoresis separations and conductivity detection (Rudasova & Masar, 2016). The repeatability and accuracy of N-acetylcysteine determination in all samples were more than satisfactory with the RSD and relative error values < 0.7% and < 1.9%, respectively, while a recovery range was achieved at 99%−101%. This work showed the analytical potential of the microchip isotachophoresis for the quantification of pharmaceutical samples that contain analyte(s) at relatively high abundances.

Taking the advantage of electrochemical detection, recent researchers also designed nontraditional microfluidic devices for drug analysis. For instance, Shiroma et al. developed a simple, cost-effective, and sensitive paper-based microfluidic device with electrochemical detection for the analysis of paracetamol and 4-aminophenol (Shiroma, Santhiago, Gobbi, & Kubota, 2012) (Fig. 7.12(a) and (b)). The separation channels of a width of 2.0 mm were created on paper via a wax printing process to define the shape of the device, while the electrochemical detection system was located at the end of the channels through sputtering, where the preseparated drugs were detected by applying a potential of 400 mV on the Au working electrode. A baseline separation of paracetamol and 4-aminophenol was obtained by injecting the sample at 12.0 mm from the working electrode which was already long enough to minimize the effect of interfering substances in the sample. Using this paper-based device, they achieved detection limits of 25.0 and 10.0 μmol/L for paracetamol and 4-aminophenol, respectively. This study provided a promising tool for lab-on-a-paper technology combining paper-based separation channels with electrochemical detection.

Besides CL and electrochemical detection, a microfluidic chip integrated to laser-induced fluorescence scanner was developed for the detection of β_2 agonist drugs like clenbuterol (Fig. 7.12(c—e)). These drugs increase muscle mass and have been often misused in farm animals (Martinez-Navarro, 1990) as well as in power sports by athletes (Delbeke, Desmet, & Debackere, 1995; Hesketh et al., 1992), making it vital to analyze them in a rapid and accurate manner. The three layers of the device consisted of a fluidic channel, a PDMS membrane, and a pneumatic control layer interspersed with many pneumatic microvalves and micropumps to enable the delivery of reagents. Glass was used to fabricate the fluidic channel and pneumatic control layer by standard lithography and etching to create microchannels. The PDMS membrane was then sandwiched between the two layers and generated pneumatic valve and pump effect due to deflection by compressed air. The drugs could be detected within 30 min and at a concentration as low as 0.088 ng/mL (Kong et al. 2009). Ho et al. developed a cost-effective and robust microfluidic system to quantify the amount of active pharmaceutical ingredients (APIs), especially artemisinin and its derivatives (Ho, Desai, & Zaman, 2015). The detection relied on an indirect way. Under alkaline condition in the presence of catalyst hematin in blood, luminol reacts with hydrogen peroxide which comes from the cleavage of artemisinin and derivatives, giving rise to a chemical compound that emits chemiluminescent signals at 425 nm. The system was able to quantify the artesunate tablets with results comparable to the conventional 96-well plate in the spectrophotometer and comparable to the conventional HPLC. More importantly, each chip could be used for 3 times given proper cleaning between the usages, thus reducing the cost per test to about $0.5. More recently, Zeid et al. developed a facile, rapid, and highly sensitive PMMA microchip-based EK chromatographic method for the simultaneous detection of two gabapentinoid drugs, gabapentin (GPN) and pregabalin (PGN) (Zeid et al., 2017). β-Cyclodextrin (β-CD) was used as the additives to optimize the separation, which enabled the analyses of both fluorescently labeled compounds. The sensitivity of the technique was enhanced by 14- and 17-fold for PGN and GPN, so that it could detect both analytes with a detection

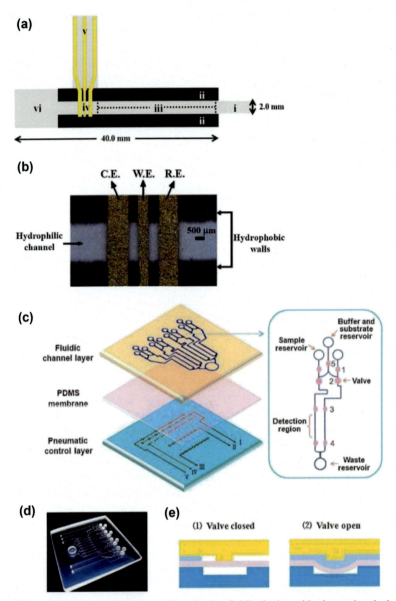

Figure 7.12 (a) Main parts of the paper-based microfluidic device with electrochemical detection: (i) eluent entrance, (ii) hydrophobic walls, (iii) region of sample addition, (iv) electrochemical detection system with three gold electrodes, (v) contact pads, and (vi) absorbent pads. (b) Photograph of the electrochemical detection system (Shiroma et al., 2012). (c) Schematic of a multilayered microfluidic device for analysis of drugs. The device comprised three layers, the top and bottom layer made of glass and a poly(dimethylsiloxane) (PDMS) membrane was sandwiched between two layers. (d) Photograph of the device. (e) Cross-sectional view of the microvalves showing closed and open position (Kong et al., 2009).

limit lower than 3 ng/mL. More importantly, the device was used for the analysis of PGN and GPN in biological fluids, with an extraction recovery rate greater than 89%.

Besides the integration of luminance/fluorescence and electrochemical based detection in microfluidic devices, other analytical techniques, including HPLC, mass spectroscopy, and SERS have also been investigated for microfluidics-based drug analysis. For example, Andreou reported a microfluidic device that detected trace concentrations of drugs of abuse in saliva samples within minutes using SERS (Andreou, Hoonejani, Barmi, Moskovits, & Meinhart, 2013) (Fig. 7.13). They utilized a flow-focusing microfluidic device to tailor the spatial arrangement and flow rate of the various streams for optimal SERS signals. The analyte, methamphetamine, was introduced into the central stream that was focused by two side streams containing Ag-NPs and salt, diffused laterally into the side streams, especially into the side

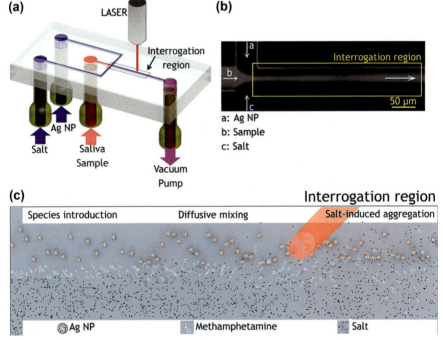

Figure 7.13 Flow-focusing microfluidic device used for controlled Ag-NP aggregation. (a) Ag-NP suspension, a saliva sample, and salt solution are loaded in the device and driven through it by a vacuum pump. (b) At the flow-focusing junction, the sample stream is enveloped by the side streams, and diffusion drives lateral mass transport between the laminar flows, here visualized with a fluorescent dye. (c) Schematic of the reaction: Ag NP, analyte, and salt solution are introduced to the channel from the left and flow toward the right. Analyte molecules resident in the focused stream diffuse laterally into the side flows. Salt ions also diffuse into the colloid stream inducing controlled nanoparticle aggregation, creating SERS (surface-enhanced Raman spectroscopy)-active clusters that convect downstream. Interrogating the region rich in colloid dimers, which provide intense plasmonic enhancement, we are able to achieve optimal SERS-based detection (Andreou et al., 2013).

containing the Ag-NPs where it may adsorb. The Ag-NPs were much bigger than any of the other chemicals involved in the process. As a result, they diffused at a slower rate than the salt ions, an aggregating agent of Ag-NPs. However, salt ions were required to travel a greater distance since they must pass through the central stream before reaching the side stream where Ag-NPs were located. This gave the analyte enough time to be adsorbed by nanoparticles before significant Ag-NP aggregation was induced. Therefore, the strongest SERS signal was only readable at a downstream location where significant aggregates (predominantly dimers and other small order aggregates) appeared. This device exhibited several advantages over conventional SERS-based techniques. It promoted the interaction between NPs and analytes in the solution along the laminar flows, while the controlled aggregation induced by the salt gave rise to a reproducible and reliable region where SERS signal was maximized. Baharfar et al. reported a microfluidic device for on-chip electromembrane extraction of trace amounts of ephedrine (EPH) and clonidine (CLO) in human urine and plasma samples, which was coupled with HPLC-UV analysis (Baharfar, Yamini, Seidi, & Karami, 2017). The device was composed of polymethylmethacrylate plates with a polypropylene sheet in between. Under the electric field, the analytes were converted to ionized form, crossed the supported liquid membrane, and then extracted into the acceptor phase. The effectiveness of the technique was determined by the analysis of real biological samples from urine and plasma. In terms of relative recoveries, a high accuracy of 94.6%−105.2% and RSD of repeatability of less than 5.1% were obtained. In addition, Zhu et al. developed a microfluidic chip based nano-HPLC integrated to tandem mass spectrometry (nano-HPLC-Chip-MS/MS) for simultaneous detection of 14 types of abused drugs and metabolites (e.g., cocaine, benzoylecgonine, cocaethylene, norcocaine, morphine, codeine, amphetamine, methamphetamine, and methadone) in the hair of drug abusers (Zhu et al., 2012). The microfluidic chip was prepared by laminating polyimide films and was coupled to an enrichment column, an analytical column and a nanospray tip. The microfluidic chip was inserted into the HPLC-Chip cube interface, which was mounted directly on the MS source for data acquisition. Similarly, Kirby et al. reported a device which incorporated microfluidics and a miniature mass spectrometer for the quantitation of drugs abuse in urine (Kirby et al., 2014) (Fig. 7.14). Apart from other microfluidic devices, this system was designed to deliver droplets of solvent to dried urine samples before conveying extracted analytes to an array of nanoelectrospray emitters for MS/MS analysis. This design increased the efficiency of drug analysis, where cocaine, benzoylecgonine, and codeine could be quantified from four samples in less than 15 min. In addition, they achieved a limit of quantitation (LOQ) for cocaine at 40 ng/mL, deeming it compatible with the performance criteria for laboratory analyses established by the United Nations Office on Drugs and Crime. Collectively, these results indicated that the technique was suitable for on-site screening, and the study became a proof of concept for integration of microfluidics with miniature mass spectrometry.

Besides the analysis of drugs in the pharmaceutical and biological samples, researchers also expanded the applications of microfluidic-based devices to the analysis of cells and artificial organs exposed to drugs in vitro. Snouber et al. reported

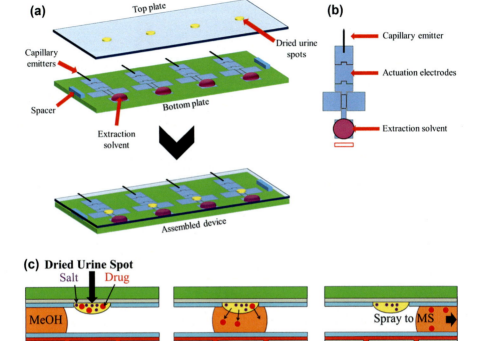

Figure 7.14 Digital microfluidic device used for extraction of drugs from dried urine. (a) Three-quarter view schematic of device, which features four independent DMF modules mated to pulled-glass capillary nanoelectrospray ionization emitters for direct analysis by tandem mass spectrometry. Urine is affixed and dried onto hydrophilic anchors located on the top plate. When assembled, the top and bottom plates are separated by a 360 μm thick spacer. (b) Top-down schematic of a single module, which features five 7 mm × 7 mm, two 2 mm × 5 mm, and one 7 mm × 5 mm actuation electrodes. The red outlined scale bar is 7 mm. (c) Side-view scheme (left-to-right) of sample cleanup illustrating the selective extraction of drug from dried urine (Kirby et al., 2014).

a "metabolomics-on-a-chip" approach to test secondary drug toxicity in bioartificial organs (Choucha Snouber et al., 2013). A microfluidic biochip was utilized to investigate the metabolic response of HepG2/C3a cells subjected to an anticancer prodrug flutamide and its active metabolite hydroxyflutamide (HF) by nuclear magnetic resonance spectroscopy to determine cell-specific molecule-response markers. The metabolic response of flutamide led to a disruption in glucose balance and mitochondrial dysfunction, illustrated by a decrease in the extracellular glucose and fructose consumptions and tricarboxylic acid cycle activity. Their findings illustrated the potential of metabolomics-on-a-chip to be used as an in vitro alternative method to predict the toxicology or function of drugs. In addition, Gao et al. reported an integrated cell-culture based microfluidic device for high-throughput drug screening with an online electrospray ionization quadrupole time-of-flight mass spectrometer (ESI-Q-TOF MS) (Gao, Li, Wang, & Lin, 2012). The multiple gradient

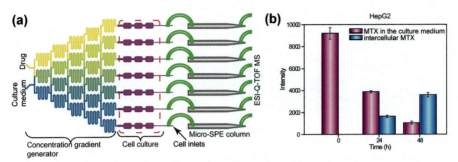

Figure 7.15 Integrated microfluidic device for drug absorption and cytotoxicity assays. (a) A schematic drawing showing the upstream concentration gradient generator, the downstream cell cultivation modules, and sample pretreatment module prior to ESI-Q-TOF MS detection. (b) Time-dependent accumulation of intracellular MTX in HepG2 cells on the microfluidic device (Gao et al., 2012).

generator was then coupled to an array of microscale cell culture chambers and on-chip solid-phase extraction (SPE) columns for sample pretreatment prior to mass analysis (Fig. 7.15). Drug absorption and cytotoxicity could be simultaneously determined using this integrated system. The device was composed of two functional parts: one part with upstream drug gradient generators and downstream cell culture chambers where liquid diffusion and mixing, cell cultivation, cell stimulation, drug absorption, and drug-induced cytotoxicity assay could be achieved, whereas the other had an integrated on-chip SPE column for sample clean-up and concentration process before the MS examination. To be a proof of concept, the absorption of methotrexate and its effects on HepG2 and Caco-2 cells were investigated, where the percentage of apoptotic cells appeared to be drug dose dependent. Comparing the results from ESI-Q-TOF MS analysis with the cytotoxicity assay, it was found that high intracellular drug concentrations increased cell cytotoxicity. Overall, this integrated system provided an easy online tool to screen drugs rapidly with low drug consumption, high throughput, and high sensitivity, thus accelerating the development of new effective and safer drugs.

In summary, microfluidic devices can play a crucial role in detecting drugs and pharmaceuticals and can be routinely used in chemical, pharmaceutical, and clinical settings with high precision and economical effectiveness.

7.3.2 Microfluidics for diagnostic purposes

The conventional diagnostic techniques based on sophisticated macroscopic equipment such as gas chromatography—mass spectrometry are only feasible in large air-conditioned laboratories, which are equipped with trained workforce and devices for sample handling, together with ample ancillary resources needed for efficient diagnosis. But, this is not attainable outside the realm of these laboratories, especially in the developing world, particularly in rural areas (Lee, Kim, Chung, Demirci, & Khademhosseini, 2010; Yager et al., 2006). Miniaturized versions of analytical platforms have been recently conceptualized, primarily based on microfluidic technology, to perform diagnostic analysis of metabolites and biomarkers associated with diseases, consuming minimal amounts of reagents, with high efficiency and speed, making the device a portable point of care, self-usable system. This not only reduces the logistic issues with sample handling and transfer but also provides patients with the luxury of testing for various markers, such as blood glucose, in the comfort of their homes, which is particularly suitable for geriatric patients. These microfluidic diagnostic devices may reduce the healthcare costs associated with diagnosis.

Microfluidic biosensors, as they are commonly known, have been fabricated for a variety of purposes. Particularly important among these are on-chip enzymatic assays. As enzymes have the potential of converting a large amount of substrate molecules into product in a fraction of a second, in a highly selective manner, they offer an exciting avenue for chemical analysis. Enzyme assay on a chip may be either homogenous or heterogeneous. In the former, all the reactants are in solution phase (Hadd, Raymond, Halliwell, Jacobson, & Ramsey, 1997) while in the latter, either of the enzyme/substrate/inhibitor needs to be immobilized on a solid surface (Krenkova & Foret, 2004; Mao, Yang, & Cremer, 2002). In some cases, enzyme immobilization is carried out on microchannel walls or onto some support inside the channels. This provides the advantages of enzyme recycling, placement of enzyme at specific locations on microchannels, and analysis in a continuous flow environment, make immobilized assays a preferable choice (Kim, Lee, & Koh, 2009).

Enzyme immobilization has been more carried out on microspheres, also known as microbeads, due to their similar size properties to microchannels, as well as large surface area for enzyme attachment (Peterson, 2005). They offer the advantage of being contained at appropriate locations by using mechanical barriers or magnetic devices. Kim et al. developed a microfluidic device for glucose detection. The device consisted of two separate chambers, for reaction and detection. In the reaction chamber, microbeads were covalently bound to enzyme, glucose oxidase and were supported by microfilters. A poly(ethylene glycol) based microarray (fabricated by photolithography) encapsulating a horseradish peroxidase formed the detection chamber. The bienzymatic reaction was used to detect the conversion of non-fluorescent substrate (Amplex Red fluorescence indicator) to a fluorescent resorufin, with glucose concentrations in the range of 1–10 mM detected successfully by fluorescence microscopy and quantified by a software (Kim et al., 2009). In a modified version, Sheng et al. used glucose oxidase modified magnetic nanoparticles, constrained in the microchannel with the aid of external magnetic field, for the amperometric analysis of glucose. The device offers a simple alternative to other such devices, as no mixing is needed, achieving higher sensitivity. Detection was linear with a range between 25 μM and 15 mM. The device also possessed a separation channel that avoided the entry of macromolecules, thereby eliminating the need to preprocess the sample. This allowed for the serum samples to be directly used for glucose analysis (Sheng, Zhang, Lei, & Ju, 2012). Other devices integrating enzyme and immunoassays were fabricated for simultaneous detection of glucose and insulin (Wang, Ibanez, & Chatrathi, 2003).

Microfluidic-based devices have been commonly used in the detection of disease biomarkers including metabolites (e.g., glutathione (GSH)), enzymes, pathogens (e.g., bacteria and DNA), and even cells. Before the widespread use of diagnostics for assessment of complex diseases, it was necessary to develop sophisticated bioassays capable of quantitatively analyzing disease biomarkers (Herr et al., 2007). GSH is an intracellular thiol-containing tripeptide which is a biomarker of oxidative stress (OS) and an important antioxidant in the cells of organisms. The rapid and accurate detection of GSH content is important for the early diagnosis and prevention of diseases. Hao et al. established an effective and rapid method based on microfluidics and LIF detection to analyze the intracellular constituents and GSH in single cells (Hao, Liu, Zhang, Li, & Jing, 2014). A hydrostatic pressure approach was utilized to inject the hepatocytes, and a low electrical potential was used to drive the single hepatocyte to the detection point. By the modification of the microfluidic device surface and optimization of injection voltage and separation, the analytes can be measured with high efficiency (e.g., 10 s for single cell analysis) smaller reagent volumes and less waste production.

Besides such small molecules, nonimmunoassays have also been employed in the diagnosis of macromolecules. Electrochemical methods of detection are recognized as one of the most sensitive as they do not involve any label tagging for studying the fate of biological compounds. Electrodes serving as sensors have found their niche in medical diagnostics due to relative ease of fabrication and integration with analytical devices. With several markers being pliable for electrochemical analysis, many methods of electrode fabrication have been pursued (Quinton et al., 2011; Wartelle, Schuhmann, Blochl, & Bedioui, 2005). Screen-printed electrodes (SPEs) based on carbon are another form of electrochemical analytical device that has been studied for the detection of chemicals like nitric oxide (Miserere et al., 2006) and biomarkers for cancer (Wan et al., 2011). They are useful for electrochemical immunosensor assays as they offer advantages such as low background current, ease of chemical modification on carbon surface, and relative inertness of carbon-based materials. A variety of materials such as nylon, glass, alumina, organic films have been used for electrode fabrication and present an interesting alternative for point-of-care testing (Miserere et al., 2006; Schuler, Asmus, Fritzsche & Moller, 2009).

Recently, Yan et al. fabricated SPEs on vegetable parchment as a substrate for disposable immunosensor fabrication in detection of prostate-specific antigen (PSA) (Fig. 7.16). Electrodes were printed from carbon and silver/silver chloride ink. The device was then integrated to a paper-based microfluidic device, to absorb detection solution and immersing the electrodes in electrolyte. The immunosensor was fabricated by coating the SPEs with a sheet of functionalized graphene, containing the enzyme-linked antibody on gold nanoparticles. The assay could detect PSA as low as 2 pg/mL and presents itself as a suitable method for detecting potential disease specific biomarkers, allowing for early diagnosis of a disease (Yan, Zang, Ge, Ge, & Yu, 2012). Shin et al. designed an aptamer-based electrochemical biosensor integrated with a microfluidic platform for online detection of secreted protein biomarkers from an organ-on-a-chip device (Shin et al., 2016). The sensor was modified with aptamers specific to a cardiac injury biomarker in extremely low abundance, the creatine kinase (CK)-MB, by electrochemical impedance spectroscopy (EIS) rather than immunoassay. Interestingly, the application of aptamers as the antigen receptors significantly

Microfluidic systems for drug discovery, pharmaceutical analysis, and diagnostic applications 301

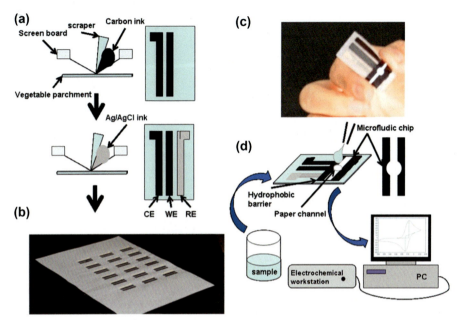

Figure 7.16 Screen printed electrodes as microfluidic platforms for immunosensor applications. (a) Carbon and silver/silver chloride electrodes were printed on a sheet of vegetable parchment, with WE, working electrode; RE, reference electrode; CE, counter electrode. (b) A sheet of vegetable parchment with 18 electrodes. (c) A hydrodynamic paper-based electrochemical sensing device for the measurement of prostate-specific antigen (PSA). (d) The detection processes of PSA (Yan et al., 2012).

increased the sensitivity and shelf life of the biosensor compared to antibody-based biosensors. They also believe that the unique microfluidic electrochemical biosensor based on the aptamer-capturing mechanism paves the way for measuring a wide variety of other biomarkers of interest.

Dried blood spot (DBS) samples on filter paper have emerged in popularity as a sampling and storage vehicle for a wide range of clinical and pharmaceutical applications. Shih et al. reported a DMF coupled to nanoelectrospray ionization mass spectrometry (nESI-MS) for the quantification of succinylacetone, a marker of hepatorenal tyrosinemia in DBS samples (Shih et al., 2012) (Fig. 7.17). The new system was fabricated by sandwiching a pulled glass capillary emitter between two DMF substrates. Droplets are driven in the DMF device by applying AC fields between electrodes on the top and bottom plates. When a droplet touches the inlet of the capillary, it spontaneously fills by capillary action in seconds. Then, a DC potential is applied between the top-plate DMF electrode and the mass spectrometer to generate a spray for MS analysis. The system was validated by application to on-chip extraction, derivatization, and analysis of succinylacetone with comparable performance to gold-standard methods.

Many bacteria-induced infectious diseases exhibit similar symptoms, such as common digestive and respiratory-borne ailments. However, it is difficult to identify

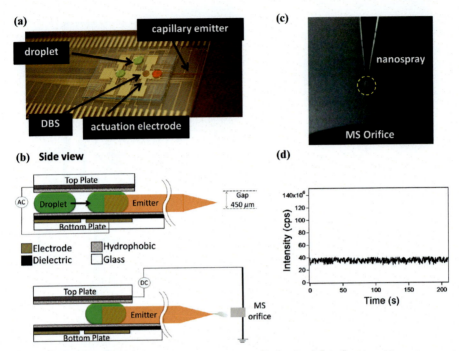

Figure 7.17 Digital Microfluidics–nanoelectrospray Ionization-Mass Spectrometry (DMF–nESI-MS) interface. (a) Image of a device (bearing colored droplets and a punched dried blood spot sample) mated to a capillary emitter. The contact pads on the sides of the device mate with a 40-pin connector for automated droplet control. (b) Side-view schematics. (top) AC electric potentials are applied between the top and bottom substrates to actuate the droplets. (bottom) DC electric potentials are applied between the top plate and the MS orifice to generate a nanoelectrospray. (c) Image of spray generated at the tip of the capillary emitter. (d) Total ion count as a function of time from a 15 μL droplet of tyrosine (5 μM). The spray was stable for >200 s, with an RSD of 7.3% (Shih et al., 2012).

the pathogenic bacteria solely based on these clinical presentations, resulting in delayed treatment and symptom deterioration. Therefore, a fast and accurate diagnostic method is critical for effectively identifying bacterial pathogens to facilitate the selection of appropriate treatment. Xia et al. has reported a rotate & react SlipChip (RnR-SlipChip) for simultaneous visual detection of multiple bacterial pathogens by LAMP (Xia et al., 2016). The device was composed of two round PDMS-glass hybrid chips that were coaxially aligned by a plastic screw-nut suite. One-step rotation after the sample loading allowed immediate mixing and reaction of multiple bacteria samples with LAMP reagents on the chip. After the optimization of LAMP conditions, a fluorescent signal-to-noise ratio of about 5-fold and a detection limit of 7.2 copies/μL genomic DNA were achieved, while five common digestive bacterial pathogens including *Bacillus cereus*, *Escherichia coli*, *Salmonella enterica*, *Vibrio fluvialis*, and *Vibrio parahaemolyticus* were visually identified in 60 min with a relatively high success rate. In addition, Hsieh et al. reported an integrated microfluidic platform for the fast, sensitive, and quantitative detection of pathogenic DNA (Hsieh, Patterson, Ferguson, Plaxco, & Soh, 2012). The platform relied on electrochemical quantitative loop-mediated isothermal amplification (MEQ-LAMP), a powerful alternative to polymerase cycling assembly (PCR) with greater sensitivity, accuracy, reaction speed, and amplicon yield. The real-time, quantitative electrochemical detection of LAMP amplification was achieved by monitoring the intercalation of DNA-binding methylene blue (MB) redox reporter molecules into newly formed DNA molecules with a set of integrated electrodes including two platinum counter and reference electrodes and a gold working electrode. Highlighting the advantages of real-time electrochemical detection and LAMP within a microfluidic device, the MEQ-LAMP method omits the usage of bulky and sophisticated optical detectors and temperature controls while ensuring robust microfluidic DNA amplification, thus making it a promising method for the diagnosis of other nucleic acid—based biomarkers, such as viral RNAs.

In contrast to antibody-free assay mentioned above, immunoassay is largely employed in the detection of macromolecular biomarkers for diagnosis purposes. Herr et al. designed a microchip-based device for the detection of disease biomarkers in human saliva. The device called microchip electrophoretic immunoassay (µCEI) was provided with molecular sieves fabricated using hydrogel, to enrich the sample, followed by electrophoretic separation to resolve a fluorescent antibody bound to an enzyme, responsible for tissue decay. Using 20 µL of saliva, they demonstrated rapid (<10 min) measurement of the collagen-cleaving enzyme matrix metalloproteinase-8 (MMP-8) in saliva from healthy and periodontally diseased samples. Using this method, they could dispense the need for using matched antibody pairs as well as to immobilize the antibody (Herr et al., 2007).

Enzyme-linked immunosorbent assay (ELISA) has been the mainstay of clinical diagnostics for detection of disease-related macromolecular biomarkers. However, the conventional macroscale ELISA protocols are laborious, sluggish, requiring multiple reagent addition and washing steps, often resulting in inconsistent results due to manual glitches. Furthermore, commercially available ELISA kits as well as instruments used are costly (Lai et al., 2004). Chip-based ELISA methods offer the advantage of faster antigen—antibody reaction with the consumption of significantly less reagents (Cesaro-Tadic et al., 2004; Murakami et al., 2004). Microfluidic ELISA platforms have been researched in great detail in the past decade (Herrmann, Veres, & Tabrizian, 2006; Holmes, She, Roach, & Morgan, 2007). Lee et al. developed a fully automatic ELISA platform for detecting antigen and antibody for hepatitis B virus, on a disposable plastic disc, made of poly(methyl methacrylate), having arrangements for conducting immunoassays from whole blood. The device had facilities for plasma separation and chambers for storage of buffers, reagents, substrates, collection of waste, mixing the reagents, and detection of the product (Fig. 7.18). Using just 150 µL of blood, the assay could be performed as opposed to double this volume in conventional methods, whereas the whole assay could be carried out in 30 min, whereas conventional well-plate based ELISA yields result in a minimum of 2 h (Lee et al., 2009). Miniaturization did not compromise the sensitivity of the device, and similar detection limit could be achieved. Recently, they developed an advanced chip to carry

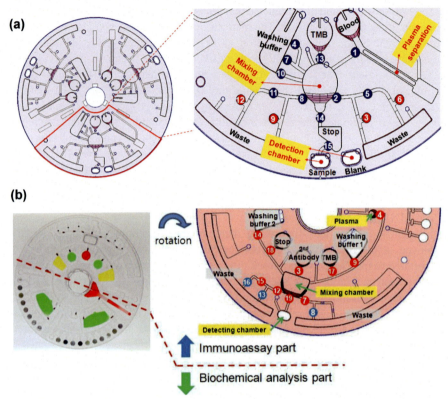

Figure 7.18 Disc-based immunoassays. (a) Disc design showing the detailed microfluidic layout and functions. The number indicates the order of the laser irradiated ferrowax microvalve (LIFM) operation (Lee et al., 2009). (b) Photograph of a disc. Detection wells on the clinical chemistry side are preloaded with lyophilized reagents. Other chambers for liquid type reagent are loaded with food dye solution for demonstration. In the right-hand side, the disc design shows the detailed microfluidic layout. The number indicates the order of the LIFM operation. The top half of the disc for the immunoassay part is rotated for easier demonstration. The blue circles with numbers are (NO)-LIFM. The other half of the disc for the clinical chemistry analysis part is shown in the bottom (Lee et al., 2011).

out the immunoassay as well as biochemical assessment of whole blood. The chip had automated arrangement for plasma separation, mixing, incubation, and detection. The freeze dried reagents for both assays were stored in dedicated compartments, and the detection was carried out by optical measurement at 10 different wavelengths to accommodate various reactions (Lee et al., 2011). Their group has also developed a multiplexed immunoassay, based on three different biomarkers to improve detection efficiency (Park, Sunkara, Kim, Hwang, & Cho, 2012).

As a basic criterion, the point-of-care diagnostic devices meant for the developing world must be inexpensive and integrated, dispensing the services of ancillary equipment (Mabey, Peeling, Ustianowski, & Perkins, 2004; Martinez et al., 2008).

In the wake of this cost consideration, paper-based microfluidic devices offer a potential alternative to glass/polymer-based open channel microsystems. These devices can also enable a multitude of sample outlets from a single inlet, ensuring simultaneous analytical assays, without the need for an external pumping device. Being light in weight and easy to stack makes their shipment logistically much easier than glass/polymer-based devices. Paper-based microfluidic devices have been researched in detail by the laboratory of George Whitesides at Harvard, termed as 3D microfluidic paper analytical devices (μPAD) (Bruzewicz, Reches, & Whitesides, 2008; Martinez, Phillips, Butte, & Whitesides, 2007; Martinez et al., 2008; Martinez, Phillips, & Whitesides, 2008). In addition, Dou et al. reported a versatile and low cost PDMS/paper-hybrid microfluidic device coupled to LAMP for the fast, sensitive, and instrument-free detection of the main meningitis-causing bacteria, *Neisseria meningitidis* (*N. meningitidis*) (Dou, Dominguez, Li, Sanchez, & Scott, 2014). The chip was composed of one top PDMS layer, one middle PDMS layer, and one glass slide for reagent delivery, LAMP reaction, and structure support, respectively. Chromatography paper was used in between as a 3D substrate for the prestorage of DNA primers for LAMP reactions to improve the detection sensitivity. This versatile hybrid system provided not only on-site qualitative diagnostic analysis but also confirmatory testing and quantitative analysis in laboratory settings with a detection limit of three copies per LAMP zone, which was relatively close to single-bacterium detection sensitivity. Furthermore, simple pathogenic microorganism detection was achieved without a laborious sample preparation process or the use of centrifuges, making it a promising point-of-care (POC) diagnosis for a broad spectrum of infectious diseases, especially for developing countries.

Noncommunicable diseases (NCDs) are now leading cause of global mortality, thus there is a growing need for cost-effective and noninvasive methods to diagnose and treat this class of disease. To this end, Warren and coworkers developed a paper-based diagnostic device with tailored synthetic biomarkers specific to colorectal cancer and thrombosis, a representative solid tumor and cardiovascular disorder, respectively (Warren, Kwong, Wood, Lin, & Bhatia, 2014). These synthetic biomarkers were composed of nanoparticles chemically modified by ligand-encoded reporters via protease-cleavable peptides. The nanoparticles passively target diseased sites in vivo, such as solid tumors or blood clots, where upregulated proteases cleaved the peptides and released reporters that were detectable by paper lateral flow assay (LFA) in the urine. LFAs utilize the sandwich complex to capture antibodies that are adsorbed onto a highly porous test strip which wicks fluids and conveys the analytes to the capture regions. The immobilized analytes are then visualized by a detection probe coupled to NPs (typically gold or latex nanospheres) that generate a colored line visible to the eye without enzymatic amplification. With over 500 proteases encoded by the human genome, this technique could be further tailored for the diagnosis of additional NCDs such as fibrosis and inflammation, as well as infectious diseases including malaria and hepatitis B to provide facile and cost-effective diagnostics for global health. Microfluidic devices have also been developed for diagnosis of lysozyme (Giuffrida, Cigliana, & Spoto, 2018), lysosomal storage disorders (Shen et al., 2012), cancer (Chen, Bai, & Chang, 2011; Das et al., 2015; Hindson et al., 2011; Lien et al., 2010; Piraino, Volpetti, Watson, & Maerkl, 2016; Tang, Vaze, & Rusling, 2012), H1N1 influenza (Lee et al., 2012), herpes simplex virus (Zubair et al., 2011), and Johne's disease in cattle (Wadhwa, Foote, Shaw, & Eda, 2012) at the molecular level. In principle, all microfluidic diagnostic devices consist of a molecular sensing unit coupled to a signal converter (transducer) that aptly reads out the results quantitatively. An elaborate review on different mechanistic approaches of biosensors is provided by Mohanty and Kougianos (2006). Since the biosensors vary greatly in their design and hence their sensitivity and efficiency, the readers are referred to a few state-of-the-art reviews for more detailed information (Choi, Goryll, Sin, Wong, & Chae, 2011; Mohammed & Desmulliez, 2011).

Beyond the molecular level, microfluidics-based systems have been widely used for the detection of cells and subcellular level vesicles (e.g., exosomes) in disease diagnosis, especially for tumors (Garcia-Cordero & Maerkl, 2020). Tumor cells can dissociate from primary and metastatic tumor sites and travel through the bloodstream in single or clusters of tumor cells, also known as circulating tumor cells (CTCs). Isolation of CTCs from the peripheral blood of patients has emerged as a valid alternative source of tumor tissue that can be utilized for molecular characterization of diseases (Kirby et al., 2012). The aim of CTC diagnostic is to retrieve single or clusters of CTCs in reasonable numbers with high purity from large volumes of whole blood (>5 mL) and at low shear stress to minimize cell damage (Garcia-Cordero & Maerkl, 2020). Initially, magnetic-based cell separation systems were widely developed and took advantage of antibody–antigen interactions to bond an antibody-decorated magnetic particle to a cell via its surface antigens. The FDA approved a macroscale immunomagnetic isolation system called CellSearch for CTCs of metastatic cancers such as breast, colorectal, and prostate cancers (Li, Stratton, Dao, Ritz, & Huang, 2013). The first microfluidic technology to capture CTCs from whole blood was called the "CTC-chip," which was reported by Nagrath and coworkers who made use of microposts coated with antibodies against EpCAM (Nagrath et al., 2007). In addition, magnetic-based microfluidic systems are more involved in the isolation and detection of CTCs. For example, Issadore and coworkers used the Hall effect to detect and count magnetically labeled CTCs (Issadore et al., 2012). A micro-Hall detector array was prepared on a substrate, while a microfluidic channel was bonded on top of the Hall detectors. A blood sample was first focused by the flow-focusing configuration of the microfluidic channel to establish a single stream of cells. As the cells moved over a Hall detector, each magnetically labeled CTC induced a Hall voltage and was, thus, counted. This device exhibited a higher CTC detection sensitivity than the CellSearch system and a high throughput of 10^7 cells per minute. A microfluidic magnetic disc has also been used to separate rare, circulating endothelial cells (CECs) from peripheral blood mononuclear cells (Chen et al., 2011). These CECs have been associated with many diseases, and the low CEC concentration in blood impedes their detection. A magnetic disc was used to trap the cells attached to immunomagnetic beads. Human umbilical vein endothelial cells (HUVECs) were used as a model for CECs and stained with anti-CD146-phycoerythrin antibody, which was tagged to antiphycoerythrin magnetic beads that attracted these cells to the magnetic disc. This magnetic disc had an inlet channel, connecting channels, and a waste reservoir. When the disc was rotated, the centrifugal force propelled away the nonmagnetic cells through the connecting channels to the waste reservoir, effectively retaining just the target cells (HUVECs) in the inlet reservoir.

Besides magnetic separation, affinity chromatography also makes use of antibody—antigen interactions to directly capture the CTCs, without the need of magnetic labeling. Generally, antibodies are conjugated to the surfaces of solid structures, which are then immersed in a fluid of biological sample where the antigens of targeted cells bond with the antibodies. To enhance the binding efficiency, the interactions between CTCs and antibody-modified surfaces have been featured by microstructures or nanostructures to one of the channel walls (Park et al., 2016; Sheng et al., 2014; Stott et al., 2010; Yoon et al., 2013).

Cells are often isolated from an ambient sample by means depending on their physical properties including stiffness, size, and density. Such physical property—based separation systems are advantageous in terms of label-free sorting, high system throughput, and low cost (Mao & Huang, 2012). Hur et al. designed a high-throughput and label-free platform for cell isolation and enrichment from heterogeneous solution using cell size as a criterion (Hur, Mach, & Di Carlo, 2011). This technique utilized a cell isolation mechanism in parallel expansion—contraction trapping reservoirs through the irreversible migration of particles into microscale vortices.

After the cell capture, CTCs were subjected to either immunostaining on-chip, analysis of surface, and intracellular signaling proteins by western blots, or release for off-chip analysis (Garcia-Cordero & Maerkl, 2020). In particular, Kirby et al. developed a geometrically enhanced differential immunocapture (GEDI) microfluidic device that coupled an antiprostate specific membrane antigen (PSMA) antibody to a 3D geometry of channel that specifically arrested CTCs with low nonspecific binding of leukocyte (Kirby et al., 2012). The GEDI device achieved higher sensitivity compared to the commercially available CellSearch system. The patient-derived CTCs were also subjected to on-chip drug treatment with docetaxel and paclitaxel, where CTCs of docetaxel-resistant patients did not show any evidence of drug activity. These measurements stood as the first functional assays of drug-target engagement in living CTCs. Chen et al. reported a novel microfluidic platform integrated with cell recognizable aptamer-encoded microwells for isolating single tumor cells with satisfied single-cell occupancy and unique bioselectivity (Chen, Wu, Zhang, Lin, & Lin, 2012). After the optimization of microwells, the single-cell occupancy was significantly increased from 0.5% to 88.2% due to the aptamer, which enabled the analysis of single-cell enzyme kinetics for the target cells in short time periods (5.0 min) and small volumes (4.5 mL). Microfluidics-based cell isolation has also been coupled to other detection techniques for facile detection. Pallaoro and coworkers reported a detection platform that combined microfluidics with SERS for the continuous identification of individual cells in a microfluidics channel (Pallaoro, Hoonejani, Braun, Meinhart, & Moskovits, 2015). They specifically designed SERS biotags (SBTs), which were based on a silver nanoparticle dimer modified by a Raman active reporter molecule and an affinity biomolecule, providing a unique label where SERS

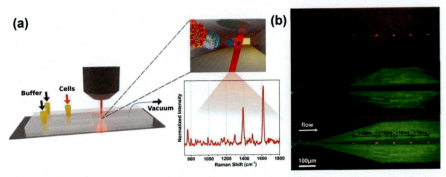

Figure 7.19 Graphical depiction of device layout and flow dynamics. (a) Schematic of setup and concept. Cells, prelabeled with a cocktail of cancer-specific (NRP) and control (UC) SBTs (the latter binding both cell types), are injected into the device, where they are flow-focused before passing through the Raman laser. (b) Simultaneous bright-field and epifluorescence (Cy3 channel, colorized orange) image of a single cell in the channel as a function of time illustrating the efficacy of flow focusing (top). Epifluorescence image (FITC channel, colorized green) of 200 nm polymer beads separately injected into the buffer channels to highlight the sheath flow (center). Montage merging the two former images (bottom), showing the overall flow dynamics in the device (Pallaoro et al., 2015).

spectrum could be deconvoluted (Fig. 7.19). SBTs were incubated with a mixture of cancerous and noncancerous prostate cells before being injected into a flow-focused microfluidic channel and forced into a single file. Cancer cells passing through the focused laser beam in the downstream were successfully identified among a large proportion of noncancerous cells by their Raman signatures. This technique achieved reliable results from all the cell mixture ratios tested, the lowest being one in 100 cells.

Exosomes are a subset of extracellular vesicles produced by tumor cells and nonmalignant cells which contain mitochondrial DNA, RNA, proteins, lipids, and metabolites (Poudineh, Sargent, Pantel, & Kelley, 2018; Simpson, Lim, Moritz, & Mathivanan, 2009). Exosomes are ubiquitous in most body fluids and are present in the circulation at early stages of cancers, making them potential cancer biomarker candidates (Dong et al., 2019). The typical exosome analysis workflow requires the isolation and quantitation of exosomes followed by the characterization of intravesicular and extravesicular contents, size, and morphology (Im et al., 2014; Zhang et al., 2018). The investigation of exosome contents at the molecular level employs a broad spectrum of techniques including western blotting, immunoassays, qRT-PCR, sequencing, flow cytometry, mass spectrometry, and many more (Garcia-Cordero & Maerkl, 2020). But current techniques for isolating exosomes (e.g., ultracentrifugation, filtration, and precipitation) are laborious due to incorporating multiple steps and are limited by low purities, especially when dealing with raw biological fluids that inherently contain a high proportion of proteins, other EVs, and cells with similar physical and/or biomolecular characteristics as exosomes (Contreras-Naranjo, Wu, & Ugaz, 2017). To this end, many studies have investigated microfluidic methods for exosome capture and analysis which are mostly based on immune-affinity (He, Crow, Roth, Zeng, & Godwin, 2014; Liu et al., 2018; Zhang et al., 2018; Zhao,

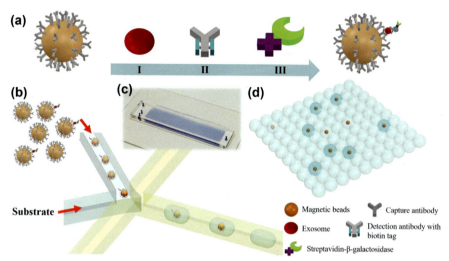

Figure 7.20 Schematic showing the droplet digital ExoELISA for exosome quantification. (a) Single exosome immunocomplex constructed on a magnetic bead. (b) Substrate and beads are coencapsulated into microdroplets. (c) Droplet digital ExoELISA chip. (d) Fluorescent readout for counting the positive droplets with the target exosomes (Liu et al., 2018).

Yang, Zeng, & He, 2016). In particular, Liu et al. reported an immunosorbent assay for digital qualification of target exosomes with the help of droplet microfluidics (Liu et al., 2018) (Fig. 7.20). The exosomes were immobilized on magnetic microbeads by forming sandwich ELISA complexes that were labeled with an enzymatic reporter producing a fluorescent signal. The microbeads were then isolated and encapsulated into enough droplets to ensure only a single bead was present in each droplet. This droplet-based single-exosome-counting enzyme-linked immunoassay (droplet digital ExoELISA) approach allowed the absolute counting of cancer-specific exosomes with an unprecedented accuracy and a minute limit of detection (LOD) of 10 exosomes per microliter ($\sim 10^{-17}$ M).

In addition to immune-affinity assay, size-based chromatography method has also been utilized in microfluidic systems for exosome isolation (Davies et al., 2012). Particularly, the herringbone chip (EVHB-Chip) is an exemplar model of microfluidic exosome isolation. This chip is capable of processing several milliliters of serum and capturing extracellular vesicles by its nanostructured surface with better performance than ultracentrifugation and magnetic beads, demonstrated by 94% tumor-extracellular vesicle (EV) specificity, a LOD of 100 EVs per μL sample, and a 10-fold increase in tumor RNA enrichment (Reategui et al., 2018). Other label-free microfluidics-based techniques include exosome trapping by nanowires (Wang et al., 2013), nanopillar-based sorting (Wunsch et al., 2016; Zeming, Thakor, Zhang, & Chen, 2016), and viscoelastic flow sorting (Liu et al., 2017), as reviewed elsewhere (Contreras-Naranjo et al., 2017). In recent years, researchers have also developed integrated microfluidic platforms for both isolation and analysis of exosomes, including overall exosome levels (Liang et al., 2017; Woo et al., 2017; Zhang, He, & Zeng, 2016) and the detection of disease specific subpopulations of exosomes (Im et al., 2014; Vaidyanathan et al., 2014), and the internal component analysis of proteins (He et al., 2014) and RNAs (Shao et al., 2015). The exosomes derived from serum, plasma, whole blood, or other biological fluids such as urine, were isolated and analyzed by surface biomarkers including CD9, CD63, CD24, CD81, and EpCAM with enhanced sensitivity as low as ~50 exosomes per μL in overall exosome level or 0.3 pg per mL for IGF-1R analysis.

In summary, microfluidic technologies have been widely applied in the diagnosis of various disease biomarkers at the molecular, subcellular, and cellular levels with great success. It is expected that microfluidic technology will play a crucial role in medical diagnostics in the coming years, essentially with the development of disposable, sample-to-result devices, making routine diagnosis a more personalized approach (Eicher & Merten, 2011; Foudeh, Fatanat Didar, Veres, & Tabrizian, 2012).

7.4 Examples of commercial microfluidic devices

The application of microfluidic devices has increased over the years as these devices now have a wide range of roles, such as examining cell behavior, studying signaling pathways and immune responses, and determining clinical efficacy of new treatments (Sinha, Subedi, & Tel, 2018). The initial designs of microfluidic chips were extremely complex, but now, numerous companies have manufactured their own version of simplified yet efficient microfluidic platforms.

Dolomite Microfluidics developed several different microfluidic platforms for drug assays. One platform is a direct write microfluidic platform with internal channels and a cloudy exterior (Shankles, Millet, Aufrecht, & Retterer, 2018). This platform requires minimal consumables to produce small-scale high-throughput screening (Gencturk, Mutlu, & Ulgen, 2017). Another platform is called the Micromixer Chip, a static mixer in a serpentine-design which generates advection. This platform exploits lamination of three input fluid flow streams which significantly decreases the mixing time required to complete diffusion of triblock copolymer and siRNA (Feldmann et al., 2017). Dolomite Microfluidics have successfully designed their products to improve reproducibility and particle size control for a wide range of users (Dolomite, 2020).

POC lab-on-a-chip devices have also improved and simplified POC diagnostics. Abbott Laboratories designed an i-STAT system device which analyzes blood chemistry by combining microfluidics and electrochemical detection (Volpatti & Yetisen, 2014). The handheld device is capable of quantifying analytes and performing immunoassays; thus the combined device increases patient satisfaction due to minimal wait times (Abbott, 2020). Claros Diagnostics Inc. have also designed a benchtop microfluidic device, consisting of three main components: a blood-collector device, disposable cartridge, and a reader. This device was created to be a time-efficient diagnostic device that can detect the elevated PSA levels in prostate cancer (Maj-Hes, Sevcenco, Szarvas, & Kramer, 2019). Only a low sample volume is required, and utilizing this device can significantly decrease the healthcare system cost and number of hospital visits required by the patient. It has now been approved to be used as a prostate cancer diagnostic test in Europe and is seeking approval from the USFDA (MIT Technology Review, 2020).

Commercial automated microfluidic products for genomic analysis are also available. Fluidigm C1 rapidly isolates, processes, and profiles individual cells, thus only requiring one tool to both extract and analyze cell activity and responses (See, Lum, Chen, & Ginhoux, 2018). This integrated microfluidic system is an automated tool with high precision and accuracy (Sinha et al., 2018). Bio-Rad has a droplet microfluidic device called ddSEQ which successfully isolates and monitors thousands of genes per cell. This device can be coupled with Illumina, a sequencing system for single cell transcriptomic experiments to produce valid reads (Romagnoli et al., 2018).

7.5 Future trends

The future of microfluidic devices for applications in drug discovery appears bright with a lot of research activity being focused on the development of miniaturized chips. However, the concern remains about the integration of these devices with ancillary equipment including electrical accessories, pressure pumps, and platforms for analysis of samples. Due to their increased acceptance and potential benefits as economical alternatives to conventional benchtop macroscale equipment, it is important to develop integrated "everything-on-a-chip" systems that are widely accepted in all stages of drug discovery and development. This may entail an interdisciplinary effort from engineers and researchers working on fluid dynamics to design micropumps, analytical equipment manufacturers to scale down analysis systems to commensurate the chip size, and finally researchers working on microfabrication to further miniaturize the platforms and making them adaptable to these ancillary systems.

Industry has played a crucial role in this respect so far. Fluidigm Corporation, a venture by Dr. Stephen Quake from Caltech, has developed various platforms for microfluidic device integration. Based on the technology known as multilayer soft lithography, three dimensional structures can be created from elastomers to form integrated valves (NanoFlex), pumps, and channels. Besides this, Caliper Life Sciences also developed several automated/semiautomated robotics controlled liquid handling systems (Zephyr) that can be potentially integrated with microfluidic devices. These microfluidic integration tools are expected to aid microfluidic-based drug discovery by improving efficiency and scalability.

With the rate of approval of new drugs declining in the past few years and the pharmaceutical industry still lacking effective tools in discovering new drugs, microfluidic platforms come with a ray of hope, chaperoning routine assays in a more efficient manner and hopefully allowing more highly efficacious and safe drugs to be discovered.

On the other hand, miniaturized devices as diagnostic kits have made inroads into the households of many diabetic patients as blood glucose monitors. Miniaturized devices for other applications not only face fabrication and technical issues of being an integrated and comprehensive system, but they also face the challenge of patient acceptance, having a direct interface with the end user. Although their acceptance is propelled by the convenience of use, the future of such devices for routine practice in other pathological conditions would rely on how the users perceive them. A sizable population, particularly in remote villages and tribal areas in developing world, lack good education, and training to use such devices might prove to be a daunting task. Moreover, it would require sincere effort on the part of clinicians and marketing professionals to persuade the patients in developed world, who have been so used to visiting a clinic to get their routine biochemical checkups, to adopt such self-usable devices. In addition, it must be ensured that such devices are safe to use and dispose, without causing any serious environmental hazards.

References

Abbott point of care i-STAT system in the hospital.(2020). Retrieved from: https://www.pointofcare.abbott/int/en/offerings/health-care-facilities/hospital. (Accessed 31 July 2020).

Alsenz, J., & Kansy, M. (2007). High throughput solubility measurement in drug discovery and development. *Advanced Drug Delivery Reviews, 59*(7), 546−567.

Andersson, M., Okeyo, G., Wilson, D., Keizer, H., Moe, P., Blount, P., et al. (2008). Voltage-induced gating of the mechanosensitive MscL ion channel reconstituted in a tethered lipid bilayer membrane. *Biosensors and Bioelectronics, 23*(6), 919−923.

Andreou, C., Hoonejani, M. R., Barmi, M. R., Moskovits, M., & Meinhart, C. D. (2013). Rapid detection of drugs of abuse in saliva using surface enhanced Raman spectroscopy and microfluidics. *ACS Nano, 7*(8), 7157−7164.

Anonymous. (2000). Signal transduction as a drug-discovery platform - (Reprinted from Nature Biotechnology, vol 16, pg 1082−1083, 1998). *Nature Biotechnology, 18*, It37−It39.

Ashburn, T. T., & Thor, K. B. (2004). Drug repositioning: Identifying and developing new uses for existing drugs. *Nature Reviews Drug Discovery, 3*(8), 673−683.

Ashraf, M. W., Tayyaba, S., & Afzulpurkar, N. (2011). Micro electromechanical systems (MEMS) based microfluidic devices for biomedical applications. *International Journal of Molecular Sciences, 12*(6), 3648−3704.

Baharfar, M., Yamini, Y., Seidi, S., & Karami, M. (2017). Quantitative analysis of clonidine and ephedrine by a microfluidic system: On-chip electromembrane extraction followed by high performance liquid chromatography. *Journal of Chromatography B: Analytical Technologies in the Biomedical and Life Sciences, 1068−1069*, 313−321.

Bange, A., Halsall, H. B., & Heineman, W. R. (2005). Microfluidic immunosensor systems. *Biosensors and Bioelectronics, 20*(12), 2488−2503.

Barbulovic-Nad, I., Yang, H., Park, P. S., & Wheeler, A. R. (2008). Digital microfluidics for cell-based assays. *Lab on a Chip, 8*(4), 519−526.

Barlow, N. E., Bolognesi, G., Flemming, A. J., Brooks, N. J., Barter, L. M., & Ces, O. (2016). Multiplexed droplet Interface bilayer formation. *Lab on a Chip, 16*(24), 4653−4657.

Battersby, B. J., & Trau, M. (2002). Novel miniaturized systems in high-throughput screening. *Trends in Biotechnology, 20*(4), 167−173.

Beebe, D. J., Mensing, G. A., & Walker, G. M. (2002). Physics and applications of microfluidics in biology. *Annual Review of Biomedical Engineering, 4*, 261−286.

Beggs, M. (2001). HTS—where next? *Drug Discovery World, 2*, 125−134.

Bogojevic, D., Chamberlain, M. D., Barbulovic-Nad, I., & Wheeler, A. R. (2012). A digital microfluidic method for multiplexed cell-based apoptosis assays. *Lab on a Chip, 12*(3), 627−634.

Bohacek, R. S., McMartin, C., & Guida, W. C. (1996). The art and practice of structure-based drug design: A molecular modeling perspective. *Medicinal Research Reviews, 16*(1), 3−50.

Braeckmans, K., De Smedt, S. C., Leblans, M., Pauwels, R., & Demeester, J. (2002). Encoding microcarriers: Present and future technologies. *Nature Reviews Drug Discovery, 1*(6), 447−456.

Brandish, P. E., Chiu, C. S., Schneeweis, J., Brandon, N. J., Leech, C. L., Kornienko, O., et al. (2006). A cell-based ultra-high-throughput screening assay for identifying inhibitors of D-amino acid oxidase. *Journal of Biomolecular Screening, 11*(5), 481−487.

Brouzes, E. (2012). Droplet microfluidics for single-cell analysis. *Methods in Molecular Biology, 853*, 105−139.

Brouzes, E., Medkova, M., Savenelli, N., Marran, D., Twardowski, M., Hutchison, J. B., et al. (2009). Droplet microfluidic technology for single-cell high-throughput screening. *Proceedings of the National Academy of Sciences of the United States of America, 106*(34), 14195−14200.

Bruzewicz, D. A., Reches, M., & Whitesides, G. M. (2008). Low-cost printing of poly (dimethylsiloxane) barriers to define microchannels in paper. *Analytical Chemistry, 80*(9), 3387−3392.

Cao, J., Kursten, D., Schneider, S., Knauer, A., Gunther, P. M., & Kohler, J. M. (2012). Uncovering toxicological complexity by multi-dimensional screenings in microsegmented flow: Modulation of antibiotic interference by nanoparticles. *Lab on a Chip, 12*(3), 474−484.

Cesaro-Tadic, S., Dernick, G., Juncker, D., Buurman, G., Kropshofer, H., Michel, B., et al. (2004). High-sensitivity miniaturized immunoassays for tumor necrosis factor a using microfluidic systems. *Lab on a Chip, 4*(6), 563−569.

Chen, J. K., Bai, B. J., & Chang, F. C. (2011). Diagnosis of breast cancer recurrence using a microfluidic device featuring tethered cationic polymers. *Applied Physics Letters, 99*(1).

Chen, H., Gao, F., He, R., & Cui, D. (2007). Chemiluminescence of luminol catalyzed by silver nanoparticles. *Journal of Colloid and Interface Science, 315*(1), 158−163.

Cheng, Y. L., Bushby, R. J., Evans, S. D., Knowles, P. F., Miles, R. E., & Ogier, S. D. (2001). Single ion channel sensitivity in suspended bilayers on micromachined supports. *Langmuir, 17*(4), 1240−1242.

Chen, P. C., Huang, Y. Y., & Juang, J. L. (2011). MEMS microwell and microcolumn arrays: Novel methods for high-throughput cell-based assays. *Lab on a Chip, 11*(21), 3619−3625.

Chen, K. C., Lee, T. P., Pan, Y. C., Chiang, C. L., Chen, C. L., Yang, Y. H., et al. (2011). Detection of circulating endothelial cells via a microfluidic disk. *Clinical Chemistry, 57*(4), 586−592.

Chen, Y. J., Roller, E. E., & Huang, X. (2010). DNA sequencing by denaturation: Experimental proof of concept with an integrated fluidic device. *Lab on a Chip, 10*(9), 1153−1159.

Chen, Q., Wu, J., Zhang, Y., Lin, Z., & Lin, J. M. (2012). Targeted isolation and analysis of single tumor cells with aptamer-encoded microwell array on microfluidic device. *Lab on a Chip, 12*(24), 5180−5185.

Cheow, L. F., Viswanathan, R., Chin, C. S., Jennifer, N., Jones, R. C., Guccione, E., et al. (2014). Multiplexed analysis of protein-ligand interactions by fluorescence anisotropy in a microfluidic platform. *Analytical Chemistry, 86*(19), 9901−9908.

Choi, S., Goryll, M., Sin, L. Y. M., Wong, P. K., & Chae, J. (2011). Microfluidic-based biosensors toward point-of-care detection of nucleic acids and proteins. *Microfluidics and Nanofluidics, 10*(2), 231−247.

Chong, K. C., Thang, L. Y., Quirino, J. P., & See, H. H. (2017). Monitoring of vancomycin in human plasma via portable microchip electrophoresis with contactless conductivity detector and multi-stacking strategy. *Journal of Chromatography A, 1485*, 142−146.

Choucha Snouber, L., Bunescu, A., Naudot, M., Legallais, C., Brochot, C., Dumas, M. E., et al. (2013). Metabolomics-on-a-chip of hepatotoxicity induced by anticancer drug flutamide and its active metabolite hydroxyflutamide using HepG2/C3a microfluidic biochips. *Toxicological Sciences, 132*(1), 8−20.

Chung, K., Rivet, C. A., Kemp, M. L., & Lu, H. (2011). Imaging single-cell signaling dynamics with a deterministic high-density single-cell trap array. *Analytical Chemistry, 83*(18), 7044−7052.

Clausell-Tormos, J., Lieber, D., Baret, J. C., El-Harrak, A., Miller, O. J., Frenz, L., et al. (2008). Droplet-based microfluidic platforms for the encapsulation and screening of Mammalian cells and multicellular organisms. *Chemical Biology, 15*(5), 427−437.

Contreras-Naranjo, J. C., Wu, H. J., & Ugaz, V. M. (2017). Microfluidics for exosome isolation and analysis: Enabling liquid biopsy for personalized medicine. *Lab on a Chip, 17*(21), 3558−3577.

Das, J., Ivanov, I., Montermini, L., Rak, J., Sargent, E. H., & Kelley, S. O. (2015). An electrochemical clamp assay for direct, rapid analysis of circulating nucleic acids in serum. *Nature Chemistry, 7*(7), 569−575.

Davies, R. T., Kim, J., Jang, S. C., Choi, E. J., Gho, Y. S., & Park, J. (2012). Microfluidic filtration system to isolate extracellular vesicles from blood. *Lab on a Chip, 12*(24), 5202−5210.

Delbeke, F. T., Desmet, N., & Debackere, M. (1995). The abuse of doping agents in competing body builders in Flanders (1988−1993). *International Journal of Sports Medicine, 16*(1), 66−70.

DeMello, A. J. (2006). Control and detection of chemical reactions in microfluidic systems. *Nature, 442*(7101), 394−402.

Dexter, J. P., & Parker, W. (2009). Parallel combinatorial chemical synthesis using single-layer poly(dimethylsiloxane) microfluidic devices. *Biomicrofluidics, 3*(3).

Ding, Y., Li, J., Xiao, W., Xiao, K., Lee, J., Bhardwaj, U., et al. (2015). Microfluidic-enabled print-to-screen platform for high-throughput screening of combinatorial chemotherapy. *Analytical Chemistry, 87*(20), 10166−10171.

Dolomite nanoparticle generation systems.(2020). Retrieved from: https://www.dolomite-microfluidics.com/microfluidic-systems/nanoparticle-generation/. (Accessed 31 July 2020).

Dong, J., Zhang, R. Y., Sun, N., Smalley, M., Wu, Z., Zhou, A., et al. (2019). Bio-inspired NanoVilli chips for enhanced capture of tumor-derived extracellular vesicles: Toward non-invasive detection of gene alterations in non-small cell lung cancer. *ACS Applied Materials and Interfaces, 11*(15), 13973−13983.

Dou, M., Dominguez, D. C., Li, X., Sanchez, J., & Scott, G. (2014). A versatile PDMS/paper hybrid microfluidic platform for sensitive infectious disease diagnosis. *Analytical Chemistry, 86*(15), 7978−7986.

Du, G., Fang, Q., & den Toonder, J. M. (2016). Microfluidics for cell-based high throughput screening platforms - a review. *Analytica Chimica Acta, 903*, 36−50.

Dunlop, J., Bowlby, M., Peri, R., Vasilyev, D., & Arias, R. (2008). High-throughput electrophysiology: An emerging paradigm for ion-channel screening and physiology. *Nature Reviews Drug Discovery, 7*(4), 358−368.

Du, G. S., Pan, J. Z., Zhao, S. P., Zhu, Y., den Toonder, J. M., & Fang, Q. (2013). Cell-based drug combination screening with a microfluidic droplet array system. *Analytical Chemistry, 85*(14), 6740−6747.

Eicher, D., & Merten, C. A. (2011). Microfluidic devices for diagnostic applications. *Expert Review of Molecular Diagnostics, 11*(5), 505−519.

El-Ali, J., Sorger, P. K., & Jensen, K. F. (2006). Cells on chips. *Nature, 442*(7101), 403−411.

Esch, M. B., King, T. L., & Shuler, M. L. (2011). The role of body-on-a-chip devices in drug and toxicity studies. *Annual Review of Biomedical Engineering, 13*, 55−72.
Evans, M., Sewter, C., & Hill, E. (2003). An encoded particle array tool for multiplex bioassays. *Assay and Drug Development Technologies, 1*(1 Pt 2), 199−207.
Feldmann, D. P., Xie, Y., Jones, S. K., Yu, D., Moszczynska, A., & Merkel, O. M. (2017). The impact of microfluidic mixing of triblock micelleplexes on in vitro/in vivo gene silencing and intracellular trafficking. *Nanotechnology, 28*(22), 224001-224001.
Fertig, N., Blick, R. H., & Behrends, J. C. (2002). Whole cell patch clamp recording performed on a planar glass chip. *Biophysical Journal, 82*(6), 3056−3062.
Foudeh, A. M., Fatanat Didar, T., Veres, T., & Tabrizian, M. (2012). Microfluidic designs and techniques using lab-on-a-chip devices for pathogen detection for point-of-care diagnostics. *Lab on a Chip - Miniaturisation for Chemistry and Biology, 12*(18), 3249−3266.
Fox, S., Farr-Jones, S., Sopchak, L., Boggs, A., Nicely, H. W., Khoury, R., et al. (2006). High-throughput screening: Update on practices and success. *Journal of Biomolecular Screening, 11*(7), 864−869.
Gao, D., Li, H., Wang, N., & Lin, J. M. (2012). Evaluation of the absorption of methotrexate on cells and its cytotoxicity assay by using an integrated microfluidic device coupled to a mass spectrometer. *Analytical Chemistry, 84*(21), 9230−9237.
Gao, J., Yin, X. F., & Fang, Z. L. (2004). Integration of single cell injection, cell lysis, separation and detection of intracellular constituents on a microfluidic chip. *Lab on a Chip, 4*(1), 47−52.
Garcia-Cordero, J. L., & Maerkl, S. J. (2020). Microfluidic systems for cancer diagnostics. *Current Opinion in Biotechnology, 65*, 37−44.
Garcia-Egido, E., Spikmans, V., Wong, S. Y., & Warrington, B. H. (2003). Synthesis and analysis of combinatorial libraries performed in an automated micro reactor system. *Lab on a Chip, 3*(2), 73−76.
Gencturk, E., Mutlu, S., & Ulgen, K. O. (2017). Advances in microfluidic devices made from thermoplastics used in cell biology and analyses. *Biomicrofluidics, 11*(5), 051502-051502.
Giuffrida, M. C., Cigliana, G., & Spoto, G. (2018). Ultrasensitive detection of lysozyme in droplet-based microfluidic devices. *Biosensors and Bioelectronics, 104*, 8−14.
Glick, Y., Ben-Ari, Y., Drayman, N., Pellach, M., Neveu, G., Boonyaratanakornkit, J., et al. (2016). Pathogen receptor discovery with a microfluidic human membrane protein array. *Proceedings of the National Academy of Sciences of the United States of America, 113*(16), 4344−4349.
Goldberg, M. D., Lo, R. C., Abele, S., Macka, M., & Gomez, F. A. (2009). Development of microfluidic chips for heterogeneous receptor-ligand interaction studies. *Analytical Chemistry, 81*(12), 5095−5098.
Gomez, F. A. (2011). Microfluidics in protein chromatography. *Methods in Molecular Biology, 681*, 137−150.
Goodnow, R. A., Jr. (2006). Hit and lead identification: Integrated technology-based approaches. *Drug Discovery Today: Technologies, 3*(4), 367−375.
Graaf, I. A. M., Groothuis, G. M. M., & Olinga, P. (2007). Precision-cut tissue slices as a tool to predict metabolism of novel drugs. *Expert Opinion on Drug Metabolism and Toxicology, 3*(6), 879−898.
Guo, M. T., Rotem, A., Heyman, J. A., & Weitz, D. A. (2012). Droplet microfluidics for high-throughput biological assays. *Lab on a Chip, 12*(12), 2146−2155.
Gurwitz, D., & Haring, R. (2003). Ligand-selective signaling and high-content screening for GPCR drugs. *Drug Discovery Today, 8*(24), 1108−1109.

Hadd, A. G., Raymond, D. E., Halliwell, J. W., Jacobson, S. C., & Ramsey, J. M. (1997). Microchip device for performing enzyme assays. *Analytical Chemistry, 69*(17), 3407−3412.

Han, M., Gao, X., Su, J. Z., & Nie, S. (2001). Quantum-dot-tagged microbeads for multiplexed optical coding of biomolecules. *Nature Biotechnology, 19*(7), 631−635.

Hao, M., Liu, R., Zhang, H., Li, Y., & Jing, M. (2014). Detection of glutathione within single mice hepatocytes using microfluidic chips coupled with a laser-induced fluorescence system. *Spectrochimica Acta Part A: Molecular and Biomolecular Spectroscopy, 125*, 7−11.

Harrison, D. J., Fluri, K., Seiler, K., Fan, Z., Effenhauser, C. S., & Manz, A. (1993). Micromachining a miniaturized capillary electrophoresis-based chemical analysis system on a chip. *Science, 261*(5123), 895−897.

Hattersley, S. M., Greenman, J., & Haswell, S. J. (2011). Study of ethanol induced toxicity in liver explants using microfluidic devices. *Biomedical Microdevices, 13*(6), 1005−1014.

He, M., Crow, J., Roth, M., Zeng, Y., & Godwin, A. K. (2014). Integrated immunoisolation and protein analysis of circulating exosomes using microfluidic technology. *Lab on a Chip, 14*(19), 3773−3780.

Herr, A. E., Hatch, A. V., Throckmorton, D. J., Tran, H. M., Brennan, J. S., Giannobile, W. V., et al. (2007). Microfluidic immunoassays as rapid saliva-based clinical diagnostics. *Proceedings of the National Academy of Sciences of the United States of America, 104*(13), 5268−5273.

Herrmann, M., Veres, T., & Tabrizian, M. (2006). Enzymatically-generated fluorescent detection in micro-channels with internal magnetic mixing for the development of parallel microfluidic ELISA. *Lab on a Chip, 6*(4), 555−560.

Hesketh, J. E., Campbell, G. P., Lobley, G. E., Maltin, C. A., Acamovic, F., & Palmer, R. M. (1992). Stimulation of actin and myosin synthesis in rat gastrocnemius muscle by clenbuterol; evidence for translational control. *Comparative Biochemistry and Physiology - Part C, 102*(1), 23−27.

Hindson, B. J., Ness, K. D., Masquelier, D. A., Belgrader, P., Heredia, N. J., Makarewicz, A. J., et al. (2011). High-throughput droplet digital PCR system for absolute quantitation of DNA copy number. *Analytical Chemistry, 83*(22), 8604−8610.

Ho, N. T., Desai, D., & Zaman, M. H. (2015). Rapid and specific drug quality testing assay for artemisinin and its derivatives using a luminescent reaction and novel microfluidic technology. *The American Journal of Tropical Medicine and Hygiene, 92*(6 Suppl. l), 24−30.

Holmes, D., She, J. K., Roach, P. L., & Morgan, H. (2007). Bead-based immunoassays using a micro-chip flow cytometer. *Lab on a Chip, 7*(8), 1048−1056.

Hosokawa, M., Asami, M., Yoshino, T., Tsujimura, N., Takahashi, M., Nakasono, S., et al. (2012). Monitoring of benzene-induced hematotoxicity in mice by serial leukocyte counting using a microcavity array. *Biosensors and Bioelectronics, 40*(1), 110−114.

Hsieh, K., Patterson, A. S., Ferguson, B. S., Plaxco, K. W., & Soh, H. T. (2012). Rapid, sensitive, and quantitative detection of pathogenic DNA at the point of care through microfluidic electrochemical quantitative loop-mediated isothermal amplification. *Angewandte Chemie International Edition in English, 51*(20), 4896−4900.

Huang, B., Wu, H., Bhaya, D., Grossman, A., Granier, S., Kobilka, B. K., et al. (2007). Counting low-copy number proteins in a single cell. *Science, 315*(5808), 81−84.

Hur, S. C., Mach, A. J., & Di Carlo, D. (2011). High-throughput size-based rare cell enrichment using microscale vortices. *Biomicrofluidics, 5*(2), 022206.

Ide, T., & Ichikawa, T. (2005). A novel method for artificial lipid-bilayer formation. *Biosensors and Bioelectronics, 21*(4), 672−677.

Imming, P., Sinning, C., & Meyer, A. (2006). Drugs, their targets and the nature and number of drug targets. *Nature Reviews Drug Discovery, 5*(10), 821−834.

Im, H., Shao, H., Park, Y. I., Peterson, V. M., Castro, C. M., Weissleder, R., et al. (2014). Label-free detection and molecular profiling of exosomes with a nano-plasmonic sensor. *Nature Biotechnology, 32*(5), 490−495.

Issadore, D., Chung, J., Shao, H., Liong, M., Ghazani, A. A., Castro, C. M., et al. (2012). Ultrasensitive clinical enumeration of rare cells ex vivo using a micro-hall detector. *Science Translational Medicine, 4*(141), 141ra192.

Javanmard, M., Babrzadeh, F., & Davis, R. W. (2010). Microfluidic force spectroscopy for characterization of biomolecular interactions with piconewton resolution. *Applied Physics Letters, 97*(17), 173704.

Jones, R., Godorhazy, L., Szalay, D., Gerencser, J., Dorman, G., Urge, L., et al. (2005). A novel method for high-throughput reduction of compounds through automated sequential injection into a continuous-flow microfluidic reactor. *QSAR and Combinatorial Science, 24*(6), 722−727.

Kachouie, N., Kang, L., & Khademhosseini, A. (2009). Arraycount, an algorithm for automatic cell counting in microwell arrays. *Biotechniques, 47*(3), x−xvi.

Kamruzzaman, M., Alam, A. M., Kim, K. M., Lee, S. H., Kim, Y. H., Kim, G. M., et al. (2012). Microfluidic chip based chemiluminescence detection of L-phenylalanine in pharmaceutical and soft drinks. *Food Chemistry, 135*(1), 57−62.

Kane, B. J., Zinner, M. J., Yarmush, M. L., & Toner, M. (2006). Liver-specific functional studies in a microfluidic array of primary mammalian hepatocytes. *Analytical Chemistry, 78*(13), 4291−4298.

Kang, L., Chung, B. G., Langer, R., & Khademhosseini, A. (2008). Microfluidics for drug discovery and development: From target selection to product lifecycle management. *Drug Discovery Today, 13*(1−2), 1−13.

Kang, L., Hancock, M. J., Brigham, M. D., & Khademhosseini, A. (2010). Cell confinement in patterned nanoliter droplets in a microwell array by wiping. *Journal of Biomedical Materials Research Part A, 93*(2), 547−557.

Kang, G., Lee, J. H., Lee, C. S., & Nam, Y. (2009). Agarose microwell based neuronal microcircuit arrays on microelectrode arrays for high throughput drug testing. *Lab on a Chip, 9*(22), 3236−3242.

Kaplowitz, N. (2005). Idiosyncratic drug hepatotoxicity. *Nature Reviews Drug Discovery, 4*(6), 489−499.

Katsuno, K., Burrows, J. N., Duncan, K., Hooft van Huijsduijnen, R., Kaneko, T., Kita, K., et al. (2015). Hit and lead criteria in drug discovery for infectious diseases of the developing world. *Nature Reviews Drug Discovery, 14*(11), 751−758.

Keng, P. Y., Chen, S., Ding, H., Sadeghi, S., Shah, G. J., Dooraghi, A., et al. (2012). Microchemical synthesis of molecular probes on an electronic microfluidic device. *Proceedings of the National Academy of Sciences of the United States of America, 109*(3), 690−695.

Khademhosseini, A., Yeh, J., Eng, G., Karp, J., Kaji, H., Borenstein, J., et al. (2005). Cell docking inside microwells within reversibly sealed microfluidic channels for fabricating multiphenotype cell arrays. *Lab on a Chip, 5*(12), 1380−1386.

Khetani, S. R., & Bhatia, S. N. (2008). Microscale culture of human liver cells for drug development. *Nature Biotechnology, 26*(1), 120−126.

Kikutani, Y., Horiuchi, T., Uchiyama, K., Hisamoto, H., Tokeshi, M., & Kitamori, T. (2002). Glass microchip with three-dimensional microchannel network for 2×2 parallel synthesis. *Lab on a Chip, 2*(4), 188−192.

Kim, D. N., Lee, Y., & Koh, W. G. (2009). Fabrication of microfluidic devices incorporating bead-based reaction and microarray-based detection system for enzymatic assay. *Sensors and Actuators B: Chemical, 137*(1), 305–312.

Kirby, B. J., Jodari, M., Loftus, M. S., Gakhar, G., Pratt, E. D., Chanel-Vos, C., et al. (2012). Functional characterization of circulating tumor cells with a prostate-cancer-specific microfluidic device. *PLoS One, 7*(4), e35976.

Kirby, A. E., Lafreniere, N. M., Seale, B., Hendricks, P. I., Cooks, R. G., & Wheeler, A. R. (2014). Analysis on the go: Quantitation of drugs of abuse in dried urine with digital microfluidics and miniature mass spectrometry. *Analytical Chemistry, 86*(12), 6121–6129.

Knight, A. R. (2000). HTS — a strategy for drug discovery. *Drug Disovery World, 1*(1), 32–38.

Kola, I., & Landis, J. (2004). Can the pharmaceutical industry reduce attrition rates? *Nature Reviews Drug Discovery, 3*(8), 711–715.

Kong, J., Jiang, L., Su, X., Qin, J., Du, Y., & Lin, B. (2009). Integrated microfluidic immunoassay for the rapid determination of clenbuterol. *Lab on a Chip, 9*(11), 1541–1547.

Kongsuphol, P., Fang, K. B., & Ding, Z. (2013). Lipid bilayer technologies in ion channel recordings and their potential in drug screening assay. *Sensors and Actuators B: Chemical, 185*, 530–542.

Kramer, J. A., Sagartz, J. E., & Morris, D. L. (2007). The application of discovery toxicology and pathology towards the design of safer pharmaceutical lead candidates. *Nature Reviews Drug Discovery, 6*(8), 636–649.

Kreir, M., Farre, C., Beckler, M., George, M., & Fertig, N. (2008). Rapid screening of membrane protein activity: Electrophysiological analysis of OmpF reconstituted in proteoliposomes. *Lab on a Chip, 8*(4), 587–595.

Krenkova, J., & Foret, F. (2004). Immobilized microfluidic enzymatic reactors. *Electrophoresis, 25*(21–22), 3550–3563.

Kumar, S. S., Chouhan, R. S., & Thakur, M. S. (2009). Enhancement of chemiluminescence for vitamin B12 analysis. *Analytical Biochemistry, 388*(2), 312–316.

Lai, S., Wang, S., Luo, J., Lee, L. J., Yang, S. T., & Madou, M. J. (2004). Design of a compact disk-like microfluidic platform for enzyme-linked immunosorbent assay. *Analytical Chemistry, 76*(7), 1832–1837.

Lal, R., & Arnsdorf, M. F. (2010). Multidimensional atomic force microscopy for drug discovery: A versatile tool for defining targets, designing therapeutics and monitoring their efficacy. *Life Sciences, 86*(15–16), 545–562.

Lee, W. G., Kim, Y. G., Chung, B. G., Demirci, U., & Khademhosseini, A. (2010). Nano/Microfluidics for diagnosis of infectious diseases in developing countries. *Advanced Drug Delivery Reviews, 62*(4–5), 449–457.

Lee, K. G., Lee, T. J., Jeong, S. W., Choi, H. W., Heo, N. S., Park, J. Y., et al. (2012). Development of a plastic-based microfluidic immunosensor chip for detection of H1N1 influenza. *Sensors, 12*(8), 10810–10819.

Lee, S. H., Lee, C. S., Kim, B. G., & Kim, Y. K. (2008). An integrated microfluidic chip for the analysis of biochemical reactions by MALDI mass spectrometry. *Biomedical Microdevices, 10*(1), 1–9.

Lee, B. S., Lee, Y. U., Kim, H. S., Kim, T. H., Park, J., Lee, J. G., et al. (2011). Fully integrated lab-on-a-disc for simultaneous analysis of biochemistry and immunoassay from whole blood. *Lab on a Chip, 11*(1), 70–78.

Lee, B. S., Lee, J. N., Park, J. M., Lee, J. G., Kim, S., Cho, Y. K., et al. (2009). A fully automated immunoassay from whole blood on a disc. *Lab on a Chip, 9*(11), 1548–1555.

Lee, C. C., Sui, G. D., Elizarov, A., Shu, C. Y. J., Shin, Y. S., Dooley, A. N., et al. (2005). Multistep synthesis of a radiolabeled imaging probe using integrated microfluidics. *Science, 310*(5755), 1793−1796.

Lew, V., Nguyen, D., & Khine, M. (2011). Shrink-induced single-cell plastic microwell array. *Journal of Laboratory Automation, 16*(6), 450−456.

Liang, L. G., Kong, M. Q., Zhou, S., Sheng, Y. F., Wang, P., Yu, T., et al. (2017). An integrated double-filtration microfluidic device for isolation, enrichment and quantification of urinary extracellular vesicles for detection of bladder cancer. *Scientific Reports, 7*, 46224.

Li, A. P., Bode, C., & Sakai, Y. (2004). A novel in vitro system, the integrated discrete multiple organ cell culture (IdMOC) system, for the evaluation of human drug toxicity: Comparative cytotoxicity of tamoxifen towards normal human cells from five major organs and MCF-7 adenocarcinoma breast cancer cells. *Chemico-Biological Interactions, 150*(1), 129−136.

Li, J., Carney, R. P., Liu, R., Fan, J., Zhao, S., Chen, Y., et al. (2018). Microfluidic print-to-synthesis platform for efficient preparation and screening of combinatorial peptide microarrays. *Analytical Chemistry, 90*(9), 5833−5840.

Lien, K. Y., Chuang, Y. H., Hung, L. Y., Hsu, K. F., Lai, W. W., Ho, C. L., et al. (2010). Rapid isolation and detection of cancer cells by utilizing integrated microfluidic systems. *Lab on a Chip, 10*(21), 2875−2886.

Lion, N., Reymond, F., Girault, H. H., & Rossier, J. S. (2004). Why the move to microfluidics for protein analysis? *Current Opinion in Biotechnology, 15*(1), 31−37.

Li, P., Stratton, Z. S., Dao, M., Ritz, J., & Huang, T. J. (2013). Probing circulating tumor cells in microfluidics. *Lab on a Chip, 13*(4), 602−609.

Liszewski, K. (2003). Broader uses for microfluidics technologies - applications expand from drug discovery to battlefield. *Genetic Engineering News, 23*(9), 40−+.

Liu, C., Guo, J., Tian, F., Yang, N., Yan, F., Ding, Y., et al. (2017). Field-free isolation of exosomes from extracellular vesicles by microfluidic viscoelastic flows. *ACS Nano, 11*(7), 6968−6976.

Liu, C., Liu, J., Gao, D., Ding, M., & Lin, J. M. (2010). Fabrication of microwell arrays based on two-dimensional ordered polystyrene microspheres for high-throughput single-cell analysis. *Analytical Chemistry, 82*(22), 9418−9424.

Liu, Y., & Singh, A. K. (2013). Microfluidic platforms for single-cell protein analysis. *Journal of Laboratory Automation, 18*(6), 446−454.

Liu, C., Wang, L., Xu, Z., Li, J. M., Ding, X. P., Wang, Q., et al. (2012). A multilayer microdevice for cell-based high-throughput drug screening. *Journal of Micromechanics and Microengineering, 22*(6).

Liu, C., Xu, X., Li, B., Situ, B., Pan, W., Hu, Y., et al. (2018). Single-exosome-counting immunoassays for cancer diagnostics. *Nano Letters, 18*(7), 4226−4232.

Li, X. J., Valadez, A. V., Zuo, P., & Nie, Z. (2012). Microfluidic 3D cell culture: Potential application for tissue-based bioassays. *Bioanalysis, 4*(12), 1509−1525.

Lok, K. S., Abdul Muttalib, S. Z., Lee, P. P., Kwok, Y. C., & Nguyen, N. T. (2012). Rapid determination of vitamin B12 concentration with a chemiluminescence lab on a chip. *Lab on a Chip, 12*(13), 2353−2361.

Lombardi, D., & Dittrich, P. S. (2010). Advances in microfluidics for drug discovery. *Expert Opinion on Drug Discovery, 5*(11), 1081−1094.

Mabey, D., Peeling, R. W., Ustianowski, A., & Perkins, M. D. (2004). Diagnostics for the developing world. *Nature Reviews Microbiology, 2*(3), 231−240.

MacBeath, G., & Schreiber, S. L. (2000). Printing proteins as microarrays for high-throughput function determination. *Science, 289*(5485), 1760−1763.

MacConnell, A. B., Price, A. K., & Paegel, B. M. (2017). An integrated microfluidic processor for DNA-encoded combinatorial library functional screening. *ACS Combinatorial Science, 19*(3), 181−192.

Maj-Hes, A., Sevcenco, S., Szarvas, T., & Kramer, G. (2019). Claros system: A rapid microfluidics-based point-of-care system for quantitative prostate specific antigen analysis from finger-stick blood. *Advances in Therapy, 36*.

Makamba, H., Hsieh, Y. Y., Sung, W. C., & Chen, S. H. (2005). Stable permanently hydrophilic protein-resistant thin-film coatings on poly(dimethylsiloxane) substrates by electrostatic self-assembly and chemical cross-linking. *Analytical Chemistry, 77*(13), 3971−3978.

Malmstadt, N., Nash, M. A., Purnell, R. F., & Schmidt, J. J. (2006). Automated formation of lipid-bilayer membranes in a microfluidic device. *Nano Letters, 6*(9), 1961−1965.

Manz, A., Graber, N., & Widmer, H. M. (1990). Miniaturized total chemical-analysis systems - a novel concept for chemical sensing. *Sensors and Actuators B: Chemical, 1*(1−6), 244−248.

Mao, X., & Huang, T. J. (2012). Exploiting mechanical biomarkers in microfluidics. *Lab on a Chip, 12*(20), 4006−4009.

Mao, H., Yang, T., & Cremer, P. S. (2002). Design and characterization of immobilized enzymes in microfluidic systems. *Analytical Chemistry, 74*(2), 379−385.

Martinez-Navarro, J. F. (1990). Food poisoning related to consumption of illicit beta-agonist in liver. *Lancet, 336*(8726), 1311.

Martinez, A. W., Phillips, S. T., Butte, M. J., & Whitesides, G. M. (2007). Patterned paper as a platform for inexpensive, low-volume, portable bioassays. *Angewandte Chemie International Edition, 46*(8), 1318−1320.

Martinez, A. W., Phillips, S. T., Carrilho, E., Thomas, S. W., 3rd, Sindi, H., & Whitesides, G. M. (2008). Simple telemedicine for developing regions: Camera phones and paper-based microfluidic devices for real-time, off-site diagnosis. *Analytical Chemistry, 80*(10), 3699−3707.

Martinez, A. W., Phillips, S. T., & Whitesides, G. M. (2008). Three-dimensional microfluidic devices fabricated in layered paper and tape. *Proceedings of the National Academy of Sciences of the United States of America, 105*(50), 19606−19611.

Maruyama, S., Hirayama, C., Abe, J., Tanaka, J., & Matsui, K. (1995). Chronic active hepatitis and liver cirrhosis in association with combined tamoxifen/tegafur adjuvant therapy. *Digestive Diseases and Sciences, 40*(12), 2602−2607.

Matsui, N., Kaya, T., Nagamine, K., Yasukawa, T., Shiku, H., & Matsue, T. (2006). Electrochemical mutagen screening using microbial chip. *Biosensors and Bioelectronics, 21*(7), 1202−1209.

Mayer, M., Kriebel, J. K., Tosteson, M. T., & Whitesides, G. M. (2003). Microfabricated teflon membranes for low-noise recordings of ion channels in planar lipid bilayers. *Biophysical Journal, 85*(4), 2684−2695.

Meagher, R. J., & Thaitrong, N. (2012). Microchip electrophoresis of DNA following preconcentration at photopatterned gel membranes. *Electrophoresis, 33*(8), 1236−1246.

Mei, Q., Fredrickson, C. K., Simon, A., Khnouf, R., & Fan, Z. H. (2007). Cell-free protein synthesis in microfluidic array devices. *Biotechnology Progress, 23*(6), 1305−1311.

Melin, J., & Quake, S. R. (2007). Microfluidic large-scale integration: The evolution of design rules for biological automation. *Annual Review of Biophysics and Biomolecular Structure, 36*, 213−231.

van Midwoud, P. M., Groothuis, G. M. M., Merema, M. T., & Verpoorte, E. (2010). Microfluidic biochip for the perifusion of precision-cut rat liver slices for metabolism and toxicology studies. *Biotechnology and Bioengineering, 105*(1), 184−194.

Miserere, S., Ledru, S., Ruille, N., Griveau, S., Boujtita, M., & Bedioui, F. (2006). Biocompatible carbon-based screen-printed electrodes for the electrochemical detection of nitric oxide. *Electrochemistry Communications, 8*(2), 238−244.

MIT technology review Claros diagnostics.(2020). Retrieved from: http://www2.technologyreview.com/tr50/clarosdx/. (Accessed 31 July 2020).

Mohammed, M. I., & Desmulliez, M. P. (2011). Lab-on-a-chip based immunosensor principles and technologies for the detection of cardiac biomarkers: A review. *Lab on a Chip, 11*(4), 569−595.

Mohanty, S. P., & Kougianos, E. (2006). Biosensors: A tutorial review. *Potentials, IEEE, 25*(2), 35−40.

Moran-Mirabal, J. M., Edel, J. B., Meyer, G. D., Throckmorton, D., Singh, A. K., & Craighead, H. G. (2005). Micrometer-sized supported lipid bilayer arrays for bacterial toxin binding studies through total internal reflection fluorescence microscopy. *Biophysical Journal, 89*(1), 296−305.

Murakami, Y., Endo, T., Yamamura, S., Nagatani, N., Takamura, Y., & Tamiya, E. (2004). On-chip micro-flow polystyrene bead-based immunoassay for quantitative detection of tacrolimus (FK506). *Analytical Biochemistry, 334*(1), 111−116.

Muster, W., Breidenbach, A., Fischer, H., Kirchner, S., Muller, L., & Pahler, A. (2008). Computational toxicology in drug development. *Drug Discovery Today, 13*(7−8), 303−310.

Nagrath, S., Sequist, L. V., Maheswaran, S., Bell, D. W., Irimia, D., Ulkus, L., et al. (2007). Isolation of rare circulating tumour cells in cancer patients by microchip technology. *Nature, 450*(7173), 1235−1239.

Nolan, J. P., & Sklar, L. A. (2002). Suspension array technology: Evolution of the flat-array paradigm. *Trends in Biotechnology, 20*(1), 9−12.

Pallaoro, A., Hoonejani, M. R., Braun, G. B., Meinhart, C. D., & Moskovits, M. (2015). Rapid identification by surface-enhanced Raman spectroscopy of cancer cells at low concentrations flowing in a microfluidic channel. *ACS Nano, 9*(4), 4328−4336.

Pampaloni, F., Reynaud, E. G., & Stelzer, E. H. K. (2007). The third dimension bridges the gap between cell culture and live tissue. *Nature Reviews Molecular Cell Biology, 8*(10), 839−845.

Park, J., Sunkara, V., Kim, T. H., Hwang, H., & Cho, Y. K. (2012). Lab-on-a-disc for fully integrated multiplex immunoassays. *Analytical Chemistry, 84*(5), 2133−2140.

Park, S. M., Wong, D. J., Ooi, C. C., Kurtz, D. M., Vermesh, O., Aalipour, A., et al. (2016). Molecular profiling of single circulating tumor cells from lung cancer patients. *Proceedings of the National Academy of Sciences of the United States of America, 113*(52), E8379−E8386.

Perrin, D., Fremaux, C., & Scheer, A. (2006). Assay development and screening of a serine/threonine kinase in an on-chip mode using caliper nanofluidics technology. *Journal of Biomolecular Screening, 11*(4), 359−368.

Peterson, D. S. (2005). Solid supports for micro analytical systems. *Lab on a Chip, 5*(2), 132−139.

Pickett, S. D., Green, D. V., Hunt, D. L., Pardoe, D. A., & Hughes, I. (2011). Automated lead optimization of MMP-12 inhibitors using a genetic algorithm. *ACS Medicinal Chemistry Letters, 2*(1), 28−33.

Piraino, F., Volpetti, F., Watson, C., & Maerkl, S. J. (2016). A digital-analog microfluidic platform for patient-centric multiplexed biomarker diagnostics of ultralow volume samples. *ACS Nano, 10*(1), 1699−1710.

Poudineh, M., Sargent, E. H., Pantel, K., & Kelley, S. O. (2018). Profiling circulating tumour cells and other biomarkers of invasive cancers. *Nature Biomedical Engineering, 2*(2), 72−84.

Pregibon, D. C., Toner, M., & Doyle, P. S. (2007). Multifunctional encoded particles for high-throughput biomolecule analysis. *Science, 315*(5817), 1393−1396.

Puckett, L. G., Dikici, E., Lai, S., Madou, M., Bachas, L. G., & Daunert, S. (2004). Investigation into the applicability of the centrifugal microfluidics development of protein-platform for the ligand binding assays incorporating enhanced green fluorescent protein as a fluorescent reporter. *Analytical Chemistry, 76*(24), 7263−7268.

Quinton, D., Girard, A., Thi Kim, L. T., Raimbault, V., Griscom, L., Razan, F., et al. (2011). On-chip multi-electrochemical sensor array platform for simultaneous screening of nitric oxide and peroxynitrite. *Lab on a Chip, 11*(7), 1342−1350.

Qureshi, Z. P., Seoane-Vazquez, E., Rodriguez-Monguio, R., Stevenson, K. B., & Szeinbach, S. L. (2011). Market withdrawal of new molecular entities approved in the United States from 1980 to 2009. *Pharmacoepidemiology and Drug Safety, 20*(7), 772−777.

Razumovitch, J., Meier, W., & Vebert, C. (2009). A microcontact printing approach to the immobilization of oligonucleotide brushes. *Biophysical Chemistry, 139*(1), 70−74.

Reategui, E., van der Vos, K. E., Lai, C. P., Zeinali, M., Atai, N. A., Aldikacti, B., et al. (2018). Engineered nanointerfaces for microfluidic isolation and molecular profiling of tumor-specific extracellular vesicles. *Nature Communications, 9*(1), 175.

Rettig, J. R., & Folch, A. (2005). Large-scale single-cell trapping and imaging using microwell arrays. *Analytical Chemistry, 77*(17), 5628−5634.

Reutlinger, M., Rodrigues, T., Schneider, P., & Schneider, G. (2014). Combining on-chip synthesis of a focused combinatorial library with computational target prediction reveals imidazopyridine GPCR ligands. *Angewandte Chemie International Edition in English, 53*(2), 582−585.

Rodríguez-Dévora, J. I., Zhang, B., Reyna, D., Shi, Z. D., & Xu, T. (2012). High throughput miniature drug-screening platform using bioprinting technology. *Biofabrication, 4*(3).

Romagnoli, D., Boccalini, G., Bonechi, M., Biagioni, C., Fassan, P., Bertorelli, R., et al. (2018). ddSeeker: a tool for processing Bio-Rad ddSEQ single cell RNA-seq data. *BMC Genomics, 19*(1), 960.

Rudasova, M., & Masar, M. (2016). Precise determination of N-acetylcysteine in pharmaceuticals by microchip electrophoresis. *Journal of Separation Science, 39*(2), 433−439.

Sahoo, H. R., Kralj, J. G., & Jensen, K. F. (2007). Multistep continuous-flow microchemical synthesis involving multiple reactions and separations. *Angewandte Chemie International Edition, 46*(30), 5704−5708.

Sandison, M. E., Zagnoni, M., & Morgan, H. (2007). Air-exposure technique for the formation of artificial lipid bilayers in microsystems. *Langmuir, 23*(15), 8277−8284.

Santos, R., Ursu, O., Gaulton, A., Bento, A. P., Donadi, R. S., Bologa, C. G., et al. (2017). A comprehensive map of molecular drug targets. *Nature Reviews Drug Discovery, 16*(1), 19−34.

Schlicht, B., & Zagnoni, M. (2015). Droplet-interface-bilayer assays in microfluidic passive networks. *Scientific Reports, 5*, 9951.

Schuler, T., Asmus, T., Fritzsche, W., & Moller, R. (2009). Screen printing as cost-efficient fabrication method for DNA-chips with electrical readout for detection of viral DNA. *Biosensors and Bioelectronics, 24*(7), 2077−2084.

Schulze, M., & Belder, D. (2012). Poly(ethylene glycol)-coated microfluidic devices for chip electrophoresis. *Electrophoresis, 33*(2), 370−378.

See, P., Lum, J., Chen, J., & Ginhoux, F. (2018). A single-cell sequencing guide for immunologists. *Frontiers in Immunology, 9*(2425).
Service, R. F. (1995). Chemistry - radio tags speed compound synthesis. *Science, 270*(5236), 577-577.
Shankles, P. G., Millet, L. J., Aufrecht, J. A., & Retterer, S. T. (2018). Accessing microfluidics through feature-based design software for 3D printing. *PLoS One, 13*(3). e0192752-e0192752.
Shao, H., Chung, J., Lee, K., Balaj, L., Min, C., Carter, B. S., et al. (2015). Chip-based analysis of exosomal mRNA mediating drug resistance in glioblastoma. *Nature Communications, 6*, 6999.
Shembekar, N., Chaipan, C., Utharala, R., & Merten, C. A. (2016). Droplet-based microfluidics in drug discovery, transcriptomics and high-throughput molecular genetics. *Lab on a Chip, 16*(8), 1314−1331.
Sheng, W., Ogunwobi, O. O., Chen, T., Zhang, J., George, T. J., Liu, C., et al. (2014). Capture, release and culture of circulating tumor cells from pancreatic cancer patients using an enhanced mixing chip. *Lab on a Chip, 14*(1), 89−98.
Sheng, J., Zhang, L., Lei, J., & Ju, H. (2012). Fabrication of tunable microreactor with enzyme modified magnetic nanoparticles for microfluidic electrochemical detection of glucose. *Analytica Chimica Acta, 709*, 41−46.
Shen, J., Zhou, Y., Lu, T., Peng, J., Lin, Z., Huang, L., et al. (2012). An integrated chip for immunofluorescence and its application to analyze lysosomal storage disorders. *Lab on a Chip, 12*(2), 317−324.
Shiddiky, M. J. A., & Shim, Y. B. (2007). Trace analysis of DNA: Preconcentration, separation, and electrochemical detection in microchip electrophoresis using Au nanoparticles. *Analytical Chemistry, 79*(10), 3724−3733.
Shih, S. C., Yang, H., Jebrail, M. J., Fobel, R., McIntosh, N., Al-Dirbashi, O. Y., et al. (2012). Dried blood spot analysis by digital microfluidics coupled to nanoelectrospray ionization mass spectrometry. *Analytical Chemistry, 84*(8), 3731−3738.
Shin, S. R., Zhang, Y. S., Kim, D. J., Manbohi, A., Avci, H., Silvestri, A., et al. (2016). Aptamer-based microfluidic electrochemical biosensor for monitoring cell-secreted trace cardiac biomarkers. *Analytical Chemistry, 88*(20), 10019−10027.
Shiroma, L. Y., Santhiago, M., Gobbi, A. L., & Kubota, L. T. (2012). Separation and electrochemical detection of paracetamol and 4-aminophenol in a paper-based microfluidic device. *Analytica Chimica Acta, 725*, 44−50.
Shi, J., Yang, T., & Cremer, P. S. (2008). Multiplexing ligand-receptor binding measurements by chemically patterning microfluidic channels. *Analytical Chemistry, 80*(15), 6078−6084.
Sikanen, T., Aura, S., Franssila, S., Kotiaho, T., & Kostiainen, R. (2012). Microchip capillary electrophoresis-electrospray ionization-mass spectrometry of intact proteins using uncoated Ormocomp microchips. *Analytica Chimica Acta, 711*, 69−76.
Simpson, R. J., Lim, J. W., Moritz, R. L., & Mathivanan, S. (2009). Exosomes: Proteomic insights and diagnostic potential. *Expert Review of Proteomics, 6*(3), 267−283.
Sinha, N., Subedi, N., & Tel, J. (2018). Integrating immunology and microfluidics for single immune cell analysis. *Frontiers in Immunology, 9*, 2373-2373.
Smith, C. (2007). Tools for drug discovery: Tools of the trade. *Nature, 446*(7132), 219−222.
Stone, H. A., Stroock, A. D., & Ajdari, A. (2004). Engineering flows in small devices: Microfluidics toward a lab-on-a-chip. *Annual Review of Fluid Mechanics, 36*(1), 381−411.
Stott, S. L., Hsu, C. H., Tsukrov, D. I., Yu, M., Miyamoto, D. T., Waltman, B. A., et al. (2010). Isolation of circulating tumor cells using a microvortex-generating herringbone-chip. *Proceedings of the National Academy of Sciences of the United States of America, 107*(43), 18392−18397.

Sui, G., Wang, J., Lee, C. C., Lu, W., Lee, S. P., Leyton, J. V., et al. (2006). Solution-phase surface modification in intact poly(dimethylsiloxane) microfluidic channels. *Analytical Chemistry, 78*(15), 5543–5551.

Sung, J. H., & Shuler, M. L. (2009). A micro cell culture analog (microCCA) with 3-D hydrogel culture of multiple cell lines to assess metabolism-dependent cytotoxicity of anti-cancer drugs. *Lab on a Chip, 9*(10), 1385–1394.

Suzuki, H., Tabata, K., Kato-Yamada, Y., Noji, H., & Takeuchi, S. (2004). Planar lipid bilayer reconstitution with a micro-fluidic system. *Lab on a Chip, 4*(5), 502–505.

Suzuki, H., Tabata, K. V., Noji, H., & Takeuchi, S. (2006). Highly reproducible method of planar lipid bilayer reconstitution in polymethyl methacrylate microfluidic chip. *Langmuir, 22*(4), 1937–1942.

Suzuki, H., Tabata, K. V., Noji, H., & Takeuchi, S. (2007). Electrophysiological recordings of single ion channels in planar lipid bilayers using a polymethyl methacrylate microfluidic chip. *Biosensors and Bioelectronics, 22*(6), 1111–1115.

Syeda, R., Holden, M. A., Hwang, W. L., & Bayley, H. (2008). Screening blockers against a potassium channel with a droplet interface bilayer array. *Journal of the American Chemical Society, 130*(46), 15543–15548.

Szita, N., Boccazzi, P., Zhang, Z. Y., Boyle, P., Sinskey, A. J., & Jensen, K. F. (2005). Development of a multiplexed microbioreactor system for high-throughput bioprocessing. *Lab on a Chip, 5*(8), 819–826.

Talwar, S., & Lynch, J. W. (2014). Phosphorylation mediated structural and functional changes in pentameric ligand-gated ion channels: Implications for drug discovery. *The International Journal of Biochemistry and Cell Biology, 53*, 218–223.

Tang, C. K., Vaze, A., & Rusling, J. F. (2012). Fabrication of immunosensor microwell arrays from gold compact discs for detection of cancer biomarker proteins. *Lab on a Chip, 12*(2), 281–286.

Tatosian, D. A., & Shuler, M. L. (2009). A novel system for evaluation of drug mixtures for potential efficacy in treating multidrug resistant cancers. *Biotechnology and Bioengineering, 103*(1), 187–198.

Terstappen, G. C., Schlupen, C., Raggiaschi, R., & Gaviraghi, G. (2007). Target deconvolution strategies in drug discovery. *Nature Reviews Drug Discovery, 6*(11), 891–903.

Thorsen, T. A. (2004). Microfluidic tools for high-throughput screening. *Biotechniques, 36*(2), 197–199.

Timm, A. C., Shankles, P. G., Foster, C. M., Doktycz, M. J., & Retterer, S. T. (2016). Toward microfluidic reactors for cell-free protein synthesis at the point-of-care. *Small, 12*(6), 810–817.

Tsuji, Y., Kawano, R., Osaki, T., Kamiya, K., Miki, N., & Takeuchi, S. (2013). Droplet-based lipid bilayer system integrated with microfluidic channels for solution exchange. *Lab on a Chip, 13*(8), 1476–1481.

Um, E., Rha, E., Choi, S. L., Lee, S. G., & Park, J. K. (2012). Mesh-integrated microdroplet array for simultaneous merging and storage of single-cell droplets. *Lab on a Chip, 12*(9), 1594–1597.

Vaidyanathan, R., Naghibosadat, M., Rauf, S., Korbie, D., Carrascosa, L. G., Shiddiky, M. J., et al. (2014). Detecting exosomes specifically: A multiplexed device based on alternating current electrohydrodynamic induced nanoshearing. *Analytical Chemistry, 86*(22), 11125–11132.

Vaino, A. R., & Janda, K. D. (2000). Euclidean shape-encoded combinatorial chemical libraries. *Proceedings of the National Academy of Sciences of the United States of America, 97*(14), 7692–7696.

Volpatti, L., & Yetisen, A. (2014). Commercialization of microfluidic devices. *Trends in Biotechnology, 32*, 347−350.

Wadhwa, A., Foote, R. S., Shaw, R. W., & Eda, S. (2012). Bead-based microfluidic immunoassay for diagnosis of Johne's disease. *Journal of Immunological Methods, 382*(1−2), 196−202.

Wan, Y., Deng, W., Su, Y., Zhu, X., Peng, C., Hu, H., et al. (2011). Carbon nanotube-based ultrasensitive multiplexing electrochemical immunosensor for cancer biomarkers. *Biosensors and Bioelectronics, 30*(1), 93−99.

Wang, J., Bao, N., Paris, L. L., Wang, H. Y., Geahlen, R. L., & Lu, C. (2008). Detection of kinase translocation using microfluidic electroporative flow cytometry. *Analytical Chemistry, 80*(4), 1087−1093.

Wang, J., Ibanez, A., & Chatrathi, M. P. (2003). On-chip integration of enzyme and immunoassays: Simultaneous measurements of insulin and glucose. *Journal of the American Chemical Society, 125*(28), 8444−8445.

Wang, Y., Shah, P., Phillips, C., Sims, C. E., & Allbritton, N. L. (2012). Trapping cells on a stretchable microwell array for single-cell analysis. *Analytical and Bioanalytical Chemistry, 402*(3), 1065−1072.

Wang, Z., Wu, H. J., Fine, D., Schmulen, J., Hu, Y., Godin, B., et al. (2013). Ciliated micropillars for the microfluidic-based isolation of nanoscale lipid vesicles. *Lab on a Chip, 13*(15), 2879−2882.

Wang, L., Yang, P., Li, Y. X., Chen, H. Q., Li, M. G., & Luo, F. B. (2007). A flow injection chemiluminescence method for the determination of fluoroquinolone derivative using the reaction of luminol and hydrogen peroxide catalyzed by gold nanoparticles. *Talanta, 72*(3), 1066−1072.

Warren, A. D., Kwong, G. A., Wood, D. K., Lin, K. Y., & Bhatia, S. N. (2014). Point-of-care diagnostics for noncommunicable diseases using synthetic urinary biomarkers and paper microfluidics. *Proceedings of the National Academy of Sciences of the United States of America, 111*(10), 3671−3676.

Wartelle, C., Schuhmann, W., Blochl, A., & Bedioui, F. (2005). Integrated compact biocompatible hydrogel-based amperometric sensing device for easy screening of drugs involved in nitric oxide production by adherent cultured cells. *Electrochimica Acta, 50*(25−26), 4988−4994.

Weltin, A., Slotwinski, K., Kieninger, J., Moser, I., Jobst, G., Wego, M., et al. (2014). Cell culture monitoring for drug screening and cancer research: A transparent, microfluidic, multi-sensor microsystem. *Lab on a Chip, 14*(1), 138−146.

Wen, Y., Zhang, X., & Yang, S. T. (2012). Medium to high throughput screening: Microfabrication and chip-based technology. *Advances in Experimental Medicine and Biology, 745*, 181−209.

Whitesides, G. M. (2003). The 'right' size in nanobiotechnology. *Nature Biotechnology, 21*(10), 1161−1165.

Whitesides, G. M. (2006). The origins and the future of microfluidics. *Nature, 442*(7101), 368−373.

Won, S. Y., Chandra, P., Hee, T. S., & Shim, Y. B. (2013). Simultaneous detection of antibacterial sulfonamides in a microfluidic device with amperometry. *Biosensors and Bioelectronics, 39*(1), 204−209.

Woo, H. K., Sunkara, V., Park, J., Kim, T. H., Han, J. R., Kim, C. J., et al. (2017). Exodisc for rapid, size-selective, and efficient isolation and analysis of nanoscale extracellular vesicles from biological samples. *ACS Nano, 11*(2), 1360−1370.

Wu, M., Gao, F., Zhang, Y., Wang, G., Wang, Q., & Li, H. (2015). Sensitive analysis of antibiotics via hyphenation of field-amplified sample stacking with reversed-field stacking in microchip micellar electrokinetic chromatography. *Journal of Pharmaceutical and Biomedical Analysis, 103*, 91−98.

Wu, M. H., Huang, S. B., & Lee, G. B. (2010). Microfluidic cell culture systems for drug research. *Lab on a Chip, 10*(8), 939−956.

Wunsch, B. H., Smith, J. T., Gifford, S. M., Wang, C., Brink, M., Bruce, R. L., et al. (2016). Nanoscale lateral displacement arrays for the separation of exosomes and colloids down to 20 nm. *Nature Nanotechnology, 11*(11), 936−940.

Wu, N., Oakeshott, J. G., Easton, C. J., Peat, T. S., Surjadi, R., & Zhu, Y. (2011). A double-emulsion microfluidic platform for in vitro green fluorescent protein expression. *Journal of Micromechanics and Microengineering, 21*(5).

Wu, H., Wheeler, A., & Zare, R. N. (2004). Chemical cytometry on a picoliter-scale integrated microfluidic chip. *Proceedings of the National Academy of Sciences of the United States of America, 101*(35), 12809−12813.

Xia, Y., Liu, Z., Yan, S., Yin, F., Feng, X., & Liu, B.-F. (2016). Identifying multiple bacterial pathogens by loop-mediated isothermal amplification on a rotate & react slipchip. *Sensors and Actuators B: Chemical, 228*, 491−499.

Xue, Q., Wainright, A., Gangakhedkar, S., & Gibbons, I. (2001). Multiplexed enzyme assays in capillary electrophoretic single-use microfluidic devices. *Electrophoresis, 22*(18), 4000−4007.

Xu, Y., Little, M. W., & Murray, K. K. (2006). Interfacing capillary gel microfluidic chips with infrared laser desorption mass spectrometry. *Journal of the American Society for Mass Spectrometry, 17*(3), 469−474.

Yager, P., Edwards, T., Fu, E., Helton, K., Nelson, K., Tam, M. R., et al. (2006). Microfluidic diagnostic technologies for global public health. *Nature, 442*(7101), 412−418.

Yamada, M., Sugaya, S., Naganuma, Y., & Seki, M. (2012). Microfluidic synthesis of chemically and physically anisotropic hydrogel microfibers for guided cell growth and networking. *Soft Matter, 8*(11), 3122−3130.

Yan, M., Zang, D., Ge, S., Ge, L., & Yu, J. (2012). A disposable electrochemical immunosensor based on carbon screen-printed electrodes for the detection of prostate specific antigen. *Biosensors and Bioelectronics, 38*(1), 355−361.

Yeo, L. Y., Friend, J. R., McIntosh, M. P., Meeusen, E. N. T., & Morton, D. A. V. (2010). Ultrasonic nebulization platforms for pulmonary drug delivery. *Expert Opinion on Drug Delivery, 7*(6), 663−679.

Yin, H. B., Pattrick, N., Zhang, X. L., Klauke, N., Cordingley, H. C., Haswell, S. J., et al. (2008). Quantitative comparison between microfluidic and microtiter plate formats for cell-based assays. *Analytical Chemistry, 80*(1), 179−185.

Yoon, H. J., Kim, T. H., Zhang, Z., Azizi, E., Pham, T. M., Paoletti, C., et al. (2013). Sensitive capture of circulating tumour cells by functionalized graphene oxide nanosheets. *Nature Nanotechnology, 8*(10), 735−741.

Zagnoni, M. (2012). Miniaturised technologies for the development of artificial lipid bilayer systems. *Lab on a Chip, 12*(6), 1026−1039.

Zeid, A. M., Kaji, N., Nasr, J. J. M., Belal, F. F., Baba, Y., & Walash, M. I. (2017). Stacking-cyclodextrin-microchip electrokinetic chromatographic determination of gabapentinoid drugs in pharmaceutical and biological matrices. *Journal of Chromatography A, 1503*, 65−75.

Zeming, K. K., Thakor, N. V., Zhang, Y., & Chen, C. H. (2016). Real-time modulated nano-particle separation with an ultra-large dynamic range. *Lab on a Chip, 16*(1), 75−85.

Zhang, P., Crow, J., Lella, D., Zhou, X., Samuel, G., Godwin, A. K., et al. (2018). Ultrasensitive quantification of tumor mRNAs in extracellular vesicles with an integrated microfluidic digital analysis chip. *Lab on a Chip, 18*(24), 3790−3801.

Zhang, P., He, M., & Zeng, Y. (2016). Ultrasensitive microfluidic analysis of circulating exosomes using a nanostructured graphene oxide/polydopamine coating. *Lab on a Chip, 16*(16), 3033−3042.

Zhang, C., & van Noort, D. (2011). Cells in microfluidics. *Topics in Current Chemistry, 304*, 295−321.

Zhao, Z., Yang, Y., Zeng, Y., & He, M. (2016). A microfluidic ExoSearch chip for multiplexed exosome detection towards blood-based ovarian cancer diagnosis. *Lab on a Chip, 16*(3), 489−496.

Zhou, X., Cai, S., Hong, A., You, Q., Yu, P., Sheng, N., et al. (2004). Microfluidic PicoArray synthesis of oligodeoxynucleotides and simultaneous assembling of multiple DNA sequences. *Nucleic Acids Research, 32*(18), 5409−5417.

Zhu, K. Y., Leung, K. W., Ting, A. K., Wong, Z. C., Ng, W. Y., Choi, R. C., et al. (2012). Microfluidic chip based nano liquid chromatography coupled to tandem mass spectrometry for the determination of abused drugs and metabolites in human hair. *Analytical and Bioanalytical Chemistry, 402*(9), 2805−2815.

Zubair, A., Burbelo, P. D., Vincent, L. G., Iadarola, M. J., Smith, P. D., & Morgan, N. Y. (2011). Microfluidic LIPS for serum antibody detection: Demonstration of a rapid test for HSV-2 infection. *Biomedical Microdevices, 13*(6), 1053−1062.

Microfluidic devices for cell manipulation

H.O. Fatoyinbo
University of Surrey, Guildford, United Kingdom

Revised by: XiuJun (James) Li
Department of Chemistry and Biochemistry, University of Texas at El Paso, El Paso, TX, United States

Guided-reading questions:

1. How many different technologies can be used for cell manipulation in microfluidic devices? What are they?
2. What is dielectrophoresis (DEP)? Why can DEP be used for cell manipulation in a microfluidic channel?

8.1 Introduction

Since the concept of microfluidic systems in the late 1970s (Terry, Jerman, & Angell, 1979), a range of microfluidic systems incorporating physical, electrical, and bio/chemical elements performing μ-processes on biological cells have been engineered and are generally referred to as laboratories-on-a-chip (LOC) or bio-microelectromechanical (Bio-MEMS) systems (Manz, Graber, & Widmer, 1990; Reyes, Iossifidis, Auroux, & Manz, 2002).

In this chapter, some key issues relating to cell behavior within microfluidic systems, including the in vitro cellular microenvironment, flow regimes, and considerations of channel networks will be discussed. Within these systems, microscale technologies engineered to act on particles dispersed in microflows can be classified in to electrical, hydrodynamic, optical, magnetic, and acoustic mechanisms. These forces acting on particles and current technological developments for processes such as separation, characterization, focusing, and trapping will be addressed. Finally, there is an overview of these technologies applied in cancer research, i.e., flow through operations and detection, with a general outlook for future trends in applications and system development will be explored.

8.1.1 Key issues

The significant reduction in system dimensions has a positive effect on performance, as characterized by various dimensionless numbers (Table 8.1), offering increased

Table 8.1 Dimensionless numbers commonly encountered in analysis of microfluidic systems.

Name	Notation	Ratio	Description	Equation
Reynolds	Re	$\dfrac{\rho u D_h}{\mu}$	$\dfrac{\text{inertial}}{\text{viscous}}$	(8.1)
Peclet	Pe	$\dfrac{D_h u}{D}$	$\dfrac{\text{convection}}{\text{diffusion}}$	(8.2)
Weissenberg	Wi	$\tau_p \dot{\gamma}$	shear rate × relax.time	(8.3)
Deborah	De	$\dfrac{\tau_p}{\tau_{\text{flow}}}$	$\dfrac{\text{relax.time}}{\text{flowtime}}$	(8.4)
Dean	Dn	$\text{Re}\left(\dfrac{D_h}{2r}\right)^{1/2}$	$\dfrac{\text{transverse flow}}{\text{longitudinal flow}}$	(8.5)
Elasticity	El	$\dfrac{\tau_p \mu}{\rho r^2}$	$\dfrac{\text{elastic effects}}{\text{inertial effects}}$	(8.6)
Knudsen	Kn	$\dfrac{L_p}{L}$	$\dfrac{\text{mean free path}}{\text{length}}$	(8.7)
Rayleigh	Ra	$\dfrac{u_b D_h}{D}$	Pe for buoyant flow	(8.8)
Grashof	Gr	$\dfrac{\rho u_b D_h}{\mu}$	Re for buoyant flow	(8.9)
Capillary	Ca	$\dfrac{\mu u}{\gamma}$	$\dfrac{\text{viscous}}{\text{interfacial}}$	(8.10)
Weber	We	$\dfrac{\rho u^2 r}{\gamma}$	$\dfrac{\text{inertial}}{\text{surface tension}}$	(8.11)
Stokes	N_{St}	$\dfrac{\mu u}{\rho g D_h^2}$	$\dfrac{\text{viscous}}{\text{gravitational}}$	(8.12)
Poiseuille	Po	$\dfrac{r^2 \Delta P}{\mu L u}$	$\dfrac{\text{pressure}}{\text{viscous}}$	(8.13)

throughput and mass parallelization of on-chip processes such as cell culturing and cellular bioassays. To tackle various issues such as system designs for biocompatibility, efficiency, and cost effectiveness, enhanced understanding of biological processes by engineers, and approaches for standardization and system integration of modular components, an interdisciplinary approach is required among physicians, scientists, and engineers.

8.2 Microenvironment on cell integrity

The ability for biological cells to maintain their functionality in vitro is critical for accurate cell-based processes. A good understanding of cell properties and factors which can contribute to cellular damage in microfluidic systems is needed in order to fabricate systems for long-term cell survival.

8.2.1 Cell structure and function

Biological cells are the functional unit of all living organisms classified as either prokaryotic or eukaryotic (Alberts et al., 1994). Structurally, they typically consist of an internal fluidic compartment (i.e., cytoplasm) dispersed with microscopic organs—organelles (e.g., cytoskeleton, mitochondria, ribosomes, etc.) of varying functional roles that maintain both internal and external microenvironments through a range of biological activities (e.g., cellular respiration, DNA replication, biochemical signaling, and protein synthesis). A semipermeable membrane surrounding the cytoplasm consists primarily of adjacent phospholipids—a hydrophilic phosphate head and two hydrophobic glyceride tails. Phospholipid heads are in contact with either the cytoplasm or the extracellular matrix (ECM), while the diglyceride tails are repelled from the cytoplasm and ECM forming the main hydrophobic region of the two-layered structure commonly referred to as the lipid bilayer. Other biological constituents of a cell membrane include ion channels, surface receptors, aquaporins, enzymes, and hormones, which all play vital roles in regulating cellular activity and structural integrity.

8.2.2 External stresses on cells

In some cell types (e.g., bacteria, fungi), a cell wall is present representing an additional structural boundary on the outer side of the cell membrane, offering rigidity and protection to mechanical stresses. For example, the cell wall of bacteria is made of peptidoglycans of varying thicknesses (10–80 nm) essential to their survival with a high (90%) or low (10%) presence of peptidoglycan signifying its' positive or negative gram strain, respectively. Yeast cells (e.g., *S. cerevisiae*) by comparison are the most common cell model for biologists in life science research and have been extensively studied down to the molecular level revealing the cell wall as a highly adaptable organelle (Klis, Boorsma, & De Groot, 2006). It has four major functions: (1) stabilization of internal osmotic conditions, (2) physical stress protection, (3) maintaining cell shape, a precondition of morphogenesis, and (4) scaffold for proteins, limiting the permeability of the cell wall to macromolecules. Physiological adaptation to changes in environmental conditions have been attributed to membrane-spanning mechanosensors detecting perturbations in the cell wall and/or plasma membrane, initiating a *cell wall integrity* (CWI) signal transduction pathway to induce gene expression for products involved in cell wall structure and remodeling (Jendretzki, Wittland, Wilk, Straede, & Heinisch, 2011). Similar transduction pathways feature in all cells, with any mutation in their component frequently associated with a type of cancer (Kim & Choi, 2010). In general, all ECMs, including fungal and bacterial cell walls, consist of proteins and polysaccharides, highly variable between taxonomic groups, providing signaling cues to cells to adjust their biophysical properties based on the external stresses placed upon them.

Mammalian cells bathed in various isoosmotic solutions possess a selectively permeable plasma membrane ($\sim$10 nm in thickness) as their outer barrier, with a resting voltage potential ranging between -100 and $+5$ mV. This membrane potential arises due to the fact that the cytoplasm of most cells is more negative with respect to the ECM or its external microenvironment (Jackson, 2006). Concentration of potassium ions along with negatively charged proteins and phosphate ions is higher inside the cell than outside, while sodium and chloride ions are more abundant outside the cell than inside. This microenvironment condition creates an electrochemical gradient across the cell membrane which is constantly regulated by ion channels to restore homeostasis. Changes in external salinity or osmolality, detected by osmosensors, have been found to initiate signaling pathways to alter the rate of protein synthesis, cell volume, and intracellular electrolyte concentrations in response (Kultz & Chakravarty, 2001). It was shown that excessive osmotic stresses on mammalian kidney cells also caused cell cycle interference and genomic damage.

Red blood cells (RBC) are *specialized* anucleated biconcave cells, ~ 8 μm in diameter and ~ 2 μm in thickness at rest (Guido & Tomaiuolo, 2009); when transported under pressure in microfluidic channels smaller in size than the cells themselves, they are physiologically suited to a high degree of mechanical stresses and the protein spectrin makes it flexible, allowing it to deform so as to exit capillaries and enter the ECM (Barshtein, Ben-Ami, & Yedgar, 2007). Osmotic deviations to normal physiological saline conditions ($\sim 0.9\%$ NaCl) cause RBCs to swell (hemolysis) in hypotonic solutions or shrink (crenate) in hypertonic solutions. This situation, "osmotic shock," can arise with all mammalian cell types when removed from their normal environment and placed within microfluidic systems of inadequate media formulations. Phenotypic change in an endothelial cell line was found to be a result of shifts in osmolarity due to water evaporation in a microfluidic cell culture platform, while it has been reported that microsystems in which a fluid-air interface exists (e.g., electrowetting-on-dielectric (EWOD), nanovial arrays, or passive pumping) have significant evaporation and loss of fluid volume issues (Berthier, Warrick, Yu, & Beebe, 2008; Heo et al., 2006).

8.3 Microscale fluid dynamics

Many classical macroscale fluid dynamic relationships can be scaled down accurately describing flow properties of solids at the microscale. Furthermore, a range of physical phenomena present themselves which are either more influential at the microscale or absent at the macroscale. In this section, a brief overview of some important hydrodynamic theory in microchannels for biological fluids is given. For a more comprehensive analysis, refer to (Beebe, Mensing, & Walker, 2002; Gad-el-Hak, 2001; Stone, Stroock, & Ajdari, 2004; Squires & Quake, 2005).

8.3.1 Dimensionless numbers

Dimensionless numbers reduce the number of variables that describe a system, thereby reducing the amount of experimental data required to make correlations of physical phenomena to scalable systems. The most common dimensionless group in fluid dynamics is the *Reynolds number* (Re), named after Osborne Reynolds who published a series of papers describing flow in pipes (Reynolds, 1883). It represents the ratio of inertial forces to viscous forces (Eq. 8.1), where ρ is the fluid density, u is average fluid velocity, D_h is cross-sectional length of the system, and μ is the dynamic fluid viscosity.

Gravesen, Branebjerg, and Jensen (1993) indicated that flow regimes within 32 different microfluidic devices analyzed were not simply laminar or turbulent but had a transitional Reynolds number, $Re_t = 30 \times (L/D_h)$, accounting for flow development, varying as a function of entrance length (L) and the hydraulic diameter (D_h). The three regimes described were based on differences in pressure drops due to inertial forces and viscous forces. Large length to hydraulic diameter ratios, greater than 70, give $Re_t > 2300$, although since none of the microsystems operated in fully developed turbulent regimes (Re $\approx$ 4000) the value had little significance. Typically, as a system is scaled down the influences of inertial forces decreases, while viscous forces become more dominant. Thus, microflows are generally characterized as laminar, with transitions to turbulent flow (Re $\geq$ 2300) rarely developing (Brody, Yager, Goldstein, & Austin, 1996; Schulte, Bardell, & Weigl, 2002). Table 8.1 defines some other common dimensionless numbers used in describing Newtonian and non-Newtonian fluid characteristics in microfluidic systems (Ruzicka, 2008).

8.3.2 Properties of biofluids

The viscosity of a fluid is related to the fluid's resistance to motion and can be determined by relating shear force and velocity gradients in a flowing fluid as described by Newton's law of viscosity (Eq. 8.14), where shear stress (τ) is defined as force per unit area, γ is the shear rate ($= du/dy$), and μ is the proportionality constant or viscosity.

$$\tau = -\mu\dot{\gamma} \quad (8.14)$$

Biological fluids are classified as non-Newtonian fluids (i.e., pseudoplastic), and their viscosity is dependent on the shear rate and shear stress ratio of the fluid. These are characterized by the power law (Eq. 8.15), where K is the consistency index and n is the flow behavior index.

$$\tau = K(\dot{\gamma})^n \quad (8.15)$$

The parameters characterize the rheology of power law fluids; when $n = 1$, the fluid type is Newtonian; $n > 1$ corresponds to dilatants; and $n < 1$ corresponds to pseudoplastics with an apparent viscosity (μ_a) that increases or decreases, respectively, with increasing shear rate. Fahraeus and Lindqvist (1931) first reported the dependence of hematocrit ($\sim$40% v/v) and relative apparent viscosity on tube radius. Subsequently, characterizing the flow behavior of RBCs in microcapillaries indicated that physical parameters such as velocity and thickness of suspending medium separating tube wall from the cell (dependent on pressure drop, capillary diameter, and RBC volume fraction) all influence the RBC's shape deformation in flow (Zharov, Galanzha, Menyaev, & Tuchin, 2006).

Media solutions bathing cells typically consist of ions, proteins, carbohydrates, gases, etc., making fluid viscosities and conductivities ($\sigma_m = \sim 1.5$ S/m) extremely high. Experiments conducted in microfluidic systems for cell manipulation tend to deviate away from the ideal suspension mixture in favor of less viscous, Newtonian solutions (i.e., aqueous solutions), ensuring (1) resistance to fluid flow and (2) saturation of technological limits are minimized. As microfluidic networks and on-chip mixing/dilutions of fluids become more complex and deviations in hydrodynamic resistance as a result of viscosity changes manifest (Pipe & McKinley, 2009), considerations of microfluidic geometries, interfaces, and integrated components need to be factored into the design process from the outset.

8.3.3 Flow dynamics in microchannels

Common methods for flow actuation within microsystems are pressure or electrokinetically driven (Stroock & Whitesides, 2003; Trietsch, Hankemeier, & van der Linden, 2011). For an incompressible fluid, the equivalent of Newton's second law ($F = ma$) can be represented by the Navier–Stokes equation (Eq. 8.16) where u is the velocity field (m/s), P is pressure (Pa), and F_b represents external body forces acting on the bulk fluid, per unit volume (e.g., ρg, magnetic, electric potential, etc.).

$$-\nabla P + \mu \nabla^2 u + F_b = \underbrace{\rho \frac{\partial u}{\partial t}}_{\text{local}} + \underbrace{\rho u \cdot \nabla u}_{\text{convective}} \qquad (8.16)$$

Microflows predominantly fall within the laminar region (Re < 1), so the nonlinear convective term in Eq. (8.16) can be neglected, along with the body forces, leaving the Stokes equation for predictable linear flow in a channel (White, 1994).

$$\rho \frac{\partial u}{\partial t} = -\nabla P + \mu \nabla^2 u \qquad (8.17)$$

Applying the mass continuity equation for incompressible fluid flow, i.e., $\nabla \cdot u = 0$, we get a linear equation in which flow is determined by pressure at low Re, with variation in pressure in the X-direction of the channel only (Brody et al., 1996).

$$\mu \nabla^2 u = \frac{dP}{dX} \qquad (8.18)$$

Steady-state flow away from the microchannel entrance, where height (h) << width (w) and length (l), is axial across the channel height (Fig. 8.1). Applying no-slip boundary conditions (i.e., $u = 0$), flow under pressure is described by Eq. (8.19). Known as Poiseuille profile flow, it has a constant negative curvature and a maximum velocity ($\mu_{\max}$) at $y = 0$.

$$u = -\frac{dP}{dx} \frac{h^2}{2\mu} \left(1 - \frac{y^2}{h^2}\right) \qquad (8.19)$$

Microfluidic devices for cell manipulation

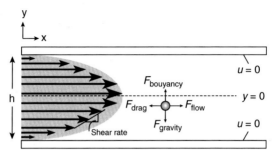

Figure 8.1 Parabolic flow profile within a microfluidic channel, where $h \ll w$. The gradient of the profile shows the shear rate, proportional to the fluid's viscosity influencing the general forces acting on a spherical particle within the flow field.

For circular channels, the average velocity, $\bar{u} = Q/A$, where Q is volumetric flow rate (m³/s) and A is cross-sectional area of the channel (m²), is often taken. Assuming no-slip conditions at the tube wall, i.e., $r = 0$ and $u = 0$, for fully developed laminar parabolic flow with a maximum velocity found at the center, the volumetric flow rate is,

$$Q = \frac{1}{2} u_{max} \pi R^2 = \frac{\pi R^4}{8\mu} \left[-\frac{d}{dX}(P + \rho g z) \right] \quad (8.20)$$

Eq. (8.20) describes Hagen–Poiseuille flow, allowing for a fluid's resistance (R_H) to flow to be described in terms of pressure drop (ΔP) for circular channels, assuming $z = 0$, i.e., horizontal channel.

$$\Delta P = \frac{8\mu L Q}{\pi R^4} = Q R_H \quad (8.21)$$

Rectangular microchannels with aspect ratios ($\alpha = w/h$) where the channel width is larger than the height (i.e., $w > h$) have flows characterized as Hele-Shaw flow (Eq. 8.22). The flow profile remains parabolic along h, but as α increases, the average velocity over the channel width becomes increasingly plug-like.

$$\Delta P = \frac{12\mu L Q}{w h^3} = Q R_H \quad (8.22)$$

For microchannels where $w < h$, Eq. (8.22) is modified to Eq. (8.23), which gives a less than 0.3% error for $\alpha < 1$ and Re < 1000 (Beebe et al., 2002; Cornish, 1928; Fuerstman et al., 2007).

$$\Delta P = \frac{12\mu L Q}{w h^3} \times \left[1 - \frac{0.63 h}{w} \tanh\left(\frac{\pi w}{2h}\right) \right]^{-1} \quad (8.23)$$

If α is unity, for a given cross-sectional area the maximum flow for a given pressure difference will exist and can be approximated to:

$$\Delta P = \frac{32\mu L Q}{h^4} \tag{8.24}$$

From Eqs. (8.21)—(8.24) we can see that pressure drops in microfluidic systems are influenced by (1) the volumetric flow rate and (2) the fluid's resistance to flow, quantities influenced by the geometry of the microchannel.

8.3.4 System design and operation

Microfluidic flow behaviors can affect cell manipulation and shear stress (Shen, Li, & Li, 2014). Computer-aided simulation (i.e., computational fluid dynamics, CFD) physical phenomena is a useful tool in design optimization of microfluidic devices (Shen et al., 2014; Shen, Li, Liu, & Li, 2017), though experimental evaluation is still performed using test particles such as commercially available nano- or micropolystyrene beads. Rapid prototyping for inexpensive microfluidic systems through techniques such as soft lithography (Whitesides, Ostuni, Takayama, Jiang, & Ingber, 2001; Zhao, Xia, & Whitesides, 1997), multilayer soft lithography (Quake & Scherer, 2000; Unger, Chou, Thorsen, Scherer, & Quake, 2000), cofabrication of multicomponent microsystems (Siegel et al., 2009), and maskless writing (Do, Zhang, & Klapperich, 2011) have had a significant impact in fabricating complex but cheap microfluidic systems, integrated with various elements required to manipulate particles.

8.3.4.1 Complex microfluidic networks

In pressure-driven laminar flow, the hydraulic-electric circuit analogy concept has been reported as a useful method for analyzing and designing complex microfluidic network systems (i.e., multiple combining or branching microchannels at a node), based solely on channel dimensions and geometry (Kim, Chesler, & Beebe, 2006; Oh, Lee, Ahn, & Furlani, 2012). The relationship between voltage, current, resistance, and conductor length in electrical circuits can be easily translated to microfluidic circuits between pressure, flow, hydraulic resistance, and channel length, respectively. In systems where fluid mixing is relatively slow and the Pe number is quite large, a boundary between the streams will develop. Fig. 8.2(a) shows a flow fraction-dependent microfluidic network, where the flow ratio of two incoming streams (Q_1 and Q_2) can be used to predict the boundary width (w) of a fully developed laminar flow a distance ($l \approx w \times \text{Re}$) away from the channel node, possessing a parabolic velocity flow profile. The fractional areas (S_1, S_2) of the parabolic profile are proportional to the volumetric flow rate of each incoming stream. In high aspect ratio microchannels, the pressure-driven flow velocity is independent of the position across the channel width, with an approximation to the boundary width realized from analysis of the ratio of incoming or outgoing volumetric flow rates (Eq. 8.25) as depicted in Fig. 8.2(b). Fig. 8.2(c) shows the equivalent electric circuit of Fig. 8.2(a).

Microfluidic devices for cell manipulation

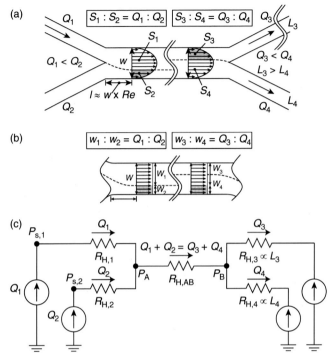

Figure 8.2 Schematic of a typical flow fraction-dependent microfluidic network when $Q_1 > Q_2$ and $Q_3 < Q_4$. There exists a boundary (*dotted lines*) between the two incoming streams or the two outgoing streams. (a) 2D model (e.g., parabolic flow profile) to estimate the boundary width. The partial areas of the parabola (S_1, and S_2, or S_3 and S_4) are proportional to the volumetric flow rates of each stream (Q_1 and Q_2, or Q_3 and Q_4). (b) 1D model (e.g., flat flow profile) to estimate the boundary width. With this rough approximation, the ratio of the boundary widths of the two incoming streams ($w_1{:}w_2$) or that of the two outgoing streams ($w_3{:}w_4$) can be estimated with the volumetric flow rate ratio of the input streams ($Q_1{:}Q_2$) or that of the output streams ($Q_3{:}Q_4$), respectively. (c) Equivalent electric circuit.
Reproduced from Oh et al. (2012), with permission of The Royal Society of Chemistry.

$$\frac{w_1}{w_2} = \frac{Q_1}{Q_2} \quad \text{or} \quad \frac{w_3}{w_4} = \frac{Q_3}{Q_4} \tag{8.25}$$

This strategy is ideally suited to aqueous solutions where tuneable concentration gradients of chemical and biochemical stimuli can be generated for cell-based studies (Sun, Wang, & Jiang, 2008). As fluid viscosity increases, hydraulic resistance of a microchannel is affected, and stream combinations at a node of differing viscosity fluids result in unpredictable flow rates and concentration profiles. Design complexity and geometric dimensions of microfluidic networks for on-chip sample preparation or cell transportation are limited and dependent on process, cell size, and cell concentration to minimize clogging. For instance, hydrodynamic filtration (HDF) setups with multiple branching microchannels of variable sizes were designed to separate highly dilute concentrations (0.3% v/v) of RBCs and leukocytes (Matsuda, Yamada, & Seki, 2011; Takagi, Yamada, Yasuda, & Seki, 2005; Yamada & Seki, 2005). Hydrodynamic focusing of particles and cells has been shown using parallel flow from two inlet buffer streams sandwiching a central stream of particles, island structures in channels to split flows, and by recombining split flows to main channels for sheath flow (Aoki, Yamada, Yasuda, & Seki, 2009; Di Carlo, Irimia, Tompkins, & Toner, 2007; Lee, Kim, Ahn, Kang, & Oh, 2009). Furthermore, PDMS (polydimethylsiloxane), a commonly used material for microfluidic channels, has a low elastic modulus, and large increases in ΔP along a microfluidic channel have resulted in channel deformations making flow rates in complex networks unpredictable (Gervais, El-Ali, Gunther, & Jensen, 2006; Sollier, Murray, Maoddi, & Di Carlo, 2011).

8.3.4.2 Bubble extraction

Gas bubble formation in microfluidic devices is regularly encountered and can cause unequal flow distribution or even inhibit flow through blockage. It arises from various sources including the device interfacing with the other modules, from the surface chemistry of the device itself, or from dead volumes upstream of fluidic channels. Elevated wall shear stresses occurring at the interfaces of bubbles and cells significantly affect the biological function of cells, causing detachment or cell membrane rupture. To enable normal device operation, strategies for eliminating gas progression have been devised and include active bubble trap and debubbler on a two-layer PDMS substrate (Skelley & Voldman, 2008) and long-term stable integrated bubble traps (IBT) for use in 10 day mammalian culturing (Zheng, Wang, Zhang, & Jiang, 2010). Lochovsky et al. recently described an in-plane bubble trap, compatible with soft lithography fabrication, where gas removal rates for nitrogen at $\Delta P = 94.6$ kPa was 0.144 µL/min and when multiple traps are operated in parallel achieved a rate of 0.6 µL/min, significantly faster and more reliable than previously reported strategies (Lochovsky, Yasotharan, & Gunther, 2012).

8.4 Manipulation technologies

Biological cells are dielectric materials with variations in electrophysiological, biophysical, and optical properties. Technologies utilizing these properties can achieve high accuracy and precision in controlling and selecting particles, while in some cases competing against hydrodynamic forces. Manipulation processes include characterization, sorting, separation, trapping, patterning, concentrating, or focusing cells in continuous flow or batch operations. As most of the technologies to be discussed have a form of "heritage" and some similarities based on field flow fractionation (FFF) operation, it is worthwhile considering this technique in a class of its own.

8.4.1 Field flow fractionation

First proposed in the 1960s, FFF is a class of "soft impact" elution techniques employed mainly to separate heterogeneous mixtures of supramolecules, proteins,

Microfluidic devices for cell manipulation

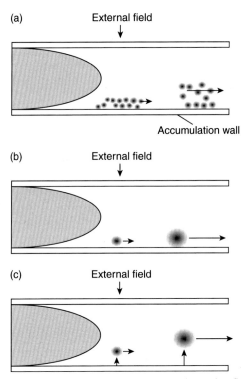

Figure 8.3 Elution modes of field flow fractionation (FFF) in a microfluidic channel with an external field acting perpendicular to the parabolic flow. (a) Normal (Brownian) FFF mode operation in which clouds of submicron particles different distances away from the accumulation wall in the parabolic flow experience different velocities. (b) Steric FFF mode separation of particles. (c) Hyperlayer FFF mode separation.

and bioparticles (<100 μm dia.) within laminar microfluidic flows (Caldwell, Cheng, Hradecky, & Giddings, 1984; Giddings, 1968). The basic principle is based on differential flow displacement along the axis of flow due to an external force field, $|F|$, applied perpendicular to the parabolic flow as in Fig. 8.3 (Giddings, 1993). Based on differences in particle mobility (i.e., physical characteristics), the field controls the equilibrium position of the particle into localized bands of laminar streamlines, varying in velocity as a function of channel height. Hence, particles positioned closest to the channel wall (the accumulation wall) are eluted slowest ($u_{wall} = 0$), while particles at the center of the channel are eluted fastest ($u_{center} = u_{max}$), resulting in different retention times. The rates at which particles move through a microchannel are governed by the retention equation, applicable to all FFF systems:

$$R = 6\lambda \left[\coth\left(\frac{1}{2\lambda}\right) - 2\lambda \right] \tag{8.26}$$

where R is the retention ratio, which for small values of λ reduces to $R = 6\lambda$. The nondimensional parameter λ is determined by the physical properties of the retained particle (Eq. 8.27), where U is the field induced velocity, D is the diffusion coefficient of the submicron particle, T is absolute temperature, k is the Boltzmann constant, and h is the channel height (Giddings, 1993).

$$\lambda = \frac{D}{Uh} = \frac{kT}{|F|h} \qquad (8.27)$$

Influences of diffusion in FFF separation mechanisms are negligible when cells or microorganisms are the object of manipulation, with retention times influenced by size, shape, density, rigidity, and surface features leading to larger bioparticles being eluted faster than smaller ones (Roda et al., 2009). Commonly referred to as "steric" and "hyperlayer" (Fig. 8.3(b) and (c)) elution modes (Chianea, Assidjo, & Cardot, 2000; Giddings & Myers, 1978), FFF mechanisms typically applied to cell manipulation include, in their broadest form, centrifugal sedimentation FFF (SdFFF) or gravitational FFF (GrFFF), flow FFF (FlFFF or F4), and electrical FFF (ElFFF) (Giddings, 1993; Kowalkowski, Buszewski, Cantado, & Dondi, 2006). Modification of the retention ratio in Eq. (8.26) takes into consideration steric exclusion of particles of radius r, where $\alpha = r/w$ from the accumulation wall, in which a reversal of the retention order of particles becomes apparent due to large particles protruding out into the flow streams (Myers & Giddings, 1982).

$$R = 6\lambda(\alpha - \alpha^2) + 6\lambda(1 - 2\alpha)\left[\coth\frac{1-2\alpha}{2\lambda} - \frac{2\lambda}{1-2\alpha}\right] \qquad (8.28)$$

For spherical particles in steric FFF mode, the factor γ accounts for particle migration issues such as hydrodynamic lift forces which increase with shear rate and increased particle diameter. Eq. (8.28) has been further simplified due to the small values of λ and α normally presented, giving a sterically controlled retention ratio of (Giddings, Chen, Wahlund, & Myers, 1987):

$$R = 6\gamma\alpha \qquad (8.29)$$

The main driving forces and subtypes applicable to FFF cell manipulation are found in Table 8.2.

8.4.2 Hydrodynamic mechanisms

8.4.2.1 Deterministic physical interactions

Deterministic lateral displacement (DLD) uses periodic arrays of asymmetric microposts of different geometries to reduce multipath zone broadening of varying sized particles (Huang, Cox, Austin, & Sturm, 2004). Processes such as separation, steering, refracting, and focusing have been demonstrated (Morton et al., 2008; Loutherback et al., 2010).

Table 8.2 Broad categorization of field flow fractionation (FFF) subtypes associated with cell manipulation.

External force	FFF subtypes	References
Cross flow (Fl)	Flow FFF (FlFFF), Hollow Fiber FlFFF, Symmetrical FlFFF (SF4), Asymmetric FlFFF (AF4)	Schmid et al. (2018)
Sedimentation (Sd)	Sedimentation FFF (SdFFF), Centrifugal SdFFF, Gravitational (GrFFF)	Roda et al. (2009a)
Electrical (El)	Electrical FFF (ElFFF), Cyclic ElFFF, Dielectrophoretic (DEP-FFF)	Kantak et al. (2006)

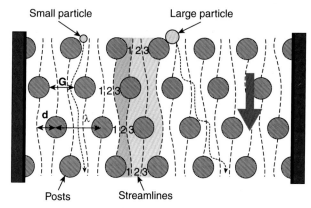

Figure 8.4 Schematic illustrating the separation by deterministic lateral displacement in an array of microposts, with an example row shift fraction of one-third. This shift creates three equal flux streamlines. The *dashed lines* are the boundaries between the streamlines, which are assigned an index in the gaps between the posts. Paths of particles both smaller and larger than the critical threshold are depicted with by their associated line paths. Small particles stay within a flow stream and large particles are displaced at each obstacle. G is the clear spacing between the gap, λ is the center-to-center postseparation, and d is the relative shift of the postcenters in adjacent rows.
Reproduced from Davis et al. (2006). Copyright 2006 National Academy of Sciences, USA.

Each row of the micropost array is shifted horizontally with respect to the previous row by a distance (d), which can be a fraction of the center-to-center distance (λ) of the micropost as in Fig. 8.4. As laminar fluid flows through the gap of adjacent microposts, it bifurcates around the micropost it meets in the next row. The gap is typically larger than the particles to avoid clogging, and based on the critical hydrodynamic diameter (D_c) of the particle, all similar sized particles follow equivalent migration paths characterized by either the zigzag mode or displacement mode. Similar to the way light rays can be redirected at the interfaces of differing materials (Fig. 8.5(a)), differences in the DLD of cells exists when compared to photons. In the zigzag mode, particles flow in

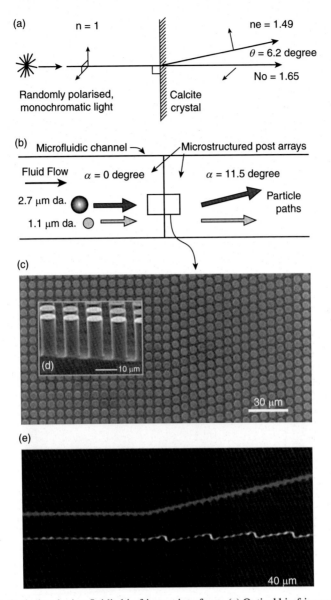

Figure 8.5 Optical and microfluidic birefringent interfaces. (a) Optical birefringence in a calcite crystal: normally incident, randomly polarized light, incident on the anisotropic crystal splits into two polarization dependent paths. Remarkably, the extraordinary ray, whose polarization is parallel to the calcite optical axis, is deflected away from the normal. (b) Schematic of particle trajectories at the interface between a neutral region and a microfluidic metamaterial element. Particles larger than a critical size follow the array asymmetry, whereas smaller particle follow the fluid flow. (c) The simplest metamaterial element is an asymmetric array of posts tilted at an angle—relative to the channel walls and bulk fluid flow. Shown is a top-view scanning electron micrograph (SEM) of the interface between a neutral array ($\alpha = 0$ degrees) and an array with array angle $\alpha = 11.3$ degrees (the gap $G = 4$ μm and postpitch $\lambda = 11$ μm are the same for both sides). (d) Cross-sectional SEM image showing the microfabricated post array. (e) Equivalent microfluidic birefringence based on particle size showing the time trace of a 2.7-μm red fluorescent (top stream) transiting the interface and being deflected from the normal. Smaller, 1.1-μm beads (bottom) stream are not deflected at the interface.
Reproduced from Morton et al. (2008). Copyright 2008 National Academy of Sciences, USA.

a cyclic procession, exiting and entering streamline lanes such as the bottom stream in Fig. 8.5(e), while in displacement mode (top stream of Fig. 8.5(e)) particles with sizes greater than D_c move at an angle determined by the ratio of micropost offset to the row-to-row spacing ($\varepsilon = d/\lambda$) (Inglis, Davis, Austin, & Sturm, 2006). As this separation technology relies on a deterministic process, faster flow rates improve the performance of the device limiting sporadic processes such as diffusional mixing. Two dimensionless numbers used to analyze fluid and particle motion in these microsystems are the Péclet number (Pe) of the particle, where $\varepsilon\lambda$ is the local characteristic length of the post where diffusion competes with fluid transport (i.e., advection), and the Reynolds number, where the traditional cross-sectional length is replaced with a characteristic length over which the fluid changes its direction. If Pe > 1, the diffusion rate is less than the advection rate at the local scale, indicating smaller particles follow the streamline path created by the posts and larger particles experience a deterministic lateral migration. Design parameters such as gap size and shift fraction e, influence D_c, and when varied in successive regions of arrays ("chirped" or "cascaded"), the dynamic range of the device is increased (Davis et al., 2006; Inglis et al., 2008).

8.4.2.2 Inertial migration

The phenomena of particle migration in Poiseuille flow macroscale and microscale systems have been observed and described (Choi, Seo, & Lee, 2011; Kim & Yoo, 2008; Segre & Silberberg, 1961, 1962). Characteristics such as particle distribution and equilibrium position have been reported to be influenced by parameters such as the channel diameter (D_h) to particle diameter (d_p) ratio, the particle volume fraction, particle density, and flow velocity (Kim & Yoo, 2012).

Particles in fluid flow are subjected to shear forces (i.e., drag) and normal forces (i.e., lift) from bound fluidic elements. Dominant inertial lift forces direct particles laterally across streamlines to equilibrium positions within microchannels, particularly when microfluidic Re is in the range of 1–100 and particle Re (Re_p) is of the order of 1, as in Eq. (8.30), where is the maximum fluid velocity and assuming $d_p/D_h \ll 1$.

$$\text{Re}_p = \frac{\rho u_{\max} d_p}{\mu D_h} = \text{Re}\left(\frac{d_p}{D_h}\right)^2 \tag{8.30}$$

Microchannel cross-sectional position influences particle migration, with randomly distributed particles seen to concentrate into narrow bands, so-called Segre and Silberberg annulus, within circular pipes (Fig. 8.6(a)). In square microchannels, particles laterally focus to equilibrium positions and subsequently accumulate near the center of each channel wall face (Fig. 8.6(b)) in a pseudo Segre and Silberberg annulus (Bhagat, Kuntaegowdanahalli, & Papautsky, 2008b; Di Carlo, 2009). Lift forces (F_L) exerted on particles in flow, scales with the intrinsic properties of the fluid, Re_p squared and the dimensionless lift coefficient f_L which is a function of the channel Re and particle position within the channel, such that at equilibrium $f_L = 0$ (Asmolov, 1999; Ho & Leal, 1974; Schonberg & Hinch, 1989).

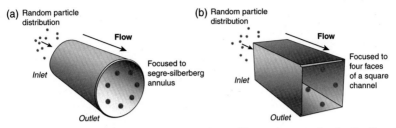

Figure 8.6 (a) In a cylindrical pipe, at moderate Reynolds numbers, randomly distributed particles are known to focus to an annulus located between the center and wall of the pipe. (b) In square channels, following the symmetry of the system, particles instead focus to four equilibrium regions centered at the faces of the channels for dilute suspensions of particles flowing at moderate Reynolds numbers.
Reproduced from Di Carlo (2009), with permission of The Royal Society of Chemistry.

$$F_L = \frac{f_L \rho U_m^2 d_p^4}{D_h^2} \tag{8.31}$$

Equilibrium positions or focusing reached by dilute suspensions of radially migrating spherical particles in microflows were attributed to the balancing of two major lateral forces: (1) inertial lift forces induced by shear-gradient fluid flow directs particles at the center region toward the channel wall and (2) wall repulsion forces at the channel wall region pushes particles toward the centerline of the fluid flow (Ho & Leal, 1974). Using Stokes' law ($F_{\text{drag}} = 3\pi\mu d_p u_p$), an expression for the particle migration velocity (u_p) from the centerline due to lift can be approximated, where $f_L = 0.5$:

$$u_P = \frac{F_L}{F_{\text{drag}}} = \frac{4\rho u_{\max}^2 d_p^3}{3\pi\mu D_h^2} f_L \tag{8.32}$$

The microchannel length (L) required for a particle to completely migrate to its equilibrium position can be calculated from Eq. (8.33), where L_p is the maximum required migration distance.

$$L = \frac{u_{\max} L_p}{U_p} = \frac{3\pi\mu D_h^2 L_p}{2\rho u_{\max} d_p^3 f_L} \tag{8.33}$$

8.4.2.3 Curved channels

Curved microchannels have been shown to have a secondary inertial effect on fluids which in turn influences particle equilibrium positions and focusing capabilities (Fig. 8.7(a–d)). The high momentum fluid at the channel center displaces the lower momentum fluid at the wall surface, causing counter-rotating vortices perpendicular to primary flow and additional drag forces on the particle from this secondary flow. The flow is characterized by two dimensionless numbers, namely Dean number and

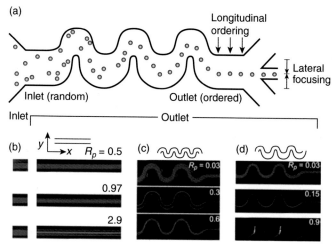

Figure 8.7 Inertial self-ordering. (a) Schematic drawing of the inertial ordering process. After flowing through a channel of a particular symmetry, precise ordering of initially scattered particles is observed both longitudinally along the direction of flow and laterally across the channel. (b) Top-down views of fluorescent streak images of flowing 9-μm-diameter particles in a square channel (50 μm) filled with water (density $\rho = 1.00$ g/mL and dynamic viscosity $\mu = 10^{-3}$ Pa s). Flow is from left to right. The inlet region is shown at the left, where the particles are initially uniformly distributed within the fluid. Longer images show the outlet 3 cm downstream for the channel Reynolds number $R_c = 15$, 30, or 90 (particle Reynolds number $R_p = 0.48, 0.97$, or 2.9). Focusing of particles into four single streamlines is observed. From above, this appears as three lines with double the intensity in the middle streak line. (c) For a symmetric curving channel, the symmetry of the system reduces focusing to two streams. Above a critical Dean number (De) focusing is perturbed. (d) For an asymmetric curving system, focusing down to a single stream is favored. Focusing is again more complex as De increases.
Reproduced from Di Carlo et al. (2007). Copyright 2008 National Academy of Sciences, USA.

the curvature ratio, $\delta = D_h/2r$ (Bhagat, Kuntaegowdanahalli, & Papautsky, 2008a). Particle focusing based on curved geometries is independent of particle density, though the ratio of Dean drag, and inertial lift is a key parameter in describing how particles behave in separation and concentration processes (Di Carlo et al., 2007; Gossett & Di Carlo, 2009).

8.4.2.4 Hydrodynamic filtering and microfluidic networks

HDF uses multiple side channels branching off a main microfluidic channel to concentrate and classify heterogeneously sized particles introduced at the system inlet (Yamada & Seki, 2005). As a particle's center cannot be present near the channel sidewall at a length equivalent to the particle radius (r_p), flow rates distributed into the side channels at a sufficiently low rate will never let particles greater than a specific diameter into the these side channels, even when the cross-sectional size of the side channel

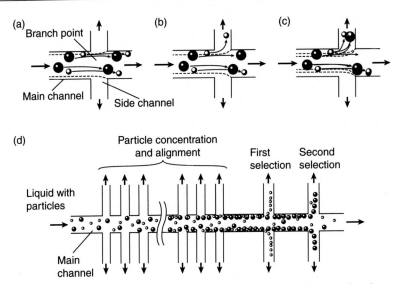

Figure 8.8 Principle of hydrodynamic filtration (a)–(c). Schematic diagrams showing particle behavior at a branch point; (a) the relative flow rates distributed into side channels are low, (b) medium, and (c) high. *Broken lines* show the virtual boundaries of the flows distributed into side and main channels. (d) Schematic diagram showing particle concentration and alignment in a microchannel having multiple branch points and side channels.
Reproduced from Yamada et al. (2005), with permission of The Royal Society of Chemistry.

is greater than the particle or the particle is flowing very close to the sidewall as depicted in Fig. 8.8(a). As fractions of pure fluid flow into upstream side channels, the concentration of particles increases downstream of the main channel, resulting in particle alignment along the sidewalls (Fig. 8.8(d)). By increasing the relative flow rates in the downstream side channels, aligned particles are collected according to size in a stepwise fashion.

The principle of pinch flow fractionation (PFF) is closely related to HDF (Nakashima, Yamada, & Seki, 2004; Yamada, Nakashima, & Seki, 2004). Two fluidic inlet streams, one with particles and one without, at differing flow rates, meet at a "pinch segment" (Fig. 8.9(a)) at which point the particle-rich fluid is focused onto one sidewall aligning particles in its stream, similar to flow FFF. Different sized particles assume characteristic positions away from the sidewall in the pinch segment, with smaller particles closest to the wall. Downstream of the pinch segment, a broadening of the microchannel (broad segment) occurs and the slight differences in positions are amplified in the spreading flow profile. The ratio of inlet flow rates and microchannel geometries affects separation efficiencies. Takagi et al. (2005) introduced asymmetric pinched flow fractionation (AsPFF) as an improvement to PFF in which multiple branching channels downstream of the pinch segment were (Fig. 8.9(b)). This offered the advantage of reduced system clogging and enhanced separation of particles through controlled flow resistance into the branched channels, achieved by adjusting channel dimensions.

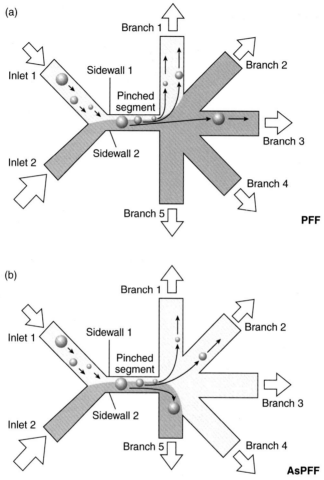

Figure 8.9 Schematic diagrams of particle separation: (a) is pinch flow fractionation (PFF) and (b) is asymmetric pinch flow fractionation (AsPFF). Liquid containing particles is light-colored, and liquid without particles is dark-colored. The size of an *arrow* represents the flow rate. In PFF, identical branch channels are arranged, and liquid flow in the pinched segment is uniformly distributed. Therefore, Branch 4 and Branch 5 are never used, and the difference in effluent positions of particles is small. In AsPFF, one branch channel (drain channel) is designed to be short and/or broad, and liquid flow is asymmetrically distributed. So all the branch channels are effectively used, and the difference in effluent positions becomes large compared with PFF.
Reproduced from Tagaki et al. (2005), with permission of The Royal Society of Chemistry.

8.4.2.5 Biomimetics

Naturally occurring hemodynamic phenomena found in microcirculatory systems, such as Zweifach−Fung (bifurcation law), margination, and plasma skimming, has been mimicked for designing microfluidic devices for blood cell separation and enrichment

(Kersaudy-Kerhoas, Dhariwal, Desmulliez, & Jouvet, 2010). RBCs tend to concentrate at the center of a blood vessel under flow, which has two consequences: (1) plasma skimming between two asymmetrical daughter vessels reduces RBC fraction in one vessel, and (2) leukocyte margination to the vessel sidewalls as a result of RBC and leukocyte collisions. This biomimetic approach of margination was demonstrated in a microfluidic system for leukocyte enrichment from blood, resulting in a 34-fold enrichment (Shevkoplyas, Yoshida, Munn, & Bitensky, 2005), while the use of multiple triangular expansions upstream (Fig. 8.10) mimicking postcapillary venules for nucleated cell margination from RBC gave a 45.75-fold enrichment (Jain & Munn, 2011). A recent demonstration of this technique was based on the blood condition sepsis where *E. coli* and *S. cerevisiae*, along with inflammatory cellular components, were removed from blood in a two stage single pass device at ~1 mL/h per channel, with realistic potential for multiplexing or parallelization for higher throughput (Hou et al., 2012).

8.4.2.6 Hydrophoresis and microstructure inclusions

Hydrophoresis is a technique whereby particles in a suspension are transported under the influence of a microstructure-induced pressure field, as illustrated in Fig. 8.11

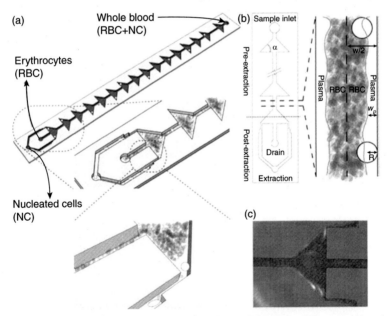

Figure 8.10 Design of nucleated cell separation unit. (a) Schematic of the separation device. The device is made using polydimethylsiloxane (PDMS) soft lithography. (b) Illustration of working principle. Whole blood enters the device at the inlet port. Nucleated cell margination is encouraged in the preextraction stage of the device. With the nucleated cells (NCs) segregated near the wall, they can then be collected into the extraction channels. Pure RBCs are also collected through the central drain channel. (c) A snapshot of the extraction region of the device. Labeled NCs can be seen entering the extraction channels at top and bottom. Reproduced from Jain and Munn (2011), with permission of The Royal Society of Chemistry.

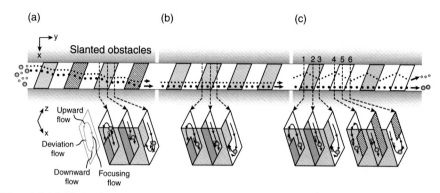

Figure 8.11 Hydrophoretic separation principle. *Shaded and lined areas* denote lower and upper slanted obstacles, respectively. A flow direction is along the *y*-axis. (a–c) Top-viewing and cross-sectional schematic diagrams of the slanted obstacles. (a) The slanted obstacles drive lateral flows across the *x*-axis by which particles are pushed to a sidewall. (b) The focused particles flow clockwise following the rotating flows generated by the bottom-side obstacles and move to the bottom of a channel. (c) The large particle is located in the area where there is no lateral pressure gradients and stays in the focused position. On the other hand, the small particle is exposed to lateral pressure gradients along the *x*-axis and deviates from its focused position.
Reproduced from Choi and Park (2007), with permission of The Royal Society of Chemistry.

(Choi & Park, 2007; Choi, Song, Choi, & Park, 2007). Stroock, Dertinger, Whitesides, and Ajdari (2002) analytically quantified the anisotropic effect oblique grooved patterns within a microchannel wall had on pressure-driven flows resulting in the movement of fluid near the structure surface in the groove direction. Fluid transverses the microchannel, interacting with opposing transverse pressure gradients creating a recirculating flow component in the cross section in addition to the principal Poiseuille flow component, with a net effect of generating helical streamlines (Stroock & Whitesides, 2003). Although this was exploited for fluid mixing, slanted obstacles on the top and bottom of a microfluidic channel were used to create transverse flows perpendicular to the main flow for size-based separation of microbeads, RBC, and microbead sheathless focusing (Choi & Park, 2007; Choi, Song, Choi, & Park, 2008). Different microstructures were reported for single-cell capture and biochemical analysis (Li & Li, 2014; Shen et al., 2014).

8.4.2.7 Hydrodynamic devices

Inertial focusing and lift hydrodynamics within asymmetric microchannels have been used to filter platelets from dilute blood cells (Di Carlo, Edd, Irimia, Tompkins, & Toner, 2008; Geislinger, Eggart, Ller, Schmid, & Franke, 2012) and isolate bacteria from human RBC at 10^8 cells/mL with >99% purity with an upper limit flow rate of 18 μL/min (Wu, Willing, Bjerketorp, Jansson, & Hjort, 2009). Kuntaegowdanahalli, Bhagat, Kumar, and Papautsky (2009) used a five-loop spiral microchannel device, as in Fig. 8.12, combining the effects of inertial and Dean

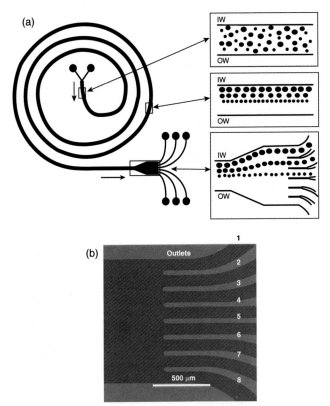

Figure 8.12 (a) Schematic of the spiral microparticle separator. The randomly dispersed particles equilibrate at different equilibrium positions along the inner wall (IW) of the spiral microchannel under the influence of lift and drag. Separation between individual particle streams is enhanced by opening the spiral channel into a wider straight channel before extracting the individual streams using a multiple outlet design. (b) The eight outlet channels of the poly(methyl methacrylate) (PMMA)-based microfluidic spiral device.
Adapted from Kuntaegowdanahalli et al. (2009), with permission from The Royal Society of Chemistry.

drag forces to focus and separate size varying polystyrene beads into separate outlet channels and subsequently neuroblastomas from glioma cells at a throughput of 1×10^6 cells/min with 80% efficiency and >90% viability. This was further adapted for sorting (~15×10^6 cells/h) of asynchronous mammalian cell lines and human mesenchymal stem cells (hMSCs) based on their phase in their cell cycle with a >95% viability (Lee et al., 2011).

HDF has been shown to generate a 29-fold enrichment of leukocytes from human blood at a flow rate of 20 μL/min using a two-step process.

An improvement on the original design was described by Yamada and Seki in which flow splitting and recombination with the main channel achieved perfect alignment of target particles along the sidewall for a more efficient separation process (Yamada & Seki, 2006) and at the center of the main channel for particle focusing

Microfluidic devices for cell manipulation

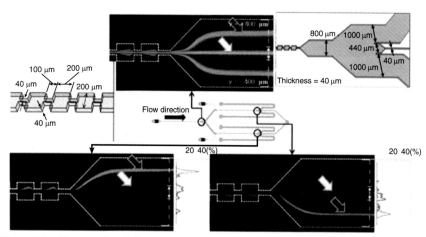

Figure 8.13 Photographs of simultaneous experiments using a mixture of the two polystyrene microspheres at Re = 85. Schematic view of multistage-multiorifice flow fractionation (MS-MOFF) and position of image captured. The top photo represents the end of first multiorifice segment. The photos represent the end of the second two multiorifice segments. *Dark arrows* indicate the 7 μm particles, and *white arrows* indicate the 15 μm particles, respectively. Dimensions of the orifice and flow broadening sections are also shown. Adapted from Sim et al. (2011), with permission from The Royal Society of Chemistry.

(Aoki et al., 2009). Size-based separation of erythrocytes from leukocytes, with up to 100 side channels, was shown to attain high levels of efficiency (Matsuda et al., 2011). Investigators recently observed the rotational behavior of spherical particles and nonspherical Janus particles at branch points and applied their findings to HDF separation based on shape (Sugaya, Yamada, & Seki, 2011), while tuning viscoelastic polymer media was demonstrated in the hydrodynamic spreading of neural and glial cells with >90% viability (Wu, Hjort, Wicher, & Svenningsen, 2008).

A multistage-multiorifice flow fractionation (MS-MOFF) (Fig. 8.13) was introduced by Jung's group, in which the combined effects of inertial lift forces with turbulent secondary Dean flow were used to separate particles based on size, through multiple series of Re constant contraction and expansion microchannels, with high purity and recovery rates demonstrated with microspheres (Park & Jung, 2009; Park, Song, & Jung, 2009; Sim, Kwon, Park, Lee, & Jung, 2011).

A tuneable hydrophoretic separation device fabricated from PDMS for elastic deformation was placed between two acrylic substrates (Choi & Park, 2009). Compressive forces applied to the substrates enabled cross-sectional tuning, allowing a range of particle diameters (2.5–7 μm), a separation criterion, to be employed without constant rebuilding of devices.

8.4.3 Electrokinetic mechanisms

H.A. Pohl described the phenomenon of dielectrophoresis (DEP) as the translational motion of a neutral particle resulting from polarization effects produced by an inhomogeneous electric field (Pohl, 1951, 1958bib_Pohl_1951bib_Pohl_1958). It was not until the late 1960s/early 1970s that experimental and theoretical reports of DEP on biological cells in suspensions began to appear (Crane & Pohl, 1968, 1972bib_Crane_and_Pohl_1968bib_Crane_and_Pohl_1972; Pohl & Crane, 1971; Pohl & Hawk, 1966). AC electrokinetic theories and the forces generated within these microsystems, are covered in depth by (Castellanos, Ramos, Gonzalez, Green, & Morgan, 2003; Hughes, 2003; Jones, 1995; Pethig, 1979, 2010bib_Pethig_1979bib_Pethig_2010; Pohl, 1978; Ramos, Morgan, Green, & Castellanos, 1998).

8.4.3.1 Dielectrophoresis

A homogenous spherical dielectric particle of radius, r, placed in a uniform electric field (E) becomes polarized due to the field's interaction, inducing a dipole moment (p) in the sphere,

$$p = 4\pi\varepsilon_m r^2 \left(\frac{\varepsilon_p - \varepsilon_m}{\varepsilon_p + \varepsilon_m}\right) E \tag{8.34}$$

where $\varepsilon_{p,m}(=\varepsilon_0\varepsilon_r)$ is the absolute permittivity of the suspending medium/particle, ε_r is the relative permittivity of the medium/particle, and ε_0 is the permittivity of free space ($\approx 8.8541878 \times 10^{-12}$ F/m). The time average DEP force acting on a polarizable particle placed in a nonuniform alternating current (AC) electrical field can be expressed in the form (Wang, Hughes, Huang, Becker, & Gascoyne, 1995),

$$\langle \overline{F}_{DEP} \rangle = 2\pi\varepsilon_m r^3 \left\{ \text{Re}(f_{CM}(\omega))\nabla E_{RMS}^2 + \text{Im}(f_{CM}(\omega))\left(E_x^2 \nabla\phi_x + E_y^2 \nabla\phi_y + E_z^2 \nabla\phi_z\right)\right\} \tag{8.35}$$

where E_{RMS} and φ are the root mean square magnitude and phase of the applied electric field in Cartesian axis (x, y, z), respectively. The polarizability (or Clausius–Mossotti) factor ($f_{CM}(\omega)$) describes the frequency-dependent dielectric characteristics of the particle and suspending medium, where the complex permittivity $\left(\varepsilon_k^*\right)$ for the medium ($k = m$) and particle ($k = p$) is described by:

$$\varepsilon_k^* = \varepsilon_k \varepsilon_0 - j\frac{\sigma_k}{\omega}, \quad j = \sqrt{-1} \tag{8.36}$$

or by a complex conductivity (σ_k^*),

$$\sigma_k^* = \sigma_k + j\omega\varepsilon_0\varepsilon_k \tag{8.37}$$

A homogeneous particle's conductivity is $\sigma_p = \sigma_b + (2K_s/r)$, where K_s is the surface conductance, σ_b is particle bulk conductivity, and ω is the angular frequency of the applied field. Thus, the complex Clausius–Mossotti factor can be expressed in terms of complex conductivities or the more common complex permittivities (Eq. 8.38).

$$f_{CM}(\omega) = \left(\frac{\varepsilon_p^* - \varepsilon_m^*}{\varepsilon_p^* + 2\varepsilon_m^*} \right) \tag{8.38}$$

In the absence of a spatially varying phased electric field, as found in traveling wave DEP (twDEP) (Masuda, Washizu, & Kawabata, 1988; Talary, Burt, Tame, & Pethig, 1996), the imaginary component (Im) of the Clausius−Mossotti factor in Eq. (8.35) equals zero, leaving the typical antiphase dielectrophoretic force, $\overline{F}_{DEP}$, originally described by Pohl (1978).

$$\langle \overline{F}_{DEP} \rangle = 2\pi\varepsilon_m r^3 \mathrm{Re}(f_{CM}(\omega)) \nabla E_{RMS}^2 \tag{8.39}$$

DEP vector response to an applied field is dictated by $\mathrm{Re}(f_{CM}(\omega))$, with $-0.5 < \mathrm{Re}(f_{CM}(\omega)) < 0$ indicating net particle movement to low intensity electrical fields (negative DEP(nDEP)) and $0 < \mathrm{Re}(f_{CM}(\omega)) < +1$ indicating movement to high intensity electrical fields (positive DEP). A null response, $\mathrm{Re}(f_{CM}(\omega)) = 0$, is referred to as the particle's crossover frequency, a parameter which has been used in DEP-based separation strategies (Fatoyinbo, Hughes, Martin, Pashby, & Labeed, 2007; Gascoyne & Vykoukal, 2004; Gascoyne, Huang, Pethig, Vykoukal, & Becker, 1992; Markx, Huang, Zhou, & Pethig, 1994). Heterogeneity in cellular structures, along with variations in size and shape (e.g., discoid, ellipsoidal, oblate) have been captured in the Clausius−Mossotti factor using the "multishell" model (van Beek, 1960; Fricke, 1924; Irimajiri, Hanai, & Inouye, 1979). Using a "smeared-out" approach, relative complex permittivities of the membrane (ε_{mem}^*) and cytoplasm (ε_{cyt}^*) for a cell of radius (r) and plasma membrane thickness (d) are evaluated and combined to obtain a particle's effective complex permittivity $(\varepsilon_p^*, \mathrm{eff})$, equivalent to a homogeneous particle, which can then replace ε_p^* in Eq. (8.38) (Huang, Holzel, Pethig, & Wang, 1992).

$$\varepsilon_{p,\mathrm{eff}}^* = \varepsilon_{men}^* \frac{\left[(r/r-d)^3 + 2\left(\left(\varepsilon_{cyt}^* - \varepsilon_{men}^* \right) / \left(\varepsilon_{cyt}^* + 2\varepsilon_{men}^* \right) \right) \right]}{\left[(r/r-d)^3 - 2\left(\left(\varepsilon_{cyt}^* - \varepsilon_{men}^* \right) / \left(\varepsilon_{cyt}^* + 2\varepsilon_{men}^* \right) \right) \right]} \tag{8.40}$$

Eq. (8.40) is useful in extracting electrophysiological properties from a cell's DEP spectrum (frequency-dependent manipulation), such as morphological changes, membrane capacitance, and conductivity, revealing ion permeability and influences of drug exposure in microfluidic cell-based assays and capturing modes within flow regimes (Coley, Labeed, Thomas, & Hughes, 2007; Fatoyinbo, Kadri, Gould, Hoettges, & Labeed, 2011; Hawkins, Huang, Arasanipalai, & Kirby, 2011; Hoettges, 2010; Labeed et al., 2011; Mulhall et al., 2011; Pethig & Talary, 2007; Sanchis et al., 2007; Unni et al., 2012; Wu, Yung, & Lim, 2012).

8.4.3.2 AC electroosmosis

In certain microelectrode configurations (e.g., coplanar electrodes), the application of an AC voltage generates fluid pumping with the direction and velocity dependent on the amplitude and frequency ($\sim 0.1-100$ kHz) of the signal (Garcia-Sanchez, Ramos, Green, & Morgan, 2006). The flow occurs due to oscillating induced charges in the double layer, present at the electrode—electrolyte interface. It is driven by the tangential component of the electric field (E_t), which produces a slip velocity (u_{slip}) characterized by the voltage drop across the double layer ($\Delta\phi_{\text{DL}}$) and the tangential electric field outside the double layer (Ramos, Morgan, Green, & Castellanos, 1999; Yeh, Seul, & Shraiman, 1997).

$$u_{\text{slip}} = \frac{1}{2}\frac{\varepsilon_m}{u}\Lambda\text{Re}[(\Delta\phi_{\text{DL}})E_t] \tag{8.41}$$

The parameter Λ is given by the ratio of the Stern layer capacitance per unit area and the capacitances per unit area of both the Stern and diffuse layers (Castellanos et al., 2003). This nonlinear electrokinetic flow of the fluid has been applied to asymmetrical electrode geometries for microfluidic pumping of fluids (Stroock & Whitesides, 2003), while others have demonstrated this technique in manipulating cells out of bulk flow and on to the electrode surfaces to enhance detection, concentration, and patterning processes (Fatoyinbo, Hoettges, Reddy, & Hughes, 2007; Melvin, Moore, Gilchrist, Grego, & Velev, 2011). A more general term describing the fluid flow, induced by electrical charges, around both metallic and dielectric surfaces in the presence of direct current (DC) and low alternating current (AC) fields is induced-charge electroosmosis (ICEO) coined by Bazant and Squires (2004, 2010).

8.4.3.3 Electrokinetic devices

Electrokinetics is a versatile technology that has benefited from advances in microelectrode fabrication technologies such as photolithography, thus an extremely large body of literature and variant technologies (based on operating strategy or electrode design) of the above principles exists. The dielectrophoretic force imparted on a cell varies with cell polarizability and volume. Applied fields can be either DC or AC; thus, the range of electrokinetic-based devices which have been designed is large and variably multifaceted or modular (Burgarella, Merlo, Dell'Anna, Zarola, & Bianchessi, 2010; Dalton & Kaler, 2007; Muller et al., 1999). The magnitude of the electric field gradient generated by 2D planar (e.g., spiral (Fig. 8.14(h)), interdigitated (Fig. 8.14(b)), interdigitated castellated (Fig. 8.14(a))) or 3D microelectrode geometries (e.g., 3-D wells (Fig. 8.12(j)), DEP-dots (Fig. 8.14(i))) decays exponentially away from the microelectrode edge (Fatoyinbo, Hoeftges, & Hughes, 2008; Green, Ramos, & Morgan, 2002; Hoettges, McDonnell, & Hughes, 2003; Morgan, Izquierdo, Bakewell, Green, & Ramos, 2001; Tsukahara & Watarai, 2003; Wang, Huang, Wang, Becker, & Gascoyne, 1997). Thus, microelectrode arrangements in DEP systems are important in generating varying morphological field gradients required to induce

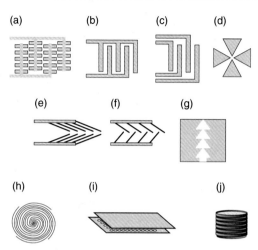

Figure 8.14 Some common microelectrode configurations for particle manipulation in electric fields. (a) Interdigitated castellated, (b) interdigitated, (c) linear quadrupole or twDEP config, (d) quadrapolar for electrorotation, (e) focusing, (f) deflectors, (g) ratchet, (h) spiral, (i) dots, and (j) wells.

motion, though consideration of the DEP force magnitude and other forces arising within the system, including, gravity, viscous drag, buoyancy, and hydrodynamic flow must be optimized accordingly for flow through operations (Hughes, 2002).

Traveling wave DEP occurs when three or more consecutively energized microelectrodes, out of phase by X degrees and summing up to 360 degrees (Fig. 8.14(c)), transport cells parallel to the substrate in a forward or backward direction depending on the sign of Im($f_{CM}(\omega)$), thus imposing variable rates of motion and retention times for different particles (Cheng, Froude, Zhu, Chang, & Chang, 2009; Green et al., 2002; Huang, Wang, Tame, & Pethig, 1993; Hughes, Pethig, & Wang, 1995; Masuda et al., 1988; Wang et al., 1997). When a quadrupolar microelectrode's (out of phase by 90 degrees as in Fig. 8.14(d)) tips are focused toward each other and pointed at a specific region, particles undergo a rotational torque (electrorotation (ROT)) with a velocity that is a function of the field frequency (Cen et al., 2004; Gimsa, 1997; Holzel, 1998). ROT is useful in probing the electrophysiology of single cells, but lacks throughput and the setup is more complex (e.g., particle drift) in comparison to DEP techniques (Hoettges et al., 2008; Hughes, 1998; Wang, Huang, Holzel, Burt, & Pethig, 1992; Wang, Pethig, & Jones, 1991).

Dielectrophoretic field flow fractionation (DEP-FFF) uses dielectric and density properties to discriminate between cells. By balancing multiple forces in hydrodynamic flow, including hydrodynamic lift, cells of different electrophysiology and density attain an equilibrium height in a microchannel through nDEP and are eluted at different rates (Gascoyne, 2009; Liao, Cheng, & Chang, 2012; Markx & Pethig, 1995; Markx, Rousselet, & Pethig, 1997; Wang et al., 2000). Microelectrodes positioned at an angle to the main flow have been used to deflect (Fig. 8.14(f)) and focus (Fig. 8.14(e)) cells to regions of a channel cross section, or into side channels, in sorting and separation processes (Doh & Cho, 2005; Kim, Qian, Kenrick, Daugherty, & Soh, 2008). As a cell approaches an angled electrode, the nDEP force can exceed drag forces, resulting in the cell traveling parallel to the electrode until the drag forces exceed the DEP force, enabling the cell to flow past the electrode in a path line specific to a cells' DEP mobility. Kim, Moon, Kwak, and Jung (2011) described a fluorescence-activated sorting system in which fluorescent microbeads were hydrodynamically focused using a sheath flow for laser excitation which was simultaneously detected by a photomultiplier tube (Fig. 8.15). Depending on the level of intensity, the beads were focused into one of three outlet channels by angled electrodes, indicating DEP's ability to sort multiple particle mixtures effectively.

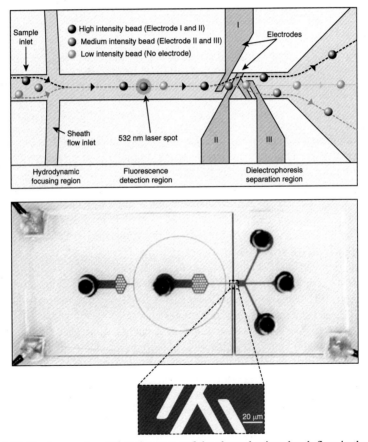

Figure 8.15 Beads were focused to the center of the channel using sheath flow in the hydrodynamic focusing region, fluorescent tags were detected in the fluorescence detection region, and beads were separated using dielectrophoretic forces in the separation region. Photographic image of the microfabricated chip; the channel has an inlet to outlet length of 21 mm, a height of 30 μm and a width 100 μm. Electrodes have a gap length of 20 μm and a width of 20 μm.
Adapted from Kim et al. (2011), with permission from Elsevier.

Insulator-based dielectrophoresis (iDEP) relies on the electric field nonuniformity being created by insulating structures/obstacles within a microfluidic channel, with a DC signal applied across these structures via two electrodes situated at either end of the channel (Chou et al., 2002; Cummings & Singh, 2000, 2003). The reduction in fabrication costs arising from complex metallization processes, a simple fluid and particle transportation mechanism through electroosmotic flow from DC signals and the reduced fouling capabilities, has made this technology an increasingly popular approach for particle trapping and concentration (Lapizco-Encinas, Davalos, Simmons, Cummings, & Fintschenko, 2005, 2004). An extension of iDEP is contactless DEP (cDEP) in which fluid electrodes are used to generate the field nonuniformities (Demierre et al., 2007; Shafiee, Caldwell, Sano, & Davalos, 2009). The fluid electrode channels containing a highly conductive solution are separated from the sample channel where insulating structures reside by thin insulating membranes, eliminating electrode—cell contact and minimizing sample contamination, joule heating, bubble formation, and electrochemical effects during cell manipulation (Henslee, Sano, Rojas, Schmelz, & Davalos, 2011; Sano, Salmanzadeh, & Davalos, 2012).

8.4.4 Acoustic mechanisms

Ultrasonic standing waves (USW) technology for fluid and particle manipulation, also referred to as acoustofluidics, is a rapidly evolving technology. Based on differences in acoustophysical properties (size, density, and compressibility), particles can be manipulated effectively using acoustic radiation forces. The most common acoustic resonator microsystem designs include (1) layered, (2) transversal, and (3) surface acoustic wave (SAW) resonators as in Figs. 8.16 and 8.17 (Lenshof, Evander, Laurell, & Nilsson, 2012). The motion of microparticles and cells in acoustic fields is aptly termed acoustophoresis (Bruus, 2012a, 2012b; Hagsater, Jensen, Bruus, & Kutter, 2007).

8.4.4.1 Acoustic radiation force

The general acoustic radiation force, F rad, for a spherical particle of radius r, immersed in a fluid in the presence of an acoustic field is given by Manneberg et al. (2009),

$$F_{\text{acoustic}} = -\left(\frac{4}{3}\pi r^3\right)\nabla\left(\gamma_1 \frac{\langle p^2 \rangle}{2\rho_m c_m^2} - \frac{3}{2}\rho_m \gamma_2 \frac{\langle u^2 \rangle}{2}\right) \quad (8.42)$$

where,

$$\gamma_1 = 1 - \frac{\rho_m c_m^2}{\rho_p c_p^2} \quad \text{and} \quad \gamma_2 = 2\frac{(\rho_p - \rho_m)}{2\rho_p + \rho_m} \quad (8.43)$$

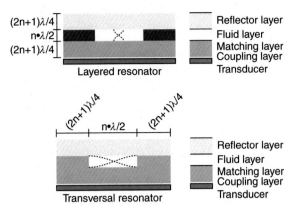

Figure 8.16 Acoustophoretic device classifications: transversal and layered resonators; the choice of material depends on what type of resonator is to be designed. The layered resonator requires carefully matched reflection and matching layers with regards to the wavelength in order to achieve a system with high Q-value. Although, as it is the system Q-value that is important here, it is possible to use materials which themselves are not acoustically optimal, such as polymers, and some losses could be acceptable as long as the system is well matched. Transversal resonators on the other hand rely more on materials with high characteristic acoustic impedance and are less sensitive to matched layers as the whole system resonates as one body. They are, thus, easier to design, but are limited to the choice of materials which can be utilized. Adapted from Lenshof et al. (2012), with permission from The Royal Society of Chemistry.

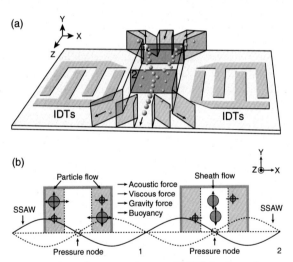

Figure 8.17 The resonance in surface acoustic wave (SAW) devices rely on waves propagating into a fluidic compartment via a wave guiding substrate. In order not to create interfering resonances, the material enclosing the fluid should be of similar characteristic acoustic impedance as the fluid, making polymers suitable. The surface waves are generated by one or more interdigitated electrode transducers positioned outside of the channel, and constructive interference of two opposite SAWs results in a standing surface acoustic wave (SSAW) in the area where the microchannel is bonded. (a) Schematic of the separation mechanism showing particles beginning to translate from the sidewall to the center of the channel due to axial acoustic forces applied to the particles when they enter the working region of the SSAW (site 1). The differing acoustic forces cause differing displacements, repositioning larger particles closer to the channel center and smaller particles farther from the center (site 2). (b) Comparison of forces (normally in pN range) acting on particles at Site 1 and Site 2, respectively.
Adapted from Shi et al. (2009), with permission from The Royal Society of Chemistry.

The pressure (p) and velocity (u) fields are time averaging, ρ and c are the density and speed of sound, for subscripts: medium (m) and particle (p). For a one dimensional plane acoustic standing wave, Eq. (8.42) reduces to:

$$F_{\text{acoustic}}(x) = 4\pi r^3 E_{\text{ac}} k \sin(2kx) \Phi \tag{8.44}$$

where E_{ac} is the acoustic energy density of wavelength λ, wavenumber $k = 2\pi/\lambda = \omega/c_m$, and the acoustophoretic contrast factor, Φ, is defined as,

$$\Phi = \gamma_1 + \frac{3}{2}\gamma_2 = \frac{5\rho_p - 2\rho_m}{2\rho_p + \rho_m} - \tilde{k} \tag{8.45}$$

From Eq. (8.45), Φ is dependent on the relative densities of the medium and particle, the relative compressibility of both materials (i.e., $\tilde{k} = k_p/k_m$), and recently included, a fluid viscosity parameter for smaller-sized particles (Settnes & Bruus, 2012). It determines the direction the acoustic force is acting on the particle in a microchannel and for the case of the simple standing half-wavelength, particles are directed toward pressure nodes for $\Phi > 0$ (central plane) or toward the antinode for $\Phi < 0$ (wall region) (Petersson, Nilsson, Jonsson, & Laurell, 2005).

8.4.4.2 Acoustophoretic devices

Acoustophoresis is not limited by high conductive fluids, surface charges, or pH, though complexities in device design, material choice, and fabrication pose challenges owing to the high quality factor (Q-value) needed for the resonator and the minimization of resonance attenuation when interfaced with channel wall forming substrates. As an alternative to the more expensive silicon substrate, isotropically wet-etched glass chips were shown to have superior performance in microfluidic acoustic cell washing and focusing also enabling visualization of cell streams (Evander, Lenshof, Laurell, & Nilsson, 2008). Acoustophoretic devices exploit half-wavelength resonators for separation, sorting, trapping, and alignment of particles (Laurell, Petersson, & Nilsson, 2007). Continuous separation of polystyrene beads on a silicon chip into multiple side channels was actuated by a 2 MHz piezoceramic plate in the first harmonic mode ($2*\lambda/2$). Separation efficiencies were found to be dependent on side channel angles branching off the main channels with a 45 degrees branch more effective than a 90 degrees branch (Nilsson, Petersson, Jonsson, & Laurell, 2004). This system was modified for the separation of 2.5% concentration of RBCs from 1% concentration of triglyceride emulsions (Petersson, Nilsson, Holm, Jonsson, & Laurell, 2004). Reducing the cross-sectional dimensions of the microchannel to a half-wavelength ($\lambda/2$), standing wave increased the acoustic force at the channel center focusing a band of RBC exiting via a central outlet channel (>70%) while lipid emulsions exited via the sides (>80%). Separation of whole blood cells from plasma in an elongated separation channel through a sequential stepwise removal of concentrated blood cells enabled subsequent plasma protein analysis (Lenshof et al., 2009). The orthogonal acoustic redistribution of particles/cells based on size in a dual-inlet laminar flow system is known as free-flow acoustophoresis (FFA) fractionation (Kumar, Feke, & Belovich, 2005; Petersson, Aberg, Sward-Nilsson, & Laurell, 2007). It can be seen from Eq. (8.46) that the particle's velocity $\upsilon_p(x)$ due to the acoustic force is proportional to the square of the particle's radius. An acoustophoretic device operating in transversal mode with multiple outlet channels and a trifurcated inlet is driven under laminar flow with buffer media injected in the central inlet and sample media from the two side inlets. As the streams flow parallel upstream in the separation channel, under the influence of an applied acoustic force, balanced by Stokes drag, large particles transverse the channel at different speeds according to size, exiting at spatially positioned outlet channels.

$$\upsilon_p(x) = \frac{2\Phi k r^2 E_{ac}}{3\mu} \sin(2kx) \tag{8.46}$$

Standing surface acoustic waves (SSAWs), where parallel interdigitated transducers (IDTs) generate lateral acoustic radiation forces on particles within the microchannel, has also recently been used to separate and focus particles in continuous flows (Fig. 8.18) (Nam, Lee, & Shin, 2011; Nam, Lim, Kim, & Shin, 2011; Shi, Huang, Stratton, Huang, & Huang, 2009; Shi et al., 2011). Acoustic tweezers in which RBCs and *E. coli* were patterned into grid-like arrays used SSAW technology as in Fig. 8.19, with the IDTs positioned orthogonally to each other (Shi et al., 2009). Although in its infancy, SSAW-based designs demonstrate versatility and lower power consumption over traditional bulk acoustic wave designs, with the potential of seamless integration of acoustic-based manipulation technologies in microfluidic systems.

8.4.5 Optical mechanisms

In the last decade, the relatively new research field of optofluidics has seen a multitude of developments for LOC systems, mainly regarding miniaturized detection systems (Cho et al., 2010bib_Cho_et_al_2010b; Mogensen & Kutter, 2009). Optofluidics can be considered as the merging of optics with microfluidic technology, i.e., the interaction of light with matter in microfluidic flow, whereas the term photophoresis has been used to describe the movement of micron-sized particles subjected to beams of light (Zhao, Koo, & Chung, 2006). The term optofluidics has been applied in a variety of ways, and it can be justifiably argued that some well-established techniques and devices (e.g., optical tweezers, surface plasmon ressonance (SPR)) have quietly been included into this technological classification (Horowitz, Awschalom, & Pennathur, 2008; Psaltis, Quake, & Yang, 2006). The basic physics of light interactions with biological materials is well understood (Svoboda & Block, 1994). Platforms for cell sorting, trapping, and manipulation in microfluidic systems, based on particle size and refractive index or fluorescence labeling, are becoming more widespread.

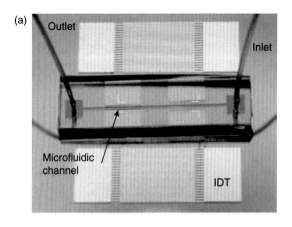

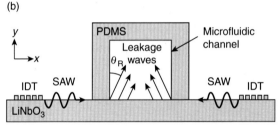

Figure 8.18 (a) A photograph a polydimethylsiloxane (PDMS) microchannel in between a pair of parallel interdigitated transducers (IDTs) used for particle focusing. (b) A cross-section schematic of the microchannel and IDTs used to generate two surface acoustic waves (SAWs) traveling in the opposite direction. The leakage waves are radiated into the liquid phase under the Rayleigh angle.
Reproduced in part from Shi et al. (2011), with permission from The Royal Society of Chemistry.

8.4.5.1 Optical devices

Cell manipulation using optical tweezers (also known as optical traps) was first demonstrated by Bell Laboratories using visible argon laser light and infrared (IR) light (Ashkin & Dziedzic, 1987; Ashkin, Dziedzic, & Yamane, 1987). Movement of a micron-sized dielectric particle is induced by the direct transfer of photon momentum to a nonabsorbing particle during refraction and reflection, i.e., the radiation pressure. The radiation pressure (optical force) from a high intensity, focused Gaussian profile laser has scattering and gradient force components, which gives a point of stable equilibrium near the beam focus. Particles are trapped transversely by the gradient force ($\sim$ pN), while the axial motion of the particle is controlled by the scattering forces (Ashkin, 1997). For cells greater than the wavelength of light ($d_p \gg \lambda$), ray optics has been used to derive the radiation force from scattering of the incident light momentum (Ashkin, 1992; Svoboda & Block, 1994).

Single beam and multiple beam configurations have been used to manipulate and trap cells in microfluidic systems with high precision and little or no damage to the cell

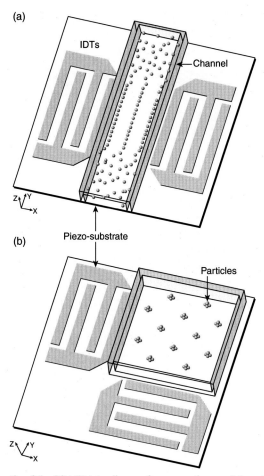

Figure 8.19 Schematic of the SSAW (standing surface acoustic wave)-based patterning devices. (a) 1D patterning using two parallel interdigitated transducers (IDTs). (b) 2D patterning using two orthogonal IDTs (the angle between the IDTs can be changed to achieve different patterns). Reproduced from Shi et al. (2009), with permission from The Royal Society of Chemistry.

integrity. Eriksson et al. (2010) assessed the impact of glucose level changes through reversible microfluidic flow on single cell *S. cerevisiae* by individually selecting and positioning them in a 5 × 5 array (1.28 mm^2) using optical tweezers. With a power density of 240 mW from the lasers, continuous cell budding indicated the cells were not adversely affected. Fig. 8.20 shows a cell sorting system using multiple microfluidic streams, optical tweezers, and an image processing methodology for recognizing fluorescence and size (Wang et al., 2011). This system uses multiple laser traps to dynamically trap and transport cells to a desired location for sorting purposes, achieving high purity factors with low sample populations. Optoelectronic tweezers (OETs) were introduced by Chiou, Ohta, and Wu (2005) where light passing through a digital micromirror display image patterned that image onto a photoconductive layer to produce virtual electrodes. When the system was energized with an AC signal, cells moved into negative or

Microfluidic devices for cell manipulation

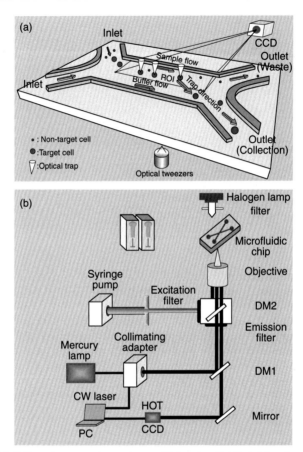

Figure 8.20 (a) Cell sorting procedure using multiple microfluidic inlet and outlet streams, optical tweezers, and an image processing methodology for recognizing fluorescence and size. (b) Cell sorter setup combined with optical tweezers and a microfluidic chip.
Reproduced from Wang et al. (2011), with permission from the Royal Society of Chemistry.

positive energy traps due to electric field gradients originating from the illuminated area. This optical platform has low power consumption and mass parallelization of single cell motion based on the combined technologies of optical tweezers and the principle of DEP manipulation. Further developments of OET technology have included integration with EWOD in which HeLa cells were either trapped or transported in microfluidic droplets via lateral droplet motion (LOET) (Shah, Ohta, Chiou, Wu, & Kim, 2009). Recently, polymer-based optically induced DEP (ODEP) devices have been developed to manipulate particles using dynamically changing virtual electrodes controlled by computer as in Fig. 8.21 or the concave curvature and flexibility of a device substrate (Lin, Hung, Jeng, Guo, & Lee, 2012; Wang, Lin, Wen, Guo, & Lee, 2010). Continuous separation of targeted single cells through optical transportation perpendicular to the flow streams, using single or multiple laser traps, have extremely low throughput, which is a significant drawback at ~ 10 cell/s compared to $\sim 10^5$ cell/s for fluorescence-activated cell sorting (FACS) technique (Murata et al., 2009).

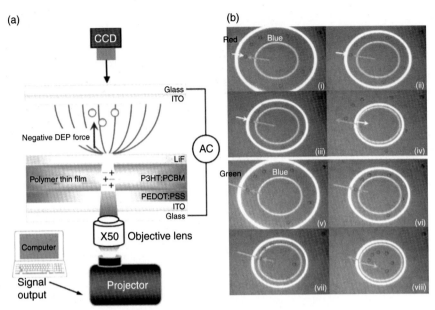

Figure 8.21 (a) Schematic illustration of polymer-based optically induced dielectrophoresis (ODEP) platform for selective manipulation of particles. (b) Series of photographs taken under an optical microscope, demonstrating the selective manipulation of polystyrene particles with a diameter of 20 μm. (i–iv) All polymer particles between the outer and inner rings are excluded as the diameter of the outer ring shrinks. (v–viii) All the polymer particles between the new outer and previous inner rings can be collected inside the inner ring as the diameter of the outer ring shrinks. Reproduced from Wang et al. (2010), with permission from the American Institute of Physics.

8.4.6 Magnetic mechanisms

Erythrocytes possess the protein hemoglobin, containing four iron atoms in a ferrous state for oxygen binding. Oxyhemoglobin and deoxyhaemoglobin are diamagnetic and paramagnetic materials, respectively. The metalloprotein methemoglobin (Fe^{3+}) is also present in erythrocytes, but in larger quantities for diseased cells, has a greater paramagnetic susceptibility than its ferrous state counterpart and malaria-infected erythrocytes (Hackett, Hamzah, Davis, & St Pierre, 2009). The first successful separation of erythrocytes from whole blood using magnetic field gradients was reported by Melville, Paul, and Roath (1975a, 1975b). The use of magnetic susceptibility as a separation parameter for magnetophoresis in laminar flow has been successfully applied directly to biological cells (Paul, Melville, Roath, & Warhurst, 1981; Takayasu, Kelland, & Minervini, 2000; Zborowski et al., 2003). Manipulating nonmagnetic cells in a high gradient magnetic field coupled with microfluidics and applications of magnetic nanoparticles in medicine and biotechnology has previously been described (Liu, Stakenborg, Peeters, & Lagae, 2009; Pamme, 2006; Pankhurst, Connolly, Jones, & Dobson, 2003).

8.4.6.1 Magnetic force

A magnetic material placed in a magnetic field (*H*) has a magnetic induction (*B*), measured in teslas (*T*), expressed by Eq. (8.44), where μ_0 is the permeability of free space ($4\pi \times 10^{-7}$ TmA^{-1}) and the magnetization, ($M = m/V$), is the magnetic moment (*m*) per unit volume (*V*) of the material (Oberteuf, 1974).

$$B = \mu_0(H + M) \tag{8.47}$$

Magnetic susceptibility (χ) is a dimensionless number relating to the degree of magnetization (A/m) of a material in response to a magnetic field.

$$M = \chi H \tag{8.48}$$

Materials classified according to their magnetic susceptibility are diamagnetic ($\chi < 0$), paramagnetic ($\chi > 0$), or ferromagnetic ($\chi \gg 0$) (Fig. 8.22). Ferromagnets, also known as permanent magnets (e.g., iron and nickel), are strongly attracted to

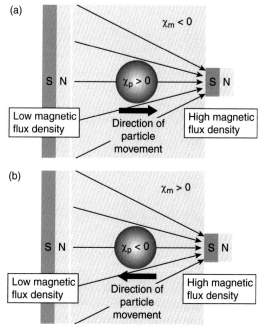

Figure 8.22 (a) Principle of magnetic attraction: a magnetic particle ($\chi_p > 0$) is suspended in a diamagnetic medium ($\chi_m < 0$), giving a Dc value greater than zero and resulting in attraction of the particle toward the magnetic field. (b) Principle of diamagnetic repulsion: a diamagnetic particle ($\chi_p < 0$) is suspended in a paramagnetic medium ($\chi_m > 0$), giving a Dc value less than zero and resulting in repulsion of the particle from the magnetic field.
Reproduced from Rodríguez-Villarreal et al. (2011), with permission from The Royal Society of Chemistry.

magnetic fields. Materials such as platinum and oxygen are considered paramagnetic and are weakly attracted and aligned in magnetic field maxima, while biological materials such as proteins, DNA, and cells are weakly diamagnetic and are repelled to magnetic field minima. Due to such factors as intrinsic structural impurities or anisotropic lattice arrangements, ferromagnetic materials on the micron scale often exhibit irreversible magnetization processes known as M-H hysteresis loops (magnetic remnant $\neq 0$), while magnetic nanoparticles display antihysteresis, a quality related to superparamagnetism—the thermally activated flipping of the net moment (Pankhurst et al., 2003). In the presence of a magnetic field, superparamagnetic (SPM) particles become magnetized, and upon removal of the magnetic field, the magnetic remnant is zero, allowing particles to disperse freely within suspending media. In medical applications, SPM beads typically consist of a magnetic iron oxide core (e.g., magnetite or maghaemite) surrounded by a biomaterial of interest for preferential functionalization, with size variations up to the micron scale.

The magnetic force ($F_{magnetic}$) on a magnetic particle in a magnetic field gradient is dependent on the particle volume (V_p) and the magnetic susceptibility difference ($\Delta\chi = \chi_p - \chi_m$) between particle and surrounding medium (Gijs, 2004; Moore et al., 2004; Zborowski, Sun, Moore, Williams, & Chalmers, 1999).

$$F_{magnetic} = \frac{V_p \Delta\chi}{\mu_0}(B \cdot \nabla)B \tag{8.49}$$

Nonzero initial magnetization (M_0) of SPM beads, observed in magnetization curves of commercial suppliers, prompted Shevkoplyas, Siegel, Westervelt, Prentiss, and Whitesides (2007) to modify the conventional expression for the magnetization force. A comparison of Eqs. (8.49) and (8.50) against experimental results of the manufacturer showed better agreement with the modified equation, enabling better prediction of bead manipulation in microfluidic systems of weaker magnetic field strengths (up to ~ 10 mT).

$$F_{magnetic} = (m_p \cdot \nabla)B = \rho V_p(M_0 \cdot \nabla)B + \frac{V_p \chi_p}{\mu_0}(B \cdot \nabla)B \tag{8.50}$$

8.4.6.2 Magnetophoretic devices

The most common approach to facilitate cell manipulation (excluding RBCs and magnetotactic bacteria (MTB)) in magnetic fields is through surface labeling with functionalized SPM particles, commercially termed magnet-activated cell sorting (MACS) by Miltenyi Biotec. However, other methods, such as endocytotic uptake of magnetic nanoparticles by inflammatory cells and separation based on their uptake capacity, have been reported (Robert et al., 2011). McCloskey, Chalmers, and Zborowski (2003) identified four parameters which significantly influenced the magnetophoretic mobility ($m_{magnetic}$) of immunomagnetically labeled cells as: (1) antibody binding capacity, (2) secondary antibody amplification, (3) interaction parameter of particle-magnetic field, and (4) cell diameter. The magnetophoretic mobility arises when Stokes drag is set to equal the magnetic force on the particle and solved for the magnetic-induced migration velocity (V_p) in a magnetic force field strength ($S_{magnetic}$), and can be used as a separation parameter between magnetically tagged and untagged cells.

$$m_{magnetic} = \frac{V_p}{S_{magnetic}} \qquad (8.51)$$

This parameter was further explored by Moore et al. (2004), in which the medium was modified with gadolinium making it paramagnetic, thus minimizing the crossover of nonspecific (i.e., untagged) particles and RBCs (repulsive-mode magnetophoresis) into the adjacent outlet stream. These studies were predominantly based around large magnets driving the high gradient magnetic fields within millimeter-sized channels. The arrangement of magnets, either permanent magnets (e.g., NdFeB) or electromagnets, varied according to channel geometry and operation; for instance, quadrupole magnet sorter (QMS) arrangements have been described for continuous separation and sorting of cells (Moore et al., 2004; Zborowski et al., 1999), and perpendicular dipole arrangements to the flow channel for fractionation, magnetophoretic mobility studies, diamagnetic repulsion flow focusing and on-chip free-flow magnetophoretic separation and sorting as shown in Fig. 8.23 (Jin et al., 2008; Pamme & Manz, 2004;

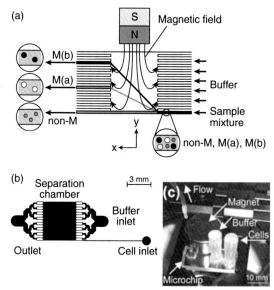

Figure 8.23 (a) Principle of free-flow magnetophoresis: laminar flow is applied in x-direction over a separation chamber, a magnetic field is applied in y-direction. Nonmagnetic material follows the direction of laminar flow, whereas magnetic particles/cells are deflected from the direction of laminar flow. (b) The microfluidic design featuring the separation chamber, one cell inlet channel and 16 buffer inlet channels. On the opposite side, there were 16 outlet channels. The structure was 30 mm deep. (c) Photograph of the microfluidic chip with cell and buffer inlet reservoirs, connection to syringe pump and NdFeB magnet.
Reproduced from Pamme and Wilhelm (2006), with permission from The Royal Society of Chemistry.

Pamme & Wilhelm, 2006; Rodriguez-Villarreal et al., 2010; Schneider et al., 2006). More complex microfabricated magnet arrangements, integrated with microsystems, have also been developed enabling localized field gradient generation for more accurate particle control and manipulation, with the aim of better integration of magnetophoretic devices into lab on a chip systems. A comprehensive overview of microelectromagnetic traps (METs), the geometries fabricated to produce magnetic field gradients which is proportional to current density and electromagnet size, and their various applications from cell manipulation and ferrofluid actuation in microchannels to biosensors was recently discussed (Basore & Baker, 2012). Using soft lithography, micromagnetic systems (Fig. 8.24(a—c)) employing current carrying circuits were used to transport 4.5 μm microbeads along the B-field maxima (Deng, Whitesides, Radhakrishnan, Zabow, & Prentiss, 2001). Two serpentine wires, shifted linearly in phase by $\pi/3$, allowed the magnetic fields to become superimposed when current flowed, trapping magnetic beads. Upon changing the input current through the wires, the field maxima changed with the microbead moving position in a zigzag path as in Fig. 8.24(d—h). Semiencapsulated planar spiral electromagnets on a glass wafer generated a magnetic field in a microchannel from a 300 mA DC current applied to the inductor enabling magnetic microbead separation (Choi, Liakopoulos, & Ahn, 2001). Continuous immunomagnetic separation of leukocytes from whole blood in a microfluidic system was achieved by inducing lateral forces from microfabricated magnetic diagonal parallel stripe arrays, which trapped and altered tagged particles' flow directions (Inglis, Riehn, Austin, & Sturm, 2004). Numerical models for the lateral magnetophoretic displacement of SPM beads and immunomagnetically labeled cells deflected in a microfluidic systems have recently been reported for a range of configurations (bead type, magnet type and orientation, binding capacity), flow rates, and channel geometries to accurately predict magnetophoretic deflection or capture (Forbes & Forry, 2012).

8.5 Manipulation of cancer cells in microfluidic systems

Microfluidics in cell biology has been applied in the manipulation and analysis of rare cells—e.g., stem, fetal, and cancer cells. The reduction in system dimensions, coupled with precise manipulation technologies, represents a positive shift toward accurate, low cost cellular bioprocesses with low sample volumes and parallelization capabilities. Of particular interest are the potential offerings these technologies can provide in advancing our knowledge and understanding in cancer biology, from the molecular mechanisms of resistance to anticancer drugs and drug discovery, through to label-less on-chip flow cytometry and microsorting operations. Although challenges are still present, microfluidic systems are fast becoming key components in many labs undertaking cancer research. See a review article for recent advances in microfluidic platforms for the applications of single-cell analysis in cancer biology, diagnostics, and therapy (Tavakoli et al., 2019).

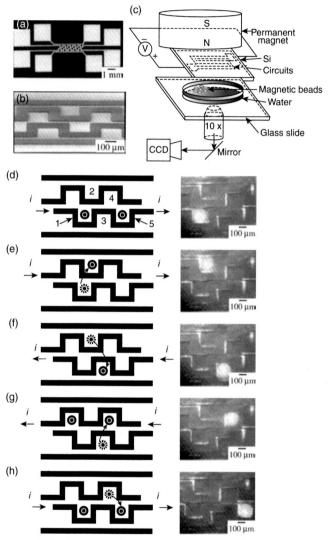

Figure 8.24 (a) Optical micrograph of micromagnetic system. The wires were ~100 μm wide and 10 μm high. The turns of the serpentine wires had an inner dimension of 200 μm × 200 μm. The closest vertical spacing between the two serpentine wires is ~50 μm. The closest horizontal distance between two turns of different wires was ~100 μm. The contact pads were 1 mm × 1 mm. (b) Magnified view of the fabricated system by SEM. (c) Setup for the manipulation of superparamagnetic microbeads using the micromagnetic system. The distance between the circuits and the air–water interface was ~50–400 μm, and the permanent magnet was 2–4 cm away from the circuits during the experiment. (d)–(h) Manipulation of magnetic microbeads in the micromagnetic system.
Reproduced from Deng et al. (2001), with permission from the American Institute of Physics.

8.5.1 Deformability and migration studies

Cancerous cells are able to change their migration mechanisms more robustly than noncancerous cells in response to changes in external stimuli. This has led to therapeutic approaches for immobilizing cancer cells via inhibition of signal transduction pathways to investigate migration mechanisms. Variations in speed and mode of migration have been identified among different cancer cell lines, with ECM-filled PDMS-microchannels designed to have predefined cell migration paths for visual quantification. Three modes of cancer migration identified include (1) mesenchymal, (2) ameboid, and (3) collective cell migration, distinguishable by their morphology and migration characteristics in response to soluble chemokines, ECM, and surface cues (Huang, Agrawal, Sun, Kuo, & Williams, 2011). An underlying cause of a cancer cell's ability to migrate through confined 3D spaces is due to its high deformability afforded by cytoskeleton compliance (Suresh, 2007). Hou et al. (2009) described the use of microfluidics to probe the deformation of benign and tumor breast cancer cells through microchannel constrictions, indicating channel entry time was faster for metastatic cells and could be used as a label-free biomarker to differentiate between healthy and nonhealthy cells. Employing inertial focusing and deformability-induced migration, Hur, Henderson-Maclennan, McCabe, and Di Carlo (2011) were able to demonstrate a passive high-throughput cell classification system, based solely on size and deformation characteristics, for targeting and enriching MCF-7 cells spiked in peripheral blood. Furthermore, cells immobilized via adhesion molecules (e.g., cadherins) coated on the surfaces of channel walls or micropillars within the channels and subjected to fluid hydrodynamic flow, applied electric fields, and different chemoattractants in gradient or diffusion based flows have been used to investigate the influences of hydrodynamic loading, chemotaxis, and electrotaxis on mechanical interactions of the substrate and the migrating cell (Cheung et al., 2009; Li & Lin, 2011; Walker et al., 2005).

8.5.2 Microfluidic separation and sorting

Tanaka et al. (2012) investigated the relationship between hematocrit and circulating tumor cancer (CTC) cell-inertial migration for designing microfluidic separators, finding cancer cell equilibrium could only be achieved at up to 10% hematocrit volume with appropriate channel lengths. This enabled a separation strategy to be developed without the need of surface cell markers, such as epithelial cell adhesion molecules (EpCAM). Human liver cancer cells (HepG2) and fibroblasts (NIH/3 T3) were separated based on their respective cell cycle phases indicating HDF's potential as a powerful damage-free separation technology in cellular genetics (Migita et al., 2010). Also, hydrophoretic sorting of an asynchronous human leukemic monocyte lymphoma population into G_0/G_1 and G_2/M cell cycle phases with 95.5% and 85.2% efficiencies, respectively, was achieved by Choi, Song, Choi, and Park (2009). Thevoz, Adams, Shea, Bruus, and Soh (2010) demonstrated acoustophoretic cell synchronization (ACS) of mammalian cells as in Fig. 8.25. An asynchronous sample of MDA-MB-231 human breast carcinoma cells was separated according to

Microfluidic devices for cell manipulation 371

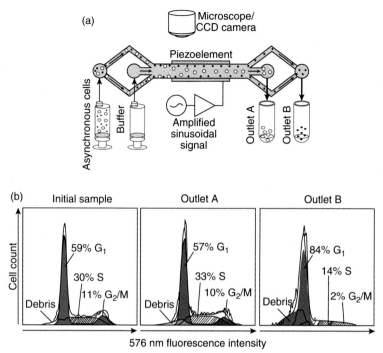

Figure 8.25 (a) Acoustophoretic cell synchronization (ACS) device and experimental setup. Asynchronous mixture of cells and buffer volumetrically pumped into the ACS device. Synchronization is achieved by fractionating the cells according to size such that larger cells (e.g., G_2) elute through outlet A whereas smaller cells (e.g., G_1) elute through outlet B. (b) Flow cytometry histograms showing cell cycle distributions before and after synchronization, based on measurements of red fluorescence centered at 576 nm, after staining the cellular DNA with propidium iodide. The populations in each phase of the cell cycle were determined by fitting cell cycle models to the histograms. The synchronized cell population at outlet B shows 84% of all cells in the G_1 phase, with 14% in the S phase and 2% in G_2/M phase. Reproduced in part from Thévoz et al. (2010), with permission from American Chemical Society.

their size-dependent phase within the cell cycle, with larger G_2/M and S-phases cells moving more rapidly to the central stream (outlet A) than the smaller G_1 phase cells (outlet B). G_1 phase synchrony at ~84% was achieved.

Magnetophoretic microfluidic devices have gained momentum in testing clinical samples to isolate, separate, and analyze CTCs, haemopoietic stem cells (HSCs), or endothelial progenitor cells (EPCs) (Plouffe, Mahalanabis, Lewis, Klapperich, & Murthy, 2012; Zborowski & Chamers, 2011). Iterative microsystem optimization through either CD133+ or MCF-7 carcinoma cell separation from human blood was performed in a disposable microfluidic chip, with applied currents of up to 1 A, producing high purity and a >96% separation efficiency. An automated cell sorting microdevice consisting of nickel pillars, magnetized externally, fabricated on PDMS and microvalves, was used to separate A549 cancer cells (Liu et al., 2007). SPM beads were efficiently trapped between magnetized pillars arrays while in situ biofunctionalization with a glycoprotein and washing of the beads took place in the vicinity of the pillars. Introduced A549 cells captured in the array, then released to the outlet, were enriched by a factor of 133, based on an original mixture ratio of 1:10 cancer to RBCs. A variation to Liu et al.'s (2007) technique was described by Saliba et al. (2010) in which biofunctionalized SPM beads self-assembled into microarray columns when magnetic traps, prepared by microcontact printing, were magnetized (Fig. 8.26). Using flow activated cell and SPM bead interaction, Jurkat and Raji cells were captured with a >94% efficiency, with successful in situ on-cell culturing carried out immediately after sorting. These systems in which biofunctionalized SPM beads were used as an immobilized bed to capture untagged cells represented a new paradigm to the freely suspended multitargeted immunomagnetic activation approach traditionally and still employed prior to sample injection in to the microchannel (Adams, Kim, & Soh, 2008).

Recently, a tuneable magnetophoretic separation device was used to separate label-free cells in a flow focused paramagnetic ionic solution (Shen, Hwang, Hahn, & Park, 2012). Although at low throughput, human lymphoma monocytes (U937) and RBCs suspended in varying concentrations of paramagnetic solution gadolinium diethylenetriamine pentaacetic acid (Gd-DTPA) were separated through repulsion forces which drove the diamagnetic particles away from the magnet at varying magnetophoretic mobility rates based on size and magnetic susceptibility properties.

8.5.3 Current challenges in sorting and detection

High-throughput microfluidic flow cytometry devices in some combination focus, count, detect, or sort cells on a single chip and rival the more complex, costly and bulkier FACS flow cytometers (e.g., BD Biosciences). Since Fu, Spence, Scherer, Arnold, and Quake (1999) introduced μFACS, an assortment of activated cell sorting microdevices relying on DEP (DACS), synthetic tags for altering complex permittivities of multitarget cells (MT-DACS), Raman spectroscopy (RACS), hydrodynamics, and magnetic susceptibilities (MACS) have been described, with some achieving throughputs as high as 10,000 cells per second or efficiencies >85% for cancerous and noncancerous separation (An, Lee, Lee, Park, & Kim, 2009; Cho, Chen, Tsai, Godin, & Lo, 2010; Hu et al., 2005; Inglis et al., 2008; Kim & Soh, 2009; Kim et al., 2008; Lau, Lee, & Chan, 2008). These new microflow cytometers have been demonstrated on cancerous cells and, except for FACS and MACS, they do not require prelabelling, relying only on the intrinsic properties (size, dielectric, deformability, refractive index) of the cells for sorting. Importantly, if any of the new microsystems is to be a serious challenger to the sheath-based, high speed quantification and sorting of FACS, issues regarding throughput, increased sensitivity, and integration of actuating mechanisms need to be fully addressed and validated before uptake in a clinical setting can be endorsed.

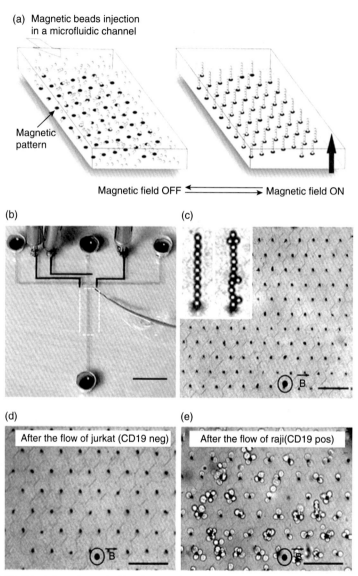

Figure 8.26 Principle and practical implementation of the Ephesia system. (a) Principle of magnetic self-assembly. A hexagonal array of magnetic ink is patterned at the bottom of a microfluidic channel. Beads coated with an antibody are injected in the channel. Beads are submitted to Brownian motion. The application of an external vertical magnetic field induces the formation of a regular array of bead columns localized on top of the ink *dots*. (b) Two level polydimethylsiloxane (PDMS) integrated microchip. Delivery and separation channels for the cells appear in the lighter shade channels. Inlets ports appear as the four dark circular reservoirs. The separation channel is the longer vertical branch. The area bearing magnetic posts is marked by the dotted white box. Channels in the upper PDMS layer, controlling the opening and closing of the

8.6 Conclusion and future trends

To begin handling clinically relevant samples, a concerted effort in combining multiple manipulation technologies is needed. It could be argued that Giddings laid down this foundation, but nowadays the rapid advances in technology has had a profound impact on engineering design and optimization of microfluidic devices for general purpose use. For example, when dealing with blood samples (~40% (v/v) hematocrit), if on-chip sample preparation units are to be incorporated for a fully automated LOC system, electrokinetic technologies with simple channel geometries would simply not cope with the high medium conductivities. Coupling of hydrodynamic technologies (e.g., HDF), through flow splitting and recombining with low ionic solutions could improve downstream electrokinetic processing operations. This approach to multitechnology coupling (MTC) integration has recently begun to become more prominent, for instance the use of complex microfluidic networks to generate conductivity gradients in DEP separation (Vahey & Voldman, 2008); the serial combination of multiorifice flow fractionation (MOFF) and DEP at high flow rates (126 µL/min) for continuous CTC separation from blood samples (Moon et al., 2011); combining acoustophoresis with DEP for focusing and preconcentration (Ravula et al., 2008); integrating acoustophoresis and magnetophoresis for multiparameter particle separation (Adams, Thevoz, Bruus, & Soh, 2009); or the apparent combination of PFF with DEP in an ApoStream flow cell for the continuous separation of CTCs from blood (Gupta et al., 2012).

8.7 Sources of further information and advice

Sources of information are predominantly in journal publications in which innovative applications of the technologies presented are used in microfluidic devices for a range of biomedical and biotechnological operations. These high impact journals include: *Lab on a chip*; *Analytical Chemistry*; *Biomedical Microdevices*; *Biomicrofluidics*; *Proceedings of the National Academy of Sciences*; *Science*; *Nature Biotechnology* and *Electrophoresis*.

Some commercial enterprises offering fabrication services of microfluidic devices for biological applications include: Fluidigm Corp (www.fluidgim.com); Dolomite Microfluidics (www.dolomite-microfluidics.com); Micralyne (www.micralyne.com), and Epigem Ltd. (www.epigem.co.uk). Companies recently established to exploit

---

inlet channels, appear as the darker shade channels. A thermocouple for in situ control of the temperature in the system is located at the top of the dotted white boundary (Scale bar: 0.5 cm). (c) Magnetically assembled array of columns of 4.5 µm beads coated with anti-CD19 mAb (specifically retaining Raji B-Lymphocytes). Typical column shapes are shown in the insets (Scale bar: 80 µm). (d) Optical micrograph of the columns after the passage of 1000 Jurkat cells, no cells seen. (e) After the passage of 400 Raji cells, numerous cells are captured and rosetted on the columns (Scale bar: 80 µm).
Reproduced from Saliba et al. (2010), Copyright 2010 National Academy of Sciences, USA.

different cell micromanipulation technologies for characterization, separation, sorting, etc., include, Optofluidics, DEPtech, ApoCell, CytonomeST with many more being created and larger biotech and pharmaceutical firms also becoming involved. Lastly, established international conferences highlighting developments in this area include µTAS, Lab on a Chip World Congress, Biodetection Technologies, and Sample Prep by the Knowledge Foundation.

References

Adams, J. D., Kim, U., & Soh, H. T. (2008). Multitarget magnetic activated cell sorter. *Proceedings of the National Academy of Sciences of the United States of America, 105*, 18165–18170.

Adams, J. D., Thevoz, P., Bruus, H., & Soh, H. T. (2009). Integrated acoustic and magnetic separation in microfluidic channels. *Applied Physics Letters, 95*, 254103–1.

Alberts, B., Bray, D., Lewis, J., Raff, M., Roberts, K., & Watson, J. D. (1994). *Molecular biology of the cell*. New York: Garland Publishing.

An, J., Lee, J., Lee, S. H., Park, J., & Kim, B. (2009). Separation of malignant human breast cancer epithelial cells from healthy epithelial cells using an advanced dielectrophoresis-activated cell sorter (DACS). *Analytical and Bioanalytical Chemistry, 394*, 801–809.

Aoki, R., Yamada, M., Yasuda, M., & Seki, M. (2009). In-channel focusing of flowing microparticles utilizing hydrodynamic filtration. *Microfluidics and Nanofluidics, 6*, 571–576.

Ashkin, A. (1992). Forces of a single-beam gradient laser trap on a dielectric sphere in the ray optics regime. *Biophysical Journal, 61*, 569–582.

Ashkin, A. (1997). Optical trapping and manipulation of neutral particles using lasers. *Proceedings of the National Academy of Sciences of the United States of America, 94*, 4853–4860.

Ashkin, A., & Dziedzic, J. M. (1987). Optical trapping and manipulation of viruses and bacteria. *Science, 235*, 1517–1520.

Ashkin, A., Dziedzic, J. M., & Yamane, T. (1987). Optical trapping and manipulation of single cells using infrared-laser beams. *Nature, 330*, 769–771.

Asmolov, E. S. (1999). The inertial lift on a spherical particle in a plane Poiseuille flow at large channel Reynolds number. *Journal of Fluid Mechanics, 381*, 63–87.

Barshtein, G., Ben-Ami, R., & Yedgar, S. (2007). Role of red blood cell flow behavior in hemodynamics and hemostasis. *Expert Review of Cardiovascular Therapy, 5*, 743–752.

Basore, J. R., & Baker, L. A. (2012). Applications of microelectromagnetic traps. *Analytical and Bioanalytical Chemistry, 403*, 2077–2088.

Bazant, M. Z., & Squires, T. M. (2004). Induced-charge electrokinetic phenomena: Theory and microfluidic applications. *Physical Review Letters, 92*, 066101.

Bazant, M. Z., & Squires, T. M. (2010). Induced-charge electrokinetic phenomena. *Current Opinion in Colloid and Interface Science, 15*, 203–213.

Beebe, D. J., Mensing, G. A., & Walker, G. M. (2002). Physics and applications of microfluidics in biology. *Annual Review of Biomedical Engineering, 4*, 261–286.

van Beek, L. K. H. (1960). Dielectric behaviour of heterogeneous systems. *Progress in Dielectrics, 7*, 69–114.

Berthier, E., Warrick, J., Yu, H., & Beebe, D. J. (2008). Managing evaporation for more robust microscale assays – Part 1. Volume loss in high throughput assays. *Lab on a Chip, 8*, 852–859.

Bhagat, A. A. S., Kuntaegowdanahalli, S. S., & Papautsky, I. (2008a). Continuous particle separation in spiral microchannels using dean flows and differential migration. *Lab on a Chip, 8*, 1906–1914.

Bhagat, A. A. S., Kuntaegowdanahalli, S. S., & Papautsky, I. (2008b). Enhanced particle filtration in straight microchannels using shear-modulated inertial migration. *Physics of Fluids, 20*, 101702.

Brody, J. P., Yager, P., Goldstein, R. E., & Austin, R. H. (1996). Biotechnology at low Reynolds numbers. *Biophysical Journal, 71*, 3430–3441.

Bruus, H. (2012a). Acoustofluidics 7: The acoustic radiation force on small particles. *Lab on a Chip, 12*, 1014–1021.

Bruus, H. (2012b). Acoustofluidics 10: Scaling laws in acoustophoresis. *Lab on a Chip, 12*, 1578–1586.

Burgarella, S., Merlo, S., Dell'Anna, B., Zarola, G., & Bianchessi, M. (2010). A modular microfluidic platform for cells handling by dielectrophoresis. *Microelectronic Engineering, 87*, 2124–2133.

Caldwell, K. D., Cheng, Z. Q., Hradecky, P., & Giddings, J. C. (1984). Separation of human and animal-cells by steric field-flow fractionation. *Cell Biophysics, 6*, 233–251.

Castellanos, A., Ramos, A., Gonzalez, A., Green, N. G., & Morgan, H. (2003). Electrohydrodynamics and dielectrophoresis in microsystems: Scaling laws. *Journal of Physics D: Applied Physics, 36*, 2584–2597.

Cen, E. G., Dalton, C., Li, Y., Adamia, S., Pilarski, L. M., & Kaler, K. V. I. S. (2004). A combined dielectrophoresis, traveling wave dielectrophoresis and electrorotation microchip for the manipulation and characterization of human malignant cells. *Journal of Microbiological Methods, 58*, 387–401.

Cheng, I. F., Froude, V. E., Zhu, Y. X., Chang, H. C., & Chang, H. C. (2009). A continuous high-throughput bioparticle sorter based on 3D traveling-wave dielectrophoresis. *Lab on a Chip, 9*, 3193–3201.

Cheung, L. S. L., Zheng, X. G., Stopa, A., Baygents, J. C., Guzman, R., Schroeder, J. A., et al. (2009). Detachment of captured cancer cells under flow acceleration in a bio-functionalized microchannel. *Lab on a Chip, 9*, 1721–1731.

Chianea, T., Assidjo, N. E., & Cardot, P. J. P. (2000). Sedimentation field-flow-fractionation: Emergence of a new cell separation methodology. *Talanta, 51*, 835–847.

Chiou, P. Y., Ohta, A. T., & Wu, M. C. (2005). Massively parallel manipulation of single cells and microparticles using optical images. *Nature, 436*, 370–372.

Cho, S. H., Chen, C. H., Tsai, F. S., Godin, J. M., & Lo, Y. H. (2010). Human mammalian cell sorting using a highly integrated micro-fabricated fluorescence-activated cell sorter (mu FACS). *Lab on a Chip, 10*, 1567–1573.

Cho, S. H., Godin, J. M., Chen, C. H., Qiao, W., Lee, H., & Lo, Y. H. (2010). Review article: Recent advancements in optofluidic flow cytometer. *Biomicrofluidics, 4*, 043001.

Choi, S., & Park, J. K. (2007). Continuous hydrophoretic separation and sizing of microparticles using slanted obstacles in a microchannel. *Lab on a Chip, 7*, 890–897.

Choi, S., & Park, J. K. (2009). Tuneable hydrophoretic separation using elastic deformation of poly(dimethylsiloxane). *Lab on a Chip, 9*, 1962–1965.

Choi, J.-W., Liakopoulos, T. M., & Ahn, C. H. (2001). An on-chip magnetic bead separator using spiral electromagnets with semi-encapsulated permalloy. *Biosensors and Bioelectronics, 16*, 409–416.

Choi, S., Song, S., Choi, C., & Park, J. K. (2007). Continuous blood cell separation by hydrophoretic filtration. *Lab on a Chip, 7*, 1532–1538.

Choi, S., Song, S., Choi, C., & Park, J. K. (2008). Sheathless focusing of microbeads and blood cells based on hydrophoresis. *Small, 4*, 634−641.

Choi, S., Song, S., Choi, C., & Park, J. K. (2009). Microfluidic self-sorting of mammalian cells to achieve cell cycle synchrony by hydrophoresis. *Analytical Chemistry, 81*, 1964−1968.

Choi, Y.-S., Seo, K.-W., & Lee, S.-J. (2011). Lateral and cross-lateral focusing of spherical particles in a square microchannel. *Lab on a Chip, 11*, 460−465.

Chou, C.-F., Tegenfeldt, J. O., Bakajin, O., Chan, S. S., Cox, E. C., Darnton, N., et al. (2002). Electrodeless dielectrophoresis of single- and double-stranded DNA. *Biophysical Journal, 83*, 2170−2179.

Coley, H. M., Labeed, F. H., Thomas, H., & Hughes, M. P. (2007). Biophysical characterization of MDR breast cancer cell lines reveals the cytoplasm is critical in determining drug sensitivity. *Biochimica et Biophysica Acta-General Subjects, 1770*, 601−608.

Cornish, R. J. (1928). Flow in a pipe of rectangular cross-section. *Proceedings of the Royal Society of London. Series A: Containing Papers of a Mathematical and Physical Character, 120*, 691−700.

Crane, J. S., & Pohl, H. A. (1968). A study of living and dead yeast cells using dielectrophoresis. *Journal of the Electrochemical Society, 115*, 584.

Crane, J. S., & Pohl, H. A. (1972). Theoretical models of cellular dielectrophoresis. *Journal of Theoretical Biology, 37*, 15−41.

Cummings, E. B., & Singh, A. K. (2000). Dielectrophoretic trapping without embedded electrodes. In C. H. Mastrangelo, & H. Becker (Eds.), *Microfluidic devices and systems iii*. Bellingham: Spie-Int Soc Optical Engineering.

Cummings, E. B., & Singh, A. K. (2003). Dielectrophoresis in microchips containing arrays of insulating posts: Theoretical and experimental results. *Analytical Chemistry, 75*, 4724−4731.

Dalton, C., & Kaler, K. V. I. S. (2007). A cost effective, re-configurable electrokinetic microfluidic chip platform. *Sensors and Actuators B: Chemical, 123*, 628−635.

Davis, J. A., Inglis, D. W., Morton, K. J., Lawrence, D. A., Huang, L. R., Chou, S. Y., et al. (2006). Deterministic hydrodynamics: Taking blood apart. *Proceedings of the National Academy of Sciences of the United States of America, 103*, 14779−14784.

Demierre, N., Braschler, T., Linderholm, P., Seger, U., van Lintel, H., & Renaud, P. (2007). Characterization and optimization of liquid electrodes for lateral dielectrophoresis. *Lab on a Chip, 7*, 355−365.

Deng, T., Whitesides, G. M., Radhakrishnan, M., Zabow, G., & Prentiss, M. (2001). Manipulation of magnetic microbeads in suspension using micromagnetic systems fabricated with soft lithography. *Applied Physics Letters, 78*, 1775−1777.

Di Carlo, D. (2009). Inertial microfluidics. *Lab on a Chip, 9*, 3038−3046.

Di Carlo, D., Edd, J. F., Irimia, D., Tompkins, R. G., & Toner, M. (2008). Equilibrium separation and filtration of particles using differential inertial focusing. *Analytical Chemistry, 80*, 2204−2211.

Di Carlo, D., Irimia, D., Tompkins, R. G., & Toner, M. (2007). Continuous inertial focusing, ordering, and separation of particles in microchannels. *Proceedings of the National Academy of Sciences of the United States of America, 104*, 18892−18897.

Doh, I., & Cho, Y.-H. (2005). A continuous cell separation chip using hydrodynamic dielectrophoresis (DEP) process. *Sensors and Actuators A: Physical, 121*, 59−65.

Do, J., Zhang, J. Y., & Klapperich, C. M. (2011). Maskless writing of microfluidics: Rapid prototyping of 3D microfluidics using scratch on a polymer substrate. *Robotics and Computer-Integrated Manufacturing, 27*, 245−248.

Eriksson, E., Sott, K., Lundqvist, F., Sveningsson, M., Scrimgeour, J., Hanstorp, D., et al. (2010). A microfluidic device for reversible environmental changes around single cells using optical tweezers for cell selection and positioning. *Lab on a Chip, 10*, 617−625.

Evander, M., Lenshof, A., Laurell, T., & Nilsson, J. (2008). Acoustophoresis in wet-etched glass chips. *Analytical Chemistry, 80*, 5178−5185.

Fahraeus, R., & Lindqvist, T. (1931). The viscosity of the blood in narrow capillary tubes. *American Journal of Physiology, 96*, 562−568.

Fatoyinbo, H. O., Hoeftges, K. F., & Hughes, M. P. (2008). Rapid-on-chip determination of dielectric properties of biological cells using imaging techniques in a dielectrophoresis dot microsystem. *Electrophoresis, 29*, 3−10.

Fatoyinbo, H. O., Hoettges, K. F., Reddy, S. M., & Hughes, M. P. (2007). An integrated dielectrophoretic quartz crystal microbalance (DEP-QCM) device for rapid biosensing applications. *Biosensors and Bioelectronics, 23*, 225−232.

Fatoyinbo, H. O., Hughes, M. P., Martin, S. P., Pashby, P., & Labeed, F. H. (2007). Dielectrophoretic separation of Bacillus subtilis spores from environmental diesel particles. *Journal of Environmental Monitoring, 9*, 87−90.

Fatoyinbo, H. O., Kadri, N. A., Gould, D. H., Hoettges, K. F., & Labeed, F. H. (2011). Real-time cell electrophysiology using a multi-channel dielectrophoretic-dot microelectrode array. *Electrophoresis, 32*, 2541−2549.

Forbes, T. P., & Forry, S. P. (2012). Microfluidic magnetophoretic separations of immunomagnetically labeled rare mammalian cells. *Lab on a Chip, 12*, 1471−1479.

Fricke, H. (1924). A mathematical treatment of the electrical conductivity of colloids and cell suspensions. *The Journal of General Physiology, 6*, 375−384.

Fuerstman, M. J., Lai, A., Thurlow, M. E., Shevkoplyas, S. S., Stone, H. A., & Whitesides, G. M. (2007). The pressure drop along rectangular microchannels containing bubbles. *Lab on a Chip, 7*, 1479−1489.

Fu, A. Y., Spence, C., Scherer, A., Arnold, F. H., & Quake, S. R. (1999). A microfabricated fluorescence-activated cell sorter. *Nature Biotechnology, 17*, 1109−1111.

Gad-el-Hak, M. (2001). Flow physics in MEMS. *Mécanique and Industries, 2*, 313−341.

Garcia-Sanchez, P., Ramos, A., Green, N. G., & Morgan, H. (2006). Experiments on AC electrokinetic pumping of liquids using arrays of microelectrodes. *IEEE Transactions on Dielectrics and Electrical Insulation, 13*, 670−677.

Gascoyne, P. R. C. (2009). Dielectrophoretic-field flow fractionation analysis of dielectric, density, and deformability characteristics of cells and particles. *Analytical Chemistry, 81*, 8878−8885.

Gascoyne, P. R. C., Huang, Y., Pethig, R., Vykoukal, J., & Becker, F. F. (1992). Dielectrophoretic separation of mammalian-cells studied by computerized image-analysis. *Measurement Science and Technology, 3*, 439−445.

Gascoyne, P. R. C., & Vykoukal, J. V. (2004). Dielectrophoresis-based sample handling in general-purpose programmable diagnostic instruments. *Proceedings of the IEEE, 92*, 22−42.

Geislinger, T. M., Eggart, B., Ller, S. B., Schmid, L., & Franke, T. (2012). Separation of blood cells using hydrodynamic lift. *Applied Physics Letters, 100*, 4.

Gervais, T., El-Ali, J., Gunther, A., & Jensen, K. F. (2006). Flow-induced deformation of shallow microfluidic channels. *Lab on a Chip, 6*, 500−507.

Giddings, J. C. (1968). Nonequilibrium theory of field-flow fractionation. *The Journal of Chemical Physics, 49*, 81.

Giddings, J. C. (1993). Field-flow fractionation − analysis of macromolecular, colloidal, and particulate materials. *Science, 260*, 1456−1465.

Giddings, J. C., Chen, X., Wahlund, K. G., & Myers, M. N. (1987). Fast particle separation by flow/steric field-flow fractionation. *Analytical Chemistry, 59*, 1957−1962.

Giddings, J. C., & Myers, M. N. (1978). Steric field-flow fractionation − new method for separating 1-μm to 100-μm particles. *Separation Science and Technology, 13*, 637−645.

Gijs, M. A. M. (2004). Magnetic bead handling on-chip: New opportunities for analytical applications. *Microfluidics and Nanofluidics, 1*, 22−40.

Gimsa, J. (1997). Particle characterization by AC-electrokinetic phenomena: 1. A short introduction to dielectrophoresis (dp) and electrorotation (ER). In D. Exerowa, & D. Platikanov (Eds.), *Surface and colloid science, July 1997* (pp. 451−460). Sofia: Elsevier.

Gossett, D. R., & Di Carlo, D. (2009). Particle focusing mechanisms in curving confined flows. *Analytical Chemistry, 81*, 8459−8465.

Gravesen, P., Branebjerg, J., & Jensen, O. S. (1993). Microfluidics − a review. *Journal of Micromechanics and Microengineering, 3*, 168−182.

Green, N. G., Ramos, A., & Morgan, H. (2002). Numerical solution of the dielectrophoretic and travelling wave forces for interdigitated electrode arrays using the finite element method. *Journal of Electrostatics, 56*, 235−254.

Guido, S., & Tomaiuolo, G. (2009). Microconfined flow behavior of red blood cells in vitro. *Comptes Rendus Physique, 10*, 751−763.

Gupta, V., Jafferji, I., Garza, M., Melnikova, V. O., Hasegawa, D. K., Pethig, R., et al. (2012). ApoStream (TM), a new dielectrophoretic device for antibody independent isolation and recovery of viable cancer cells from blood. *Biomicrofluidics, 6*, 024133.

Hackett, S., Hamzah, J., Davis, T. M. E., & St Pierre, T. G. (2009). Magnetic susceptibility of iron in malaria-infected red blood cells. *Biochimica et Biophysica Acta-Molecular Basis of Disease, 1792*, 93−99.

Hagsater, S. M., Jensen, T. G., Bruus, H., & Kutter, J. P. (2007). Acoustic resonances in microfluidic chips: Full-image micro-PIV experiments and numerical simulations. *Lab on a Chip, 7*, 1336−1344.

Hawkins, B. G., Huang, C., Arasanipalai, S., & Kirby, B. J. (2011). Automated dielectrophoretic characterization of *Mycobacterium smegmatis*. *Analytical Chemistry, 83*, 3507−3515.

Henslee, E. A., Sano, M. B., Rojas, A. D., Schmelz, E. M., & Davalos, R. V. (2011). Selective concentration of human cancer cells using contactless dielectrophoresis. *Electrophoresis, 32*, 2523−2529.

Heo, Y. S., Cabrera, L. M., Song, J. W., Futai, N., Tung, Y.-C., Smith, G. D., et al. (2006). Characterization and resolution of evaporation-mediated osmolality shifts that constrain microfluidic cell culture in poly(dimethylsiloxane) devices. *Analytical Chemistry, 79*, 1126−1134.

Hoettges, K. F. (2010). Dielectrophoresis as a cell characterisation tool. In M. P. Hughes, & K. F. Hoettges (Eds.), *Microengineering in biotechnology*. Totowa, NJ: Humana Press Inc.

Hoettges, K. F., Hubner, Y., Broche, L. M., Ogin, S. L., Kass, G. E. N., & Hughes, M. P. (2008). Dielectrophoresis-activated multiwell plate for label-free high-throughput drug assessment. *Analytical Chemistry, 80*, 2063−2068.

Hoettges, K. F., McDonnell, M. B., & Hughes, M. P. (2003). Use of combined dielectrophoretic/electrohydrodynamic forces for biosensor enhancement. *Journal of Physics D: Applied Physics, 36*, L101−L104.

Ho, B. P., & Leal, L. G. (1974). Inertial migration of rigid spheres in 2-dimensional unidirectional flows. *Journal of Fluid Mechanics, 65*, 365−400.

Holzel, R. (1998). Nystatin-induced changes in yeast monitored by time resolved automated single cell electrorotation. *Biochimica et Biophysica Acta, 1425*, 311−318.

Horowitz, V. R., Awschalom, D. D., & Pennathur, S. (2008). Optofluidics: Field or technique? *Lab on a Chip, 8*, 1856−1863.

Hou, H. W., Gan, H. Y., Bhagat, A. A. S., Li, L. D., Lim, C. T., & Han, J. (2012). A microfluidics approach towards high-throughput pathogen removal from blood using margination. *Biomicrofluidics, 6*, 024115.

Hou, H. W., Li, Q. S., Lee, G. Y. H., Kumar, A. P., Ong, C. N., & Lim, C. T. (2009). Deformability study of breast cancer cells using microfluidics. *Biomedical Microdevices, 11*, 557−564.

Huang, Y., Agrawal, B., Sun, D. D., Kuo, J. S., & Williams, J. C. (2011). Microfluidics-based devices: New tools for studying cancer and cancer stem cell migration. *Biomicrofluidics, 5*, 013412.

Huang, L. R., Cox, E. C., Austin, R. H., & Sturm, J. C. (2004). Continuous particle separation through deterministic lateral displacement. *Science, 304*, 987−990.

Huang, Y., Holzel, R., Pethig, R., & Wang, X. B. (1992). Differences in the AC electrodynamics of viable and non-viable yeast cells determined through combined dielectrophoresis and electrorotation studies. *Physics in Medicine and Biology, 37*, 1499−1517.

Huang, Y., Wang, X. B., Tame, J. A., & Pethig, R. (1993). Electrokinetic behavior of colloidal particles in traveling electric-fields − studies using yeast-cells. *Journal of Physics D: Applied Physics, 26*, 1528−1535.

Hu, X. Y., Bessette, P. H., Qian, J. R., Meinhart, C. D., Daugherty, P. S., & Soh, H. T. (2005). Marker-specific sorting of rare cells using dielectrophoresis. *Proceedings of the National Academy of Sciences of the United States of America, 102*, 15757−15761.

Hughes, M. P. (1998). Computer aided analysis of conditons for optimizing practical electrorotation. *Physics in Medicine and Biology, 43*, 3639−3648.

Hughes, M. P. (2002). Strategies for dielectrophoretic separation in laboratory-on-a-chip systems. *Electrophoresis, 23*, 2569−2582.

Hughes, M. P. (2003). *Nanoelectromechanics in engineering and biology*. Boca Raton, FL: CRC Press.

Hughes, M. P., Pethig, R., & Wang, X.-B. (1995). Dielectrophoretic forces on particles in travelling electric fields. *Journal of Physics D: Applied Physics, 29*, 474−482.

Hur, S. C., Henderson-Maclennan, N. K., McCabe, E. R. B., & Di Carlo, D. (2011). Deformability-based cell classification and enrichment using inertial microfluidics. *Lab on a Chip, 11*, 912−920.

Inglis, D. W., Davis, J. A., Austin, R. H., & Sturm, J. C. (2006). Critical particle size for fractionation by deterministic lateral displacement. *Lab on a Chip, 6*, 655−658.

Inglis, D. W., Davis, J. A., Zieziulewicz, T. J., Lawrence, D. A., Austin, R. H., & Sturm, J. C. (2008). Determining blood cell size using microfluidic hydrodynamics. *Journal of Immunological Methods, 329*, 151−156.

Inglis, D. W., Riehn, R., Austin, R. H., & Sturm, J. C. (2004). Continuous microfluidic immunomagnetic cell separation. *Applied Physics Letters, 85*, 5093−5095.

Irimajiri, A., Hanai, T., & Inouye, A. (1979). Dielectric theory of multi-stratified shell-model with its application to a lymphoma cell. *Journal of Theoretical Biology, 78*, 251−269.

Jackson, M. B. (2006). *Molecular and cellular biophysics*. Cambridge, UK: Cambridge University Press.

Jain, A., & Munn, L. L. (2011). Biomimetic postcapillary expansions for enhancing rare blood cell separation on a microfluidic chip. *Lab on a Chip, 11*, 2941−2947.

Jendretzki, A., Wittland, J., Wilk, S., Straede, A., & Heinisch, J. J. (2011). How do I begin? Sensing extracellular stress to maintain yeast cell wall integrity. *European Journal of Cell Biology, 90*, 740−744.

Jin, X., Zhao, Y., Richardson, A., Moore, L., Williams, P. S., Zborowski, M., et al. (2008). Differences in magnetically induced motion of diamagnetic, paramagnetic, and superparamagnetic microparticles detected by cell tracking velocimetry. *Analyst, 133*, 1767−1775.

Jones, T. B. (1995). *Electromechanics of particles*. Cambridge, UK: Cambridge University Press.

Kantak, A., Merugu, S., & Gale, B. K. (2006). Improved theory of cyclical electrical field flow fractionation. *Electrophoresis, 27*, 2833−2843.

Kersaudy-Kerhoas, M., Dhariwal, R., Desmulliez, M. P. Y., & Jouvet, L. (2010). Hydrodynamic blood plasma separation in microfluidic channels. *Microfluidics and Nanofluidics, 8*, 105−114.

Kim, D., Chesler, N. C., & Beebe, D. J. (2006). A method for dynamic system characterization using hydraulic series resistance. *Lab on a Chip, 6*, 639−644.

Kim, E. K., & Choi, E.-J. (2010). Pathological roles of MAPK signaling pathways in human diseases. *Biochimica et Biophysica Acta - Molecular Basis of Disease, 1802*, 396−405.

Kim, H. J., Moon, H. S., Kwak, B. S., & Jung, H. I. (2011). Microfluidic device to separate micro-beads with various fluorescence intensities. *Sensors and Actuators B: Chemical, 160*, 1536−1543.

Kim, U., Qian, J., Kenrick, S. A., Daugherty, P. S., & Soh, H. T. (2008). Multitarget dielectrophoresis activated cell sorter. *Analytical Chemistry, 80*, 8656−8661.

Kim, U., & Soh, H. T. (2009). Simultaneous sorting of multiple bacterial targets using integrated dielectrophoretic-magnetic activated cell sorter. *Lab on a Chip, 9*, 2313−2318.

Kim, Y. W., & Yoo, J. Y. (2008). The lateral migration of neutrally-buoyant spheres transported through square microchannels. *Journal of Micromechanics and Microengineering, 18*, 065015.

Kim, Y. W., & Yoo, J. Y. (2012). Transport of solid particles in microfluidic channels. *Optics and Lasers in Engineering, 50*, 87−98.

Klis, F. M., Boorsma, A., & De Groot, P. W. J. (2006). Cell wall construction in *Saccharomyces cerevisiae*. *Yeast, 23*, 185−202.

Kowalkowski, T., Buszewski, B., Cantado, C., & Dondi, F. (2006). Field-flow fractionation: Theory, techniques, applications and the challenges. *Critical Reviews in Analytical Chemistry, 36*, 129−135.

Kultz, D., & Chakravarty, D. (2001). Maintenance of genomic integrity in mammalian kidney cells exposed to hyperosmotic stress. *Comparative Biochemistry and Physiology A: Molecular and Integrative Physiology, 130*, 421−428.

Kumar, M., Feke, D. L., & Belovich, J. M. (2005). Fractionation of cell mixtures using acoustic and laminar flow fields. *Biotechnology and Bioengineering, 89*, 129−137.

Kuntaegowdanahalli, S. S., Bhagat, A. A. S., Kumar, G., & Papautsky, I. (2009). Inertial microfluidics for continuous particle separation in spiral microchannels. *Lab on a Chip, 9*, 2973−2980.

Labeed, F. H., Lu, J., Mulhall, H. J., Marchenko, S. A., Hoettges, K. F., Estrada, L. C., et al. (2011). Biophysical characteristics reveal neural stem cell differentiation potential. *PLoS One, 6*, e25458.

Lapizco-Encinas, B. H., Davalos, R. V., Simmons, B. A., Cummings, E. B., & Fintschenko, Y. (2005). An insulator-based (electrodeless) dielectrophoretic concentrator for microbes in water. *Journal of Microbiological Methods, 62*, 317−326.

Lapizco-Encinas, B. H., Simmons, B. A., Cummings, E. B., & Fintschenko, Y. (2004). Dielectrophoretic concentration and separation of live and dead bacteria in an array of insulators. *Analytical Chemistry, 76*, 1571−1579.

Lau, A. Y., Lee, L. P., & Chan, J. W. (2008). An integrated optofluidic platform for Raman-activated cell sorting. *Lab on a Chip, 8*, 1116−1120.

Laurell, T., Petersson, F., & Nilsson, A. (2007). Chip integrated strategies for acoustic separation and manipulation of cells and particles. *Chemical Society Reviews, 36*, 492−506.

Lee, W. C., Bhagat, A. A. S., Huang, S., van Vliet, K. J., Han, J., & Lim, C. T. (2011). High-throughput cell cycle synchronization using inertial forces in spiral microchannels. *Lab on a Chip, 11*, 1359−1367.

Lee, K., Kim, C., Ahn, B., Kang, J. Y., & Oh, K. W. (2009). Hydrodynamically focused particle filtration using an island structure. *Biochip Journal, 3*, 275−280.

Lenshof, A., Ahmad-Tajudin, A., Jaras, K., Sward-Nilsson, A. M., Aberg, L., Marko-Varga, G., et al. (2009). Acoustic whole blood plasmapheresis chip for prostate specific antigen microarray diagnostics. *Analytical Chemistry, 81*, 6030−6037.

Lenshof, A., Evander, M., Laurell, T., & Nilsson, J. (2012). Acoustofluidics 5: Building microfluidic acoustic resonators. *Lab on a Chip, 12*, 684−695.

Liao, S. H., Cheng, I. F., & Chang, H. C. (2012). Precisely sized separation of multiple particles based on the dielectrophoresis gradient in the z-direction. *Microfluidics and Nanofluidics, 12*, 201−211.

Li, X. J., & Li, P. C. H. (2014). Cytosolic calcium measurement for single-cell drug efficacy and cardiotoxicity evaluations using microfluidic biochips. *Canadian Journal of Pure and Applied Sciences, 8*, 2663−2669.

Li, J., & Lin, F. (2011). Microfluidic devices for studying chemotaxis and electrotaxis. *Trends in Cell Biology, 21*, 489−497.

Lin, S. J., Hung, S. H., Jeng, J. Y., Guo, T. F., & Lee, G. B. (2012). Manipulation of microparticles by flexible polymer-based optically-induced dielectrophoretic devices. *Optics Express, 20*, 583−592.

Liu, Y. J., Guo, S. S., Zhang, Z. L., Huang, W. H., Baigl, D., Xie, M., et al. (2007). A micropillar-integrated smart microfluidic device for specific capture and sorting of cells. *Electrophoresis, 28*, 4713−4722.

Liu, C. X., Stakenborg, T., Peeters, S., & Lagae, L. (2009). Cell manipulation with magnetic particles toward microfluidic cytometry. *Journal of Applied Physics, 105*, 102014.

Lochovsky, C., Yasotharan, S., & Gunther, A. (2012). Bubbles no more: In-plane trapping and removal of bubbles in microfluidic devices. *Lab on a Chip, 12*, 595−601.

Loutherback, K., Chou, K. S., Newman, J., Puchalla, J., Austin, R. H., & Sturm, J. C. (2010). Improved performance of deterministic lateral displacement arrays with triangular posts. *Microfluidics and Nanofluidics, 9*, 1143−1149.

Manneberg, O., Hagsater, S. M., Svennebring, J., Hertz, H. M., Kutter, J. P., Bruus, H., et al. (2009). Spatial confinement of ultrasonic force fields in microfluidic channels. *Ultrasonics, 49*, 112−119.

Manz, A., Graber, N., & Widmer, H. M. (1990). Miniaturized total chemical analysis systems: A novel concept for chemical sensing. *Sensors and Actuators B: Chemical, 1*, 244−248.

Markx, G. H., Huang, Y., Zhou, X. F., & Pethig, R. (1994). Dielectrophoretic characterization and separation of microorganisms. *Microbiology-UK, 140*, 585−591.

Markx, G. H., & Pethig, R. (1995). Dielectrophoretic separation of cells: Continuous separation. *Biotechnology and Bioengineering, 45*, 337−343.

Markx, G. H., Rousselet, J., & Pethig, R. (1997). DEP-FFF: Field-flow fractionation using non-uniform electric fields. *Journal of Liquid Chromatography and Related Technologies, 20*, 2857−2872.

Masuda, S., Washizu, M., & Kawabata, I. (1988). Movement of blood cells in liquid by nonuniform traveling field. *IEEE Transactions on Industry Applications, 24*, 217−222.

Matsuda, M., Yamada, M., & Seki, M. (2011). Blood cell classification utilizing hydrodynamic filtration. *Electronics and Communications in Japan, 94*, 1−6.
McCloskey, K. E., Chalmers, J. J., & Zborowski, M. (2003). Magnetic cell separation: Characterization of magnetophoretic mobility. *Analytical Chemistry, 75*, 6868−6874.
Melville, D., Paul, F., & Roath, S. (1975a). Direct magnetic separation of red-cells from whole-blood. *Nature, 255*, 706.
Melville, D., Paul, F., & Roath, S. (1975b). High gradient magnetic separation of red-cells from whole-blood. *IEEE Transactions on Magnetics, 11*, 1701−1704.
Melvin, E. M., Moore, B. R., Gilchrist, K. H., Grego, S., & Velev, O. D. (2011). On-chip collection of particles and cells by AC electroosmotic pumping and dielectrophoresis using asymmetric microelectrodes. *Biomicrofluidics, 5*, 034113.
Migita, S., Funakoshi, K., Tsuya, D., Yamazaki, T., Taniguchi, A., Sugimoto, Y., et al. (2010). Cell cycle and size sorting of mammalian cells using a microfluidic device. *Analytical Methods, 2*, 657−660.
Mogensen, K. B., & Kutter, J. P. (2009). Optical detection in microfluidic systems. *Electrophoresis, 30*, S92−S100.
Moon, H. S., Kwon, K., Kim, S. I., Han, H., Sohn, J., Lee, S., et al. (2011). Continuous separation of breast cancer cells from blood samples using multiorifice flow fractionation (MOFF) and dielectrophoresis (DEP). *Lab on a Chip, 11*, 1118−1125.
Moore, L. R., Milliron, S., Williams, P. S., Chalmers, J. J., Margel, S., & Zborowski, M. (2004). Control of magnetophoretic mobility by susceptibility-modified solutions as evaluated by cell tracking velocimetry and continuous magnetic sorting. *Analytical Chemistry, 76*, 3899−3907.
Morgan, H., Izquierdo, A. G., Bakewell, D., Green, N. G., & Ramos, A. (2001). The dielectrophoretic and travelling wave forces generated by interdigitated electrode arrays: Analytical solution using fourier series. *Journal of Physics D: Applied Physics, 34*, 1553−1561.
Morton, K. J., Loutherback, K., Inglis, D. W., Tsui, O. K., Sturm, J. C., Chou, S. Y., et al. (2008). Hydrodynamic metamaterials: Microfabricated arrays to steer, refract, and focus streams of biomaterials. *Proceedings of the National Academy of Sciences of the United States of America, 105*, 7434−7438.
Mulhall, H. J., Labeed, F. H., Kazmi, B., Costea, D. E., Hughes, M. P., & Lewis, M. P. (2011). Cancer, pre-cancer and normal oral cells distinguished by dielectrophoresis. *Analytical and Bioanalytical Chemistry, 401*, 2455−2463.
Muller, T., Gradl, G., Howitz, S., Shirley, S., Schnelle, T., & Fuhr, G. (1999). A 3-D microelectrode system for handling and caging single cells and particles. *Biosensors and Bioelectronics, 14*, 247−256.
Murata, M., Okamoto, Y., Park, Y. S., Kaji, N., Tokeshi, M., & Baba, Y. (2009). Cell separation by the combination of microfluidics and optical trapping force on a microchip. *Analytical and Bioanalytical Chemistry, 394*, 277−283.
Myers, M. N., & Giddings, J. C. (1982). Properties of the transition from normal to steric field-flow fractionation. *Analytical Chemistry, 54*, 2284−2289.
Nakashima, M., Yamada, M., & Seki, M. (2004). Pinched flow fractionation (PFF) for continuous particle separation in a microfluidic device. In *MEMS 2004: 17th IEEE international conference on micro electro mechanical systems, technical digest*. New York: IEEE.
Nam, J., Lee, Y., & Shin, S. (2011). Size-dependent microparticles separation through standing surface acoustic waves. *Microfluidics and Nanofluidics, 11*, 317−326.

Nam, J., Lim, H., Kim, D., & Shin, S. (2011). Separation of platelets from whole blood using standing surface acoustic waves in a microchannel. *Lab on a Chip, 11*, 3361−3364.

Nilsson, A., Petersson, F., Jonsson, H., & Laurell, T. (2004). Acoustic control of suspended particles in micro fluidic chips. *Lab on a Chip, 4*, 131−135.

Oberteuf, J. A. (1974). Magnetic separation − review of principles, devices, and applications. *IEEE Transactions on Magnetics, MA10*, 223−238.

Oh, K. W., Lee, K., Ahn, B., & Furlani, E. P. (2012). Design of pressure-driven microfluidic networks using electric circuit analogy. *Lab on a Chip, 12*, 515−545.

Pamme, N. (2006). Magnetism and microfluidics. *Lab on a Chip, 6*, 24−38.

Pamme, N., & Manz, A. (2004). On-chip free-flow magnetophoresis: Continuous flow separation of magnetic particles and agglomerates. *Analytical Chemistry, 76*, 7250−7256.

Pamme, N., & Wilhelm, C. (2006). Continuous sorting of magnetic cells via on-chip free-flow magnetophoresis. *Lab on a Chip, 6*, 974−980.

Pankhurst, Q. A., Connolly, J., Jones, S. K., & Dobson, J. (2003). Applications of magnetic nanoparticles in biomedicine. *Journal of Physics D: Applied Physics, 36*, R167−R181.

Park, J. S., & Jung, H. I. (2009). Multiorifice flow fractionation: Continuous size-based separation of microspheres using a series of contraction/expansion microchannels. *Analytical Chemistry, 81*, 8280−8288.

Park, J. S., Song, S. H., & Jung, H. I. (2009). Continuous focusing of microparticles using inertial lift force and vorticity via multi-orifice microfluidic channels. *Lab on a Chip, 9*, 939−948.

Paul, F., Melville, D., Roath, S., & Warhurst, D. C. (1981). A bench top magnetic separator for malarial parasite concentration. *IEEE Transactions on Magnetics, 17*, 2822−2824.

Petersson, F., Aberg, L., Sward-Nilsson, A. M., & Laurell, T. (2007). Free flow acoustophoresis: Microfluidic-based mode of particle and cell separation. *Analytical Chemistry, 79*, 5117−5123.

Petersson, F., Nilsson, A., Holm, C., Jonsson, H., & Laurell, T. (2004). Separation of lipids from blood utilizing ultrasonic standing waves in microfluidic channels. *Analyst, 129*, 938−943.

Petersson, F., Nilsson, A., Jonsson, H., & Laurell, T. (2005). Carrier medium exchange through ultrasonic particle switching in microfluidic channels. *Analytical Chemistry, 77*, 1216−1221.

Pethig, R. (1979). *Dielectric and electronic properties of biological materials*. Chichester, UK: John Wiley & Sons.

Pethig, R. (2010). Review article-dielectrophoresis: Status of the theory, technology, and applications. *Biomicrofluidics, 4*, 35.

Pethig, R., & Talary, M. S. (2007). Dielectrophoretic detection of membrane morphology changes in Jurkat T-cells undergoing etoposide-induced apoptosis. *IET Nanobiotechnology, 1*, 2−9.

Pipe, C. J., & McKinley, G. H. (2009). Microfluidic rheometry. *Mechanics Research Communications, 36*, 110−120.

Plouffe, B. D., Mahalanabis, M., Lewis, L. H., Klapperich, C. M., & Murthy, S. K. (2012). Clinically relevant microfluidic magnetophoretic isolation of rare-cell populations for diagnostic and therapeutic monitoring applications. *Analytical Chemistry, 84*, 1336−1344.

Pohl, H. A. (1951). The motion and precipitation of suspensoids in divergent electric fields. *Journal of Applied Physics, 22*, 869−871.

Pohl, H. A. (1958). Some effects of nonuniform fields on dielectrics. *Journal of Applied Physics, 29*, 1182−1188.

Pohl, H. A. (1978). *Dielectrophoresis*. Cambridge, UK: Cambridge Unviersity Press.

Pohl, H. A., & Crane, J. S. (1971). Dielectrophoresis of cells. *Biophysical Journal, 11*, 711−727.

Pohl, H. A., & Hawk, I. (1966). Separation of living and dead cells by dielectrophoresis. *Science, 152*, 647.

Psaltis, D., Quake, S. R., & Yang, C. H. (2006). Developing optofluidic technology through the fusion of microfluidics and optics. *Nature, 442*, 381–386.

Quake, S. R., & Scherer, A. (2000). From micro- to nanofabrication with soft materials. *Science, 290*, 1536–1540.

Ramos, A., Morgan, H., Green, N. G., & Castellanos, A. (1998). Ac electrokinetics: A review of forces in microelectrode structures. *Journal of Physics D: Applied Physics, 31*, 2338–2353.

Ramos, A., Morgan, H., Green, N. G., & Castellanos, A. (1999). AC electric-field-induced fluid flow in microelectrodes. *Journal of Colloid and Interface Science, 217*, 420–422.

Ravula, S. K., Branch, D. W., James, C. D., Townsend, R. J., Hill, M., Kaduchak, G., et al. (2008). A microfluidic system combining acoustic and dielectrophoretic particle preconcentration and focusing. *Sensors and Actuators B: Chemical, 130*, 645–652.

Reyes, D. R., Iossifidis, D., Auroux, P. A., & Manz, A. (2002). Micro total analysis systems. 1. Introduction, theory, and technology. *Analytical Chemistry, 74*, 2623–2636.

Reynolds, O. (1883). An experimental investigation of the circumstances which determine whether the motion of water shall be direct or sinuous, and the law of resistance in parallel channels. *Philosophical Transactions of the Royal Society of London, 174*, 935–982.

Robert, D., Pamme, N., Conjeaud, H., Gazeau, F., Iles, A., & Wilhelm, C. (2011). Cell sorting by endocytotic capacity in a microfluidic magnetophoresis device. *Lab on a Chip, 11*, 1902–1910.

Roda, B., Zattoni, A., Reschiglian, P., Moon, M. H., Mirasoli, M., Michelini, E., et al. (2009). Field-flow fractionation in bioanalysis: A review of recent trends. *Analytica Chimica Acta, 635*, 132–143.

Rodriguez-Villarreal, A. I., Tarn, M. D., Madden, L. A., Lutz, J. B., Greenman, J., Samitier, J., et al. (2010). Flow focussing of particles and cells based on their intrinsic properties using a simple diamagnetic repulsion setup. *Lab on a Chip, 11*, 1240–1248.

Ruzicka, M. C. (2008). On dimensionless numbers. *Chemical Engineering Research and Design, 86*, 835–868.

Saliba, A. E., Saias, L., Psychari, E., Minc, N., Simon, D., Bidard, F. C., et al. (2010). Microfluidic sorting and multimodal typing of cancer cells in self-assembled magnetic arrays. *Proceedings of the National Academy of Sciences of the United States of America, 107*, 14524–14529.

Sanchis, A., Brown, A. P., Sancho, M., Martinez, G., Sebastian, J. L., Munoz, S., et al. (2007). Dielectric characterization of bacterial cells using dielectrophoresis. *Bioelectromagnetics, 28*, 393–401.

Sano, M. B., Salmanzadeh, A., & Davalos, R. V. (2012). Multilayer contactless dielectrophoresis: Theoretical considerations. *Electrophoresis, 33*, 1938–1946.

Schmid, M., Häusele, B., Junk, M., Brookes, E., Frank, J., & Cölfen, H. (2018). High-resolution asymmetrical flow field-flow fractionation data evaluation via Richardson–Lucy-based fractogram correction. *Analytical Chemistry, 90*(23), 13978–13986.

Schneider, T., Moore, L. R., Jing, Y., Haam, S., Williams, P. S., Fleischman, A. J., et al. (2006). Continuous flow magnetic cell fractionation based on antigen expression level. *Journal of Biochemical and Biophysical Methods, 68*, 1–21.

Schonberg, J. A., & Hinch, E. J. (1989). Inertial migration of a sphere in Poiseuille flow. *Journal of Fluid Mechanics, 203*, 517–524.

Schulte, T. H., Bardell, R. L., & Weigl, B. H. (2002). Microfluidic technologies in clinical diagnostics. *Clinica Chimica Acta, 321*, 1–10.

Segre, G., & Silberberg, A. (1961). Radial particle displacements in Poiseuille flow of suspensions. *Nature, 189*, 209.

Segre, G., & Silberberg, A. (1962). Behaviour of macroscopic rigid spheres in Poiseuille flow. 2. Experimental results and interpretation. *Journal of Fluid Mechanics, 14*, 136−157.

Settnes, M., & Bruus, H. (2012). Forces acting on a small particle in an acoustical field in a viscous fluid. *Physical Review E, 85*, 12.

Shafiee, H., Caldwell, J. L., Sano, M. B., & Davalos, R. V. (2009). Contactless dielectrophoresis: A new technique for cell manipulation. *Biomedical Microdevices, 11*, 997−1006.

Shah, G. J., Ohta, A. T., Chiou, E. P. Y., Wu, M. C., & Kim, C. J. (2009). EWOD-driven droplet microfluidic device integrated with optoelectronic tweezers as an automated platform for cellular isolation and analysis. *Lab on a Chip, 9*, 1732−1739.

Shen, F., Hwang, H., Hahn, Y. K., & Park, J. K. (2012). Label-free cell separation using a tunable magnetophoretic repulsion force. *Analytical Chemistry, 84*, 3075−3081.

Shen, F., Li, X., & Li, P. C. H. (2014). Study of flow behaviors on single-cell manipulation and shear stress reduction in microfluidic chips using computational fluid dynamics simulations. *Biomicrofluidics, 8*, 014109.

Shen, F., Li, Y., Liu, Z., & Li, X. (2017). Study of flow behaviors of droplet merging and splitting in microchannels using Micro-PIV measurement. *Microfluidics and Nanofluidics, 21*, 66.

Shevkoplyas, S. S., Siegel, A. C., Westervelt, R. M., Prentiss, M. G., & Whitesides, G. M. (2007). The force acting on a superparamagnetic bead due to an applied magnetic field. *Lab on a Chip, 7*, 1294−1302.

Shevkoplyas, S. S., Yoshida, T., Munn, L. L., & Bitensky, M. W. (2005). Biomimetic autoseparation of leukocytes from whole blood in a microfluidic device. *Analytical Chemistry, 77*, 933−937.

Shi, J. J., Ahmed, D., Mao, X., Lin, S. C. S., Lawit, A., & Huang, T. J. (2009). Acoustic tweezers: Patterning cells and microparticles using standing surface acoustic waves (SSAW). *Lab on a Chip, 9*, 2890−2895.

Shi, J. J., Huang, H., Stratton, Z., Huang, Y. P., & Huang, T. J. (2009). Continuous particle separation in a microfluidic channel via standing surface acoustic waves (SSAW). *Lab on a Chip, 9*, 3354−3359.

Shi, J. J., Yazdi, S., Lin, S. C. S., Ding, X. Y., Chiang, I. K., Sharp, K., et al. (2011). Three-dimensional continuous particle focusing in a microfluidic channel via standing surface acoustic waves (SSAW). *Lab on a Chip, 11*, 2319−2324.

Siegel, A. C., Tang, S. K. Y., Nijhuis, C. A., Hashimoto, M., Phillips, S. T., Dickey, M. D., et al. (2009). Cofabrication: A strategy for building multicomponent microsystems. *Accounts of Chemical Research, 43*, 518−528.

Sim, T. S., Kwon, K., Park, J. C., Lee, J. G., & Jung, H. I. (2011). Multistage-multiorifice flow fractionation (MS-MOFF): Continuous size-based separation of microspheres using multiple series of contraction/expansion microchannels. *Lab on a Chip, 11*, 93−99.

Skelley, A. M., & Voldman, J. (2008). An active bubble trap and debubbler for microfluidic systems. *Lab on a Chip, 8*, 1733−1737.

Sollier, E., Murray, C., Maoddi, P., & Di Carlo, D. (2011). Rapid prototyping polymers for microfluidic devices and high pressure injections. *Lab on a Chip, 11*, 3752−3765.

Squires, T. M., & Quake, S. R. (2005). Microfluidics: Fluid physics at the nanoliter scale. *Reviews of Modern Physics, 77*, 977−1026.

Stone, H. A., Stroock, A. D., & Ajdari, A. (2004). Engineering flows in small devices: Microfluidics toward a lab-on-a-chip. *Annual Review of Fluid Mechanics, 36*, 381−411.

Stroock, A. D., Dertinger, S. K., Whitesides, G. M., & Ajdari, A. (2002). Patterning flows using grooved surfaces. *Analytical Chemistry, 74*, 5306−5312.

Stroock, A. D., & Whitesides, G. M. (2003). Controlling flows in microchannels with patterned surface charge and topography. *Accounts of Chemical Research, 36*, 597−604.

Sugaya, S., Yamada, M., & Seki, M. (2011). Observation of nonspherical particle behaviors for continuous shape-based separation using hydrodynamic filtration. *Biomicrofluidics, 5*, 13.

Sun, K., Wang, Z. X., & Jiang, X. Y. (2008). Modular microfluidics for gradient generation. *Lab on a Chip, 8*, 1536−1543.

Suresh, S. (2007). Biomechanics and biophysics of cancer cells. *Acta Biomaterialia, 3*, 413−438.

Svoboda, K., & Block, S. M. (1994). Biological applications of optical forces. *Annual Review of Biophysics and Biomolecular Structure, 23*, 247−285.

Takagi, J., Yamada, M., Yasuda, M., & Seki, M. (2005). Continuous particle separation in a microchannel having asymmetrically arranged multiple branches. *Lab on a Chip, 5*, 778−784.

Takayasu, M., Kelland, D. R., & Minervini, J. V. (2000). Continuous magnetic separation of blood components from whole blood. *IEEE Transactions on Applied Superconductivity, 10*, 927−930.

Talary, M. S., Burt, J. P. H., Tame, J. A., & Pethig, R. (1996). Electromanipulation and separation of cells using travelling electric fields. *Journal of Physics D: Applied Physics, 29*, 2198−2203.

Tanaka, T., Ishikawa, T., Numayama-Tsuruta, K., Imai, Y., Ueno, H., Yoshimoto, T., et al. (2012). Inertial migration of cancer cells in blood flow in microchannels. *Biomedical Microdevices, 14*, 25−33.

Tavakoli, H., Zhou, W., Ma, L., Perez, S., Ibarra, A., Xu, F., et al. (2019). Recent advances in microfluidic platforms for single-cell analysis in cancer biology, diagnosis and therapy. *TrAC Trends in Analytical Chemistry, 117*, 13−26.

Terry, S. C., Jerman, J. H., & Angell, J. B. (1979). A gas chromatographic air analyzer fabricated on a silicon wafer. *IEEE Transactions on Electron Devices, 26*, 1880−1886.

Thevoz, P., Adams, J. D., Shea, H., Bruus, H., & Soh, H. T. (2010). Acoustophoretic synchronization of mammalian cells in microchannels. *Analytical Chemistry, 82*, 3094−3098.

Trietsch, S. J., Hankemeier, T., & van der Linden, H. J. (2011). Lab-on-a-chip technologies for massive parallel data generation in the life sciences: A review. *Chemometrics and Intelligent Laboratory Systems, 108*, 64−75.

Tsukahara, S., & Watarai, H. (2003). Dielectrophoresis of microbioparticles in water with planar and capillary quadrupole electrodes. *IEE Proceedings - Nanobiotechnology, 150*, 59−65.

Unger, M. A., Chou, H. P., Thorsen, T., Scherer, A., & Quake, S. R. (2000). Monolithic microfabricated valves and pumps by multilayer soft lithography. *Science, 288*, 113−116.

Unni, H. N., Hartono, D., Yung, L. Y. L., Ng, M. M. L., Lee, H. P., Khoo, B. C., et al. (2012). Characterization and separation of Cryptosporidium and Giardia cells using on-chip dielectrophoresis. *Biomicrofluidics, 6*, 012805.

Vahey, M. D., & Voldman, J. (2008). An equilibrium method for continuous-flow cell sorting using dielectrophoresis. *Analytical Chemistry, 80*, 3135−3143.

Walker, G. M., Sai, J. Q., Richmond, A., Stremler, M., Chung, C. Y., & Wikswo, J. P. (2005). Effects of flow and diffusion on chemotaxis studies in a microfabricated gradient generator. *Lab on a Chip, 5*, 611−618.

Wang, X. L., Chen, S. X., Kong, M., Wang, Z. K., Costa, K. D., Li, R. A., et al. (2011). Enhanced cell sorting and manipulation with combined optical tweezer and microfluidic chip technologies. *Lab on a Chip, 11*, 3656−3662.

Wang, X.-B., Huang, Y., Holzel, R., Burt, J. P., & Pethig, R. (1992). Theoretical and experimental investigations of the interdependence of the dielectric, dielectrophoretic and electrorotational behaviour of colloidal particles. *Journal of Physics D: Applied Physics, 26*, 312−322.

Wang, X. B., Huang, Y., Wang, X., Becker, F. F., & Gascoyne, P. R. (1997). Dielectrophoretic manipulation of cells with spiral electrodes. *Biophysical Journal, 72*, 1887−1899.

Wang, X. B., Hughes, M. P., Huang, Y., Becker, F. F., & Gascoyne, P. R. C. (1995). Non-uniform spatial distributions of both the magnitude and phase of AC electric fields determine dielectrophoretic forces. *Biochimica et Biophysica Acta- General Subjects, 1243*, 185−194.

Wang, W., Lin, Y. H., Wen, T. C., Guo, T. F., & Lee, G. B. (2010). Selective manipulation of microparticles using polymer-based optically induced dielectrophoretic devices. *Applied Physics Letters, 96*, 113302.

Wang, X.-B., Pethig, R., & Jones, T. B. (1991). Relationship of dielectrophoretic and electrorotational behaviour exhibited by polarized particles. *Journal of Physics D: Applied Physics, 25*, 905−912.

Wang, X. B., Yang, J., Huang, Y., Vykoukal, J., Becker, F. F., & Gascoyne, P. R. C. (2000). Cell separation by dielectrophoretic field-flow-fractionation. *Analytical Chemistry, 72*, 832−839.

White, F. M. (1994). *Fluid mechanics*. New York: McGraw-Hill Inc.

Whitesides, G. M., Ostuni, E., Takayama, S., Jiang, X. Y., & Ingber, D. E. (2001). Soft lithography in biology and biochemistry. *Annual Review of Biomedical Engineering, 3*, 335−373.

Wu, Z. G., Hjort, K., Wicher, G., & Svenningsen, A. F. (2008). Microfluidic high viability neural cell separation using viscoelastically tuned hydrodynamic spreading. *Biomedical Microdevices, 10*, 631−638.

Wu, Z. G., Willing, B., Bjerketorp, J., Jansson, J. K., & Hjort, K. (2009). Soft inertial microfluidics for high throughput separation of bacteria from human blood cells. *Lab on a Chip, 9*, 1193−1199.

Wu, L. Q., Yung, L. Y. L., & Lim, K. M. (2012). Dielectrophoretic capture voltage spectrum for measurement of dielectric properties and separation of cancer cells. *Biomicrofluidics, 6*, 014113.

Yamada, M., Nakashima, M., & Seki, M. (2004). Pinched flow fractionation: Continuous size separation of particles utilizing a laminar flow profile in a pinched microchannel. *Analytical Chemistry, 76*, 5465−5471.

Yamada, M., & Seki, M. (2005). Hydrodynamic filtration for on-chip particle concentration and classification utilizing microfluidics. *Lab on a Chip, 5*, 1233−1239.

Yamada, M., & Seki, M. (2006). Microfluidic particle sorter employing flow splitting and recombining. *Analytical Chemistry, 78*, 1357−1362.

Yeh, S. R., Seul, M., & Shraiman, B. I. (1997). Assembly of ordered colloidal aggregates by electric-field-induced fluid flow. *Nature, 386*, 57−59.

Zborowski, M., & Chamers, J. J. (2011). Rare cell separation and analysis by magnetic sorting. *Analytical Chemistry, 83*, 8050−8056.

Zborowski, M., Ostera, G. R., Moore, L. R., Milliron, S., Chalmers, J. J., & Schechter, A. N. (2003). Red blood cell magnetophoresis. *Biophysical Journal, 84*, 2638−2645.

Zborowski, M., Sun, L. P., Moore, L. R., Williams, P. S., & Chalmers, J. J. (1999). Continuous cell separation using novel magnetic quadrupole flow sorter. *Journal of Magnetism and Magnetic Materials, 194*, 224−230.

Zhao, B. S., Koo, Y. M., & Chung, D. S. (2006). Separations based on the mechanical forces of light. *Analytica Chimica Acta, 556*, 97−103.
Zhao, X. M., Xia, Y. N., & Whitesides, G. M. (1997). Soft lithographic methods for nanofabrication. *Journal of Materials Chemistry, 7*, 1069−1074.
Zharov, V. P., Galanzha, E. I., Menyaev, Y., & Tuchin, V. V. (2006). In vivo highspeed imaging of individual cells in fast blood flow. *Journal of Biomedical Optics, 11*, 4.
Zheng, W., Wang, Z., Zhang, W., & Jiang, X. (2010). A simple PDMS-based microfluidic channel design that removes bubbles for long-term on-chip culture of mammalian cells. *Lab on a Chip, 10*, 2906−2910.

Microfluidic devices for immobilization and micromanipulation of single cells and small organisms

Peng Pan [1,2], Pengfei Song [1,3], Xianke Dong [1,2], Weize Zhang [2], Yu Sun [1,4], Xinyu Liu [1,4]

[1]Department of Mechanical and Industrial Engineering, University of Toronto, Toronto, Ontario, Canada; [2]Department of Mechanical Engineering, McGill University, Montreal, Quebec, Canada; [3]Department of Electrical and Electronic Engineering, Xi'an Jiaotong-Liverpool University, Suzhou, Jiangsu, China; [4]Institute of Biomedical Engineering, University of Toronto, Toronto, Ontario, Canada

Guided-reading questions:

- What are the major types of micromanipulation on single cells and small organisms?
- How can microfluidic devices facilitate robotic manipulation of single cells and small organisms?
- What are the biological and biomedical applications of cell and organism manipulation?

9.1 Introduction

Cells are the basic structural and functional unit of living creatures (Alberts et al., 2002). This small organizational unit contains a highly complex and hierarchical architecture of interconnected molecular networks and represents life and its related consciousness (Anselmetti, 2009). As for the cells derived from a mother cell or the same type of cells under similar external stimuli, there may exist cell-to-cell differences in terms of size, growth rate, and morphology (Buettner et al., 2015; Junker & van Oudenaarden, 2014; Spudich & Koshland, 1976). This heterogeneity within the same population of cells needs to be studied through single cell analysis. In addition, single cell analysis techniques can also be used to identify differences between individual cells at different stages and conditions. Therefore, single cell analysis is not only an efficient way to probe the cell heterogeneity but also a promising means to detect disease and test medicine. Moreover, single cell microsurgery is widely used in many applications such as intracytoplasmic sperm injection—ICSI

(Lu et al., 2011; Rubino, Viganò, Luddi, & Piomboni, 2016), RNA interference (Schluep et al., 2017), drug discovery (Huang, Teng, Chen, Tang, & He, 2010), generation of transgenic animals (Adams, Pathak, Shao, Lok, & Pires-daSilva, 2019), biopsy for preimplantation genetic screening (PGS) (Mastenbroek & Repping, 2014; Sermon, Van Steirteghem, & Liebaers, 2004; Zimmerman et al., 2016), and so on.

Apart from the single cells, many small organisms such as the nematode worm *Caenorhabditis elegans* (roundworm), *Drosophila melanogaster* (fruit fly), and *Danio rerio* (zebrafish) are widely used for studying human physiological development and diseases (Brenner, 1974; Flinn, Bretaud, Lo, Ingham, & Bandmann, 2008; Jennings, 2011; Paquet et al., 2009; Pisharath, Rhee, Swanson, Leach, & Parsons, 2007; Ramesh et al., 2010; Sternberg, 2001; Taylor, 2006), drug discovery, and toxicology (Barros, Alderton, Reynolds, Roach, & Berghmans, 2008; Chakraborty, Hsu, Wen, Lin, & Agoramoorthy, 2009; Giacomotto & Ségalat, 2010; Pardo-Martin et al., 2010; Saito & van den Heuvel, 2002; Ségalat, 2007). There are many reasons for their utility. First, it has been demonstrated recently that there is a remarkable degree of similarity in the developmental mechanisms of these model organisms and humans (Council, 2000). Not only individual genes and proteins but also entire pathways of signaling and response and their functions in developing embryos appear highly conserved throughout evolution (Council, 2000). The utility of these small organisms for biomedical research mitigates the ethical, economical, and experimental barriers associated with the use of mammalian models for biological studies. In particular, due to their small body sizes, optically transparent or translucent bodies, short life cycles, and ease of cultivation, these model organisms greatly facilitates many types of biological studies (Mondal, Ahlawat, & Koushika, 2012). Similar to single cell manipulation, conventional manipulation and immobilization techniques for small organisms also have certain limitations that hamper cell and organism-based studies.

Over the past few decades, robotic micromanipulation provides a better way to study the physical interaction with biological samples when compared with the conventional manual manipulation. Leveraging techniques including robotics, automation, advanced control laws, and microelectromechanical systems (MEMS) (Pan, Wang, Ru, Sun, & Liu, 2017), robotic micromanipulation systems have been increasingly accurate, efficient, intelligent, and capable of performing manipulation tasks on biological samples ranging from single cells to small model organisms (Cheah, Li, Yan, & Sun, 2013; Hu & Sun, 2011; Lu et al., 2011; Nakajima et al., 2012; Thakur et al., 2014; Wang, Liu, Gelinas, Ciruna, & Sun, 2007). Due to its unprecedented capabilities, robotic micromanipulation techniques such as automated cell injection and mechanical cell/organism stimulation have been widely used in a variety of biological and biomedical areas such as genetics, cell development, drug screen, and in-vitro fertilization. In applications like cell/organism injection and characterization, a target object needs to be positioned to a desired place and sometimes immobilized mechanically before manipulation. Conventionally, a holding pipette is usually used to immobilize a cell at a time for further manipulation. For small organisms like the nematode worm *C. elegans* and *Drosophila* larvae, they always move around, which makes it more difficult to position and immobilize them. Usually, they are manually placed on a glass slide or agar plate and immobilized through surface adhesion. These protocols are tedious, time-consuming, and inconsistent, which limits the high-throughput studies of cells and organisms that involve micromanipulation.

With advances in the field of microfluidics (Dragone, Sans, Rosnes, Kitson, & Cronin, 2013; Fiorini & Chiu, 2005; Stirman, Harker, Lu, & Crane, 2014), the cell/organism positioning and immobilization have been significantly facilitated by microfluidic devices, and the related microfluidic techniques have enabled the high-speed robotic micromanipulation of cells and organisms. In particular, microfluidics provides new devices suitable for patterning cells at predetermined positions for high-throughput robotic injection. Moreover, microfluidic devices enable the immobilization of many organisms at the same time or the loading of individual organisms sequentially to significantly facilitate the robotic micromanipulation tasks for accurate, automated, high-throughput operations.

In this chapter, we will discuss three microfluidic devices we previously developed for immobilization and robotic micromanipulation of single cells and small organisms. First, we will introduce a glass microfluidic device for rapid single cell immobilization in robotic mouse zygote microinjection. Then, we will describe the development of a novel microfluidic device that enables fully automated, high-speed microinjection of *C. elegans*. The microfluidic device is automatically regulated by on-chip pneumatic valves and allows rapid loading, immobilization, injection, and downstream sorting of single *C. elegans*. Finally, we will briefly discuss a microfabricated device for immobilizing single *Drosophila* larvae for mechanotransduction studies.

9.2 Glass microfluidic device for rapid single cell immobilization and microinjection

Microinjection is a commonly used method to introduce materials into cells for reproductive studies, genetics, and molecule screening. There are mainly two types of cells that usually requires microinjection: adherent cells (e.g., most of the cells derived from tissues) and suspended cells (e.g., oocytes and embryos). For suspended cell injection, a target cell usually needs to be immobilized by a holding micropipette for subsequent injection, and the search and immobilization of each cell is highly skill-dependent and time-consuming. Although robotics promises automated microinjection at a high speed with high reproducibility, the use of a holding micropipette for cell immobilization is a hurdle for further improving the injection speed. The development of a microfluidic device that is capable of rapidly immobilizing many suspended cells into a regular pattern can facilitate both manual and robotic microinjection of these cells. Since differential interference contrast (DIC) microscopy is most commonly used in microinjection for cell imaging, glass should be chosen as the material for the construction of cell immobilization devices (Murphy, 2002).

Until now, many cell trapping techniques have been reported including dielectrophoresis (Voldman, Gray, Toner, & Schmidt, 2002), surface chemistry (Chen, Mrksich, Huang, Whitesides, & Ingber, 1997), optical tweezers (Jordan et al., 2005), ultrasonic trapping (Haake et al., 2005), magnetic trapping (Ino et al., 2008), and mechanical confinements (Carlborg, Haraldsson, Stemme, & van der Wijngaart, 2007; Di Carlo, Wu, & Lee, 2006; Rettig & Folch, 2005; Suzuki et al., 2007; Tan & Takeuchi, 2007). Among these existing techniques, only mechanical confinements can provide enough forces to immobilize cells for microinjection. These mechanical confinement structures include microwells (Rettig & Folch, 2005), hydrodynamic traps (Di Carlo et al., 2006; Tan & Takeuchi, 2007), and vacuum-based confinements (Carlborg et al., 2007; Suzuki et al., 2007). Microwells do not provide secured immobilization during cell penetration as the trapped cell can slightly move inside the microwell (Rettig & Folch, 2005). The hydrodynamic traps inside closed microchannels (Di Carlo et al., 2006; Tan & Takeuchi, 2007) prevent an injection micropipette from accessing the trapped cells. As for vacuum-based confinements, they employ an array of micrometer-sized through-holes connected to a vacuum chamber for immobilizing individual cells. In vacuum-based confinements, fabrication of through-holes (e.g., 2–50 μm) on a substrate is a critical fabrication step. Although through-holes have been formed on different materials (e.g., silicon, polydimethylsiloxane—PDMS, and photoresist) (Carlborg et al., 2007; Matthews & Judy, 2006; Suzuki et al., 2007), forming through-holes with a diameter ≤50 μm on a glass substrate remains a challenge. Although laser micromachining can be used to drill high-aspect-ratio through-holes on glass substrates (Gattass & Mazur, 2008), laser micromachined through-holes have rough surfaces along vertical walls, and the minute amount of debris on the vertical wall can cause shadows around through-holes in imaging.

In this section, we present the design and microfabrication of a glass microfluidic device with through-holes for rapid immobilization of single mouse zygotes (i.e., single-cell embryos) in robotic microinjection (Liu & Sun, 2009). As shown in Fig. 9.1, the cell holding device has a top glass layer with an array of through-holes inside a cell holding cavity, a bottom glass layer, and a PDMS spacer for forming a vacuum chamber. Taking into consideration the size of mouse oocytes/zygotes (∼100 μm), the size of the through-holes was designed to be 35–40 μm. As DIC microscopy was used for imaging during mouse zygote microinjection, glass was chosen as the material to meet the imaging requirement. Standard cover slips (size: 22 mm × 60 mm, thickness: ∼180 μm, Fisher Scientific) were used as the top glass layer. The bottom glass layer is a regular microscope slide (size: 76 mm × 26 mm, thickness: 1 mm, Fisher Scientific).

The device fabrication process is shown in Fig. 9.2(a), which mainly consists of: (i) double-side wet etching of the top glass cover slip and (ii) bonding of the top cover slip and the bottom glass slide using a thin PDMS layer. For wet etching of the cover slip, evaporated metal layers of Cr/Au (30/800 nm) plus hard-baked positive photoresist (S1818, Shipley) were used as etch mask. One side of the cover slip was first etched by using 14.3% hydrofluoric acid (HF) to form the ∼155 μm deep cell holding cavity and leave a ∼25 μm thick layer of glass. Then, the cover slip was etched from its backside to form an array of 3×3 or 5×5 through-holes of 35–40 μm in diameter. After that, a ∼100 μm thick PDMS layer was spin-coated and cured on the bottom glass slide, and then cut by a scalpel to form a central square window. Finally, the bottom glass slide was bonded with the top cover slip through the PDMS layer by using oxygen plasma treatment. A cell immobilization device is shown in Fig. 9.2(b).

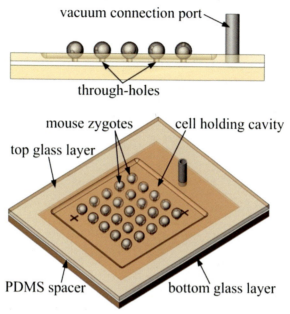

Figure 9.1 Schematic of the vacuum-based cell holding device.
Reprinted with permission from X. Liu and Sun (2009). Copyright 2009 Springer Nature.

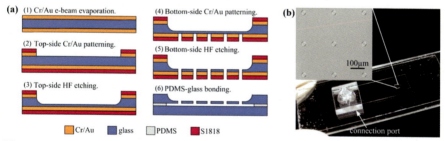

Figure 9.2 (a) Microfabrication process and (b) photograph of the glass cell immobilization device. The inlet in (b) shows the zoomed-in view of a 3×3 array of through-holes on the top glass cover slip.
Adapted with permission from Springer. Reprinted with permission from X. Liu and Sun (2009). Copyright 2009 Springer Nature.

Fig. 9.3 shows the zygote immobilization process by a cell immobilization device with 5×5 through-holes. A batch of mouse zygotes were first transferred to the cell holding cavity (Fig. 9.3(a)). As a negative pressure was applied, each through-hole trapped a single cell. The immobilization process costed approximately 10 s. Extra untrapped cells were removed using a transfer pipette (Fig. 9.3(c)). The complete process including the removal of extra cells typically takes 31 s for devices with an array of 5×5 through-holes.

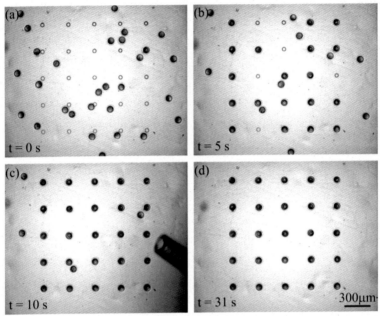

Figure 9.3 Immobilization on a 5×5 array of mouse zygotes. (a) 30 mouse zygotes were transferred to the cell holding cavity. (b) With the application of a low sucking pressure (1.8 kPa), through-holes trapped individual cells. 19 cells were immobilized within 5 s. (c) 25 cells were immobilized within 10 s. A transfer pipette was used to remove extra untrapped zygotes. (d) The immobilized 5×5 array of mouse zygotes. The complete process including removal of extra untrapped cells typically takes 31 s.
Reprinted with permission from X. Liu and Sun (2009). Copyright 2009 Springer Nature.

After the zygotes were trapped by the through-holes, we controlled the robotic system, shown in Fig. 9.4, to perform automated microinjection. The details of the robotic microinjection system can be found in Liu et al. (2011). Fig. 9.5(a) shows a zygote penetrated with the micropipette tip at the cytoplasm center. An injection speed of 200 μm/s and a retraction speed of 500 μm/s were used in the experiments, which have proven to be optimal in terms of minimizing injection-induced cell lysis. The robotic system injected a total of 200 mouse zygotes (Institute of Cancer Research (ICR) strain)) at a speed of 9 cells/min. The injected zygotes were thereafter cultured in potassium-supplemented simplex optimized medium (KSOM) medium (Specialty Media) for 72 h (37°C, 5% CO_2) to allow the zygotes to develop into blastocysts. Fig. 9.5(b) shows robotically injected zygotes that successfully developed to the blastocyst stage. Based on the 200 injected mouse zygotes, the cell holding device and the robotic injection system produced a survival rate of 89.8%, higher than the best survival rate (~80%) achieved by a proficient injection technician with over 12-year experience using a holding micropipette and an injection micropipette. The result demonstrates that, compared to conventional manual microinjection, the cell holding devices do not produce additional negative impact on embryonic development.

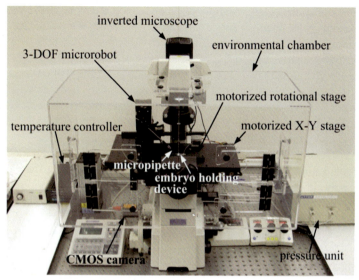

Figure 9.4 A robotic system for automated mouse zygote microinjection. A cell holding device is used to immobilize an array of mouse zygotes.
Reprinted with permission from X. Liu and Sun (2009). Copyright 2009 Springer Nature.

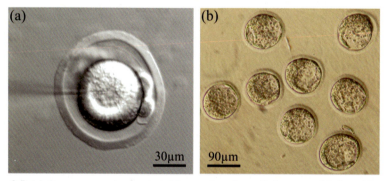

Figure 9.5 (a) A mouse zygote penetrated by a micropipette before material deposition. The micropipette injects a cell in a diagonal direction. (b) Robotically injected mouse zygotes developing into blastocysts.
Reprinted with permission from X. Liu and Sun (2009). Copyright 2009 Springer Nature.

9.3 Microfluidic device for automated, high-speed microinjection of *C. elegans*

Caenorhabditis elegans is an excellent model organism widely used in different types of biological research such as aging, development, drug screening, genetics, and neuroscience (Bargmann, 1993; Brenner, 1974; Ellis & Horvitz, 1986; Ewbank &

Zugasti, 2011; Hendricks, Ha, Maffey, & Zhang, 2012; Kenyon, 2010; Van Raamsdonk & Hekimi, 2010; Wang, Yang, Chai, Shi, & Xue, 2002; Wen et al., 2012; Zhang, Lu, & Bargmann, 2005). Despite its simple body structure, 60%−80% of *C. elegans* genes have counterparts in human genes, and many of these genes are relevant to human diseases (Artal-Sanz, de Jong, & Tavernarakis, 2006; Hillier et al., 2005; Nussbaum-Krammer & Morimoto, 2014). In addition to many well-known advantages of *C. elegans* such as short life cycle, transparency, ease and low cost of cultivation, and small size, *C. elegans* is the first animal with its genome completely sequenced, providing a powerful gene information library (Blaxter, 1998; Hillier et al., 2008; Hulme & Whitesides, 2011). These merits make *C. elegans* as a popular model organism for whole animal−based drug testing and screening, and its complete genomic resources greatly simplify the drug screen and identification of gene function (Bargmann & Horvitz, 1991; Kaletta & Hengartner, 2006; O'Reilly, Luke, Perlmutter, Silverman, & Pak, 2014).

For the worm-based drug testing experiments, there are several methods to expose *C. elegans* to drug solutions such as perfusion, feeding, or microinjection. Among these methods, microinjection is the only way capable of precise control over delivering small volumes of drugs to specific intrabody sites. Microinjection is particularly useful for testing water-insoluble drugs for which the perfusion or feeding method is not feasible; it consumes a less amount of drug than other methods, which could be a favorable feature for early-stage drug development where drug candidates are precious (Avery & Horvitz, 1990; Leung et al., 2008; Liu, Yang, Chen, & Wang, 2012; Mohan, Chen, Hsieh, Wu, & Chang, 2010; Nakajima et al., 2012, 2011; Nakanishi et al., 2013). Besides drug testing/screening applications, microinjection has also been widely used to deliver generic materials (e.g., DNA, morpholino, and RNAi) into the gonad of *C. elegans* to create transgenetic animals (Evans, 2006).

The conventional microinjection of *C. elegans* is performed manually, which is labor-intensive and inconsistent. In addition, it leads to a low throughput and uncertainties in results (Kimble, Hodgkin, Smith, & Smith, 1982). To conduct injection of a *C. elegans*, it should be immobilized first for subsequent body penetration by a micropipette. The conventional immobilization method is to manually place *C. elegans* on an agarose plate by using a worm picker, which is time-consuming and can easily damage the worm due to lengthy and inaccurate manual operations. These limitations of manual manipulation significantly restrict the use of the microinjection technique in large-scale studies of *C. elegans*.

Recently, different types of microfluidic devices have been developed to significantly facilitate *C. elegans* handling and advancing worm biology research (Ai, Zhuo, Liang, McGrath, & Lu, 2014; Bakhtina & Korvink, 2014; Chronis, 2010; Chung, Crane, & Lu, 2008; Chung et al., 2011; Crane et al., 2012; Lockery et al., 2008; Rohde, Zeng, Gonzalez-Rubio, Angel, & Yanik, 2007; Shi, Qin, Ye, & Lin, 2008; Song et al., 2015). In some microfluidic device designs, worms were immobilized in enclosed channels (Chung et al., 2008; Crane et al., 2012; Hulme, Shevkoplyas, Apfeld, Fontana, & Whitesides, 2007; Krajniak & Lu, 2010). However, a micropipette is not allowed to access the worm body for material injection. Two microfluidic devices have been reported to facilitate manual *C. elegans* microinjection.

R. Ghaemi (2013) used a narrowed microfluidic channel for immobilizing a *C. elegans* for subsequent injection. The precise control of worm body position inside the immobilization channel is realized by adjusting the loading pressure, which is less controllable. Zhao et al. (2013) designed a microfluidic device with an open chamber to immobilize single *C. elegans* via negative pressure suction from channels on the side wall of the open chamber. This design does provide open space for a micropipette to access the worm body for injection. However, both aforementioned microfluidic devices (Ghaemi, 2013; Zhao et al., 2013) lack on-chip pneumatic valves for continuous worm loading and immobilization, and no automated *C. elegans* injection was demonstrated. In addition, Hwang, Krajniak, Matsunaga, Benian, and Lu (2014) proposed a worm immobilization method based on sol–gel transition of a worm-carrying hydrogel to immobilize worms for imaging and injection. This method has been further integrated into a microinjection platform for automated worm injection (Gilleland, Falls, Noraky, Heiman, & Yanik, 2015). However, the sol–gel translation is relatively slow and thus unsuitable for use in high-speed microinjection of *C. elegans*.

In this section, we present a pneumatic valve–regulated microfluidic device for automated loading, immobilization, and microinjection of single *C. elegans* (Song, Dong, & Liu, 2016). The device design allows individual worms to be sequentially loaded into a microchannel, and the worm handling process is automatically controlled by on-chip pneumatic valves. The microfluidic device is integrated with a robotic system and custom-made control algorithms coordinate operations of the whole system for full automation. As a proof-of-concept experiment, we use the system to inject 200 *C. elegans* and characterize the system performance. The system demonstrates an injection speed of 6.6 worm/min and a presorting success rate of 77.5% (postsorting success rate: 100%), both much higher than the performance of manual operation (speed: 1 worm/4 min and success rate: ~30%).

As schematically illustrated in Fig. 9.6(a), this device consists of two microchannel layers: (i) the top fluid-channel layer (blue, 45 μm thick) for worm loading, transferring, immobilization, and (ii) the bottom pneumatic-valve layer (red, 30 μm thick) for regulating flows in the top layer. In the top layer, a micropillar array was designed inside the worm loading chamber for filtering out debris in the fluid to avoid channels blocking. An immobilization channel (30 μm wide and 800 μm long) connected to the worm loading chamber is small enough to securely immobilize a young adult worm (~40 μm in diameter). Once a worm is immobilized inside the channel, fluid resistance of the immobilization channel will significantly increase and thereby the pressure drop at the inlet of the immobilization channel becomes low, keeping the second worm from loading (Shen, Li, & Li, 2014). An injection channel (420 μm wide) connected to the side of the immobilization channel has an open end that allows a micropipette to access the immobilized worm (Fig. 9.6(b)). A row of micropillars is arranged at the connection of the immobilization and injection channels, which restricts the worm from swimming into the injection channel. A separate flush channel (Fig. 9.6(a)) is connected to the upstream of the immobilization channel and is responsible for flushing the immobilized worm out of the immobilization channel once the injection is completed. Bifurcated downstream sorting channels collect the successfully injected worms into the collection outlet. Multiple pneumatic microvalves (Fig. 9.6(a)) are

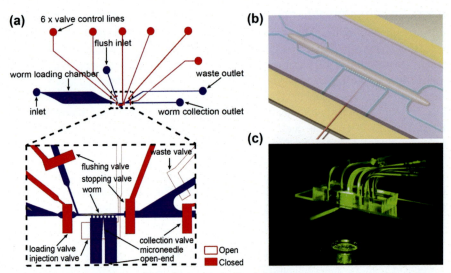

Figure 9.6 Microfluidic device for high-speed microinjection of *C. elegans*. (a) Schematic layout of the microfluidic device. (b) Blowup of the injection area on the device. (c) Photograph of an injection device during fluorescence imaging of the injected worm.
Reprinted with permission from Song et al. (2016). Copyright 2016 AIP Publishing.

used to regulate the fluid flows in the immobilization channel, flush channel, and the downstream sorting channels, and are coordinately controlled by custom-made control software.

The microfluidic device was fabricated through standard soft lithography, and then integrated with a robotic system for automated *C. elegans* microinjection. The system setup, as shown in Fig. 9.7, mainly consists of an inverted microscope (10×; IX-83, Olympus), a custom-made 16-channel solenoid valve controller, a motorized XY stage (ProScan III, Prior), a glass micropipette, a three-degree-of-freedom (3-DOF) micromanipulator (MP285, Sutter), a complementary metal-oxide semiconductor (CMOS) camera (Basler, A601f), and a host computer. The glass micropipette, with a tip

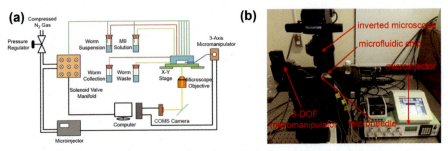

Figure 9.7 System setup for automated *C. elegans* injection. (a) Schematic layout and (b) photograph of the system (Song et al., 2016).
Reprinted with permission from Song et al. (2016). Copyright 2016 AIP Publishing.

diameter of 5 μm, is mounted on and automatically controlled by the micromanipulator. The computer-controlled, pressure-driven microinjector (Narishige, IM 300) is connected to the micropipette for precisely regulating the volume of the material injected into the worm body. The valve controller is used to automatically regulate the nitrogen gas pressure and thus to coordinate the operations of the on-chip pneumatic valves, as shown in Table 9.1, for automated *C. elegans* microinjection.

Fig. 9.8 shows the image sequence of *C. elegans* loading, immobilization, injection, and downstream sorting. 85 pL of fluorescein isothiocyanate (FITC) dye was injected into a worm to demonstrate the feasibility of worm microinjection. After injection, we found that the worm body expanded along its length upon material delivery. In the meanwhile, the fluorescence imaging showed that the fluorescence intensity of the worm body was much higher in the proximity of injection location (Fig. 9.9), indicating that the fluorescence dye had been successfully injected into the worm body without flowing out. We repeated this examination for 20 worms and did not found any false positive case (that is, a worm expanded upon material delivery, but no fluorescent dye was observed in the worm body).

Using the robotic system, 200 *C. elegans* were injected automatically. The results confirm that the microfluidic device is capable of rapid loading, immobilization, injection, and sorting of *C. elegans* with an injection speed of 6.6 worm/min and a presorting success rate of 77.5%. Different from existing microfluidic devices for *C. elegans* injection, this device requires minimal human intervention, is operated automatically, and provides significantly improved injection speed and success rate over conventional manual injection.

9.4 Microfabricated device for immobilization and mechanical stimulation of *Drosophila* larvae

Drosophila has been used as a model organism for studying sensory mechanotransduction and neural basis of behavior (Ernstrom & Chalfie, 2002; Jarman, 2002). A recent study demonstrated that millinewton-level mechanical touches at the anterior segment of a *Drosophila* larva induced the larva's reorientation and selection of a new path for forward movement (Pan et al., 2018; Zhou, Cameron, Chang, & Rao, 2012). In the follow-up neural circuit studies, researchers found that a set of 50 interconnected neurons expressing the cell-surface protein *Turtle* (*Tutl*) were involved in the adjustment of moving direction. These exciting findings shed light on the unknown mechanisms controlling navigational behaviors in response to mechanical stimulation, and further dissection of the *Tutl*-positive neural circuitry is needed. Through the simultaneous mechanical stimulation of *Drosophila* larvae and fluorescent calcium imaging of transmissions in the *Tutl*-positive neural circuits, it is possible to examining the role of individual *Tutl*-positive neurons in regulation of the touch-induced movement adjustments. Previously, a fine eyebrow was employed to apply the touch force to a *Drosophila* larva to mimic the real scenario where an object hits the larva body (Zhou et al., 2012). However, it cannot be used to study the response of individual neurons to

Table 9.1 Inlet/valve operation states.

Inlet/valve states Device states	Loading inlet	Flushing inlet	Loading valve	Flushing valve	Injection valve	Stopping valve	Waste valve	Collection valve
Worm loading	On	Off	On	Off	Off	Partial off	On	Off
Worm immobilization/injection	Off	Off	Off	Off	On	Fully off	On	Off
Worm collection	Off	On	Off	On	Off	Fully open	On/off	Off/on

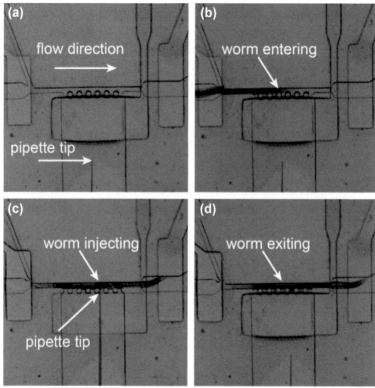

Figure 9.8 Image frame sequence of the injection area of the microfluidic device during worm injection. (a) Before worm loading. (b) A worm entering the immobilization channel. (c) The worm being injected. (d) The worm being flushed away (Song et al., 2016).
Reprinted with permission from Song et al. (2016). Copyright 2016 AIP Publishing.

the mechanical stimulation as the *Drosophila* larva was not immobilized. In addition, the gentle touch is applied manually. The inconsistent touching forces manually applied led to variations in results obtained from different experiments.

Recently, microfluidic devices have been used to immobilize *Drosophila* larvae and perform fluorescence imaging at the same time (Ghannad-Rezaie, Wang, Mishra, Collins, & Chronis, 2012; Mondal, Ahlawat, Rau, Venkataraman, & Koushika, 2011). However, in these devices, *Drosophila* larvae were fixed inside the enclosed microfluidic chambers, which does not allow a pipette to apply a gentle touch to the anterior segment (nose) of the larva body. In this study, a simple *Drosophila* larva immobilization device was designed and microfabricated for rapidly immobilizing single larvae with their noses exposed outside the device for mechanical stimulation (Zhang et al., 2015). As schematically illustrated in Fig. 9.10(a), this PDMS device

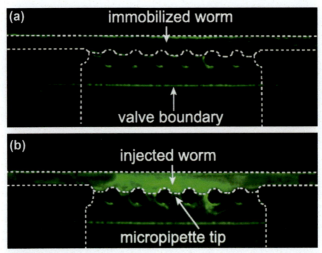

Figure 9.9 Experimental validation of the worm body expansion as a reliable indication for successful injection. The dashed lines show the boundaries of the worm and the PDMS channel. (a) An immobilized worm before injection of fluorescence dye. No obvious fluorescence signal was observed in the worm body. (b) The worm after injection of fluorescence dye. The injected fluorescence dye was observed in the proximity of the injection site, which correlates the worm body expansion observed during injection.
Reprinted with permission from Song et al. (2016). Copyright 2016 AIP Publishing.

consists of four separate modules for immobilizing four third-instar larvae. Each module has a 130 μm-thick microchannel fabricated by the regular soft lithography. The microchannel thickness ensures the body of a third-instar larva to be firmly compressed once the PDMS layer was bonded with a glass substrate. Each microchannel has a 0.75 mm opening formed via manual cutting after soft lithography. The standard deviation of the opening size was ±0.08 mm (n = 4).

To use the PDMS device to immobilize a *Drosophila* larva, a double-sided transparent tape was first attached to a glass slide, and four larvae were transferred onto the adhesive tape with their body positions aligned in a row and their noses oriented toward the same direction. Then, four PDMS modules were used to fix the four larva bodies in the microchannels, and the adhesive tape forms reversible bonding with the PDMS module. After larva immobilization, the device was mounted onto a robotic system for force-controlled mechanical stimulation and quantitative fluorescence imaging of *Drosophila* larvae. To automatically perform larva touching experiments, customized image processing and force control algorithms were integrated into the robotic system. Touch forces of 5 mN were applied to the larva nose and fluoresce images of the *Tutl*-positive neurons were obtained.

Fluorescent photographs of a larva body before and after the 5 mN touch were shown in Fig. 9.11(a) and (b), respectively. The glowing spots in the larva body are

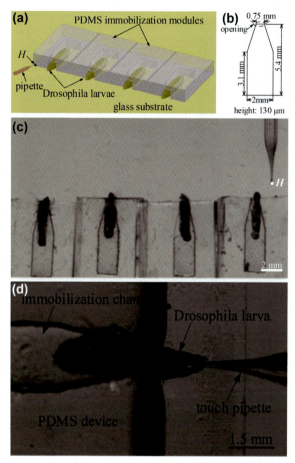

Figure 9.10 *Drosophila* larva immobilization device. (a) Schematic of the device with four separate immobilization modules. (b) Dimensions of the microchannel in each module. (c) Microscopic photograph of four immobilized larvae in the device. (d) A bright-field snapshot of an immobilized *Drosophila* larva being touched by a glass pipette at the force level of 5 mN. Reprinted with permission from W. Zhang, Sobolevski, Li, Rao, and Liu (2015). Copyright 2016 IEEE.

groups of the green fluorescent protein (GFP)-expressing *Tutl*-positive neurons. Among them, three groups of *Tutl*-positive neurons (the ones in areas 1–3) were chosen for further analysis. Fig. 9.11(c) shows the dynamic changes of fluorescence intensity in area 1 in six consecutive frames (exposure time: 400 ms) upon touching. One can see that the fluorescent intensity in area 1 started to increase once the force was applied and stabilizes after 2 s. In Fig. 9.11(d), average fluorescence intensity values of the three areas in five consecutive image frames were presented. The whole manipulation process of a single larva (from positioning the larva into the field-of-view to completion of touching and imaging) took 15 s, yielding a speed of 4 larvae/min. In comparison, a proficient human operator typically has a speed of 1 larva per 5 min.

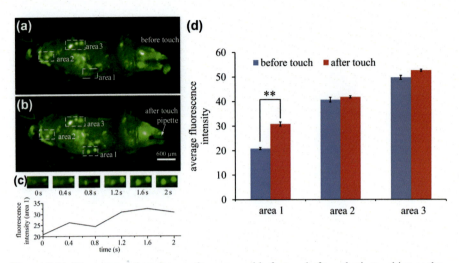

Figure 9.11 Fluorescence imaging results measured before and after robotic touching at the level of 5 mN. (a) and (b) Fluorescent images of a *Drosophila* larva taken (a) before and (a) after the 5 mn touch. The average fluorescence intensity values of areas 1–3 that included *Tutl*-positive neurons were quantified offline. (c) Consecutive image frames and fluorescence intensity values showing dynamic change in the calcium signal of area 1 upon touching. (d) Quantitative data of the average fluorescence intensity values of areas 1–3 measured from five consecutive image frames before and after touching (n = 5). $^*P < .05$ as compared to the intensity values measured before touching.
Reprinted with permission from W. Zhang et al. (2015). Copyright 2016 IEEE.

9.5 Conclusions and outlook

Automated robotic micromanipulation such as microinjection and mechanical stimulation has found applications in a variety of fields such as genetics, development, pathology, drug screen, and in vitro fertilization. Conventionally, the immobilization of cells and small organisms is performed manually. Although robotics promises automated micromanipulation at a high speed with high reproducibility, manual immobilization/positioning is a hurdle for system automation, which limits large-scale biological studies. With advances in microfluidics, microfluidic devices have been used in cell/organism positioning and immobilization, which significantly facilitate robotic cell/organism manipulation. This chapter introduces three microfluidic devices we developed for the immobilization and robotic micromanipulation of three typical biological samples: mouse embryos/zygotes, *C. elegans*, and *Drosophila* larvae. The devices have been proven to be more efficient for immobilizing their corresponding samples, which greatly facilitates the robotic micromanipulation of these samples. These microfluidic devices and their associated robotic systems will find important applications in a variety of biological and biomedical studies such as drug testing/screening, genetics, mechanotransduction, and neuroscience.

Despite many advances made in the past few decades, there are still many exciting topics requiring further investigation. It is noted that most of the existing microfluidic devices were developed for single task of cell/small organism manipulation. It would be desirable to integrate different functions into a microfluidic device for realizing multistep manipulation procedures of single cells/small organisms. In addition, some improvements are still needed to increase the automation and efficiency of cells/organism manipulation. The marriage of robotics and microfluidics provides a better route to smart, high-throughput, and high-consistency manipulation of single cells and small organisms. What is more, microfluidic devices have rewarded biological researchers with vast amounts of data but not necessarily the ability to analyze complex data effectively for further manipulation. There is a trend to develop artificial intelligence (AI)-based methods to improve data processing capability. Finally, one should note that the practical use of these microfluidic devices in real biological researches is still relatively limited. We should try to improve the microfluidic device designs to make them easier to make and use, low cost, and reliable to operate, which will increase their adoption in biological and biomedical research.

References

Adams, S., Pathak, P., Shao, H., Lok, J. B., & Pires-daSilva, A. (2019). Liposome-based transfection enhances RNAi and CRISPR-mediated mutagenesis in non-model nematode systems. *Scientific Reports, 9*(1), 1−12.

Ai, X., Zhuo, W., Liang, Q., McGrath, P. T., & Lu, H. (2014). A high-throughput device for size based separation of *C. elegans* developmental stages. *Lab on a Chip, 14*(10), 1746−1752.

Alberts, B., Johnson, A., Lewis, J., Raff, M., Roberts, K., Walter, P., et al. (2002). *Molecular biology of the cell. New York: Garland science; 2002. Classic textbook now in its* (5th ed.).

Anselmetti, D. (2009). *Single cell analysis: Technologies and applications.* John Wiley & Sons.

Artal-Sanz, M., de Jong, L., & Tavernarakis, N. (2006). Caenorhabditis elegans: A versatile platform for drug discovery. *Biotechnology Journal: Healthcare Nutrition Technology, 1*(12), 1405−1418.

Avery, L., & Horvitz, H. R. (1990). Effects of starvation and neuroactive drugs on feeding in *Caenorhabditis elegans. Journal of Experimental Zoology, 253*(3), 263−270.

Bakhtina, N. A., & Korvink, J. G. (2014). Microfluidic laboratories for *C. elegans* enhance fundamental studies in biology. *RSC Advances, 4*(9), 4691−4709.

Bargmann, C. I. (1993). Genetic and cellular analysis of behavior in *C. elegans. Annual Review of Neuroscience, 16*(1), 47−71.

Bargmann, C. I., & Horvitz, H. R. (1991). Chemosensory neurons with overlapping functions direct chemotaxis to multiple chemicals in *C. elegans. Neuron, 7*(5), 729−742.

Barros, T. P., Alderton, W. K., Reynolds, H. M., Roach, A. G., & Berghmans, S. (2008). Zebrafish: An emerging technology for in vivo pharmacological assessment to identify potential safety liabilities in early drug discovery. *British Journal of Pharmacology, 154*(7), 1400−1413.

Blaxter, M. (1998). *Caenorhabditis elegans* is a nematode. *Science, 282*(5396), 2041−2046.

Brenner, S. (1974). The genetics of *Caenorhabditis elegans. Genetics, 77*(1), 71−94.

Buettner, F., Natarajan, K. N., Casale, F. P., Proserpio, V., Scialdone, A., Theis, F. J., et al. (2015). Computational analysis of cell-to-cell heterogeneity in single-cell RNA-sequencing data reveals hidden subpopulations of cells. *Nature Biotechnology, 33*(2), 155–160.

Carlborg, C. F., Haraldsson, T., Stemme, G., & van der Wijngaart, W. (2007). Reliable batch manufacturing of miniaturized vertical vias in soft polymer replica molding. In *11th international conference on miniaturized systems for chemistry and life sciences (microTAS 2007), Paris, France, 7–11 Oct, 2007* (pp. 527–529).

Chakraborty, C., Hsu, C. H., Wen, Z. H., Lin, C. S., & Agoramoorthy, G. (2009). Zebrafish: A complete animal model for in vivo drug discovery and development. *Current Drug Metabolism, 10*(2), 116–124.

Cheah, C. C., Li, X., Yan, X., & Sun, D. (2013). Observer-based optical manipulation of biological cells with robotic tweezers. *IEEE Transactions on Robotics, 30*(1), 68–80.

Chen, C. S., Mrksich, M., Huang, S., Whitesides, G. M., & Ingber, D. E. (1997). Geometric control of cell life and death. *Science, 276*(5317), 1425–1428.

Chronis, N. (2010). Worm chips: Microtools for *C. elegans* biology. *Lab on a Chip, 10*(4), 432–437.

Chung, K., Crane, M. M., & Lu, H. (2008). Automated on-chip rapid microscopy, phenotyping and sorting of *C. elegans*. *Nature Methods, 5*(7), 637.

Chung, K., Zhan, M., Srinivasan, J., Sternberg, P. W., Gong, E., Schroeder, F. C., et al. (2011). Microfluidic chamber arrays for whole-organism behavior-based chemical screening. *Lab on a Chip, 11*(21), 3689–3697.

National Research Council (US) Committee on Developmental Toxicology. (2000). *Scientific frontiers in developmental toxicology and risk assessment*. National Academies Press.

Crane, M. M., Stirman, J. N., Ou, C.-Y., Kurshan, P. T., Rehg, J. M., Shen, K., et al. (2012). Autonomous screening of *C. elegans* identifies genes implicated in synaptogenesis. *Nature Methods, 9*(10), 977.

Di Carlo, D., Wu, L. Y., & Lee, L. P. (2006). Dynamic single cell culture array. *Lab on a Chip, 6*(11), 1445–1449.

Dragone, V., Sans, V., Rosnes, M. H., Kitson, P. J., & Cronin, L. (2013). 3D-printed devices for continuous-flow organic chemistry. *Beilstein Journal of Organic Chemistry, 9*(1), 951–959.

Ellis, H. M., & Horvitz, H. R. (1986). Genetic control of programmed cell death in the nematode *C. elegans*. *Cell, 44*(6), 817–829.

Ernstrom, G. G., & Chalfie, M. (2002). Genetics of sensory mechanotransduction. *Annual Review of Genetics, 36*(1), 411–453.

Evans, T. C. (2006). Transformation and microinjection. *Worm, 10*.

Ewbank, J. J., & Zugasti, O. (2011). *C. elegans*: Model host and tool for antimicrobial drug discovery. *Disease Models and Mechanisms, 4*(3), 300–304.

Fiorini, G. S., & Chiu, D. T. (2005). Disposable microfluidic devices: Fabrication, function, and application. *Biotechniques, 38*(3), 429–446.

Flinn, L., Bretaud, S., Lo, C., Ingham, P. W., & Bandmann, O. (2008). Zebrafish as a new animal model for movement disorders. *Journal of Neurochemistry, 106*(5), 1991–1997.

Gattass, R. R., & Mazur, E. (2008). Femtosecond laser micromachining in transparent materials. *Nature Photonics, 2*(4), 219–225.

Ghaemi, R. (2013). In *In paper presented at the17th international conference on miniaturized systems for chemistry and life sciences (MicroTAS 2013)*.

Ghannad-Rezaie, M., Wang, X., Mishra, B., Collins, C., & Chronis, N. (2012). Microfluidic chips for in vivo imaging of cellular responses to neural injury in *Drosophila* larvae. *PLoS One, 7*(1).

Giacomotto, J., & Ségalat, L. (2010). High-throughput screening and small animal models, where are we? *British Journal of Pharmacology, 160*(2), 204−216.

Gilleland, C. L., Falls, A. T., Noraky, J., Heiman, M. G., & Yanik, M. F. (2015). Computer-assisted transgenesis of *Caenorhabditis elegans* for deep phenotyping. *Genetics, 201*(1), 39−46.

Haake, A., Neild, A., Kim, D.-H., Ihm, J.-E., Sun, Y., Dual, J., et al. (2005). Manipulation of cells using an ultrasonic pressure field. *Ultrasound in Medicine and Biology, 31*(6), 857−864.

Hendricks, M., Ha, H., Maffey, N., & Zhang, Y. (2012). Compartmentalized calcium dynamics in a *C. elegans* interneuron encode head movement. *Nature, 487*(7405), 99−103.

Hillier, L. W., Coulson, A., Murray, J. I., Bao, Z., Sulston, J. E., & Waterston, R. H. (2005). Genomics in *C. elegans*: So many genes, such a little worm. *Genome Research, 15*(12), 1651−1660.

Hillier, L. W., Marth, G. T., Quinlan, A. R., Dooling, D., Fewell, G., Barnett, D., et al. (2008). Whole-genome sequencing and variant discovery in *C. elegans*. *Nature Methods, 5*(2), 183.

Huang, X., Teng, X., Chen, D., Tang, F., & He, J. (2010). The effect of the shape of mesoporous silica nanoparticles on cellular uptake and cell function. *Biomaterials, 31*(3), 438−448.

Hulme, S. E., Shevkoplyas, S. S., Apfeld, J., Fontana, W., & Whitesides, G. M. (2007). A microfabricated array of clamps for immobilizing and imaging *C. elegans*. *Lab on a Chip, 7*(11), 1515−1523.

Hulme, S. E., & Whitesides, G. M. (2011). Chemistry and the worm: *Caenorhabditis elegans* as a platform for integrating chemical and biological research. *Angewandte Chemie International Edition, 50*(21), 4774−4807.

Hu, S., & Sun, D. (2011). Automatic transportation of biological cells with a robot-tweezer manipulation system. *The International Journal of Robotics Research, 30*(14), 1681−1694.

Hwang, H., Krajniak, J., Matsunaga, Y., Benian, G. M., & Lu, H. (2014). On-demand optical immobilization of *Caenorhabditis elegans* for high-resolution imaging and microinjection. *Lab on a Chip, 14*(18), 3498−3501.

Ino, K., Okochi, M., Konishi, N., Nakatochi, M., Imai, R., Shikida, M., et al. (2008). Cell culture arrays using magnetic force-based cell patterning for dynamic single cell analysis. *Lab on a Chip, 8*(1), 134−142.

Jarman, A. P. (2002). Studies of mechanosensation using the fly. *Human Molecular Genetics, 11*(10), 1215−1218.

Jennings, B. H. (2011). *Drosophila*−a versatile model in biology & medicine. *Materials Today, 14*(5), 190−195.

Jordan, P., Leach, J., Padgett, M., Blackburn, P., Isaacs, N., Goksör, M., et al. (2005). Creating permanent 3D arrangements of isolated cells using holographic optical tweezers. *Lab on a Chip, 5*(11), 1224−1228.

Junker, J. P., & van Oudenaarden, A. (2014). Every cell is special: Genome-wide studies add a new dimension to single-cell biology. *Cell, 157*(1), 8−11.

Kaletta, T., & Hengartner, M. O. (2006). Finding function in novel targets: *C. elegans* as a model organism. *Nature Reviews Drug Discovery, 5*(5), 387−399.

Kenyon, C. J. (2010). The genetics of ageing. *Nature, 464*(7288), 504−512.

Kimble, J., Hodgkin, J., Smith, T., & Smith, J. (1982). Suppression of an amber mutation by microinjection of suppressor tRNA in *C. elegans*. *Nature, 299*(5882), 456−458.

Krajniak, J., & Lu, H. (2010). Long-term high-resolution imaging and culture of *C. elegans* in chip-gel hybrid microfluidic device for developmental studies. *Lab on a Chip, 10*(14), 1862−1868.

Leung, M. C. K., Williams, P. L., Benedetto, A., Au, C., Helmcke, K. J., Aschner, M., et al. (2008). *Caenorhabditis elegans*: An emerging model in biomedical and environmental toxicology. *Toxicological Sciences, 106*(1), 5−28.

Liu, X., Fernandes, R., Gertsenstein, M., Perumalsamy, A., Lai, I., Chi, M., et al. (2011). Automated microinjection of recombinant BCL-X into mouse zygotes enhances embryo development. *PLoS One, 6*(7).

Liu, X., & Sun, Y. (2009). Microfabricated glass devices for rapid single cell immobilization in mouse zygote microinjection. *Biomedical Microdevices, 11*(6), 1169.

Liu, J.-H., Yang, S.-T., Chen, X.-X., & Wang, H. (2012). Fluorescent carbon dots and nanodiamonds for biological imaging: Preparation, application, pharmacokinetics and toxicity. *Current Drug Metabolism, 13*(8), 1046−1056.

Lockery, S. R., Lawton, K. J., Doll, J. C., Faumont, S., Coulthard, S. M., Thiele, T. R., et al. (2008). Artificial dirt: Microfluidic substrates for nematode neurobiology and behavior. *Journal of Neurophysiology, 99*(6), 3136−3143.

Lu, Z., Zhang, X., Leung, C., Esfandiari, N., Casper, R. F., & Sun, Y. (2011). Robotic ICSI (intracytoplasmic sperm injection). *IEEE Transactions on Biomedical Engineering, 58*(7), 2102−2108. https://doi.org/10.1109/TBME.2011.2146781

Mastenbroek, S., & Repping, S. (2014). Preimplantation genetic screening: Back to the future. *Human Reproduction, 29*(9), 1846−1850.

Matthews, B., & Judy, J. W. (2006). Design and fabrication of a micromachined planar patch-clamp substrate with integrated microfluidics for single-cell measurements. *Journal of Microelectromechanical Systems, 15*(1), 214−222.

Mohan, N., Chen, C.-S., Hsieh, H.-H., Wu, Y.-C., & Chang, H.-C. (2010). In vivo imaging and toxicity assessments of fluorescent nanodiamonds in *Caenorhabditis elegans*. *Nano Letters, 10*(9), 3692−3699.

Mondal, S., Ahlawat, S., & Koushika, S. P. (2012). Simple microfluidic devices for in vivo imaging of *C. elegans*, *Drosophila* and zebrafish. *Journal of Visualized Experiments, 67*, e3780.

Mondal, S., Ahlawat, S., Rau, K., Venkataraman, V., & Koushika, S. P. (2011). Imaging in vivo neuronal transport in genetic model organisms using microfluidic devices. *Traffic, 12*(4), 372−385.

Murphy, D. B. (2002). *Fundamentals of light microscopy and electronic imaging*. John Wiley & Sons.

Nakajima, M., Hirano, T., Kojima, M., Hisamoto, N., Homma, M., & Fukuda, T. (2011). Direct nano-injection method by nanoprobe insertion based on E-SEM nano robotic manipulation under hybrid microscope. In *2011 IEEE international conference on robotics and automation* (pp. 4139−4144).

Nakajima, M., Hirano, T., Kojima, M., Hisamoto, N., Nakanishi, N., Tajima, H., et al. (2012). Local nano-injection of fluorescent nano-beads inside *C. elegans* based on nanomanipulation. In *2012 IEEE/RSJ international conference on intelligent robots and systems* (pp. 3241−3246).

Nakanishi, N., Nakajima, M., Hisamoto, N., Takeuchi, M., Homma, M., & Fukuda, T. (2013). Local drug micro-injection to Ca enorhabdi ti s el eg ans with micro-gel beads. In *MHS2013* (pp. 1−4).

Nussbaum-Krammer, C. I., & Morimoto, R. I. (2014). *Caenorhabditis elegans* as a model system for studying non-cell-autonomous mechanisms in protein-misfolding diseases. *Disease Models and Mechanisms, 7*(1), 31−39.

O'Reilly, L. P., Luke, C. J., Perlmutter, D. H., Silverman, G. A., & Pak, S. C. (2014). *C. elegans* in high-throughput drug discovery. *Advanced Drug Delivery Reviews, 69*, 247−253.

Pan, P., Qu, J., Zhang, W., Dong, X., Wei, W., Ru, C., et al. (2018). Robotic stimulation of freely moving *Drosophila* larvae using a 3D-printed micro force sensor. *IEEE Sensors Journal, 19*(8), 3165−3173.

Pan, P., Wang, W., Ru, C., Sun, Y., & Liu, X. (2017). MEMS-based platforms for mechanical manipulation and characterization of cells. *Journal of Micromechanics and Microengineering, 27*(12), 123003.

Paquet, D., Bhat, R., Sydow, A., Mandelkow, E.-M., Berg, S., Hellberg, S., et al. (2009). A zebrafish model of tauopathy allows in vivo imaging of neuronal cell death and drug evaluation. *Journal of Clinical Investigation, 119*(5), 1382−1395.

Pardo-Martin, C., Chang, T.-Y., Koo, B. K., Gilleland, C. L., Wasserman, S. C., & Yanik, M. F. (2010). High-throughput in vivo vertebrate screening. *Nature Methods, 7*(8), 634.

Pisharath, H., Rhee, J. M., Swanson, M. A., Leach, S. D., & Parsons, M. J. (2007). Targeted ablation of beta cells in the embryonic zebrafish pancreas using *E. coli* nitroreductase. *Mechanisms of Development, 124*(3), 218−229.

Ramesh, T., Lyon, A. N., Pineda, R. H., Wang, C., Janssen, P. M. L., Canan, B. D., et al. (2010). A genetic model of amyotrophic lateral sclerosis in zebrafish displays phenotypic hallmarks of motoneuron disease. *Disease Models and Mechanisms, 3*(9−10), 652−662.

Rettig, J. R., & Folch, A. (2005). Large-scale single-cell trapping and imaging using microwell arrays. *Analytical Chemistry, 77*(17), 5628−5634.

Rohde, C. B., Zeng, F., Gonzalez-Rubio, R., Angel, M., & Yanik, M. F. (2007). Microfluidic system for on-chip high-throughput whole-animal sorting and screening at subcellular resolution. *Proceedings of the National Academy of Sciences, 104*(35), 13891−13895.

Rubino, P., Viganò, P., Luddi, A., & Piomboni, P. (2016). The ICSI procedure from past to future: A systematic review of the more controversial aspects. *Human Reproduction Update, 22*(2), 194−227.

Saito, R. M., & van den Heuvel, S. (2002). Malignant worms: What cancer research can learn from *C. elegans*. *Cancer Investigation, 20*(2), 264−275.

Schluep, T., Lickliter, J., Hamilton, J., Lewis, D. L., Lai, C.-L., Lau, J. Y. N., et al. (2017). Safety, tolerability, and pharmacokinetics of ARC-520 injection, an RNA interference-based therapeutic for the treatment of chronic hepatitis B virus infection. In , *Clinical pharmacology in drug development: Vol. 6. Healthy volunteers* (pp. 350−362) (4).

Ségalat, L. (2007). Invertebrate animal models of diseases as screening tools in drug discovery. *ACS Chemical Biology, 2*(4), 231−236.

Sermon, K., Van Steirteghem, A., & Liebaers, I. (2004). Preimplantation genetic diagnosis. *The Lancet, 363*(9421), 1633−1641.

Shen, F., Li, X., & Li, P. C. H. (2014). Study of flow behaviors on single-cell manipulation and shear stress reduction in microfluidic chips using computational fluid dynamics simulations. *Biomicrofluidics, 8*(1), 14109.

Shi, W., Qin, J., Ye, N., & Lin, B. (2008). Droplet-based microfluidic system for individual *Caenorhabditis elegans* assay. *Lab on a Chip, 8*(9), 1432−1435.

Song, P., Dong, X., & Liu, X. (2016). A microfluidic device for automated, high-speed microinjection of *Caenorhabditis elegans*. *Biomicrofluidics, 10*(1), 11912.

Song, P., Zhang, W., Sobolevski, A., Bernard, K., Hekimi, S., & Liu, X. (2015). A microfluidic device for efficient chemical testing using *Caenorhabditis elegans*. *Biomedical Microdevices, 17*(2), 38.

Spudich, J. L., & Koshland, D. E. (1976). Non-genetic individuality: Chance in the single cell. *Nature, 262*(5568), 467−471.

Sternberg, P. W. (2001). Working in the post-genomic *C. elegans* world. *Cell, 105*(2), 173−176.

Stirman, J. N., Harker, B., Lu, H., & Crane, M. M. (2014). Animal microsurgery using microfluidics. *Current Opinion in Biotechnology, 25*, 24−29.

Suzuki, T., Yamamoto, H., Ohoka, M., Okonogi, A., Kabata, H., Kanno, I., et al. (2007). High throughput cell electroporation array fabricated by single-mask inclined UV lithography exposure and oxygen plasma etching. In *TRANSDUCERS 2007-2007 international solid-state sensors, actuators and microsystems conference* (pp. 687−690).

Tan, W.-H., & Takeuchi, S. (2007). A trap-and-release integrated microfluidic system for dynamic microarray applications. *Proceedings of the National Academy of Sciences, 104*(4), 1146−1151.

Taylor, M. V. (2006). Comparison of muscle development in *Drosophila* and vertebrates. In *Muscle development in* Drosophila (pp. 169−203). Springer.

Thakur, A., Chowdhury, S., Švec, P., Wang, C., Losert, W., & Gupta, S. K. (2014). Indirect pushing based automated micromanipulation of biological cells using optical tweezers. *The International Journal of Robotics Research, 33*(8), 1098−1111.

Van Raamsdonk, J. M., & Hekimi, S. (2010). Reactive oxygen species and aging in *Caenorhabditis elegans*: Causal or casual relationship? *Antioxidants and Redox Signaling, 13*(12), 1911−1953.

Voldman, J., Gray, M. L., Toner, M., & Schmidt, M. A. (2002). A microfabrication-based dynamic array cytometer. *Analytical Chemistry, 74*(16), 3984−3990.

Wang, W., Liu, X., Gelinas, D., Ciruna, B., & Sun, Y. (2007). A fully automated robotic system for microinjection of zebrafish embryos. *PLoS One, 2*(9).

Wang, X., Yang, C., Chai, J., Shi, Y., & Xue, D. (2002). Mechanisms of AIF-mediated apoptotic DNA degradation in *Caenorhabditis elegans*. *Science, 298*(5598), 1587−1592.

Wen, Q., Po, M. D., Hulme, E., Chen, S., Liu, X., Kwok, S. W., et al. (2012). Proprioceptive coupling within motor neurons drives *C. elegans* forward locomotion. *Neuron, 76*(4), 750−761.

Zhang, Y., Lu, H., & Bargmann, C. I. (2005). Pathogenic bacteria induce aversive olfactory learning in *Caenorhabditis elegans*. *Nature, 438*(7065), 179−184.

Zhang, W., Sobolevski, A., Li, B., Rao, Y., & Liu, X. (2015). An automated force-controlled robotic micromanipulation system for mechanotransduction studies of *Drosophila* larvae. *IEEE Transactions on Automation Science and Engineering, 13*(2), 789−797.

Zhao, X., Xu, F., Tang, L., Du, W., Feng, X., & Liu, B.-F. (2013). Microfluidic chip-based *C. elegans* microinjection system for investigating cell–cell communication in vivo. *Biosensors and Bioelectronics, 50*, 28−34.

Zhou, Y., Cameron, S., Chang, W.-T., & Rao, Y. (2012). Control of directional change after mechanical stimulation in *Drosophila*. *Molecular Brain, 5*(1), 39.

Zimmerman, R. S., Jalas, C., Tao, X., Fedick, A. M., Kim, J. G., Pepe, R. J., et al. (2016). Development and validation of concurrent preimplantation genetic diagnosis for single gene disorders and comprehensive chromosomal aneuploidy screening without whole genome amplification. *Fertility and Sterility, 105*(2), 286−294.

Microfluidic devices for developing tissue scaffolds

L.T. Chau, J.E. Frith, R.J. Mills, D.J. Menzies, D.M. Titmarsh, J.J. Cooper−White
The University of Queensland, Brisbane, QLD, Australia

Revised by: Yu Zhou
R&D, Siemens, Tarrytown, NY, United States

Guided reading questions

1. What are the key issues and technical challenges for successful tissue engineering?
2. What does microfluidics technology contribute to research and development of successful tissue engineering?

10.1 Introduction

In *vivo* tissue repair and regeneration are substantially facilitated by recruited stem cells from peripheral blood or from those resident in most, if not all, tissues (Sakamoto, Ohashi, & Sato, 2006). Their depletion within an organ system may lead to full or partial loss of function (Palsson & Bhatia, 2004), indicating their critical role in tissue repair and replacement. Cells within tissues are surrounded by a three dimensional (3D) microenvironment of three (principle) "support" systems: vasculature, other cells (including stem cells), and cell-secreted extracellular matrix (ECM). Constitutionally, tissues vary from being cell-dense (1×10^9 cells/cm^3), vascularized, and extracellular matrix-poor structures, in the case of, for example muscle and fat tissue, through to cell-poor (1×10^6 cells/cm^3), avascular, and extracellular matrix-rich structures, in the case of cartilage.

The field of tissue engineering aims to bring together key design principles of engineering and our understanding of cell biology and tissue genesis to invoke local repair or regeneration of damaged or diseased tissue. Researchers utilize a variety of cell sources, depending on their tissue end point or target, including mature (fully differentiated), progenitor, and stem cells. Through their combination with biomaterials and in vitro culture environments, cells are encouraged to generate functional tissues. However, the significant regenerative potential and clinical translation of tissue engineering practices, especially those using stem cells or progenitor cells, remains largely untapped. This is due largely to deficiencies in our knowledge of what microenvironments must be provided to the chosen cell types to facilitate the development of tissues that are not only composed of the appropriate cell types and phenotypes but that also are functionally equivalent to the lost or damaged tissue. This chapter discusses the current status of microfluidic device—based research attempting to address and overcome these deficiencies, with the aim of ultimately enabling clinical translation of cell-based tissue engineering therapies.

10.2 Key issues and technical challenges for successful tissue engineering

While there are many alternative paths or approaches being taken by researchers to achieve what are intrinsically complex outcomes in order to produce a functional, engineered tissue, there remain a number of key challenges or hurdles to achieving such directed tissue genesis, both in vitro and in vivo, from available cell sources. They are: (1) obtaining clinically relevant numbers, through ex vivo expansion and/or differentiation (e.g., from pluripotent or multipotent stem cells to fully differentiated end points) of the targeted cell types for implantation with the chosen scaffold; (2) encouraging effective and efficient cell seeding and scaffold colonization within both in vitro (for extended culture prior to implantation) and in vivo (involving active recruitment of endogenous cells) contexts; and (3) rapid vascularization of the cell-laden scaffold postimplantation to avoid necrosis and encourage further tissue growth and maturation. We will now explore each of these challenges in more detail.

10.2.1 Clinically relevant cell numbers: from stem cells through to mature, fully differentiated cells

It is estimated that in a myocardial infarction, approximately one billion cardiomyocytes (the functional "beating" cells in heart tissue) can be lost. Unfortunately, mature human cardiomyocytes are nonproliferative, and hence, in order to invoke functional repair of damaged heart tissue through cardiomyocyte repopulation, the human body needs assistance. One of the current approaches which has significant potential is the implantation of human cardiomyocytes into this damaged site that have been generated in vitro from human pluripotent stem cell (hPSC) sources (human embryonic stem cells (hESCs) and induced pluripotent stem cells (iPSCs)). However, the progression of a stem cell from a pluripotent, multipotent, or early progenitor stage into a range of terminally differentiated, mature cells that form adult tissues involves differentiation through quite a number of intermediate populations. For example, in specifying contractile cardiomyocytes from hPSCs, cells must pass from the pluripotent phenotype through a primitive streak-like population, to precardiac mesoderm, to cardiac progenitors, to cardiomyocytes, then to functional, mature cardiomyocytes, as a minimum set of developmental stages (there may be more undiscovered complexity within those stages). Current protocols for deriving cardiomyocytes from hPSCs quote 1—1.5 cardiomyocytes per input hPSC; therefore, $\sim 1 \times 10^9$ hPSCs would be required as a starting point, requiring $\sim 20 \times 10^3$ cm^2 of starting culture area (as an estimate based on some monolayer protocols). It is clear, then, that the problem of arriving at a clinical dose of functional cells is a significant challenge.

This is particularly true for therapies involving adult stem cells, which are typically rare cell populations and have a more limited potential for expansion than their pluripotent counterparts. For example, mesenchymal stem cells (MSCs) make up between just 0.01% and 0.001% of mononuclear cells in the bone marrow and, therefore, require significant expansion in order to generate clinically relevant numbers (Pittenger et al., 1999). However, comparisons of MSCs shortly after isolation to those that have undergone several passages show a dramatic increase in population doubling time and a diminished ability to differentiate along the osteo-, adipo-, and chondrogenic lineages (Banfi et al., 2000). As a result, there is a significant drive to develop methods for expansion that retain the beneficial properties of the cells in a manner that is reproducible, fully defined, and amenable to the scale-up that will be required for translation to the clinic.

An alternative strategy to using stem cells is to "transdifferentiate" a resident cell in the damaged tissue site (or periphery) that is nonfunctional into a functional cell type, for example, in the case of cardiac tissue, transdifferentiation of cardiac fibroblasts (nonfunctional in terms of beating) into functional cardiomyocytes has been proven to be possible (both in vitro and in vivo) (Kou et al., 2011). However, for transdifferentiation (also known as direct reprogramming) approaches, the reprogramming method or process is itself a long and inefficient process (some can take place over a few weeks), with poor understanding of the molecular events and cellular changes that occur before arriving at the reprogrammed cell type, usually with a low efficiency. Producing enough cells for functional tissue recovery is, thus, still a significant challenge.

Ensuring that significant cell numbers of the target phenotype are present at the output of any bioprocess is, thus, essential for their successful use in the intended tissue engineering endpoint application. This can be achieved in several ways:

- Increasing the number of starting point cells (e.g., stem cells);
- Increasing efficiency of differentiation to intermediate and target phenotypes;
- Increasing the efficiency of direct reprogramming/transdifferentiation; or
- Selection processes (sorting, density gradient centrifugation, antibiotic selection, sub-culturing).

10.2.2 Effective cell seeding and scaffold colonization

One of the major challenges still confronting the application of tissue-engineered scaffolds in the clinic is inadequate cell colonization. Previous strategies have generally suffered from high cell colonization at the periphery and little to none within the center of the constructs. To achieve sufficient cell colonization, an effective cell seeding methodology that allows homogenous cell seeding needs to be employed, and the seeded cells need sufficient nutrients and oxygen in order to survive, proliferate, and regenerate the required tissue.

Cell colonization of a biomaterial scaffold is influenced by its physical, spatial, and biochemical properties (Fig. 10.1). Physical cues, including stiffness and topography,

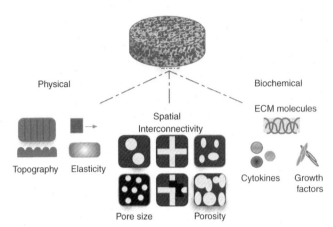

Figure 10.1 Physical, spatial, and biochemical properties that influence cell colonization.

can have a profound effect on cell adhesion and migration (Diehl, Foley, Nealey, & Murphy, 2005; Doyle, Wang, Matsumoto, & Yamada, 2009; Isenberg, Dimilla, Walker, Kim, & Wong, 2009; Kaiser, Reinmann, & Bruinink, 2006; Lo, Wang, Dembo, & Wang, 2000; Pelham & Wang, 1997), while pore size (Cao et al., 2006; Chu, Orton, Hollister, Feinberg, & Halloran, 2002; Malda et al., 2005; Oh, Park, Kim, & Lee, 2007; O'Brien, Harley, Yannas, & Gibson, 2005; Tsuruga, Takita, Itoh, Wakisaka, & Kuboki, 1997; van Tienen et al., 2002; Zmora, Glicklis, & Cohen, 2002), porosity (Baker et al., 2008; Karageorgiou & Kaplan, 2005; Silva et al., 2006; Spiteri, Pilliar, & Kandel, 2006), and interconnectivity (Griffon, Sedighi, Schaeffer, Eurell, & Johnson, 2006; Melchels et al., 2010) are examples of important spatial parameters that can similarly have substantial impacts. The material that the scaffold is made from will also affect colonization by altering the specific cell-material interactions (for example those mediated by integrins) with subsequent effects on cell adhesion and migration (Lawrence & Madihally, 2008). More recently, there has been a wider appreciation of the variation in modes of cell migration and scaffold colonization observed in two dimensional (2D) and 3D environments, where the degradation rate of the material is a relevant parameter in determining the movement of cells into and within the scaffold. All of these factors must be taken into account during scaffold design in order to promote optimal cell colonization.

Traditionally, three seeding methodologies have been used: static, dynamic, and perfusion bioreactor cultures. Of these, static seeding methods are the simplest but perhaps the least effective. Using such methods, a high-density suspension of cells is added to the surface of the scaffold, where it is hoped they will adhere and migrate through to the center. This may be aided by seeding several sides of the construct. Dynamic seeding methodologies can take many forms; however, one common example is the use of a spinner flask, which encourages movement of culture medium laden with cells through the pores of the scaffold. Such methods have been used to seed MSCs into calcium phosphate scaffolds for bone tissue engineering, resulting in an enhanced proportion of the cells adhering to the material and improved penetration throughout the construct (Griffon, Abulencia, Ragetly, Fredericks, & Chaieb, 2011). Under perfusion, culture medium is passed through scaffolds from one direction to the other. This may occur with constant provision of fresh culture medium or may exist in a closed loop with the medium passing across the construct multiple times. As with dynamic cell seeding strategies, the movement of the medium through the scaffold has been shown to aid both the efficiency of seeding and has also been shown to promote uniform tissue development across the construct (Zhao & Ma, 2005). For both dynamic and perfusion cultures, the rate of media flow through the scaffold is crucial, as it is necessary to balance the rate of provision of nutrients and removal of waste products while at the same time minimizing the shear forces applied to cells to maximize viability and allow their initial adhesion to the presented biomaterial surface. Additional strategies, such as those involving growth factor incorporation, may be used to promote migration into the center of the scaffold. Growth factors, such as vascular endothelial growth factor (VEGF), may also be used to promote vascularization, which in turn will bring cells into the scaffold, as well as providing an environment in which nutrients such as oxygen and glucose are available and where waste products are readily removed.

Effective cell seeding and colonization of scaffolds remain a significant challenge, and limitations in our knowledge and understanding of the relevant parameter space mean that seeding strategies must currently be optimized for each individual situation. It is particularly difficult to separate out the effects of each individual factor on the final result, and more information is required in order to enable the rational design guidelines for effective colonization of any given biomaterial construct.

10.2.3 Vascularization

Vascularization is the process of growing blood vessels into a tissue to improve oxygen and nutrient supply. It remains an overriding limiting factor in tissue engineering large 3D constructs, either during in *vitro* preculture or in vivo postimplantation. In the absence of a vascular network, metabolite supply and cell viability in a scaffold are compromised when diffusion distances are greater than 150–200 μm (Folkman & Hochberg, 1973) (Fig. 10.2). As a result, tissue engineering has been largely limited to thin or avascular tissues such as skin (Kremer, Lang, & Berger, 2000) or cartilage (Vacanti & Upton, 1994). Engineering a large complex tissue, thus, necessitates growing a physiologically relevant vasculature that promotes cell survival, tissue organization, and rapid vascularization following implantation. The incorporation of a functional microcirculatory network into the scaffold prior to implantation is, therefore, essential. In addition, in order for the large 3D construct to remain viable, the microcirculatory network is required to mimic natural vasculature and carry out angiogenesis, a process where new capillaries are formed from preexisting blood vessels (Patan, 2000).

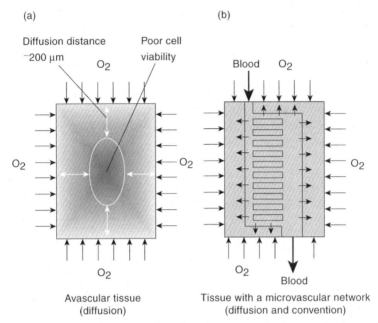

Figure 10.2 Distribution of oxygen and nutrients in an avascular tissue and a tissue with a microvascular network. (a) In an avascular tissue, diffusion alone can only supply metabolite sufficiently within the first 200. This is assuming that the surface of the tissue is exposed to fresh blood supply via the flanking capillary network. As a result, cells which are at a distance of greater than 200 μm from this supply will be compromised. (b) In a tissue with a microvascular network, metabolite supply is both by convection and diffusion. Therefore, cells can be nourished and sustained throughout the tissue construct.

Many methods have been developed to fabricate microvasculature for prevascularization of scaffolds. Early studies often involved fibers, synthetic, or natural, as "sacrificial" or temporary microvessel templates (Chrobak, Potter, & Tien, 2006; Ko & Iwata, 2001; Neumann, Nicholson, & Sanders, 2003; Migliore, Vozzi, Vozzi, & Ahluwalia, 2008; Takei, Sakai, Ono, Ijima, & Kawakami, 2006). However, these approaches either resulted in a multichannelled microvascular construct without a common inlet and outlet (Ko & Iwata, 2001) or multiple single micronscale vessels (Chrobak, Potter, & Tien, 2006; Migliore et al., 2008; Neumann et al., 2003; Takei et al., 2006), making them impractical and technically challenging for surgical implantation.

Researchers later fabricated larger complex 3D microvascular networks. These involved sacrificial "cotton candy" sugar structures in polymeric (poly-dimethylsiloxane (PDMS), epoxy, or polycarbonate) matrices (Bellan et al., 2009), and random assemblies of discrete, micron-scale gelatin components to form a large modular tissue–engineered construct (McGuigan & Sefton, 2007a, 2007b). However, while these methods are novel, there is limited control over the hydrodynamics of the random networks formed. Control over hydrodynamics in a microvascular network construct is important to ensure adequate delivery of nutrients to all cells, along with appropriate levels of shear stress for normal cell function.

Microfabrication is another method that has been commonly used in the development of artificial microvasculature. The main advantages of microfabrication technology over other methods include being able to achieve resolutions of 10 μm, which are on the same length scale as capillaries (Borenstein et al., 2002; Kaihara et al., 2000) and the ability to invoke structural uniformity in such microvascular networks. Several investigators have recently used microfabrication to establish and optimize microvascular network designs and create microcirculatory networks with varying levels of success.

We will now highlight some of the past and present approaches utilizing microfluidic technology to overcoming the above listed hurdles to translation and clinical uptake of tissue-engineered products.

10.3 Microfluidic device platforms

Recent advances in microfluidic technology offer unprecedented control over fluid (both single phase and multiphase) flow, interface dynamics, droplet and particle size and size distribution, heat transfer, and reaction conditions. This control results largely from the imposition of laminar flow and the domination of surface forces in the inherently small length scales within these devices. Microfluidic technologies are also ideally suited for parallelization or scale-up. It is for these reasons that researchers have turned to microfabrication and microfabricated in vitro environs to probe cellular behaviors that are otherwise difficult to investigate within standard cell culture methods. For instance, Kitsara et al. surveyed the micro- and nanofabrication methods used for cardiac tissue engineering (Kitsara et al., 2018, Heart on a chip: Micro-nanofabrication and microfluidics steering the future of cardiac tissue engineering). Further, such platforms permit the investigation, and real-time readout in some cases, of the impacts of varying microenvironmental conditions, including both biochemical factors (such as media exchange, oxygen concentration, pH, factor, and ligand concentration) and biophysical factors (such as substrate mechanics, scaffold geometry, pore size, and connectivity), on cell fate choices, such as morphology, migration, proliferation, differentiation, and apoptosis. Ultimately, these choices determine the success or failure of our attempts at directed tissue genesis from any cell type, whether terminally differentiated or pluripotent. We now provide a review of some of the more recent examples of microdevices that have been designed to probe such complex parameter space in order to provide the necessary insight required to ensure successful tissue engineering outcomes.

10.3.1 Microdevices for optimization of microenvironments for cell/stem cell expansion and differentiation

Stem cells and their differentiated sublineages are important components in tissue-engineered constructs, either from the perspective of incorporation within the construct or design of the construct in order to recruit and support native cells. Control of cell phenotype through isolation, expansion of a stem cell population, and specification and maintenance of differentiated lineages of interest are, therefore, essential in ensuring the quality and efficacy of cells incorporated or targeted in tissue-engineered constructs.

Fortunately, microscale technologies are expanding the repertoire of assay platforms in investigating features of stem cell and stem cell—derived populations, including their expansion and differentiation (Salieb-Beugelaar, Simone, Arora, Philippi, & Manz, 2010). Because of several advantageous capabilities, including high parallelization, continuous fluid flow, and reduced culture dimensions, microscale (and particularly microfluidic) systems can provide opportunities for high-fidelity screening of stem cell culture processes under well-controlled microenvironmental conditions. Stem cells can sense and respond to a variety of stimuli, such as soluble factors, ECM proteins, cell—cell contacts, mechanical forces, and properties (shear, strain, elastic, and viscous moduli) and electrical stimulation, and further can be manipulated by introduction of genetic material and pharmacological agents, etc. Microtechnologies such as biomolecule spotting, surface micropatterning, and microfluidic systems are ideal platforms for screening these stimuli, as has been recently reviewed (Titmarsh, Chen, Wolvetang, & Cooper-White, 2012a). While biomolecule spotting platforms have been applied more thoroughly for investigating combinations of ECM proteins for stem cells, microfluidic technologies in particular have made inroads into examining the physical, soluble factor, paracrine factor, and coculture cues that drive stem cell expansion and differentiation, which we will now summarize.

Medium flow rate in continuous flow microfluidic systems affects biochemical and biophysical parameters (medium turnover, shear stress, etc.). Microbioreactor arrays have been developed to supply a logarithmic range of flow rates and assess mouse embryonic stem cell (mESC) growth, which improved with increasing flow rate (Kim, Vahey, Hsu-Yi, & Voldman, 2006). For hESCs, a device with a much narrower, linear range of flow rates showed they were more sensitive, as they expanded best in a small window of flow rates and were limited outside this window (Titmarsh, Hidalgo, Turner, Wolvetang, & Cooper-White, 2011). Fluidic resistance allowed control of fluid flow in these microfluidic systems. Instead of continuous flow, other systems have used programmed medium exchange to investigate temporal stimulation of mESCs (Ellison, Munden, & Levchenko, 2009) and HSCs (Lecault et al., 2011) with various factors.

Microfluidic systems are also ideal for controlled introduction of soluble factors and screening their effects on the expansion or differentiation of stem cell populations. Moreover, this can be done in a semi-high throughput manner due to the parallelization that can be achieved with microfabrication. For example, a multiplexed microbioreactor array platform recently enabled full factorial screening of exogenous and paracrine factors in hESC differentiation to a primitive streak-like population (Titmarsh et al., 2012b).

A fully automated microfluidic system based on pneumatic valve control was developed to screen 96 discrete, individually addressable microbioreactor chambers, which could be fed with arbitrary mixtures of up to 16 medium components or soluble factors. This system has been utilized for automated screening of culture environments for MSC growth and differentiation (Gómez-Sjöberg, Leyrat, Pirone, Chen, & Quake, 2007). Importantly, the application of continuous medium perfusion in closed microfluidic stem cell culture systems has identified autocrine/paracrine effects as critical regulators of stem cell populations (Blagovic, Kim, & Voldman, 2011; Moledina et al., 2012). A recent review highlighted the way microfluidic technologies are providing new avenues to assess and manipulate paracrine effects (Przybyla & Voldman, 2012).

10.3.2 Microdevices for studying the effects of substrate and ligand type, pore geometry, and scaffold architecture on cell migration, scaffold colonization, and tissue development

Investigating the numerous parameters that influence scaffold colonization and tissue development within a 3D biomaterial is difficult. This is predominantly due to the inability to systematically investigate, and independently change, scaffold properties, and the ever-present immune response when performing in vivo studies. As such, microdevices have recently been used to introduce a high degree of control over the cellular microenvironment. The development of these devices has allowed the methodical evaluation of various scaffold parameters, including the substrate or ligand type, pore geometry, and architecture on scaffold development.

Studying cell migration not only provides an insight into the fundamentals of cell biology, but it is also useful in assessing the suitability of various substrates and materials as a tissue engineering construct. Numerous microdevices have been developed to overcome the deficiencies associated with traditional methodologies and have allowed investigation into the cell motility in response to chemokines (Lin & Butcher, 2006; Saadi, Wang, Lin, & Jeon, 2006), ligands (Doran,Mills, Parker, Landman, & Cooper-White, 2009), coculture (Chung et al., 2009), mechanical constraints (Irimia & Toner, 2009), and pore architecture (Mills, Frith, Hudson, & Cooper-White, 2011). These devices not only allow precise microenvironmental control but can also elucidate results that are indiscernible using conventional assays or techniques.

A traditional assay to assess cell migration in response to a substrate is the wound healing or scrape assay. This involves creating a "wound" within a confluent cell monolayer (generally by scraping the cell with a pipette tip) and observing the closure of the "wound" edges to quantify cell migration rates. While this method is relatively straightforward, the outcomes are confounded by a number of factors, including the ambiguity of the substrate, as a result of the wound generation removing the desired surface or fouling due to cellular secretions, and the damage to cells at the wound edge, which impacts cell migration.

A number of different microdevices have been developed to overcome the problems associated with techniques such as the wound healing assay and allow a more systematic investigation into cell migration. One of the earliest of these microdevices developed by Nie et al. (2007) uses a laminar flow of trypsin to generate a well-defined "wound" edge. While this method elicits only minor damage to cells on the wound edge, the surface onto which the cells will migrate remains ambiguous. Poujade et al. also developed an eloquent PDMS-based stencil tool, in which a PDMS stencil is applied to a surface prior to cell seeding. The stencil is then peeled off, allowing cell migration to begin (Poujade et al., 2007). Although this approach overcomes many of the problems associated with the classical wound healing assay, even this solution potentially compromises surface composition, as the PDMS stencil must be fixed on top of the virgin surface until the cell monolayer is established.

More recently, a microdevice developed by Doran et al. (2009) has allowed the maintenance of a defined surface with no cellular damage during the initiation of cell migration. This device consists of a main inoculation chamber with perpendicular protruding migration channels (Fig. 10.3). In operation, cells are seeded into the main

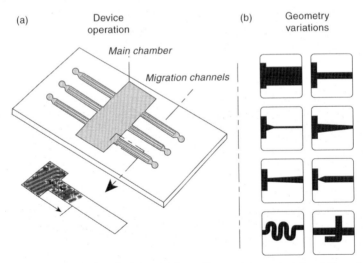

Figure 10.3 Schematic of microdevice operation and geometric constraint variations. (a) Once a cell monolayer is established within the main chamber, migration is initiated via backfilling of the migration channels. Migration can then be quantified by measuring cell progression into the channel. (b) This format can be used to study the effect of various substrates, or by incorporating geometry variations (as shown) along the length of the migration channels, can be used to determine how different cell types interpret architectural aspects of a tissue-engineered scaffold. These parameters include various pore sizes, contractions, expansions, junctions, and tortuosity.

chamber, but the cell suspension does not enter the migration channels due to the presence of a fluid meniscus at each channel entrance, a result of the channel dimensions (100 s of microns) and high (relative) fluid surface tension. This allows a confluent monolayer to be established within the central chamber with a "cell edge" at the interface between this chamber and the migration channel. Cell migration is then initiated via backfilling the migration channels, to effectively "break" the fluid meniscus and allow cells to access the channel. This microdevice, thus, allows the assessment of cell migration without the confounding issues of cellular damage or surface ambiguity, providing a rapid and robust tool to assess the influence of substrate biochemistry on cell migration, and, thus, cell colonization of space.

The flexibility of this device also allows the presentation of 2D geometrical challenges to mimic the architectural aspects and characteristics of 3D porous scaffolds. This adaption allows for the assessment of cell migration in response to geometrical challenges that mimic the architectural aspects and characteristics of 3D porous scaffolds in a 2D arrangement. This device has been utilized to investigate the influence of varying channel widths, degrees of channel tortuosity, the presence of contractions or expansions, and channel junctions on the migration of NIH 3 T3 mouse fibroblasts and human bone marrow—derived mesenchymal stromal cell (hMSC) (Mills et al., 2011). Data gained from this device showed that these 2 cell types have vastly different migration characteristics; 3 T3 fibroblasts migrate as a collective cell front, whereas hMSCs migrate as single cells. This resulted in 3 T3 fibroblasts displaying significant differences in migration depending on the type of geometrical constraint, while hMSCs were only influenced by channel width when it approached that of the length scale of a single cell, characteristics that would have a significant influence on the scaffold colonization by these two different cell populations. This clearly demonstrates the use of a microdevice to provide the necessary insight into how certain cell types, as a result of their migration characteristics, encounter and deal with different geometric constraints that may exist within biomaterial constructs, thereby highlighting the utility of microdevices to provide biological insights, relevant to tissue engineering, which could not be obtained using traditional techniques.

10.3.3 Microdevices for studying cell mechanics and impacts of shear stress on endothelial and smooth muscle cell function

Shear stress is known to influence the morphology, and even the fate, of many cell types (Gosgnach, Challah, Coulet, Michel, & Battle, 2000; Gutierrez et al., 2008; Kou et al., 2011; Lu et al., 2004; Qazi, Shi, & Tarbell, 2011; Shi & Tarbell, 2011), including endothelial and smooth muscle cells (Song et al., 2005; Sakamoto et al., 2006; Plouffe et al., 2007; Chau, Doran, & Cooper-White, 2009; Tkachenko, Gutierrez, Ginsberg, & Groisman, 2009; Wang et al.,2010). As blood flows through a vessel, shear stress is generated and directly sensed by endothelial cells lining the vascular wall. Endothelial cells may act as a mediator between flow conditions and smooth muscle cell functions. Physiologically, smooth muscle cells exist below the endothelial cell lining and are protected from the shear stress. However, in pathological conditions involving endothelial injury, smooth muscle cells can become exposed to shear stress (Palumbo et al., 2000; Shi, Abraham, & Tarbell, 2010; Shi & Tarbell, 2011). Therefore, understanding cell mechanics and impacts of shear stress on endothelial and smooth muscle cell function is important in vascular studies and tissue engineering.

Many shear microdevices have been developed. In general, they were fabricated using conventional microfabrication techniques and their designs involved an inlet channel branching into multiple channels of varying dimensions, which allowed multiple shear forces to be studied simultaneously (Chau et al., 2009; Gutierrez et al., 2008; Kou et al., 2011; Li, Ku, & Forest, 2012a; Song et al., 2005; Tkachenko, Gutierrez, Ginsberg, & Groisman, 2009). These microdevices have been used to study shear-dependent platelet aggregation (Li et al., 2012a) and adhesion to various ECM proteins (Gutierrez et al., 2008), and effects of shear stress on osteoblasts (Kou et al., 2011), fibroblasts (Lu et al., 2004), and endothelial cells (Chau et al., 2009; Song et al., 2005; Tkachenko et al., 2009).

A number of microdevices have been used for studying cell mechanics and shear stress on endothelial cell function. These include a multishear microfluidic device that allowed the simultaneous evaluation of 10 shear stresses covering physiological shear range (0.7–130 dyn/cm^2, 0.07–13 Pa) (Chau et al., 2009) (Fig. 10.4), a shear culture system composed of microfluidic channels interfaced with computer-controlled piezoelectric pins on a Braille display that can generate pulsatile flow and shear stresses up to 12 dyn/cm^2 (1.2 Pa) (Song et al., 2005), and a microfluidic perfusion device with a magnetic clamp to secure an unsealed PDMS microfluidic chip against cover glasses with endothelial monolayers tested at a shear range of 0.07–9 dyn/cm^2 (0.007–0.9 Pa) (Tkachenko et al., 2009). All three studies confirmed cell elongation and alignment in the direction of shear over time.

Impacts of direct shear stress on smooth muscle cells have not been studied as extensively as on endothelial cells. This is likely due to smooth muscle cells not normally (at least in healthy tissue) being exposed to shear stress in vivo. However, after endothelial damage, shear stress can be sensed directly by smooth muscle cells, triggering many complex mechanotransduction pathways and influencing cell properties and functions (Palumbo et al., 2000; Shi et al., 2010; Shi & Tarbell, 2011). Shear studies for smooth muscle cells have been conducted with endothelial cells in a parallel-plate flow chamber (Gosgnach et al., 2000; Chiu et al., 2003; Sakamoto et al., 2006; Ekstrand, Razuvaev, Folkersen, Roy, & Hedin, 2010; Wang et al., 2010), a cone-and-plate apparatus (Palumbo et al., 2000), a rotating shear rod (Shi et al., 2010), and a microfluidic device (Plouffe et al., 2007). Murthy et al. (Plouffe et al., 2007) used a tapered channel microfluidic design to induce varying shear forces (1.9, 2.9 and 3.9 dyn/cm^2, 0.19, 0.29 and 0.39 Pa) and showed peptide-mediated selective adhesion of smooth muscle, endothelial cells, and fibroblast cells under shear flow. All in all, the impacts of shear stress on smooth muscle and endothelial cells, and the interactions between these cells under fluid flow are highly complex, and further investigations are required.

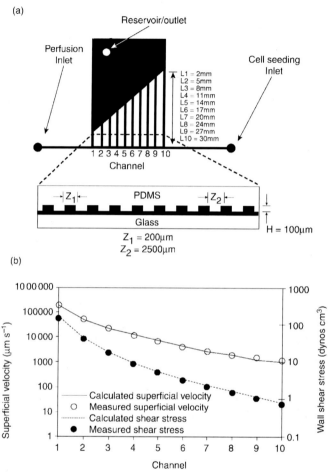

Figure 10.4 A multishear microdevice for the study of cell mechanics. The device delivers multiple physiologically relevant shear stresses, spanning over two orders of magnitude for any one flow rate. (a) Schematic of the device. (b) Measured and calculated superficial velocities and shear stresses for the multishear device at an inlet flow rate of 20 mL/h. Reproduced from Chau et al., 2009 with permission from The Royal Society of Chemistry.

10.3.4 Microdevices for the creation of microcirculatory networks

Microcirculatory network formation is a significant and challenging goal in the engineering of large 3D artificial structures. As mentioned in Section 10.2.3, microfabrication has been commonly used to fabricate microdevices for creating microcirculatory networks. It provides both the required resolution and ability to control uniformity of microvascular network structures. In general, these microdevices can be used in vitro as platforms for vascular studies or in vivo as tissue-engineered microvascular constructs.

A well-designed vascular network is essential in microdevices for microcirculatory network formation. Over the past decade, several investigators have attempted to establish and optimize microvascular network designs (Borenstein et al., 2002; Shin et al., 2004; Weinberg, Borenstein, Kaazempur-Mofrad, Orrick, & Vacanti, 2004; Fidkowski et al., 2005; Wang & Hsu, 2006; Chau, Rolfe, & Cooper-White, 2011). In general, they recognized the need for the network design to mimic natural vasculature dimensions and fluid dynamics, with a single inlet and outlet (Borenstein et al., 2002; Chau et al., 2011; Fidkowski et al., 2005; Shin et al., 2004; Wang & Hsu, 2006; Weinberg et al., 2004). Furthermore, each of the branches in the microvascular network design needs to have similar velocity profiles in order for oxygen and nutrients to be uniformly transported to all cells in the network and allow uniform cell seeding, more rapid achievement of confluent coatings, and better control over cell behavior for in vitro and in vivo studies (Chau et al., 2011; Wang & Hsu, 2006).

It is important that a well-designed vascular network also needs to be coupled with suitable flow and shear profiles required by the cells (Chau et al., 2011). Cells from diverse tissues and different parts of the vascular tree are heterogeneous with respect to their surface phenotype and protein expression, such that they can express different markers and generate different responses to the same stimulus (Augustin, Kozian, & Johnson, 1994; Jackson & Nguyen, 1997; McCarthy, Kuzu, Gatter, & Bicknell, 1991). Mismatches between flows and cells will lead to problems with endothelization, which seemed to be the case for some early microdevices (Fidkowski et al., 2005; Shin et al., 2004). Recognizing this, Chau et al. (2011) incorporated suitable flows for culturing human umbilical vein endothelial cells (HUVECs) in microchannels, previously elucidated in a "multishear" device (Chau et al., 2009), into a "ladder-like" microvascular network design and showed the development, in less than 28 h, of a fully patent, microcirculatory network, composed of a contiguous monolayer of HUVECs (Fig. 10.5).

Similar to a number of other studies (Borenstein et al., 2002; Shin et al., 2004; Wang & Hsu, 2006), this microvascular network structure (Chau et al., 2011) was generated from a commonly used material in microfabrication, PDMS. However, while PDMS is ubiquitous and inexpensive, it is not biodegradable and has limited biocompatibility. Furthermore, the high stiffness of PDMS (580 kPa) (Galan et al., 2007) compared to natural solid tissues ($\sim 0.1-100$ kPa) (Engler, Sen, Sweeny, & Discher, 2006) may impede vascular sprouting or angiogenesis, the formation of new capillaries from preexisting blood vessels (Patan, 2000). Therefore, these microdevices are limited as tissue-engineered constructs for implantation.

Problems of biocompatibility with synthetic materials eventually led researchers to explore the use of native ECM proteins and hydrogels in microfabrication. For examples, Golden & Tien (2007) fabricated a microfluidic system comprised collagen Type I or fibrin, and Paguirigan & Beebe (2006, 2007) crosslinked gelatin with the naturally

Microfluidic devices for developing tissue scaffolds 427

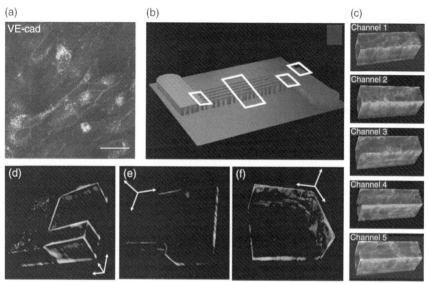

Figure 10.5 Endothelial cells fully lining the walls and corners of an artificial microvascular network after 24 h of culture. (a) The endothelial cells formed a monolayer with stable cell—cell adhesions, with the presence of VE-cadherin (the major adherens junction protein in endothelial cells) throughout the network after immunostaining. (b) A schematic of the microvascular network to show areas where 3D images were obtained. (c) Tilted 3D images of endothelial cells in microchannels with a height of 200 μm and width of 100 μm. The cells were immunostained for von Willebrand factor, actin stress fibers, and nuclei and found to form a confluent monolayer on all walls and corners of all channels of the network. Confocal Z-stacks: 40 slices, 5 μm spacing. (d, e, f) Tilted 3D images of endothelial cells at sections of the microvascular network. The cells were immunostained for von Willebrand factor, actin stress fibers, and nuclei. Scale bars are shown as white arrows in x, y, and z axes. Scale bars are only an estimation: (d) 100 μm, (e) 50 μm, and (f) 50 μm. Confocal Z-stacks: (d) 40 slices, 5 μm spacing, (e) 30 slices, 2 μm spacing, and (f) 30 slices, 3.5 μm spacing.
Reprinted with permission from *Biomicrofluidics*, 5, 034115 (2011); Copyright 2011 American Institute of Physics.

occurring enzyme transglutaminase to produce microfluidic devices. The vascular network design of Chau et al. (2011) has also been reported to be moved from PDMS into a gelatin system and they observed HUVECs self-assembling after 24 h of perfusion and sprouting after 5 days of perfusion (Chau, 2010). Stroock and his team also developed a hydrogel microfluidic system using alginate (Cabodi et al., 2005; Choi et al., 2007) and recently moved onto collagen Type 1 (Zheng et al., 2012) to show the establishment of an artificial microcirculatory network. Recent review on the state-of-the-art developments in vascularization of microtissues, limitations of current systems and potential future strategies were reported (Osaki, Sivathanu, & Kamm 2018, Vascularized microfluidic organ-chips for drug screening, disease models, and tissue engineering).

10.4 Conclusion and future trends

As evidenced from the discussion above, there have been substantial developments in the past decade utilizing microbioreactors and microfluidic devices to probe cell behaviors in synthetic culture environments. These device platforms have been designed to: optimize culture outcomes in readiness for scaffold seeding and colonization; study parameters relevant to common scaffold characteristics (including surface chemistry or composition, pore size, connectivity, mechanical property); create "tissue-like" environments that mimic diffusion and convective length scales in tissues, the magnitudes of shear stress, and perfusion rates "seen" by cells in tissues, the ECM composition of tissues, and the geometric challenges presented to cells when they "invade" a synthetic microenvironment; and develop functional, microvascular tissue constructs that may 1 day be surgically integrated into the host environment to provide immediate support for a cell-laden scaffold. These device platforms and their associated outcomes will continue to contribute to an ever-evolving set of design guidelines that will ultimately assist tissue engineers in achieving one of the major goals for the field: directed tissue genesis.

To date, much of the work related to the investigation of (stem) cell behavior and optimization of the cells' microenvironment (for example, the stem-cell niche) within microfluidic devices has in essence been performed with cells interacting with 2D substrates or surfaces, even though they may be enclosed within a 3D fluidic environment. However, all cells (including stem cells) are known to behave vastly differently in their native 3D environment, and in the future we are likely to see a significant trend away from 2D substrates. A recent review of testing of various microfluidic approaches for stem cell—based neural tissue engineering was reported (Karimi et al., 2016, Microfluidic systems for stem cell-based neural tissue engineering). Bulk hydrogel scaffold systems, often thought to be a closer mimic of the native ECM, are currently being used to investigate the impact of a 3D microenvironment on a host of cell behaviors, such as migration, growth, and differentiation. Microfluidic devices have only recently been utilized to move these bulk hydrogel systems into cell-laden microgel particles, with the significant advantages of uniform size, controlled physical and chemical properties, degradation rate, and encapsulated cell density. Some examples of materials used to generate hydrogel-based microparticles in microfluidic devices include alginate (Sugiura et al., 2005; Hong, Shin, Lee, Wong, & Cooper-White, 2007; Tan & Takeuchi, 2007) and collagen (Bruzewicz, McGuigan, & Whitesides, 2008; Hong, Hsu, Kaunas, & Kameoka, 2012), agarose (Kumachev et al., 2011) and poly(ethylene glycol) (Tumarkin et al., 2012), which were crosslinked via chemical, thermal, and photo stimuli, respectively. The use of microfluidic devices to encapsulate cells in hydrogel particles or to otherwise provide 3D microenvironments (for a recent review see Li, Valadez, Zuo, & Nie, 2012b) has, however, only just begun, as this methodology provides to researchers a high throughput means to investigate a number of environmental variables on cell viability, proliferation, and differentiation capabilities, such as mechanical properties, porosity, chemistry, the presentation of specific proteins and biochemical cues, encapsulated cell density, and rate of degradation of the encapsulating material.

Cells within tissues respond to changes in their local (3D) microenvironment through actively remodeling ECM, the secretion of soluble factors, and through cell—cell mediated interactions. With the continual, rapid advancement in our capabilities to fabricate microdevices from a multitude of material systems, with high resolution and fidelity, inclusive of advanced measurement, sensing, and control, we will in the near future have the capacity to develop in vitro device platforms or systems that mimic *simultaneously* many aspects of the in vivo extracellular (and intracellular) environment. In a highly controlled and tunable manner, with such device platforms, we will be able to decipher, manipulate, and ultimately invoke control over critical contributors to tissue repair and remodeling that have previously been elusive to tissue engineers, bioengineers, and biologists, such as cell—cell communication, paracrine—autocrine signaling, and tissue patterning.

References

Augustin, H. G., Kozian, D. H., & Johnson, R. C. (1994). Differentiation of endothelial cells: Analysis of the constitutive and activated endothelial cell phenotypes. *BioEssays, 16*, 901—906.

Baker, B. M., Gee, A. O., Metter, R. B., Nathan, A. S., Marklein, R. A., Burdick, J. A., et al. (2008). The potential to improve cell infiltration in composite fiber-aligned electrospun scaffolds by the selective removal of sacrificial fibers. *Biomaterials, 29*, 2348—2358.

Banfi, A., Muraglia, A., Dozin, B., Mastrogiacomo, M., Cancedda, R., & Quarto, R. (2000). Proliferation kinetics and differentiation potential of ex vivo expanded human bone marrow stromal cells: Implications for their use in cell therapy. *Experimental Hematology, 28*, 707—715.

Bellan, L. M., Singh, S. P., Henderson, P. W., Porri, T. J., Craighead, H. G., & Spector, J. A. (2009). Fabrication of an artificial 3-dimensional vascular network using sacrificial sugar structures. *Soft Matter, 5*, 1297—1540.

Blagovic, K., Kim, L. Y., & Voldman, J. (2011). Microfluidic perfusion for regulating diffusible signaling in stem cells. *PloS One, 6*, e22892.

Borenstein, J. T., Terai, H., King, K. R., Weinberg, E. J., Kaazempur-Mofrad, M. R., & Vacanti, J. P. (2002). Microfabrication technology for vascularized tissueengineering. *Biomedical Microdevices, 4*, 167—175.

Bruzewicz, D. A., McGuigan, A. P., & Whitesides, G. M. (2008). Fabrication of a modular tissue construct in a microfluidic chip. *Lab on a Chip, 8*, 663—671.

Cabodi, M., Choi, N. W., Gleghorn, J. P., Lee, C. S., Bonassar, L. J., & Stroock, A. D. (2005). A microfluidic biomaterial. *Journal of the American Chemical Society, 127*, 13788—13789.

Cao, Y., Mitchell, G., Messina, A., Price, L., Thompson, E., Penington, A., et al. (2006). The influence of architecture on degradation and tissue ingrowth into three-dimensional poly(lactic-co-glycolic acid) scaffolds in vitro and in vivo. *Biomaterials, 27*, 2854—2864.

Chau, L. (2010). *Ex vivo tissue vascularisation. Doctor of philosophy*. PhD Thesis. The University of Queensland.

Chau, L., Doran, M., & Cooper-White, J. (2009). A novel multishear microdevice for studying cell mechanics. *Lab on a Chip, 9*, 1897−1902.

Chau, L. T., Rolfe, B. E., & Cooper-White, J. J. (2011). A microdevice for the creation of patent, three-dimensional endothelial cell-based microcirculatory networks. *Biomicrofluidics, 5*(3), 034115-1-034115-14.

Chiu, J. J., Chen, L. J., Lee, P. L., Lee, C. I., Lo, L. W., Usami, S., et al. (2003). Shear stress inhibits adhesion molecule expression in vascular endothelial cells induced by coculture with smooth muscle cells. *Blood, 101*, 2667−2674.

Choi, N. W., Cabodi, M., Held, B., Gleghorn, J. P., Bonassar, L. J., & Stroock, A. D. (2007). Microfluidic scaffolds for tissue engineering. *Nature Materials, 6*, 908−915.

Chrobak, K. M., Potter, D. R., & Tien, J. (2006). Formation of perfused, functional microvascular tubes in vitro. *Microvascular Research, 71*, 185−196.

Chung, S., Sudo, R., Mack, P. J., Wan, C.-R., Vickerman, V., & Kamm, R. D. (2009). Cell migration into scaffolds under co-culture conditions in a microfluidic platform. *Lab on a Chip, 9*, 269−275.

Chu, T. M. G., Orton, D. G., Hollister, S. J., Feinberg, S. E., & Halloran, J. W. (2002). Mechanical and in vivo performance of hydroxyapatite implants with controlled architectures. *Biomaterials, 23*, 1283−1293.

Diehl, K. A., Foley, J. D., Nealey, P. F., & Murphy, C. J. (2005). Nanoscale topography modulates corneal epithelial cell migration. *Journal of Biomedical Materials Research Part A, 75A*, 603−611.

Doran, M. R., Mills, R. J., Parker, A. J., Landman, K. A., & Cooper-White, J. J. (2009). A cell migration device that maintains a defined surface with no cellular damage during wound edge generation. *Lab on a Chip, 9*, 2364−2369.

Doyle, A. D., Wang, F. W., Matsumoto, K., & Yamada, K. M. (2009). One-dimensional topography underlies three-dimensional fibrillar cell migration. *The Journal of Cell Biology, 184*, 481−490.

Ekstrand, J., Razuvaev, A., Folkersen, L., Roy, J., & Hedin, U. (2010). Tissue factor pathway inhibitor-2 is induced by fluid shear stress in vascular smooth muscle cells and affects cell proliferation and survival. *Journal of Vascular Surgery, 52*, 167−175.

Ellison, D., Munden, A., & Levchenko, A. (2009). Computational model and microfluidic platform for the investigation of paracrine and autocrine signaling in mouse embryonic stem cells. *Molecular BioSystems, 5*, 1004−1012.

Engler, A. J., Sen, S., Sweeny, H. L., & Discher, D. E. (2006). Matrix elasticity directs stem cell lineage specification. *Cell, 126*, 677−689.

Fidkowski, C., Kaazempur-Mofrad, M. R., Borenstein, J., Vacanti, J. P., Langer, R., & Wang, Y. (2005). Endothelialized microvasculature based on a biodegradable elastomer. *Tissue Engineering, 11*, 302−309.

Folkman, J., & Hochberg, M. (1973). Self-regulation of growth in three dimensions. *Journal of Experimental Medicine, 138*, 745−753.

Galan, I., Deleon, J. A., Diaz, L., Hong, J. S., Khalek, N., Munoz-Fernandez, M. A., et al. (2007). Effect of a bone marrow microenvironment on the ex-vivo expansion of umbilical cord blood progenitor cells. *The International Journal of Literary Humanities, 29*, 58−63.

Golden, A. P., & Tien, J. (2007). Fabrication of microfluidic hydrogels using molded gelatin as a sacrificial element. *Lab on a Chip, 7*, 720−725.

Gómez-Sjöberg, R., Leyrat, A. A., Pirone, D. M., Chen, C. S., & Quake, S. R. (2007). Versatile, fully automated, microfluidic cell culture system. *Analytical Chemistry, 79*, 8557−8563.

Gosgnach, W., Challah, M., Coulet, F., Michel, J. B., & Battle, T. (2000). Shear stress induces angiotensin converting enzyme expression in cultured smooth muscle cells: Possible involvement of bFGF. *Cardiovascular Research, 45*, 486−492.

Griffon, D. J., Abulencia, J. P., Ragetly, G. R., Fredericks, L. P., & Chaieb, S. (2011). A comparative study of seeding techniques and three-dimensional matrices for mesenchymal cell attachment. *Journal of Tissue Engineering and Regenerative Medicine, 5*, 169−179.

Griffon, D. J., Sedighi, M. R., Schaeffer, D. V., Eurell, J. A., & Johnson, A. L. (2006). Chitosan scaffolds: Interconnective pore size and cartilage engineering. *Acta Biomaterialia, 2*, 313−320.

Gutierrez, E., Petrich, B. G., Shattil, S. J., Ginsberg, M. H., Groisman, A., & Kasirer-Friede, A. (2008). Microfluidic devices for studies of shear-dependent platelet adhesion. *Lab on a Chip, 8*, 1486−1495.

Hong, S., Hsu, H.-J., Kaunas, R., & Kameoka, J. (2012). Collagen microsphere production on a chip. *Lab on a Chip, 12*, 3277−3280.

Hong, J. S., Shin, S. J., Lee, S., Wong, E., & Cooper-White, J. (2007). Spherical and cylindrical microencapsulation of living cells using microfluidic devices. *Korea-Australia Rheology Journal, 19*(3), 157−164.

Irimia, D., & Toner, M. (2009). Spontaneous migration of cancer cells under conditions of mechanical confinement. *Integrative Biology, 1*, 506−512.

Isenberg, B. C., Dimilla, P. A., Walker, M., Kim, S., & Wong, J. Y. (2009). Vascular smooth muscle cell durotaxis depends on substrate stiffness gradient strength. *Biophysical Journal, 97*, 1313−1322.

Jackson, C. J., & Nguyen, M. (1997). Human microvascular endothelial cells differ from macrovascular endothelial cells in their expression of matrix metalloproteinases. *The International Journal of Biochemistry and Cell Biology, 29*, 1167−1177.

Kaihara, S., Borenstein, J., Koka, R., Lalan, S., Ochoa, E. R., Ravens, M., et al. (2000). Silicon micromachining to tissue engineer branched vascular channels for liver fabrication. *Tissue Engineering, 6*, 105−117.

Kaiser, J.-P., Reinmann, A., & Bruinink, A. (2006). The effect of topographic characteristics on cell migration velocity. *Biomaterials, 27*, 5230−5241.

Karageorgiou, V., & Kaplan, D. (2005). Porosity of 3D biomaterial scaffolds and osteogenesis. *Biomaterials, 26*, 5474−5491.

Karimi, M., & Bahrami, S. (2016). Microfluidic systems for stem cell-based neural tissue engineering. *Lab Chip, 16*(14), 2551−2571. https://doi.org/10.1039/c6lc00489j.

Kim, L., Vahey, M. D., Hsu-Yi, L., & Voldman, J. (2006). Microfluidic arrays for logarithmically perfused embryonic stem cell culture. *Lab on a Chip, 6*, 394−406.

Kitsara, M., Kontziampasis, D., Agbulut, O., & Chen, Y. (2018). Heart on a chip: Micro-nanofabrication and microfluidics steering the future of cardiac tissue engineering. *Microelectron. Eng.* https://doi.org/10.1016/j.mee.2018.11.001.

Ko, I. K., & Iwata, H. (2001). An approach to constructing three-dimensional tissue. *Annals of the New York Academy of Sciences, 944*, 443−455.

Kou, S., Pan, L., Noort, D., Meng, G., Wu, X., Sun, H., et al. (2011). A multishear microfluidic device for quantitative analysis of calcium dynamics in osteoblasts. *Biochemical and Biophysical Research Communications, 408*, 350−355.

Kremer, M., Lang, E., & Berger, A. C. (2000). Evaluation of dermal-epidermal skin equivalents ('composite-skin') of human keratinocytes in a collagen-glycosaminoglycan matrix(Integra artificial skin). *British Journal of Plastic Surgery, 53*, 459–465.

Kumachev, A., Greener, J., Tumarkin, E., Eiser, E., Zandstra, P. W., & Kumacheva, E. (2011). High-throughput generation of hydrogel microbeads with varying elasticity for cell encapsulation. *Biomaterials, 32*, 1477–1483.

Lawrence, B. J., & Madihally, S. V. (2008). Cell colonization in degradable 3D porous matrices. *Cell Adhesion and Migration, 2*, 9–16.

Lecault, V., Vaninsberghe, M., Sekulovic, S., Knapp, D., Wohrer, S., Bowden, W., et al. (2011). High-throughput analysis of single hematopoietic stem cell proliferation in microfluidic cell culture arrays. *Nature Methods, 8*, 581–586.

Li, M., Ku, D., & Forest, C. (2012). Microfluidic system for simultaneous optical measurement of platelet aggregation at multiple shear rates in whole blood. *Lab on a Chip, 12*, 1355–1362.

Lin, F., & Butcher, E. C. (2006). T cell chemotaxis in a simple microfluidic device. *Lab on a Chip, 6*, 1462–1469.

Li, X.-J., Valadez, A. V., Zuo, P., & Nie, Z. (2012). Microfluidic 3D cell culture: Potential application for tissue-based bioassays. *Bioanalysis, 4*(12), 1509–1525.

Lo, C.-M., Wang, H.-B., Dembo, M., & Wang, Y.-L. (2000). Cell movement is guided by the rigidity of the substrate. *Biophysical Journal, 79*, 144–152.

Lu, H., Koo, L. Y., Wang, W. M., Lauffenburger, D. A., Griffith, L. G., & Jensen, K. F. (2004). Microfluidic shear devices for quantitative analysis of cell adhesion. *Analytical Chemistry, 76*, 5257–5264.

Malda, J., Woodfield, T. B. F., van der Vloodt, F., Wilson, C., Martens, D. E., Tramper, J., et al. (2005). The effect of PEGT/PBT scaffold architecture on the composition of tissue engineered cartilage. *Biomaterials, 26*, 63–72.

McCarthy, S. A., Kuzu, I., Gatter, K. C., & Bicknell, R. (1991). Heterogeneity of the endothelial cell and its role in organ preference of tumour metastasis. *Trends in Pharmacological Sciences, 12*, 462–467.

McGuigan, A. P., & Sefton, M. V. (2007). Design criteria for a modular tissue-engineered construct. *Tissue Engineering, 13*, 1079–1089.

McGuigan, A. P., & Sefton, M. V. (2007). Modular tissue engineering: Fabrication of a gelatin-based construct. *Journal of Tissue Engineering and Regenerative Medicine, 1*, 136–145.

Melchels, F. P. W., Barradas, A. M. C., van Blitterswijk, C. A., de Boer, J., Feijen, J., & Grijpma, D. W. (2010). Effects of the architecture of tissue engineering scaffolds on cell seeding and culturing. *Acta Biomaterialia, 6*, 4208–4217.

Migliore, A., Vozzi, F., Vozzi, G., & Ahluwalia, A. (2008). Controlled in vitro growth of cell microtubes: Towards the realisation of artificial microvessels. *Biomedical Microdevices, 10*, 81–88.

Mills, R. J., Frith, J. E., Hudson, J. E., & Cooper-White, J. J. (2011). Effect of geometric challenges on cell migration. *Tissue Engineering Part C Methods, 17*, 999–1010.

Moledina, F., Clarke, G., Oskooei, A., Onishi, K., Gunther, A., & Zandstra, P. W. (2012). Predictive microfluidic control of regulatory ligand trajectories in individual pluripotent cells. *Proceedings of the National Academy of Sciences, 109*, 3264–3269.

Neumann, T., Nicholson, B. S., & Sanders, J. E. (2003). Tissue engineering of perfused microvessels. *Microvascular Research, 66*, 59–67.

Nie, F. Q., Yamada, M., Kobayashi, J., Yamato, M., Kikuchi, A., & Okano, T. (2007). On-chip cell migration assay using microfluidic channels. *Biomaterials, 28*, 4017−4022.

Oh, S. H., Park, I. K., Kim, J. M., & Lee, J. H. (2007). In vitro and in vivo characteristics of PCL scaffolds with pore size gradient fabricated by a centrifugation method. *Biomaterials, 28*, 1664−1671.

O'Brien, F. J., Harley, B. A., Yannas, I. V., & Gibson, L. J. (2005). The effect of pore size on cell adhesion in collagen-GAG scaffolds. *Biomaterials, 26*, 433−441.

Osaki, T., Sivathanu, V., & Kamm, R. D. (2018). Vascularized microfluidic organ-chips for drug screening, disease models and tissue engineering. *Current Opinion in Biotechnology, 52*, 116−123. https://doi.org/10.1016/j.copbio.2018.03.011.

Paguirigan, A., & Beebe, D. J. (2006). Gelatin based microfluidic devices for cell culture. *Lab on a Chip, 6*, 407−413.

Paguirigan, A. L., & Beebe, D. J. (2007). Protocol for the fabrication of enzymatically cross-linked gelatin microchannels for microfluidic cell culture. *Nature Protocols, 2*, 1782−1788.

Palsson, B., & Bhatia, S. (2004). *Tissue engineering*. New Jersey: Pearson Prentice Hall.

Palumbo, R., Gaetano, C., Melillo, G., Toschi, E., Remuzzi, A., & Capogrossi, M. C. (2000). Shear stress downregulation of platelet-derived growth factor receptor-beta and matrix metalloprotease-2 is associated with inhibition of smooth muscle cell invasion and migration. *Circulation, 102*, 225−230.

Patan, S. (2000). Vasculogenesis and angiogenesis as mechanisms of vascular network formation, growth and remodeling. *Journal of Neurooncology, 50*, 1−15.

Pelham, R. J., & Wang, Y.-L. (1997). Cell locomotion and focal adhesions are regulated by substrate flexibility. *Proceedings of the National Academy of Sciences, 94*, 13661−13665.

Pittenger, M. F., Mackay, A. M., Beck, S. C., Jaiswal, R. K., Douglas, R., Mosca, J. D., et al. (1999). Multilineage potential of adult human mesenchymal stem cells. *Science, 284*, 143−147.

Plouffe, B. D., Njoka, D. N., Harris, J., Liao, J., Horick, N. K., Radisic, M., et al. (2007). Peptide-mediated selective adhesion of smooth muscle and endothelial cells in microfluidic shear flow. *Langmuir, 23*, 5050−5055.

Poujade, M., Grasland-Mongrain, E., Hertzog, A., Jouanneau, J., Chavrier, P., Ladoux, B., et al. (2007). Collective migration of an epithelial monolayer in response to a model wound. *Proceedings of the National Academy of Sciences of the United States of America, 104*, 15988−93.

Przybyla, L., & Voldman, J. (2012). Probing embryonic stem cell autocrine and paracrine signaling using microfluidics. *Annual Review of Analytical Chemistry, 5*, 293−315.

Qazi, H., Shi, Z. D., & Tarbell, J. M. (2011). Fluid shear stress regulates the invasive potential of glioma cells via modulation of migratory activity and matrix metalloproteinase expression. *PloS One, 6*, e20348.

Saadi, W., Wang, S.-J., Lin, F., & Jeon, N. (2006). A parallel-gradient microfluidic chamber for quantitative analysis of breast cancer cell chemotaxis. *Biomedical Microdevices, 8*, 109−118.

Sakamoto, N., Ohashi, T., & Sato, M. (2006). Effect of fluid shear stress on migration of vascular smooth muscle cells in cocultured model. *Annals of Biomedical Engineering, 34*, 408−415.

Salieb-Beugelaar, G. B., Simone, G., Arora, A., Philippi, A., & Manz, A. (2010). Latest developments in microfluidic cell biology and analysis systems. *Analytical Chemistry, 82*, 4848−4864.

Shi, Z. D., Abraham, G., & Tarbell, J. M. (2010). Shear stress modulation of smooth muscle cell marker genes in 2-D and 3-D depends on mechanotransduction by heparan sulfate proteoglycans and ERK1/2. *PloS One, 5*, e12196.

Shin, M., Matsuda, K., Ishii, O., Terai, H., Kaazempur-Mofrad, M., Borenstein, J., et al. (2004). Endothelialized networks with a vascular geometry in microfabricated poly(dimethyl siloxane). *Biomedical Microdevices, 6*, 269−278.

Shi, Z. D., & Tarbell, J. M. (2011). Fluid flow mechanotransduction in vascular smooth muscle cells and fibroblasts. *Annals of Biomedical Engineering, 39*, 1608−1619.

Silva, M. M. C. G., Cyster, L. A., Barry, J. J. A., Yang, X. B., Oreffo, R. O. C., Grant, D. M., et al. (2006). The effect of anisotropic architecture on cell and tissue infiltration into tissue engineering scaffolds. *Biomaterials, 27*, 5909−5917.

Song, J. W., Gu, W., Futai, N., Warner, K. A., Nor, J. E., & Takayama, S. (2005). Computer-controlled microcirculatory support system for endothelial cell culture and shearing. *Analytical Chemistry, 77*, 3993−3999.

Spiteri, C. G., Pilliar, R. M., & Kandel, R. A. (2006). Substrate porosity enhances chondrocyte attachment, spreading, and cartilage tissue formation in vitro. *Journal of Biomedical Materials Research, 78A*, 676−683.

Sugiura, S., Oda, T., Izumida, Y., Aoyagi, Y., Satake, M., Ochiai, A., et al. (2005). Size control of calcium alginate beads containing living cells using micro-nozzle array. *Biomaterials, 26*, 3327−3331.

Takei, T., Sakai, S., Ono, T., Ijima, H., & Kawakami, K. (2006). Fabrication of endothelialized tube in collagen gel as starting point for self-developing capillary-like network to construct three-dimensional organs in vitro. *Biotechnology and Bioengineering, 95*, 1−7.

Tan, W. H., & Takeuchi, S. (2007). Monodisperse alginate hydrogel microbeads for cell encapsulation. *Advanced Materials, 19*, 2696−2701.

van Tienen, T. G., Heijkants, R. G. J. C., Buma, P., de Groot, J. H., Pennings, A. J., & Veth, R. P. H. (2002). Tissue ingrowth and degradation of two biodegradable porous polymers with different porosities and pore sizes. *Biomaterials, 23*, 1731−1738.

Titmarsh, D. M., Chen, H., Wolvetang, E. J., & Cooper-White, J. J. (2012). Arrayed cellular environments for stem cells and regenerative medicine. *Biotechnology Journal, 8*(2), 167−179. https://doi.org/10.1002/biot.201200149.

Titmarsh, D., Hidalgo, A., Turner, J., Wolvetang, E., & Cooper-White, J. (2011). Optimization of flowrate for expansion of human embryonic stem cells in perfusion microbioreactors. *Biotechnology and Bioengineering, 108*, 2894−2904.

Titmarsh, D. M., Hudson, J. E., Hidalgo, A., Elefanty, A. G., Stanley, E. G., Wolvetang, E. J., et al. (2012). Microbioreactor arrays for full factorial screening of exogenous and paracrine factors in human embryonic stem cell differentiation. *PloS One, 7*(12), e52405.

Tkachenko, E., Gutierrez, E., Ginsberg, M. H., & Groisman, A. (2009). An easy to assemble microfluidic perfusion device with a magnetic clamp. *Lab on a Chip, 9*, 1085−1095.

Tsuruga, E., Takita, H., Itoh, H., Wakisaka, Y., & Kuboki, Y. (1997). Pore size of porous hydroxyapatite as the cell-substratum controls BMP-induced osteogenesis. *Journal of Biochemistry, 121*, 317−324.

Tumarkin, E., Tzadu, L., Csaszar, E., Seo, M., Zhang, H., Lee, A., et al. (2012). High-throughput combinatorial cell co-culture using microfluidics. *Integrative Biology, 3*, 653−662.

Vacanti, C. A., & Upton, J. (1994). Tissue-engineered morphogenesis of cartilage and bone by means of cell transplantation using synthetic biodegradable polymer matrices. *Clinics in Plastic Surgery, 21*, 445−462.

Wang, G. J., & Hsu, Y. F. (2006). Structure optimization of microvascular scaffolds. *Biomedical Microdevices, 8*, 51–58.

Wang, Y. H., Yan, Z. Q., Qi, Y. X., Cheng, B. B., Wang, X. D., Zhao, D., et al. (2010). Normal shear stress and vascular smooth muscle cells modulate migration of endothelial cells through histone deacetylase 6 activation and tubulin acetylation. *Annals of Biomedical Engineering, 38*, 729–737.

Weinberg, E. J., Borenstein, J. T., Kaazempur-Mofrad, M. R., Orrick, B., & Vacanti, J. P. (2004). Design and fabrication of a constant shear microfluidic network for tissue engineering. *Materials Research Society Proceedings, 820*. O5.4.1/W9.4.1-O5.4.6/W9.4.6.

Zhao, F., & Ma, T. (2005). Perfusion bioreactor system for human mesenchymal stem cell tissue engineering: Dynamic cell seeding and construct development. *Biotechnology and Bioengineering, 91*, 482–493.

Zheng, Y., Chen, J., Craven, M., Choi, N. W., Totorica, S., Diaz-Santana, A., et al. (2012). In vitro microvessels for the study of angiogenesis and thrombosis. In *Proceedings of the national academy of sciences of the United States of America* (Vol. 109, pp. 9342–9347).

Zmora, S., Glicklis, R., & Cohen, S. (2002). Tailoring the pore architecture in 3-D alginate scaffolds by controlling the freezing regime during fabrication. *Biomaterials, 23*, 4087–4094.

Microfluidic devices for stem cell analysis

D.-K. Kang, J. Lu, W. Zhang, E. Chang, M.A. Eckert, M.M. Ali, W. Zhao
University of California, Irvine, CA, United States

Revised by: XiuJun (James) Li
Department of Chemistry and Biochemistry, University of Texas at El Paso, El Paso, TX, United States

Guided-reading questions:

1. Why is the microfluidic technology beneficial to stem cell studies?
2. What are the major applications of microfluidic technology in stem cell studies?

11.1 Introduction

Over the past decades, stem cells have demonstrated great potential to treat diseases ranging from paralysis to heart failure to liver disease. Recently, the relatively new field of microfluidics has provided tools to study stem biology in novel, previously impossible ways that promise to hasten the translation of stem cells from the bench to the bedside.

11.1.1 Stem cells: the current status

Stem cells are defined as cells that can unlimitedly regenerate while maintaining the ability to become one or more specialized cell types through the process called differentiation. There are two kinds of stem cells that have been isolated from mammals: (1) embryonic stem cells (ESCs) that are derived from the inner cell mass of blastocysts, an early stage embryo (Thomson et al., 1998) and (2) adult stem cells that are found in various tissues and bone marrow. The primary difference between ESCs and adult stem cells is their differentiation potencies in vivo. ESCs are categorized as pluripotent stem cells that can differentiate into almost any cell lineage within the three germ layers (endoderm, mesoderm, and ectoderm). In contrast, adult stem cells include lineage-restricted stem cells such as hematopoietic stem cells (HSCs) (Muller-Sieburg, Cho, Thoman, Adkins, & Sieburg, 2002), mesenchymal stem cells (MSCs) (Jiang et al., 2002), endothelial stem cells (Gehling et al., 2000), neural stem cells (NSCs) (Altman, & Das, 1965; Alvarez-Buylla, Seri, & Doetsch, 2002), mammary stem cells (Liu, Dontu, & wicha, 2005), intestinal stem cells (van der Flier & Clevers, 2009), olfactory adult stem cells (Roisen et al., 2001), and neural crest stem cells

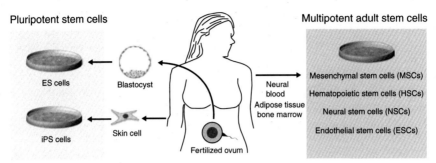

Figure 11.1 Derivation and differentiation of human stem cells for cell-based therapies. Embryonic stem cells (ESCs) are usually derived from the inner cell mass of a blastocyst. Induced pluripotent stem cells (iPSCs) are produced by in vitro reprogramming of adult cells so that they enter an ESC-like state. Both ES and iPSCs are pluripotent—they can be differentiated into a wide range of specialized cell types via multipotent intermediate cells. Adult stem cells can be collected from a variety of sources, including bone marrow, peripheral blood, adipose tissue, and neural tissue. They are generally believed to be multipotent, with the ability to differentiate into specialized cell types belonging to the organ from which they were derived.

(Fig. 11.1) (Clewes et al., 2011; Dupin & Coelho-Aguiar, 2012). On the other hand, adult stem cells are classified as multipotent stem cells that can only differentiate into their closely related progeny. For instance, NSCs can only differentiate into neurons, astrocytes, and oligodendrocytes while HSCs can only repopulate cells existing in blood, such as T-lymphocytes, B-lymphocytes, natural killer cells, monocytes, macrophages, granulocytes, platelets, and erythrocytes. Despite the differences in their fate potencies as well as their origins, both ESCs and adult stem cells possess great potential to impact human health. Currently induced pluripotent stem cells (iPSCs), derived from adult skin, liver, and stomach cells, have the capability to differentiate into all of the cells of the adult body (Takahashi & Yamanaka, 2006).

With their extraordinary abilities to repopulate specific cells of therapeutic interest, stem cells have attracted attention as potential therapeutic agents in regenerative medicine, a process of replacing or regenerating damaged cells, tissues, or organs to restore or establish normal function (Mason & Dunnill, 2008). In the past decade, substantial progress has been made in the fields of adult stem cells and ESCs. For instance, HSCs have been used to improve the treatment of autoimmune diseases (Burt et al., 2008; Sykes & Nikolic, 2005), and MSCs have been used in regeneration or treatment of damaged heart tissues, neurological disorders, vascular disease, kidney disease, diabetes, lung injury, osteogenesis imperfecta, cartilage injury, bone injury, spinal cord injury, autoimmune diseases, and others (Phinney & Prockop, 2007). Recently in Canada, MSCs have been approved for the treatment of children who suffer from graft-versus-host disease, a potentially deadly complication of bone marrow transplantation. Additionally, a recent study led by Notta et al. (2011) demonstrated that isolated HSCs are capable of long-term multilineage engraftment, which indicates the potential of using HSCs as an in vitro source of red blood cells for transfusion (Migliaccio, Whitsett, Papayannopoulou, & Sadelain, 2012). NSC-based transplantation studies have been reported for brain injury (Nakatomi et al., 2002) and various untreatable central nervous system (CNS) disorders such as stroke, Parkinson's disease, Huntington's disease, multiple sclerosis, and spinal cord injury (SCI) (Martino & Pluchino, 2006). ESCs have been shown to benefit patients who suffer from intractable epilepsy (Noebels et al., 2012), and aid the process of cardiac regeneration (Boheler, 2010; Shiba et al., 2012). With all the promising scientific progress in the stem cell field, several adult and ESC-based treatments are in clinical trials to prove their safety and efficacy.

11.1.2 Stem cells culture and analysis: conventional approaches

The most valuable trait of stem cells is their potency, the ability to turn into specific tissues in addition to those from which they were derived. Although this unique property could potentially transform current medicine and shape the future of regenerative medicine, it is also a problem that impedes the development of stem cell therapeutics. While stem cell scientists continually work on the discovery and development of new approaches to analyze and derive cells for therapeutic applications, the major challenge in developing these therapeutics is controlling the fate of the cells when scaling up the stem cell culture techniques for clinical usage (Serra, Brito, Correia, & Alves, 2012; Sharma, Raju, Sui, & Hu, 2011). Insufficient understanding of stem cell biology is the major bottleneck. Thus, developing not only a new cell culture platform but also new technologies for stem cell analysis is essential for furthering our understanding of stem cell biology.

To overcome this hurdle, it is important to recognize the problems associated with conventional approaches that are used for stem cell culture and analysis. *In vivo*, stem cells reside in a three-dimensional (3D) dynamic microenvironment, where they interact with the surrounding cells and extracellular matrix (ECM) and are exposed to low oxygen content and growth factor gradients. The crosstalk between stem cells and their environmental cellular niche provides signals that modulate the cellular response, such as self-renewal, differentiation, and apoptosis. Each cellular response of stem cells in vivo pertains to a unique environmental signal. For example, the environmental signal to each stem cell is spatially and dynamically different. In addition, there are physiological factors in *in vivo* systems that a culture dish or an incubator cannot fully mimic. In conventional in vitro approaches, such as two-dimensional (2D) adhesion cultures, stem cells are grown on Petri dishes or flasks in humidity, temperature, and CO_2 controlled incubators, which are not the exact mimic of the natural physiological environment. Furthermore, physiological fluid flow (Csete, 2010) and shear stresses (Csete, 2010) are impossible to introduce to a culture dish. Without a precisely controlled microenvironment in the in vitro culture, it is impossible to decipher the biological mechanism that modulates stem cell plasticity in vitro. Moreover, failure to maintain these key niche factors may trigger unexpected differentiation, and cell death and may lead to inaccurate results. A detailed understanding of the variant microenvironmental interactions and signaling pathways of stem cells in vivo will allow many stem cell–based therapeutic approaches to become possible.

11.1.3 Emerging technologies for cell research: microfluidics

Over the past decade, miniaturized devices known as "micro total analysis systems" (μTAS) or "lab-on-a-chip" devices have been continuously developed for cell manipulation and analysis. Soft lithography introduced in the late 1990s has become the most common method for fabrication of miniaturized devices, due to its advantages, which include low cost, fast fabrication time, and physical characteristics of the materials. Specific advantages in microdevice-based cell research include: (1) single-cell manipulation, (2) high throughput, (3) reduction of reagent consumption and the number of cells required, (4) tight control of signal gradients and flow in space and time, (5) tight control of physical and chemical factors, and (6) automation. Miniaturized devices present enormous opportunities to analyze, characterize, and manipulate cells (Zhang, Wei, Zeng, Xu, & Li, 2017; Li, Valadez, Zuo, & Nie, 2012; Qi, Huang, & Han, 2016).

In this chapter, we will first describe several microfluidic technologies that have advanced the molecular and cellular analysis of stem cells, including cell culture platforms, novel biosensor development, and microtechnologies that have potential to enable stem cell analysis. Then, we will discuss state-of-the-art microfabricated devices that have revealed new insights into stem cell biology. Finally, we will discuss microfabricated devices that have potential to impact the stem cell field and its future trends. We believe that this chapter will stimulate new directions for future development and use of microfabricated devices for stem cell analysis and regenerative medicine.

11.2 Technologies used in stem cell analysis

"Lab-on-a-chip" is a miniaturized multifunction apparatus; various microdevices have been developed, such as microchannels, gradient generators, microdroplet generators, dilution chambers, cell capture devices, microwells, microvalves, mixers, and microelectrodes. Recently, various applications have been developed that possess substantial potential to advance analytical assays on cells. Examples include "microfabricated cell culture platforms" for deciphering the niche environment to cellular responses (Fig. 11.2), concentration generating microfluidics devices to regulate biochemical/biological components (Fig. 11.3), "single-cell and high-throughput polymerase chain reaction (PCR)" to identify gene expression (Fig. 11.4), microfabricated cell sorters (Fig. 11.5), cell separator (Figs. 11.6 and 11.7), and novel biosensor development.

11.2.1 Miniaturized devices for cell culture

In vitro mammalian cell culture has played a fundamental role in facilitating the development of biotechnology and accelerating our understanding of cell biology. However, the microenvironment, and the role it plays in homeostasis, is still poorly understood because it comprises a complex array of biochemical and physical cues localized both temporally and spatially that alters the behavior of cells (Davenport, 2005). To effectively improve cell analysis, decoupling the interaction between the

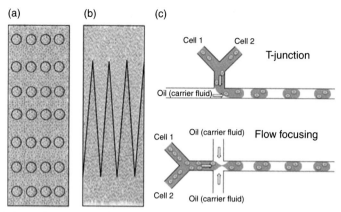

Figure 11.2 Emerging microfluidic platforms for advancing cell analysis. Microfluidics cell culture platform. (a) Microwell chip for cell culture (Khademhosseini et al., 2006a). (b) Silicon comb structured microdevice for studying the dynamics of intercellular communication between hepatocytes and supportive stromal cells in coculture (Hui & Bhatia, 2007). (c) Droplet microfluidics device for cell analysis. The compartmentalizing of cells can be accomplished with microfluidics using T-junctions (top) or Flow-focusing (bottom).

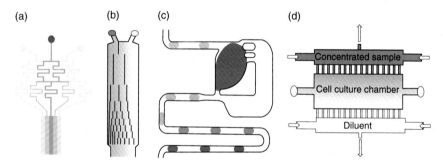

Figure 11.3 Microfluidics concentration gradient generators. (a) "Christmas tree" structured concentration gradient generator (Jeon et al., 2000). (b) Universal microfluidic gradient generator (Irimia et al., 2006). (c) Microdroplet dilutor (Niu, Gielen, Edel, & Demello, 2011). (d) Sink/source chamber (Shamloo, Ma, Poo, Sohn, & Heilshorn, 2008). Showing positions of source and sink (reagent) channels and cell culture chamber.

microenvironment and cellular response is critical. Microfluidic cell culture systems create new opportunities for the spatial and temporal control of cell growth and stimuli by combining surfaces that mimic the complex biochemistries and geometries of the ECM within microfluidic channels with the ability to transport of fluids and soluble factors (El-Ali, Sorger, & Jensen, 2006; Meyvantsson & Beebe, 2008) in controlled manner. These systems not only provide more accurate control over environmental cues, including cell—cell interaction, precise soluble factor control, and cell—ECM interaction (Csete, 2010); but they can also be used to manipulate physiological

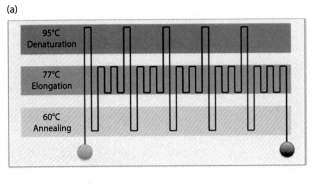
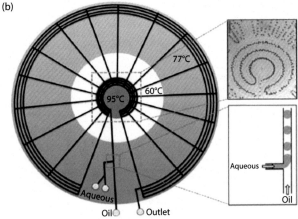

Figure 11.4 Microfluidics-based polymerase chain reaction (PCR) (Kopp, de Mello, & Manz, 1998). (a) Continuous microfluidics PCR. (b) Droplet microfluidics PCR. Reprinted and reproduced by permission of Schaerli et al. (2009).

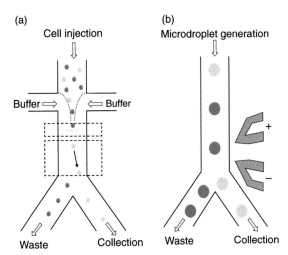

Figure 11.5 Fluorescence-activated sorting. (a) Optical switching sorter. (b) Microelectrode-based sorter (Baret et al., 2009).

Microfluidic devices for stem cell analysis

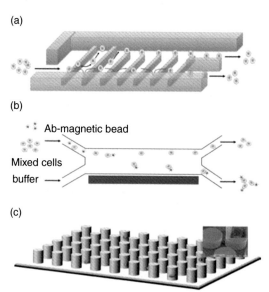

Figure 11.6 Cell surface marker targeting cell sorter. (a) Scalable parallel sorting device (Choi et al., 2012). Deterministic cell rolling based cell sorting (cell surface marker targeting). (b) Micromagnetic microfluidics cell sorter (Yung, Fiering, Mueller, & Ingber, 2009). Based on magnetic isolation, target cells or pathogens can be isolated from complex mixtures or whole blood. (c) Micropost cell sorter. Microposts coated with antibodies against target cells such as circulating cancer cells (CTC).
Reprinted and reproduced by permission of Nagrath et al. (2007).

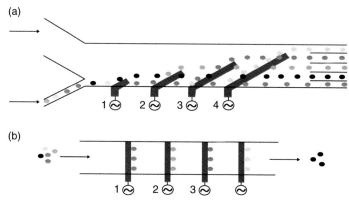

Figure 11.7 Dielectrophoresis (DEP) based cell sorter. At a particular frequency, cells move either away from the electrode (negative DEP) (Hu et al., 2005) (a) or toward the electrode (positive DEP) (b) (Flanagan et al., 2008).

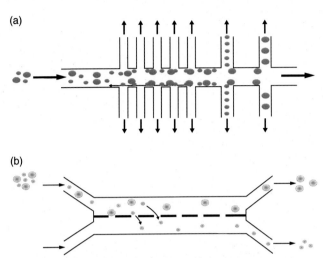

Figure 11.8 Size-based cell sorting. (a) Hydrodynamic filtration based cell sorter (Yamada & Seki, 2005). (b) Microfiltration based cell sorter (Wei et al., 2011). Porous membrane integrated microfluidics device can be used to separate different sized particles or cells.

stresses (Csete, 2010) and in vivo microenvironmental factors in a precise way. Several recently developed miniaturized cell culture devices have the ability to mimic precise niche environments and serve as tools to further improve cell analysis, including control over cell–cell (Hui & Bhatia, 2007), cell–soluble (Dahan, Bize, Lehnert, Horisberger, & Gijs, 2008; Chen, Wo, & Jong, 2012; Kim, Kim, & Jeon, 2010), and cell–ECM (Roach, Parker, Gadegaard, & Alexander, 2010) cues in both 2D and 3D microenvironments and the manipulation of mechanical characteristics of the cell niche (Fig. 11.9) (Vanapalli, Duits, & Mugele, 2009). Stem cell fate and function is regulated by a combination of intrinsic programs and signals from the microenvironment. Intrinsic determinants can consist of both genetic and epigenetic components. In addition, the importance of environmental signals in stem cell function has been highlighted by the identification of distinct stem cell niches in a wide range of organ systems. Overall, high-throughput analysis of stem cells, utilizing both controlled cellular microenvironments and perturbations of intrinsic elements, can provide substantial insight into the factors governing stem cell biology.

11.2.1.1 Biophysical regulation

For capturing and growing cells within microfluidic channels, Khademhosseini and his colleagues introduced microwell integrated microfluidic devices (Fig. 11.2a) (Khademhosseini et al., 2004). Poly(ethylene glycol) (PEG)-based microwells were fabricated by the polydimethylsiloxane (PDMS) stamping method, and NIH3T3 fibroblasts were adhered and cultured on the microwell in the microfluidics device. After the introduction of microwell-based microfluidics, there have been developments to

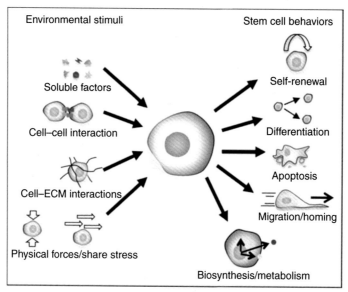

Figure 11.9 Microfluidics-based stem cell culture platform to mimic the in vivo culture condition in vitro. Combination of various factors involved in controlling stem cell fate and behavior in the stem cell niche.
Reproduced by permission from Underhill and Bhatia (2007).

control the fabrication of cell aggregates of uniform shape from differentiated cell lines (Fukuda et al., 2006) to control the interaction of ESCs with other cells (Khademhosseini et al., 2006) and to control size, shape, and homogeneity of embryoid bodies (EBs) (Karp et al., 2007). In addition, it is increasingly recognized that cells behave very differently when surrounded by a 3D ECM compared to anchored 2D substrate. Modeling the in vivo microenvironment typically involves placing cells in a 3D ECM in a physiologically relevant context with respect to other cells. Microfluidic perfusion coculture devices for 3D microenvironments act as systems for investigating cell–cell and cell–ECM interactions (Huang et al., 2009). Huang and colleagues utilized this system to construct a multicellular 3D culture for investigating the behaviors of metastatic breast cancer cells and tumor-derived macrophages in spatially, well-defined geometries. They demonstrated the versatility and potential of this new microfluidic platform to engineer 3D microscale architectures. Furthermore, tremendous progress has been made in the context of organ on a chip systems, including lung-on-a-chip (Huh et al., 2010), blood-vessel-on-a-chip (Bellan et al., 2009; Song et al., 2009), and liver-on-a-chip (Van Midwoud, Verpoorte, & Groothuis, 2011). Nevertheless, microfluidic cell culture systems provide a great opportunity to decipher cellular responses to the niche microenvironment.

11.2.1.2 Cell—cell interaction

To study cell—cell interactions in a microsystem and control cell—cell crosstalk in 2D, microfabricated devices with silicon comb structures were developed (Hui & Bhatia, 2007). Hui and Bhatia developed a microdevice consisting of two silicon combs that could be separated and brought into close contact with each other for precise cellular positioning to study the dynamics of intercellular communication between hepatocytes and supportive stromal cells in coculture (Fig. 11.2b). Using this microfabricated device, they demonstrated, with micrometer-scale precision, the dynamic regulation of cell—cell interactions via direct manipulation of adherent cells. As a proof-of-concept study, they utilized this tool in deconstructing the dynamics of intercellular communication between hepatocytes and supportive stromal cells in coculture. They concluded that preservation of hepatocyte viability and liver-specific functions in coculture depends on an initial contact-mediated signal followed by a sustained short-range soluble signal from fibroblasts to hepatocytes. This platform enables the investigation of dynamic cell—cell interaction in a multitude of applications and shows the potential in deciphering part of the stem cell niche.

Hydrogel, a type of material widely used as synthetic ECM, has been integrated in microfluidic devices to investigate cell—cell interactions (Lanza, Hayes, & Chick, 1996). Various hydrogel materials are available for cell encapsulation such as collagen, gelatin, fibrin, alginate, and agarose (Wan, 2012). With precise manipulation, droplet microfluidics technologies are able to encapsulate the cells into the picoliter-sized droplets for growing and analyzing them (Fig. 11.2c and d). Due to their ability to control the size, shape, and morphology, microfluidics have become one of the most promising approaches for cell encapsulation. For instance, Tumarkin et al. (2011) developed a microfluidic platform for the high-throughput generation of hydrogel microbeads for cell coculture. The platform was used to coencapsulate factor-dependent and responsive blood progenitor cell lines (MBA2 and M07e cells, respectively) at varying ratios and demonstrated that in-bead paracrine secretion can modulate the viability of the factor-dependent cells. Microgel encapsulation platforms are tools that help to determine how different cell types communicate with each other while minimizing the barriers of complex paracrine interactions that are seen in conventional cell culture techniques.

11.2.1.3 Biochemical regulation

To mimic the biochemical microenvironment in vivo, Jeon and colleagues introduced the first microfluidics gradient generator based on a "Christmas Tree structure" to dilute chemical/biological samples for a concentration-dependent experiment (Fig. 11.3a) (Jeon et al., 2000). *In vivo*, a wide range of biological processes, including proliferation, migration, differentiation, wound healing, cancer metastasis, inflammation, and stem cell development, are governed by a gradient of specific molecular cues. Thus, generating concentration differences in both growth factors and transcription factors in vitro plays a critical role in reconstituting the niche environments.

The microfluidics device was composed of a network of channels consisting of horizontal channels, vertical channels (serpentine), and a branching point. At the branching point, highly concentrated samples met with buffer and moved to the serpentine channel where they can be mixed. After mixing in the serpentine channel, the fluid splits into two side horizontal channels and the split fluid meets other fluids of both higher concentration and lower concentration. After several generations of branched systems, each fluid stream may achieve different concentration gradients. Because of the importance of concentration gradients for cell biological analysis, various microfluidic-based gradient generators have been developed after the introduction of the "Christmas Tree" structured device for both 2D and 3D cell culture. In particular, microjet devices (Keenan, Hsu, & Folch, 2006), universal gradient generators (Fig. 11.3b) (Irimia, Geba, & Toner, 2006), source/sink gradient generators (Abhyankar, Lokuta, Huttenlocher, & Beebe, 2006), osmotic pump gradient generators (Park, Hwang, Lee, & Lee, 2007), and microdroplet dilutors (Fig. 11.3c) (Niu et al.) have been developed and used in cell signaling assays (Abhyankar et al., 2006), cell migration assays (Lin et al., 2005), differentiation studies (Chung et al., 2005, 2007; Park et al., 2007, 2009), chemotaxis assays (Lin et al., 2005), and drug toxicity tests (Toh et al., 2009).

11.2.2 Miniaturized conventional technologies for cell analysis

The critical advantage of microfluidic technology over traditional assays is its high sensitivity in the micrometer scale. Several miniaturized technologies have been developed to perform accurate analytical gene/protein assays, such as microfluidic PCR. Additionally, microfluidic technologies, such as the miniaturized cell sorters, have been developed to enhance the performance of existing technologies.

Microfluidic PCR technologies are great examples of improved analytical assays using microtechnology. In the early 1990s, microfabricated PCR devices were first introduced by Northrup and colleagues (Northrup, Ching, & Watson, 1993). Manz and colleagues then introduced a continuous-flow microfluidics-based PCR system in which a channel (40 m deep and 90 m wide) was fabricated in glass with a total length of 2.2 m for 20 cycles (Kopp et al.) (Fig. 11.4a). The temperature was controlled with heated copper blocks (60°C, 77°C, 95°C) that were integrated under the microfluidics channels for denaturation, annealing, and extension. This pioneering work has since inspired the development of a broad range of chip-based microfluidic PCR devices (Bu, Melvin, Ensell, Wilkinson, & Evans, 2003; Crews, Wittwer, & Gale, 2008; Schneegass, Brautigam, & Kohler, 2001; Sun, Yamaguchi, Ishida, Matsuo, & Misawa, 2002). In 2009, Hollfelder and colleagues developed a droplet-based microfluidics PCR (microdroplet PCR) device in which an oil inlet joined two aqueous inlet channels to form a droplet at a T-junction (Fig. 11.4b). Generated droplets passed through the inner circles of the hot zone to denature the template. Then, as the droplets travel through the device, annealing and template extension occurs until the droplets finally exit the device after 34 cycles (Schaerli et al., 2009). This microdroplet PCR device allows efficient amplification from a single molecule of DNA per droplet. Since then, microdroplet-based PCR devices have been rapidly developing (Markey, Mohr, & Day, 2010; Schaerli et al., 2009; Taly, Kelly, & Griffiths, 2007; Tewhey et al., 2009). (See Chapter 13 for more information about PCR techniques.)

Miniaturized cell sorters are another great example of existing technologies that were redesigned to perform on the micrometer scale (Fu, Spence, Scherer, Arnold, & Quake, 1999). The first miniaturized cell sorter was the fluorescence-activated cell sorter (FACS), the gold standard in conventional cell isolation processes. Basing their technology on targeting cell surface markers, Fu and colleagues introduced microfabricated FACS (ìFACS), which was fabricated by soft lithography. Cells expressing green fluorescent protein (GFP) were sorted out using ìFACS (Fig. 11.5a and b). Moreover, miniaturized magnetic-activated cell sorters (MACS) have also been developed (Fig. 11.6b). These cell sorters are advantageous because they have a short operating time, are user-friendly, can be fabricated a low cost, are less labor-intensive, and have reduced sample/reagent consumption. Ingber and colleagues introduced microfabricated high-gradient magnetic field concentrator (HGMC; microneedle) integrated microfluidic devices to remove bacteria from blood. HGMCs generate a stronger magnetic field gradient across the microchannel in which bacteria could be isolated by anti *E. coli* antibody-coated paramagnetic microparticles within the magnetic field (Xia et al., 2006) (Fig. 11.6b). Taking advantage of the higher surface to volume ratio present at microscales, micropost microfluidics device was developed to isolate circulating tumor cells (CTCs) from the bloodstream based on specific surface protein (Nagrath et al., 2007). CTC-targeting antibodies (Anti-EpCAM) were coated onto microposts in microfluidic channels and CTCs were captured from the peripheral blood of cancer patients (Fig. 11.6c). Cell rolling properties were also utilized to isolate the cells using microfluidics. Karnik and his colleagues introduced a cell rolling microfluidics device in which the microfluidic channels were coated with P-selectin to guide the target cells into an isolating chamber (Fig. 11.6a) (Choi, Karp, & Karnik, 2012; Lee, Bose, van Vliet, Karp, & Karnik, 2011). In addition to the surface protein targeting strategy, Huang and colleagues introduced microfluidic size-based particle separation (Huang, Cox, Austin, & Sturm, 2004). Size differences between the particles have become one of the most important parameters that are used to isolate the particles using microfluidics (Fig. 11.8a). For instance, various devices have been developed to isolate CTCs from blood based on size differences between blood components and CTCs (RBC: ~8 ìm, WBC: 10−15 m, and CTC:16−20 m) (Fig. 11.8b) (Hosokawa et al., 2010; Hur, Henderson-MacLennan, McCabe, & di Carlo, 2011; Mach, Kim, Arshi, Hur, & di Carlo, 2011; Mohamed, Murray, Turner, & Caggana, 2009; Tan, Yobas, Lee, Ong, & Lim, 2009; Zheng et al., 2007). Additionally, there are reports of microfluidic devices that continuously monitor a patient's inflammatory response during cardiac surgery involving cardiopulmonary bypass (CPB) procedures (Aran et al., 2011) and remove bacteria from human blood (Aran et al., 2011; Mach & Di Carlo, 2010; Wu, Willing, Bjerketorp, Jansson, & Hjort, 2009b). The development of novel, microscale cell sorting strategies, such as microfluidics-based cell sorters, have paved the way to a better understanding of cell biology.

11.2.3 Emerging microfluidics technologies

We have demonstrated that we can mimic in vivo environments of cellular niches and enhance the sensitivity of existing technologies through microfluidic devices. In the following section, we will discuss the development of emerging technologies that investigate transport phenomena in microscale cell analysis.

The concept of droplet microfluidics was first introduced by Song and colleagues (Song, Tice, & Ismagilov, 2003) to address issues in cross-contamination, Taylor dispersion, solute—surface interactions, and the need for substantial volumes of reagents and relatively long channel lengths for continuous flow in microfluidics. Since then, various droplet-based microfluidic devices have been developed. By combining two immiscible phases (typically water and oil) in microfluidic channels (two main channel geometries are T-junction and flow focusing), picoliter-sized droplets can be generated and served as compartments for reactions (Fig. 11.2c and d). The rate of droplet formation in microfluidic channels can reach up to millions per second, and the concentration of encapsulated molecules can also be precisely controlled by manipulating the concentration of ingredients and speed of the fluid injections. With high accuracy and high-throughput potential, droplet microfluidics permits multiple reactions to be performed by varying the reaction conditions (Song, Chen, & Ismagilov, 2006). Various chemical and biological samples including DNA/RNA, protein, mammalian cells, bacteria, and worms have been manipulated and analyzed using droplet microfluidics. Furthermore, gene/protein expression, enzyme kinetics, cell proliferation, cell differentiation, cell signaling, protein crystallization, cytotoxicity assays, and organic synthesis have been achieved in droplet microfluidics. It has been shown that droplet microfluidics could satisfy demands that are not met by continuous-microfluidic devices (deMello, 2006; Solvas & deMello, 2011).

The integration of electrokinetics in microfluidics has also created systems with the potential to reveal important cellular traits (Markx & Davey, 1999; Pethig, Lee, & Talary, 2004). Electrical analyses of biological cells that detect dielectric properties represent a powerful tool for label-free analysis, characterization, and manipulation of biological cells (Fuhr et al., 1994; Gagnon, 2011; Pethig, 1996). To measure the dielectric characteristic of cells, two different techniques have been used: impedance spectroscopy and dielectrophoresis (DEP) (Fig. 11.7a and b). So far, the electrokinetic analysis of cells using microfluidics has revealed significant cellular behaviors, including cell cycle (Kim et al., 2007), proliferation (Lu et al., 2012), differentiation (Bagnaninchi & Drummond, 2011; Park et al., 2011; Reitinger, Wissenwasser, Kapferer, Heer, & Lepperdinger, 2012), and apoptosis induced by both chemical and physical impact (Patela & Markxb, 2008). By realizing that cells have distinct behaviors under exposure to an electric field, Becker and colleagues introduced DEP-based cancer cell isolation from blood (Becker et al., 1995). Additionally, Fiedler and colleagues first introduced a DEP-based cell sorter in microfluidics (Fiedler, Shirley, Schnelle, & Fuhr, 1998). Moreover, isolation of pathogens (such as bacteria) (Hu et al., 2005) and CTCs (Moon et al., 2011) from human blood has been achieved using DEP-based microfluidics. Based on the examples provided here, it is evident that electrokinetics-based microfluidics will contribute to the advancement of stem cell analysis.

11.3 Examples of microfluidic platform for stem cell analysis: stem cell culture platform—mimicking in vivo culture conditions in vitro

In the above sections, we introduced various platform technologies in microfluidics, including miniaturized cell culture systems, miniaturized analytical tools, and cell separators/sorters. Furthermore, we introduced microfluidic devices with specific functions, such as microelectrophoresis, single-cell analysis, and gene expression profiling. Recently, microdevices have also been used as tools for understanding stem cell behavior and have shown great potential in analysis of stem cells (Blagovic, Kim, & Voldman, 2011), such as stem cell culture, stem cell purification, labeling detection, cell separation, gene discrimination, and cell identification. Additionally, integration of microchannels with nanoelectrospray emitters allows for sample preparation for mass spectrometry in high-throughput and proteomics analysis.

Stem cell behavior is extremely sensitive to environmental stimuli, as depicted in Fig. 11.9; the stimuli are difficult to manipulate, demonstrate, and quantify with traditional methods. Schofield first proposed the "niche" hypothesis, to describe the physiologically limited microenvironment which supports stem cells (Schofield, 1978). The stem cell niche is a reservoir of multipotent stem cells that can maintain normal, injured, or aged organs and tissues, in response to signals that regulate whether they should remain quiescent, undergo self-renewal, or differentiate (Vazin & Schaffer, 2010). Recently, engineers have been able to create microfluidic microenvironments that can qualitatively and quantitatively emulate several key properties of the stem cell niche in *vitro*, thus enabling reductionist studies of their influences on stem cell behavior, including both biochemical and biophysical regulation. Previously, Gupta et al. (2010); Toh, Blagović, and Voldman (2010) have summarized the engineered miniaturized cell culture platforms and microfluidics-based approaches that can be translated to address particular issues in stem cell research. Wu, Lin, and Lee (2011) have provided a comprehensive review of papers published in recent years studying stem cells using microtechnologies. Here, we will emphasize the state-of-the-art miniaturized stem cell culture platforms that have contributed to understanding the relationship between microenvironmental cues and stem cell behavior in vivo, with an emphasis on biochemical regulation, cell–cell interactions, and biophysical regulation.

11.3.1 Biochemical regulation

In vivo, cells frequently respond to spatially distinct profiles of a variety of morphogens, growth factors, and other biochemical cues. In order to study the biochemical regulation of environmental cues, mimicking those biochemical profiles in vivo is critical. Distinct approaches have been developed in microfluidics to help identify the biochemical regulators that affect stem cell behavior, including external molecular gradients, paracrine and autocrine signaling, and spatially distinct microenvironments for stem cell manipulation.

11.3.1.1 Spatially distributed gradient generation

The molecular gradients generated by microfluidic devices are precise and comparable to in vivo systems (Csete, 2010). Gradient characteristics such as slope and concentrations can be quantified and correlated. With an increased *in vivo*—like chemotactic gradient in the microchannels, migration of stem cells can be studied on a single-cell basis instead of in mass cultures using Boyden chambers. An interesting study led by Chung and his colleagues investigated neural stem/progenitor cells (NSPCs) differentiation in response to a combinational gradient consisting of fibroblast growth factor 2 (FGF2), platelet-derived growth factor (PDGF), and epidermal growth factor (EGF). They demonstrated that human NSPCs (hNSPC) can be grown in microfluidic devices and can be induced to differentiate into other cells depending on the specific growth factor concentration gradients (Fig. 11.10a) (Chung et al., 2005). Similarly, Park et al. (2009) cultured an enriched population of neural progenitors derived from human ESCs in a microfluidic chamber for 8 days with continuous cytokine gradients (sonic hedgehog, fibroblast growth factor 8, and bone morphogenetic protein 4). They found that the average numbers of both neuronal cell body clusters and neurite bundles were directly proportional to sonic hedgehog concentrations in the gradient chip. Both studies showed that gradient-generating microfluidic devices are useful systems for both basic and translational research, with straightforward mechanisms and operational schemes.

11.3.1.2 Spatially distinct biochemical profile exposure

As we discussed previously, microfluidic technologies enable the possibility of precisely manipulating spatially distinct molecular profiles and dynamic fluidic environments. Fung, Beyzavi, Abgrall, Nguyen, and Li (2009) developed a Y-channel device with two inlets for two different culture media. An EB, a transient state of ESC to multipotent stem cells, was immobilized between the two streams. They demonstrated that by independently cultivating the two halves of an EB in two separate media, from laminar coflow in a microchannel, cell differentiation could be induced in half of the EB while retaining the other half of the EB in an uninduced stage.

11.3.1.3 Adhesive ligands (extracellular matrix) regulation

Signals that promote the anchoring or localization of stem cells to their proper niches are critical for maintaining their ability to self-renew and differentiate (Guilak et al., 2009; Scadden, 2006). Contrary to the combinatorial nature of ECM in vivo, it is difficult to investigate the influence of adhesive ligands on stem cell phenotypes. Anderson, Levenberg, and Langer (2004) introduced a polymer array synthesis approach

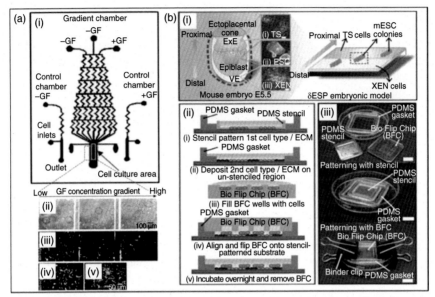

Figure 11.10 Microfluidics-based biochemical regulation (a) "Christmas tree" structured concentration gradient generator. (i) Schematic design of the microfluidic device showing the gradient chamber and two control chambers. Cells are loaded into the chambers via inlet ports (top of panel). Human neural stem cells (NSCs) cultured in the gradient chamber (ii, iii) for 7 days differentiated into astrocytes (stained with antibody against GFAP). Phase contrast images (ii) and fluorescence micrographs (iii, iv, v) showing stained nuclei (Hoechst) to identify all cells in the field. Astrocytic differentiation occurred more readily in the low GF compartment (iii). (b) Reconstituting proximal-distal (PD) epiblast patterning in vitro with Differential Environmental Spatial Patterning (dESP). (i) Conceptual design. (ii) Operation of SESP (iii) Components and assembly of SESP; middle and bottom panels show the assembly of components during the stenciling and flipping steps of SESP, respectively. Scale bar = 1 cm.
Reprinted by permission from Chung et al. (2005); Toh et al. (2011).

for rapid, nanoliter-scale synthesis of biomaterials, and characterization of their interactions with cells. As a proof-of-principle experiment, over 1700 human ESC (hESC)–material interactions were investigated. They identified various levels of hESC attachment and spreading, cell-type specific growth, growth factor–specific proliferation, and differentiation into cytokeratin-positive cells. This microarray approach offers new levels of control over hESC behavior.

The introduction of microprinting technologies in microfluidics represents another approach that has enabled our understanding of the role of ECM components on stem cell phenotypes in a high-throughput and combinatorial manner. Flaim, Chien, and Bhatia (2005) first developed an ECM microarray platform for the culture of patterned cells atop a combinatorial matrix mixture. This platform is used to investigate stem cell differentiation in response to a multitude of adhesive ligands in parallel. They observed mouse ESCs (mESC) on multiple unique combinations of multiple ECMs, which indicated that differentiation toward the hepatic fate is influenced in a combinatorial and complex dose-dependent manner. They further extended the platform to study human neural precursors in which they demonstrated how ECM components affect self-renewal and differentiation into neurons and glia (Flaim, Teng, Chien, & Bhatia, 2008). This platform facilitates the study of almost any insoluble ligand in a combinatorial fashion. Though we have only discussed a few examples, there are several microfluidic devices that have been developed to cultivate stem cells and to investigate the relationship between adhesive ligands and stem cell regulation (Chin et al., 2004; Lanfer et al., 2009; Solanki et al., 2010).

In addition to the development of microfluidics as a tool for understanding the interactions between adhesive molecules and stem cells, Toh, Blagovic, Yu, and Voldman (2011) introduced a spatially organized stem cell developmental model to interrogate the role of space in fate specification using micropatterning (Fig. 11.10b). They introduced "spatially organized stem cell developmental models" to interrogate the role of space in fate specification. Specifically, they developed differential environmental spatial patterning (dESP) to organize different microenvironments around single ESC colonies via sequential micropatterning. This study demonstrates the potential of using microfluidic devices to mimic the developmental progression of stem cell in vivo.

11.3.2 Cell—cell interaction

Cell—cell signaling via membrane protein contact or paracrine/autocrine signaling is crucial for maintaining stem cell homeostasis. For example, ESCs must be cultured in clumps in order for them to survive in vitro. To understand the influence of cell—cell interactions on stem cell homeostasis, three different approaches have been adapted in microfluidics, including controlling paracrine/autocrine signals and the development of cell coculture systems.

11.3.2.1 Paracrine and autocrine signaling control

Autocrine and paracrine signaling mechanisms are traditionally difficult to investigate due to limited technology and the submicromolar concentrations that are involved. Ellison, Munden, and Levchenko (2009) developed a computational model and a microfluidic cell culture platform that could control the removal of molecular factors secreted by cells into the surrounding media. With this system, they investigated the influence of paracrine and autocrine signaling in mESCs. They proved that the existence of soluble autocrine/paracrine factors, secreted by mESCs, contributes to their viability in in *vitro* culture conditions. Moreover, Blagovic and colleagues utilized the microfluidic perfusion system to investigate the biological role of autocrine and paracrine signals (Blagovic et al., 2011) (Fig. 11.11a). They developed a multiplex microfluidic platform to continuously remove cell-secreted (autocrine/paracrine) factors to downregulate diffusible signaling. By comparing cell growth and differentiation in side-by-side chambers with or without added cell-secreted factors, they isolated the effects of diffusible signaling from artifacts such as shear, nutrient depletion, and

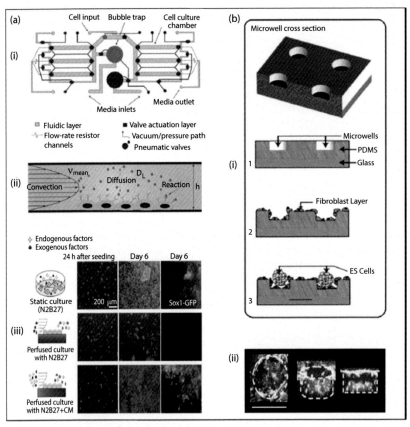

Figure 11.11 Microfluidics-based cell—cell interaction study. (a) Paracrine and autocrine signaling control. (i) Schematic of the perfusion device. Gray and black outlines represent fluidic and control layers, respectively. (ii) Microfluidic perfusion systems use flow to fine-tune the relative significance of convection, diffusion, and reaction. (iii) Monoculture neuroectodermal differentiation and comparison of differentiation makers in static and perfusion systems (upper, middle, bottom). (b) Microwell chip—based EB formation and EB size controlling. (i) Schematic representation of the coculture system formed by human embryonic stem (hES) and mouse embryonic fibroblast (MEF) cells. Polydimethylsiloxane (PDMS) was cured on a silicon master to produce microwell-patterned surfaces. Surfaces were treated with fibronectin and seeded with MEFs to create a monolayer for ES culture. (ii) 3D confocal reconstruction of hES—MEF cocultures within a microwell on day 1 rotated at 45°C intervals. In all figures, scale bars correspond to 200 μm.
Reprinted by permission from Blagovic et al. (2011); Khademhosseini et al. (2006).

microsystem effects, and found that cell-secreted growth factor(s) are required during neuroectodermal specification. Then, they induced FGF4 signaling in minimal chemically defined medium (N2B27) and inhibited FGF signaling in fully supplemented differentiation medium with cell-secreted factors to determine that the non-FGF cell-secreted factors are required to promote growth of differentiating mESCs.

From this study, they found that autocrine/paracrine signaling drives neuroectodermal commitment of mESCs through both FGF4-dependent and FGF4-independent pathways, and demonstrated that microfluidic perfusion systems are able to alter diffusible signaling of mESCs.

11.3.2.2 Controlling cell shape: EB formation and size control

Currently, there are two major approaches for culturing hESCs. The first method, also the most traditional way, is to coculture hESCs with a feeder layer consisting of mitotically inactivated murine embryonic fibroblasts (MEFs). MEFs supply a microenvironment for hESCs by maintaining the growth and health conditions necessary to maintain the undifferentiated status of hESCs. The second approach is to culture hESCs under feeder-free conditions such as Matrigel. Nevertheless, the common problem in both of these approaches is that they generate variable sized aggregates of cells. Large cell clusters tend to differentiate at the borders and small clusters of cells hinder proliferation and recovery of hESCs in culture. In addition, different sizes of EBs might lead to different cell lineage differentiation. For example, it has been reported that sufficient blood formation in EBs requires from 500 to 1000 cells. EBs with higher cell numbers were not able to form erythroid lineages (Ng, 2005). Therefore, controlling the size of cell aggregates is important for controlling the homogeneity of the cultures.

Recently, microfabrication-based approaches have become powerful tools for controlling the cellular microenvironment as well as the size of cell aggregates. Immobilizing cells on micropatterned surfaces in a microfluidic device allows cell shape and differentiation to be controlled. It has been reported that if hESCs/MEFs are cocultured in a microwell system, and the hESC aggregates are removed afterward, then 26% of the EBs had an area between 10,000 and 21,000 μm^2. These results show that it is possible to generate EBs with controllable sizes (Khademhosseini et al., 2006). In comparison, EBs that were prepared from hESC aggregates without the microwell system had variable sizes and less homogeneity than those prepared with the microwell system (Fig. 11.11b).

11.3.3 Biophysical regulation

In addition to biochemical factors, the stem cell niche environment also has unique mechanical properties that play an important role in regulating stem cell differentiation (Reilly & Engler, 2010). Microfluidic devices have been engineered to study the mechanical interactions between stem cells and their microenvironment. These devices facilitate our understanding of how mechanical signals (the mechanical interaction between the cell and its matrix) regulate stem cell behavior. Recently developed microfluidic devices have the ability to control microscale biophysical factors such as stiffness of the ECM, the geometry and shape of the cells, and the external shear stress experienced by the cells.

11.3.3.1 Controlling environmental mechanical influence

The stiffness of the ECM has been recognized as an influential component in stem cell differentiation. A landmark study led by Engler, Sen, Sweeney, and Discher (2006) has shown that the elasticity of the ECM can direct MSC's lineage specification. Alexander and his colleagues introduced stem cell encapsulation in hydrogel microbeads (agarose gel) to study the effects of variable cellular microenvironment elasticity on stem cell fate (Fig. 11.13) (Kumachev et al., 2011). The mESCs were encapsulated within the agarose microgels and different elastic moduli were obtained by injecting, into a microfluidic droplet generator, two streams of agarose solutions, one with a high concentration of agarose and the other with a low concentration of agarose, at varying relative volumetric flow rates.

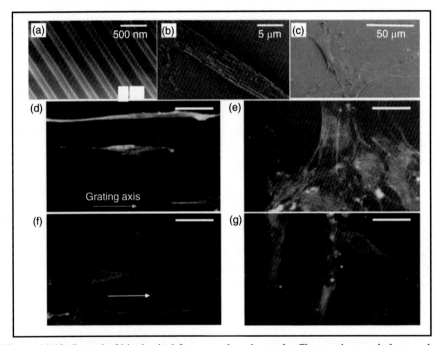

Figure 11.12 Control of biophysical factors at the microscale. Changes in morphology and proliferation of human mesenchymal stem cells (hMSC) cultured on nanogratings. Scanning electron micrographs of (a) polydimethylsiloxane (PDMS) nanopatterned by replica molding; hMSCs cultured on (b) nanopatterned PDMS and (c) unpatterned PDMS. Confocal micrographs of F-actin-stained hMSCs on (d) nanopatterned PDMS and (e) unpatterned PDMS in hMSC proliferation medium; (f) nanopatterned PDMS and (g) unpatterned PDMS cultured in presence of 1 μm of retinoic acid (RA). Bar = 500 nm for (i), 5 μm for B, 50 μm for C-G.
Reprinted by permission from Yim et al. (2007).

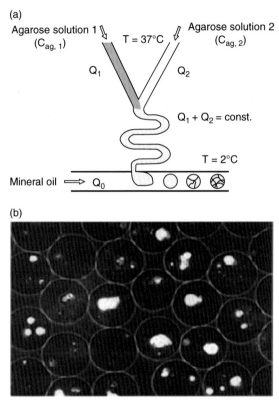

Figure 11.13 Microfluidics-based single stem cell analysis. Fluorescence optical microscopy images of agarose microgels encapsulating R1 mES cells in HBSS buffer.
Reprinted by permission from Kumachev et al. (2011).

Not only does the stiffness of the ECM affect stem cell differentiation, but also the geometry and the shape of the cells also exert a force on cells, which regulates stem cell behavior. To address the relationship between cell shape and stem cell behaviors, Yim, Pang, and Leong, (2007) utilized a nanoimprinting technique to create nanostructures to further our understanding of the role of topography on stem cell phenotypes (Fig. 11.12a). They found that the combination of nanotopography and biochemical cues, such as retinoic acid, further enhances the upregulation of neuronal marker expression. However, nanotopography showed a stronger effect, compared to retinoic acid alone, on an unpatterned surface. This study demonstrated the significance of nanotopography in understanding the differentiation mechanisms of adult stem cells.

11.3.3.2 Controlling external shear stress

Evidence of mechanically induced stem cell differentiation has been reported using several types of mechanical forces including stretch, strain, compression, and shear stress (Stolberg & McCloskey, 2009). Even though the mechanism on how cells sense and translate mechanical signals into a biological response remains poorly characterized, recently developed microfluidic cell culture devices have been used as tools to study the influence of shear stress on stem cell behavior. Toh and colleagues designed a multiplex logarithmic microfluidics array to directly screen perfusion effects across a wide range of flow rates, corresponding to 1000 times variation in applied shear stress in a single device (Toh & Voldman, 2011). They found flow-induced shear stress specifically upregulates the epiblast marker Fgf5. Epiblast-state transition in mESCs involves heparin sulfate proteoglycans, which have also been shown to transduce shear stress in endothelial cells. This study demonstrates that self-renewing mESCs possess the molecular machinery to sense shear stress.

11.4 Examples of microfluidic platform for stem cell analysis: single stem cell analysis

The fundamental goal of cell biology is to understand how cells operate, communicate with each other, and regulate their behaviors. Traditionally, 10^3-10^6 cells are used for cell biology experiments such as cell signaling, proliferation, migration, and invasion assays. However, cell behavior is dictated by their microenvironment, including soluble factors, ECM, and other cells. Specifically, stem cells and their fates are controlled by various niche factors, such as other cells within the niche, with stem cell behavior and differentiation dependent on the microenvironment (Moore & Lemischka, 2006). In addition, fundamental misunderstandings of the heterogeneity of stem cells have hindered development of clinically effective cell-based therapies; heterogeneity in cell populations poses a major obstacle in understanding complex biological processes (Lecault et al., 2011). As a result, high-throughput, single stem cell analysis is essential to expand our understanding of the heterogeneity within complex cell populations. Based on phenotype (protein expression) and genotype (gene expression), various microfluidic-based single-cell analytical methods have been developed recently (Guo, Rotem, Heyman, & Weitz, 2012; Zare & Kim, 2010).

11.4.1 Single-cell culture platform

Single cells can be cultured or controlled in microfabricated devices such as microdroplet- (Fig. 11.13) or microwell-based devices. Lecault et al. (2011) introduced microfluidics-based platforms for analysis of single HSC proliferation (Fig. 11.14). They fabricated PDMS-based microfluidic devices featuring 1600 cell culture chambers, each with a volume of 4.1 nL, and integrated microvalves for automated control and exchange of cell culture media. The effect of steel factor (SF) concentrations on survival and proliferation of HSCs, at a single-cell level, was defined and the growth rates of all clones (single cells) could be monitored and compared in real time.

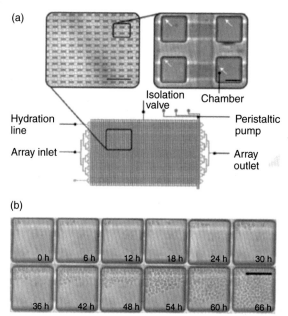

Figure 11.14 High-throughput analysis of single hematopoietic stem cell (HSC) proliferation in microfluidic. (a) Schematic of the device with micrographs as insets. The cell culture layer contains 1600 chambers connected by flow channels (gray). Arrows indicate single cells. Scale bars, 1 mm (left) and 100 μm (right). (b) Time-lapse automated imaging of clonal ND13 cell expression in a chamber. Scale bar, 100 μm.
Reprinted by permission from Lecault et al. (2011).

11.4.2 Cell cycle analysis

Recently, Kobel et al. (2012) introduced a single-cell cytometric microfluidics device. The microfluidic device consisted of 2048 arrayed single-cell traps and was utilized to quantify the spatial distribution of single cell for automatic tracking of dividing HSCs at single-cell level (Fig. 11.15). By using the "Fluorescence Ubiquitination Cell Cycle Indicator" (FUCCI) system, HSCs were transfected to regenerate red fluorescence (in G1 or G0 phase) or green fluorescence signal (in S/G2-M phase). Transfected cells were introduced and trapped in an image-based cytometry chip on a single-cell level. Then, the microfluidics chip was imaged using an automated microscope to analyze cell cycle phase. This approach should allow on-chip cytometry of diverse single-cell behaviors in long-term microfluidics culture.

11.4.3 Gene expression profiling

To characterize the heterogeneity within stem cells, microfluidics-based single-cell analysis has been employed on a variety of stem cell populations, including HSCs and ESCs. Glotzbach et al. (2011) developed a microfluidic RT (Reverse

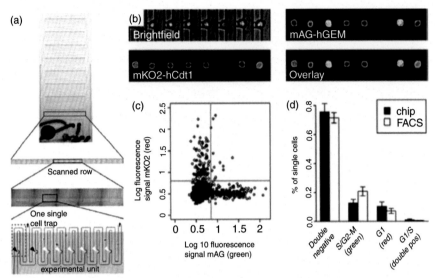

Figure 11.15 Cell cycle analysis of single stem cells with microfluidics. (a) Image-based cytometry on a microfluidic chip. (b) Micrographs of trapped hematopoietic stem cells (HSCs). S/G2-M (marked in gray, left bottom panel) and G1 (marked in white, right top panel). (c) The populations of S/G2-M and G1 phase HSCs (marked in gray and white) on the microfluidic chip. (d) Comparison of microfluidic chip and flow cytometry for the analysis of the cell cycle phases.
Reprinted by permission from Kobel et al. (2012).

Transcription)-PCR platform to investigate the heterogeneity of HSCs (Fig. 11.16). Murine HSCs were sorted by FACS into each well of a 96-well plate with RT-PCR reagents preloaded in each well. To create cDNA for each gene target within each individual cell, low-cycle RT-PCR was performed. Single-cell cDNA was then loaded into a microfluidic device, along with the primer-probe sets for each gene target, and qPCR was performed for each cell across all 48 gene targets in parallel by using the BioMark instrument (Glotzbach et al., 2011). This resulted in 2304 data points for each chip run. Using this microfluidics-based approach, 43 gene expressions (known to be highly relevant to hematopoiesis) were successfully measured from 300 individual HSCs. In addition, Zhong et al. (2007) developed microfluidic processors to profile single hESC expression through extraction of single-cell mRNA; synthesis of the cDNA was accomplished using the same device. The group concluded that whole population gene expression does not represent the gene expression present in individual cells. Using the unique advantages of microfluidics, it is possible to profile the gene expression of individual cells in the same niche that is otherwise considered heterogeneous using conventional gene expression methods.

Increasing numbers of miniaturized technologies have been developed to investigate the single-cell gene profile. Yet, none of these technologies has been applied to the stem cell field (Cai, Friedman, & Xie, 2006; Dhof, Wernig, Citri, Pang, & Malenka, 2011; White et al., 2011). Especially, White et al. developed RT-qPCR, which

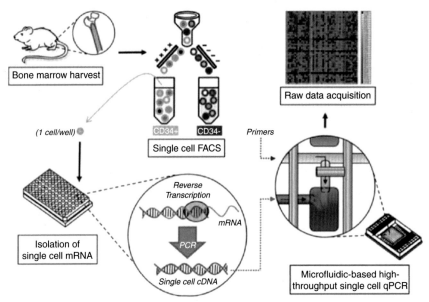

Figure 11.16 Single-cell gene expression analysis demonstrates transcriptional variation in murine long-term hematopoietic stem cells (LT-HSCs). Schematic of high-throughput microfluidic chip-based single-cell transcriptional analysis. A single-cell is sorted by fluorescence-activated cell sorter (FACS) into each well of a 96-well plate preloaded with reverse transcription–polymerase chain reaction (RT-PCR) reagents. A low-cycle RT-PCR preamplification step creates cDNA for each gene target within each individual cell. Single-cell cDNA and primer-probe sets for each target gene are then loaded onto the microfluidics chip. The BioMark machine performs qPCR for each cell across all 48 gene targets in parallel, resulting in 2304 data points for each chip run.
Reprinted by permission from Glotzbach et al. (2011).

can measure gene expression from hundreds of single cells (Fig. 11.17). This technology was applied to 3300 single-cell measurements of (i) miRNA expression in K562 cells, (ii) coregulation of a miRNA and one of its target transcripts during differentiation in ESCs, and (iii) single nucleotide variant detection in primary lobular breast cancer cells. However, it is expected that these miniaturized technologies will pave the way to fully understanding stem cell heterogeneity in gene/protein expression levels and will help realize the potential of stem cells in regenerative medicine in the near future.

11.5 Microdevices for label-free and noninvasive monitoring of stem cell differentiation

Because the interest in utilizing stem cells for therapeutic purposes is increasing, it becomes even more critical to develop technologies that track the cellular status of

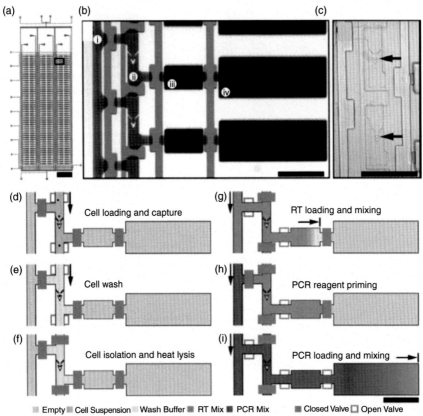

Figure 11.17 Design and operation of the microfluidic device for single-cell gene expression analysis. (a) Schematic of microfluidic device. Scale bar: 4 mm. The device features six sample input channels, each divided into 50 compound reaction chambers for a total of 300 reverse transcription–quantitative polymerase chain reaction (RT-qPCR) reactions using approximately 20 μL of reagents. The rectangular box indicates the region depicted in (b). (b) Optical micrograph of array unit. For visualization, the fluid paths and control channels are loaded with blue (marked in dark gray) and red (marked in gray) dyes, respectively. Each unit consists of (i) a reagent injection line, (ii) a 0.6 nL cell capture chamber with integrated cell traps, (iii) a 10 nL RT chamber, and (iv) a 50 nL PCR chamber. Scale bar: 400 μm. (c) Optical micrograph of 2 cell capture chambers with trapped single cells indicated by black arrows. Each trap includes upstream deflectors to direct cells into the capture region. Scale bar: 400 μm. (d–i) Device operation. (d) A single-cell suspension is injected into the device. (e) Cell traps isolate single cells from the fluid stream and permit washing of cells to remove extracellular RNA. (f) Actuation of pneumatic valves results in single-cell isolation prior to heat lysis. (g) Injection of reagent (gray) for RT reaction (10 nL). (i) Reagent injection line is flushed (dark gray) for PCR. (ii) Reagent for qPCR (black) is combined with RT product in 50 nL qPCR chamber. Scale bar for (d–i): 400 μm.
Reprinted by permission from White et al. (2011).

cells in vitro without the need for cell labeling. Intrinsic dielectric properties of cells have been proven as a new label-free approach in characterizing and monitoring stem cells (Pethig, 2010). The cell's dielectric characteristics can be attributed to the plasma membrane and the cytoplasm. The dielectric characteristics are defined by two parameters, capacitance and conductance. The majority of microfluidic studies have focused on the dielectric properties of the plasma membrane because of technical limitations (Bagnaninchi & Drummond, 2011; Fatoyinbo, Hoettges, & Hughes, 2008). Specific membrane capacitance (Cspec) is the measurement of a membrane's capacity to hold charges, which reveals the level of membrane folding and composition. Specific membrane conductance (Gspec), in contrast, is the membrane's ability to deliver charges, which reflects the expressions of ion channels. Several groups have successfully integrated electrokinetics in microtechnologies and have developed platforms to either track stem cell differentiation without the need for cell surface markers using DEP (Fatoyinbo et al., 2008; Hoettges et al., 2008; Patela & Markxb, 2008), or to distinguish subpopulations of stem cell progeny using single-cell impedance cytometry (Figs. 11.18−11.21).

Among the studies utilizing DEP to reveal the distinct dielectric signatures existing among stem cell populations, Flanagan et al. (2008) first identified that the dielectric response of NSPC to a nonuniform electric field is different from the response from differentiated mouse astrocytes and mouse neurons in a single DEP trapping device (Fig. 11.18). They also observed distinct dielectric responses existing between NSPCs isolated from different embryonic stages (E12, E16 for day 12 and day 16, respectively) with similar cell surface protein expression patterns (Nestin and GFAP protein expression). They further identified that the intrinsic dielectric characterization could be used to reveal the heterogeneity of NSPCs within the culture. Labeed et al. (2011) exploited another DEP-well system to further verify if the difference in NSPCs isolated from distinct embryonic stages is attributed to the dielectric properties of the membrane components or cytoplasmic components (Fig. 11.19). By measuring the dielectric properties of both the cell membrane and the cytoplasm, they identified the specific membrane capacitance (Cspec) as a novel biophysical marker to reflect the neuronal fate potential of NSPCs. They confirmed these findings by measuring Cspec of NSPCs with a distinct neuronal fate (human NSPCs isolated from distinct regions of brain with similar developmental stage and mouse NSPCs isolated from cortical brain regions from distinct developmental stage). Furthermore, the Cspec of cells dynamically changes as NSPCs lose their neuronal fate potential by passaging the cells in vitro over 20 times. In addition, DEP has also been applied to other adult stem cell fields. Vykoukal, Gascoyne, and Vykoukal 2009 utilized a simple approach method, called the conductivity method, to extract the dielectric properties of subpopulations of HSCs (Fig. 11.20). They used cell size verse Cspec plots as a way to discriminate the complete mononuclear and polymorphonuclear blood cell subpopulations from each other. These studies provide evidence that the dielectric signature of the cell membrane can be used as a label-free marker in reflecting the fate potential and differentiation progression of stem cells.

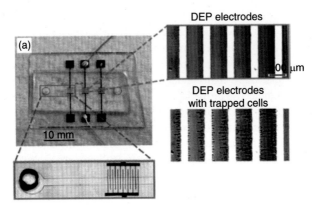

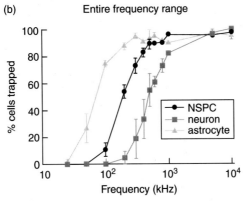

Figure 11.18 Microdevices for label-free and noninvasive monitoring of stem cell differentiation. Dielectrophoresis (DEP) microfluidics device based stem cell isolation by using distinct dielectric properties of stem cells. (a) Image of the DEP device. The top right panel is enlarged to show a higher-magnification view of the electrodes in the channel, and the bottom right panel shows a higher-magnification view of the electrodes when the DEP force is applied and cells are trapped. (b) DEP trapping efficiency curves distinguish embryonic day 12.5 mouse neural stem/progenitor cells (NSPCs), neurons, and astrocytes. NSPCs, neurons, and astrocytes showed distinct trapping efficiency curves.
Reprinted by permission from Flanagan et al. (2008).

In addition to monitoring Cspec of cells using DEP, impedance spectroscopy has recently been developed to monitor the differentiation of stem cells in real time (Bagnaninchi & Drummond, 2011; Park et al., 2011; Reitinger et al., 2012). For instance, Bagnaninchi & Drummond (2011) identified that the differentiation of adipose-derived stem cells along osteogenic and adipogenic lineages can be monitored based on their Cspec measurements. Park et al. (2011) found that neural differentiation of MSCs can be monitored using impedance sensing. Although those studies were not using microfluidics-based approaches, it extended the applicability of using dielectric signatures of cells as markers for MSCs. Recently, single-cell impedance cytometry

Microfluidic devices for stem cell analysis 465

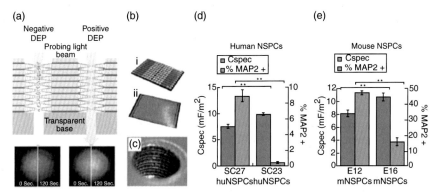

Figure 11.19 DEP (dielectrophoresis)-well system used to measure cellular dielectric properties by correlating the cellular dielectric response to light transmission through a microwell system. (a) The electrodes are energized at a range of frequencies, eliciting the response of particles contained within the well of either positive or negative DEP. The intensity of light passing through the well indicates the magnitude and sign of the force. (b) The DEP-well formats devised are (i) the smaller spectra-chip (size 37 × 23.5 mm^2), which can be energized by up to 19 parallel frequencies on four wells each, and (ii) the larger 1536-well plate (size 127 × 86 mm^2) on a standard well-plate template. (c) Close inspection of the inside of a 1.2 mm diameter well reveals the gold-plated conducting electrode "stripes" that surround the inside of each well. (d) The specific membrane capacitance (Cspec, mF = milliFarad) of SC27 and SC23 human neural stem/progenitor cells (huNSPCs). (e) The specific membrane capacitance of E12 and E16 mouse NSPCs (mNSPC) (**$P < .01$, $n = 3$ or more separate experiments with different sets of cells).
Reprinted by permission from Hoettges et al. (2008); Labeed et al. (2011).

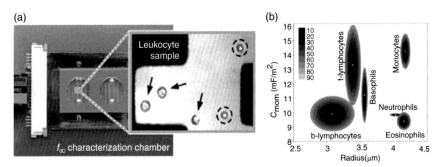

Figure 11.20 Dielectric characterization of complete mononuclear and polymorphonuclear blood cell subpopulations by label-free discrimination. (a) Photograph of cell characterization device with dielectrophoresis (DEP) microelectrode, fluidic reservoirs, electrical interconnect, and signal input. (insert) Eosinophil preparation on castellated electrode; eosinophils are indicated by arrows while erythrocytes are circled. (b) Scattergram of leukocyte subpopulation properties as determined during DEP crossover frequency analysis.
Reprinted by permission from Vykoukal et al. (2009).

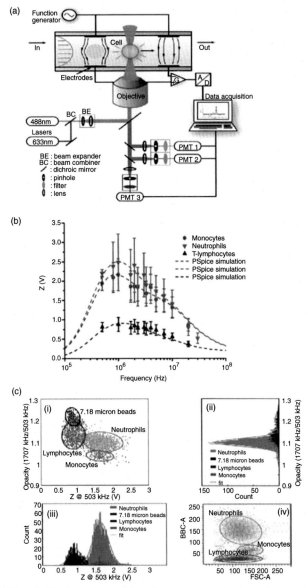

Figure 11.21 Microfluidic impedance cytometry to measure the impedance of single cells at two frequencies. (a) Schematic diagram of the microimpedance cytometer system, including the confocal-optical detection setup. Dual laser excitation and three color detection are implemented along with dual frequency impedance measurement. The cell flows through the microchannel and passes between two pairs of electrodes and the optical detection region. The fluorescence properties and impedance of the cell are measured simultaneously, allowing comparison of the electrical and optical properties of single cells. (b) Magnetic-activated cell sorters (MACS) purified populations of T-lymphocytes, monocytes, and neutrophils.
Reprinted by permission from Holmes et al. (2009).

represents an alternative approach to measuring cell dielectric characteristics (Sun & Morgan, 2010) on a micrometer scale. Holmes et al. (2009) developed a microfluidic impedance cytometry device to measure the impedance of a single cell at two frequencies (Fig. 11.21). They found that the low frequency (503 kHz) impedance magnitude, a measure of cell size, enables discrimination of the T-lymphocyte population from the larger cells that make up the monocyte and neutrophil populations. Dual frequency measurements enabled discrimination of the cells according to both membrane capacitance and size and allowed them to distinguish monocytes, neutrophils, and lymphocytes from each other at the same time. These studies indicate that single-cell impedance cytometry devices have potential to track stem cell differentiation without the need for cell labeling or genetic manipulation, which is beneficial for the development of stem cell—based regenerative medicine.

One of the concerns in integrating electrokinetics in microtechnologies for stem cell research is the potential adverse effect that electric field exposures can have on stem cell plasticity or differentiation potential. To address this issue, Lu et al. (2012) completed a comprehensive study investigating the impact of AC electric field exposures on stem cells that are required for DEP and impedance measurements. No adverse impact on cell viability, proliferation, or fate potential of NSPCs was noticed for the time that was required for the dielectric property measurements. This study indicated that monitoring stem cell differentiation using DEP and impedance spectroscopy in vitro is noninvasive and has the potential to advance stem cell research.

11.6 Microfluidics stem cell separation technology

The detection, isolation, and sorting of specific subpopulations of stem cells are important in both fundamental research and clinical applications of stem cell—based therapeutics. Advances in microfluidic cell sorting devices have enabled scientists to attain improved separation with comparative ease and considerable timesaving (Baret et al., 2009; Kiermer, 2005). Based on the detection method utilized, microfluidic cell sorting devices can be classified as either marker-dependent or label-free (Figs. 11.22—11.26). The marker-dependent approach relies on the identification of specific cell surface protein expression levels. For example, thermoresponsive microfluidics has been used to selectively release captured cells from blood (Fig. 11.22) (Gurkan et al., 2011). In this case, the authors used anti-CD4 and anti-CD34 antibodies immobilized in a microfluidic device to capture CD4+ and CD34+ cells from blood. Cooling the microchip below 32°C led to release of the collected cells. 195 CD4+ cells and 19 CD34+ cells per million blood cells were successfully quantified without labeling using this affinity microfluidics device. Optical switching based fluorescence-activated microfluidic cell sorters have been also developed to isolate GFP expressing cells (Fig. 11.23) (Wang et al., 2004). When GFP expressing cells are detected and determined to be a target cell, the optical switch is activated, and a focused laser spot deflects the cell to the

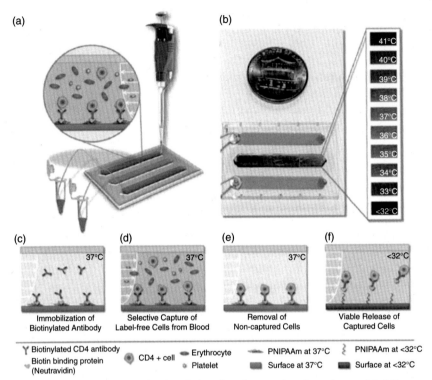

Figure 11.22 Microfluidic cell sorting devices based on marker-dependent or label-free approaches. Thermo-responsive microfluidic chip developed for releasing selectively captured cells from blood. (a) The microfluidic chip is composed of three parallel channels (4 × 22 × 80 mm), one of which (middle channel) is used as the temperature indicator channel. Blood is introduced into the top and bottom release channels with manual pipetting. (b) The middle channel is coated with temperature sensitive liquid crystal dye, which is responsive to temperatures between 35 and 40°C. The target temperature is maintained in the middle channel. (c–f) Schematic of the working principle of label-free selective capture from whole blood and controlled release of cells in thermoresponsive microfluidic channels. Reprinted by permission from Gurkan et al. (2011).

target output channel. The laser spot is translated at a speed matched to the flow velocity and at a small angle relative to the axis of the flow to maximize the interaction time between the laser and the cell. The resulting lateral displacement of the cell across the flow stream is sufficient to ensure that it will be directed toward the target output channel. In addition, MACS has been achieved in microfluidics for stem cell extraction (Fig. 11.24) (Tan et al., 2005). Anti-CD31 (PECAM1) monoclonal antibody-conjugated magnetic beads were introduced into the microfluidics device to remove human umbilical cord vein endothelial cells (HUVEC) from a mixture of HUVEC

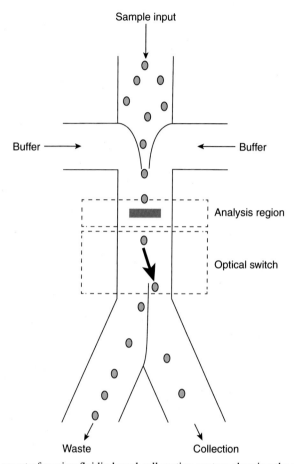

Figure 11.23 Layout of a microfluidic-based cell sorting system showing the sorting junction and optical switch. Cells in the sample are aligned to the center of the channel by flow focusing. Fluorescently labeled target cells are analyzed and detected by turning on the optical switch. Target cells are directed by the laser to the collection output while all other cells flow to the waste output.
Reprinted by permission from Wang et al. (2005).

and hMSC cells introduced into the device at the same time through the other channel. The two streams are completely mixed in the micromixer and the cell—bead complexes separated into the buffer fluid by an external magnetic field. For the label-free approach, unique biophysical characterizations, such as size and electrophysiological properties of the membrane, are required to enable the label-free cell separation in microfluidic devices. Various microfluidics-based cell sorters that are used to isolate stem cells are summarized in Table 11.1.

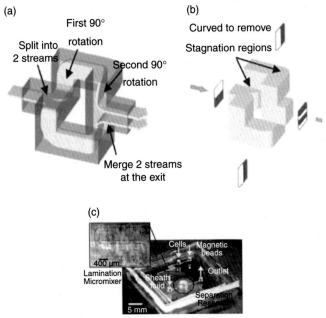

Figure 11.24 Micromagnetic separators for stem cell sorting. (a) Lamination micromixer with 180 degrees rotation. (b) Geometry of a single mixer unit. (c) Prototype μ-IMCS. Reprinted by permission from Tan et al. (2005).

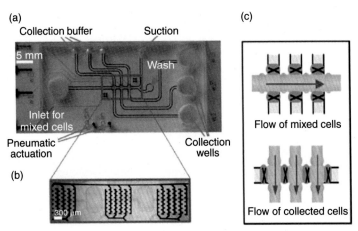

Figure 11.25 Dielectrophoresis (DEP)-based microfluidics cell sorter. (a) Polydimethylsiloxane (PDMS)-glass microfluidic device for DEP trapping. (b) The device has three trapping sites with castellated electrodes that can be independently addressed. The initial mixture of cells flows through all three trapping sites. (c) The collection is done with three perpendicular flows after isolating each trapping zone by closing adjacent pneumatic valves.
Reprinted by permission from Prieto et al. (2012).

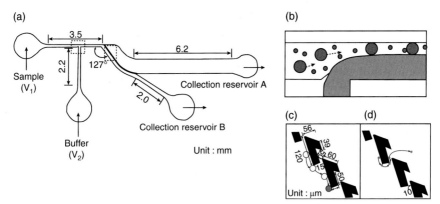

Figure 11.26 Microfluidic device for separation of amniotic fluid mesenchymal stem cells (AF MSCs) utilizing louver-array structures. (a) Schematic illustration of the cell separation chip. (b) Detailed view showing that beads or cells can be focused to form a narrow stream. (c) and (d) Detailed dimensions of the chip and cell separation mechanism. (c) The larger beads or cells are separated by the louver-like structures. (d) The smaller beads or cells flow through the gap between the louver-like structures.
Reprinted by permission from Wu et al. (2009a,b).

11.6.1 Marker-dependent approach

11.6.1.1 Fluorescence-activated stem cell sorting

FACS, the golden standard for conventional stem cell separation, has also been developed in microfluidics to isolate rare cells. Although developing a practical technology for microfluidic-based FACS has proved challenging, Wang et al. (2004) took a unique approach to developing this technology by first integrating an optical switching system for the rapid (2–4 ms), active control of cell routing on a microfluidics chips (Fig. 11.23). Using all-optical switching, a fluorescence-activated microfluidic cell sorter has been implemented and evaluated. This study suggests the possibility of integrating FACS on a microfluidic chip to allow more precise analysis of stem cells in real time.

11.6.1.2 Magnetic-activated stem cell sorting

MACS, one of the most popular conventional cell isolation methods, has recently been developed in microfluidics to isolate rare cells. Tan et al. (2005) first introduced micromagnetic separators for stem cell sorting (Fig. 11.24). A 3D mixer was integrated in a microfluidic channel to achieve lamination with 180-degree rotations and rapid mixing between cells and magnetic beads. To isolate the target cell from the mixture, magnetic beads conjugated with CD31 antibodies were used to remove CD31+ endothelial cells with an external magnetic field. Up to 90.2% of hMSCs were isolated and recovered. In addition, Souse and colleagues introduced a two-inlet/two-outlet microfluidics

Table 11.1 Microfluidics devices for stem cell isolation/separation.

Isolation method	Details of isolation	Targeted cells	Carrier medium and control cells	% Recovery	% purity/fold increase	Marker-dependent	Label-free	References
Cell affinity	Anti-EPCs marker antibody immobilized microfluidics channel (CD23, VEGFR-2, CD31, and CD146)	EPCs	MSCs, VSMCs, VECs	N/A	N/A	Yes	Yes	(Plouffe et al., 2009; Gurkan et al., 2011)
Cell affinity	CD34 antibody immobilized PNIPAAm microfluidics channel	EPCs	Whole blood	N/A	19 cells/10^6 blood cells (EPCs/WBCs + RBCs)	Yes	Yes	(Liu et al., 2005)
Magnetic microbead	CD31 antibody-conjugated magnetic bead	CD31-hMSCs (hMSCs)	HUVEC	90.2	N/A	Yes	Yes	(Miwa et al., 2005a)
Magnetic microbead	Anti-SSEA1 antibody-conjugated magnetic bead.	SSEA-1+ mESCs	Heterogeneous mESCs (SSEA-1+ mESCs and SSEA-1− mESCs)	N/A	95–99.5	Yes	Yes	(Sousa et al., 2011)

DEP-based microfluidics	N/A	Hematopoietic CD34+ stem cells	Bone marrow and peripheral blood stem cell harvests	N/A	5-fold enrichment	Yes	Yes	(Talary et al., 1995)
DEP-based microfluidics	N/A	NG2+ cells and Nestin + cells (putative progenitor cells)	Nucleated cell fraction isolated from adipose tissue and the bulk of the erythrocytes	N/A	(1.9 % × 28 %)/ 14-fold increase	Yes	Yes	(Vykoukal et al., 2008)
DEP-based microfluidics	N/A	Neurons	Neurons and NSPCs,	N/A	1.4-fold enrichment to neuron culture	Yes	Yes	(Prieto et al., 2012)
Size	Louver-array structure	AFMSCs	Endothelial cells in amniotic fluid	97.1%	N/A	No	Yes	(Wu et al., 2009a)
Size	Porous membrane integrated microfluidics	HSCs	Bone marrow	98%	N/A	No	Yes	(Schirhagl et al., 2011)

device to isolate mouse mESCs using superparamagnetic particles. To isolate specific embryonic antigen 1 positive (SSEA-1+) mESCs from a heterogeneous population of mESCs, anti-SSEA-1 antibodies were conjugated onto superparamagnetic beads and mixed with the cell mixture. Once the mixture was injected into the microfluidics channel and the magnetic field was applied, SSEA-1+ mESCs were deviated from the direction of laminar flow according to their magnetic susceptibility and were, thus, separated from SSEA-1$^-$ mESCs.

11.6.1.3 Cell affinity—based stem cell isolation

Affinity chromatography is one of the most popular methods for separation, isolation, and purification of target biomolecules from whole mixtures based on highly sensitive and specific interactions between antigen and antibody, or receptor and ligand. Brian and colleagues developed microfluidics-based cell affinity devices that have the capability of capturing circulating endothelial progenitor cells (EPCs) (Plouffe, Kniazeva, Mayer, Murthy, & Sales, 2009), suggesting its potential application for MSC isolation. Gurkan et al. (2011) developed a thermoresponsive microfluidics device for selectively releasing captured cells from blood (Fig. 11.22). Antihuman CD34+ antibodies were immobilized in a PNIPAAm microfluidics channel at 37°C; when blood containing CD34+ stem cells was injected into the channel (e.g., to capture CD34+ EPCs), the CD34+ cells were successfully captured from the whole blood. To release the captured cells, the microfluidics device was then cooled down below 32°C. The released cells displayed greater than 90% viability by a live/dead assay.

11.6.2 Label-free approach

11.6.2.1 Electrophysiological properties

Isolating specific progenies and progenitor cells based on their distinct behavior under the exposure of an AC electric field represents a new approach in the stem cell field. Contrary to conventional techniques, which rely on the presence of specific cell surface markers, DEP separates cells based on cells' intrinsic dielectric characteristics without the need of labeling. Talary, Mills, Hoy, Burnett, and Pethig 1995 first demonstrated the potential usage of DEP in an HSC sorter. By applying a sinusoidal AC electric field (6 V peak—peak at 5 kHz), they found a 5.9-fold enrichment of CD34+ cells (0.84%—4.97%) trapped in the integrated castellated electrode. Similarly, Stephens and colleagues utilized the same platform to isolate CD34+ cells directly from the diluted peripheral blood stem cell harvests. They demonstrated a nearly five-fold increase in the frequency of the CD34+ cells populations in the fractions collected within the 50—10 kHz range. They further confirmed that the isolated CD34+ cells were capable of forming colonies using a colony formation assay. These two studies demonstrate the possibility of exploiting DEP as a noninvasive and label-free sorting approach in the stem cell field.

Recently, Prieto, Lu, Nourse, Flanagan, and Lee 2012 developed a dielectrophoretic assisted cell sorting (DACS) array, which consists of a DEP electrode array with three multiplexed trapping regions that can be independently activated at different frequencies. This device was used to separate a mixture of NSPCs and differentiated neurons (Fig. 11.25). They reported the first statistically significant neural cell sorting using DACS to enrich neurons from a heterogeneous population of mouse derived NSPCs and differentiated neurons. A 1.4-fold neuronal enrichment was achieved. In addition, Vykoukal, Vykoukal, Freyberg, Alt, and Gascoyne (2008) developed a dielectrophoretic field-flow fractionation separator (DEP-FFF) using a novel microfluidics—microelectronic hybrid flex-circuit fabrication approach. They applied DEP-FFF to separation putative stem cells (NG2+) from adipose tissue. In this study, a nucleated cell fraction from cell debris and the bulk of the erythrocyte population was first isolated from adipose tissue. By introducing the cell fraction into the DEP-FFF, they found a 14-fold enrichment in the NG2+ cell population (2%—28% purity). They further identified that NG2+ cell enrichment is coincident with Nestin + cell enrichment, indicating that the isolation of the cells occurred in the early developmental stage. These studies imply that the intrinsic dielectric characteristic of cells could be used as a label-free approach for stem cell isolation for transplantation.

11.6.2.2 Size differences

Size difference between distinct cell types and between subpopulations of HSCs has been well recognized and could be used as a parameter for stem cell sorting. For example, the presence of MSCs in amniotic fluid (AF) is an attractive cell source, as MSCs do not have the same ethical issues that surround ESCs. A variety of cells are present in the AF, including stem cells, amniotic cells, and many dead epithelial cells with diameters of 4—6 µm, 15—20 µm, and 40—60 µm, respectively. Taking this into consideration, Wu, Lin, Hwang, and Lee (2009a) developed a microfluidic device to isolate MSCs from AF using a combination of a T-junction focusing structure and a louver-like structure to isolate amniotic fluid MSCs (AFMSCs) (Fig. 11.26). Another example of size-based stem cell isolation was introduced recently by Schirhagl, Fuereder, Hall, Medeiros, and Zare (2011) Their layered microfluidics device was fabricated to generate a sorter that could simultaneously valve and filter. The top and bottom layers contained channels and pressure valves, while the middle layer was a PDMS porous membrane (pore size: 10, 15, or 20 µm). The porous membrane was fabricated using soft lithography, and it was integrated between the microfluidics layers. Because HSCs are larger in size than other cells present in bone marrow, with the exception of monocytes, HSCs were successfully isolated from human bone marrow samples without any sample pretreatment. At smaller pore sizes (≤ 15 µm), stem cell isolation efficiency was significantly increased.

11.7 Conclusion and future trends

For practical therapeutic purposes, ESCs hold greater therapeutic potential compared to adult stem cells due to their multipotency in vivo, as they are an unlimited source of any kind of adult stem cells. However, the ethical implications surrounding the way in which ESCs are obtained prevent ESC-based therapeutics reaching their full potential as a viable option for clinical applications. To circumvent this issue, Takahashi and Yamanaka (2006) discovered a process in 2006, called dedifferentiation, to reprogram differentiated adult fibroblasts back to an embryonic-like state by introducing four transcriptional factors, Oct3/4, Sox2, c-Myc, and Klf4, under ES cell culture conditions. These derived stem cells were designated as iPSCs—adult stem cells that not only exhibit the morphology and growth properties of ESCs but also express ES cell marker genes. Because of the similarities between ESCs and iPS cells in differentiation potential and the absence of ethical issues that surround human ES research, iPS cells have great clinical potential in regenerative medicine. Microfluidics will certainly play a role in the development of the iPS field in the future. In particular, microfluidics offers unique opportunities to assess the viability, differentiation potential, and heterogeneity of these cells in a high-throughput manner. In addition, the fine control of chemical and physical gradients allowed with microfluidic techniques also offer great utility in regulating the differentiation and understanding the biology of iPS cells.

Ethical issues are not the only concerns surrounding stem cell research. Because stem cell biology is not completely understood, their use in clinical applications remains uncertain. Stem cell migration and homing are mechanisms that are continually investigated, as the exact mechanisms of stem cell recruitment and migration is vastly unknown. Nevertheless, microfluidic devices have enabled new discoveries in identifying some of the key mechanisms involved in stem cell recruitment and migration. In response to injury or inflammation, stem cells may be mobilized into the circulatory system; to migrate to these areas, they must interact with the local endothelium and extravasate into the surrounding tissue. Recently, vascular microenvironments were mimicked in microfluidic devices by cultivating endothelial cells in the microfluidic channels. The microenvironment of a blood vessel, including shear stress, cellular interactions between multiple cocultured cells, and microstructures could be incorporated into the device. Based on microfluidic artificial blood vessels (MABV), various cell migration and cell invasion assays were developed. Kamm et al. developed a cocultivating microfluidics device in which cancer and endothelial cells were cocultured. After coculturing both cells for 4 days, endothelial cells migrated toward MTLn3 cells, a highly invasive breast adenocarcinoma cell line (Chung et al., 2009). Similar coculture microfluidic devices were also constructed to investigate hepatocyte-induced blood vessel formation (angiogenesis) in microfluidics (Chung et al., 2009). Unfortunately, we do not yet have an example of stem cell migration research using MABVs, although these devices hold great potential to yield tremendous opportunities in understanding stem cell migration and homing mechanisms.

Specifically, through microfluidics-based vasculature research, critical roles of endothelial selectins (P and E) and vascular cell adhesion molecule-1 (VCAM-1) have been identified in hematopoietic progenitor cells (HPCs) homing to the BM (Frenette, Subbarao, Mazo, von Andrian, & Wagner, 1998; Mazo et al., 1998). Recently microfluidics-based cell rolling has been achieved with by coating the device with a molecule, P-selectin, which stimulates cell rolling (Choi et al., 2012). The P-selectin coated microfluidic channels have repetitive slant ridges with trenches in between. The target cells roll through the slant ridges via interaction between the P-selectin on slant ridges and the ligand on the cell surface. The cells eventually roll through the trenches and flow into a collecting chamber. In the future, we anticipate that similar devices will be used to both understand the normal interactions of other stem cells with endothelial adhesion ligands as well as engineer therapies that maximize these interactions for therapeutic interventions.

During injury and inflammation, adult stem cells are mobilized to the circulatory system (Roufosse, Direkze, Otto, & Wright, 2004). Specifically, multiple groups have observed an increase in MSC populations in the vasculature following injury. Although the functional role of these circulating MSCs remains poorly understood, similar processes may underlie MSC recruitment to tumors and inflamed tissues (Karnoub et al., 2007). Unfortunately, current techniques make studying the individual steps underlying this phenomenon difficult. In particular, current intravital microscopy techniques are difficult to apply to the processes of intravasation into the bloodstream and extravasation into distant organs. Understanding the fundamental biology of stem cell recruitment and homing has major implications for influencing therapeutic applications of these cells as they become more widely used in diverse clinical settings (Karp & Teol, 2009).

In recent years, the concept of the cancer stem cell (CSC) has become a new paradigm for understanding cancer initiation, progression, and response to therapies (Visvader & Lindeman, 2012). The fundamental hypothesis is that a cellular subpopulation of the tumor possesses both self-renewal abilities and the capacity to give rise to other, differentiated cells in the tumor. Recent observations have suggested that CSCs themselves are responsible for the spread of cancer cells to other organs in the process of metastasis (Baccelli & Trumpp, 2012). As metastasis involves intravasation into the bloodstream, tropism to cancer-specific secondary organs, and eventual extravasation into those organs, microfluidics offers numerous opportunities to reveal the biology underlying CSC-driven metastasis (Valastyan & Weinberg, 2011). The central role of CSCs in sustaining tumor growth and progression suggests that therapies specifically targeting the CSC or its associated niche could more effectively treat cancer. Microfluidics again offers opportunities to accelerate the identification of novel pathways and targets through novel drug screening platforms. In addition, microfluidics has a clear role to play in the isolation of CSCs from the heterogeneous cell population of primary tumors. As current markers for CSCs vary widely between cancers types, the label-free technologies described above, including DEP, will be interesting to apply to the detection and isolation of CSCs.

Additionally, future trends in microfluidic-based stem cell research will be focused on developing technologies to effectively screen drug candidates, investigate stem cell differentiation, and test the efficacy of engineered stem cells in an in vitro model that closely mimics human biology (Zhang et al., 2017). Microfluidics could be used to assess potential drugs for pregnant women as drugs can be harmful to the fetus in the womb, microfluidics can be a useful tool to safely screen side effects of the drug candidates on ESCs. Furthermore, drug companies could use this platform to further enhance their stringency tests during drug development. Alternatively, microfluidics can be used to differentiate, analyze, and sort stem cells for the purposes of cell therapy. Ultimately, through investigating stem cells with microfluidic devices, it may be possible to control stem cell differentiation to develop artificial organs/tissues and to repair damaged internal body systems. In the future, integration of multiple "organs on a chip" to generate microfluidic systems that mimic the full range of physiology of humans may be useful for understanding normal biology, disease processes, and the role of stem cells in these processes. For these reasons, companies such as Aldagen (http://www.aldagen.com) and Innovative Micro Technology (IMT, http://www.imtmems.com/) focus on the development of microfluidic devices dealing with stem cells. In the near future, microfluidic-based systems will become a powerful platform not only for fundamental stem cell research but also for stem cell—based clinical applications.

11.8 Sources of further information and advice

Sun, Y. B., Weng, S. and Fu, J. P. (2012). Microengineered synthetic cellular microenvironment for stem cells. *Wiley Interdisciplinary Reviews-Nanomedicine and Nanobiotechnology*, 4, 414—427.
Lutolf, M. P. and Blau, H. M. (2009). Artificial stem cell niches. *Advances in Materials, 21*, 3255—3268.
Ashton, R. S., Keung, A. J., Peltier, J. and Schaffer, D. V. (2011). Progress and prospects for stem cell engineering. *Annual Review of Chemical Biomolecular Engineering, 2*, 479—502.
Gossett, D. R., Weaver, W. M., Mach, A. J., Hur, S. C., Tse, H. T., Lee, W., et al (2010). Label-free cell separation and sorting in microfluidic systems. *Analytical and Bioanalytical Chemistry, 397*, 3249—3267.
Squires, T. M. and Quake, S. R. (2005). Microfluidics: Fluid physics at the nanoliter scale. *Reviews of Modern Physics, 77*, 977—1026.
Beebe, D. J., Mensing, G. A. and Walker, G. M. (2002). Physics and applications of microfluidics in biology. *Annual Review of Biomedical Engineering, 4*, 261—286.

References

Abhyankar, V. V., Lokuta, M. A., Huttenlocher, A., & Beebe, D. J. (2006). Characterization of a membrane-based gradient generator for use in cell-signaling studies. *Lab on a Chip, 6*, 389—393.
Altman, J., & Das, G. D. (1965). Autoradiographic and histological evidence of postnatal hippocampal neurogenesis in rats. *The Journal of Comparative Neurology, 124*, 319—335.
Alvarez-Buylla, A., Seri, B., & Doetsch, F. (2002). Identification of neural stem cells in the adult vertebrate brain. *Brain Research Bulletin, 57*, 751—758.
Anderson, D. G., Levenberg, S., & Langer, R. (2004). Nanoliter-scale synthesis of arrayed biomaterials and application to human embryonic stem cells. *Nature Biotechnology, 22*, 863—866.

Aran, K., Fok, A., Sasso, L. A., Kamdar, N., Guan, Y. L., Sun, Q., et al. (2011). Microfiltration platform for continuous blood plasma protein extraction from whole blood during cardiac surgery. *Lab on a Chip, 11*, 2858−2868.

Baccelli, I., & Trumpp, A. (2012). The evolving concept of cancer and metastasis stem cells. *The Journal of Cell Biology, 198*, 281−293.

Bagnaninchi, P. O., & Drummond, N. (2011). Real-time label-free monitoring of adipose-derived stem cell differentiation with electric cell-substrate impedance sensing. *Proceedings of the National Academy of Sciences of the United States of America, 108*, 6462−6467.

Baret, J.-C., Miller, O. J., Taly, V., Ryckelynck, M., El-Harrak, A., Frenz, L., et al. (2009). Fluorescence-activated droplet sorting (FADS): Efficient microfluidic cell sorting based on enzymatic activity. *Lab on a Chip, 9*, 1850−1858.

Becker, F. F., Wang, X. B., Huang, Y., Pethig, R., Vykoukal, J., & Gascoyne, P. R. C. (1995). Separation of human breast-cancer cells from blood by differential dielectric affinity. *Proceedings of the National Academy of Sciences of the U S A, 92*, 860−864.

Bellan, L. M., Singh, S. P., Henderson, P. W., Porri, T. J., Craighead, H. G., & Spector, J. A. (2009). Fabrication of an artificial 3-dimensional vascular network using sacrificial sugar structures. *Soft Matter, 5*, 1354.

Blagovic, K., Kim, L. Y., & Voldman, J. (2011). Microfluidic perfusion for regulating diffusible signaling in stem cells. *PloS One, 6*, e22892.

Boheler, K. R. (2010). Pluripotency of human embryonic and induced pluripotent stem cells for cardiac and vascular regeneration. *Thrombosis and Haemostasis, 104*, 23−29.

Bu, M. Q., Melvin, T., Ensell, G., Wilkinson, J. S., & Evans, A. G. R. (2003). Design and theoretical evaluation of a novel microfluidic device to be used for PCR. *Journal of Micromechanics and Microengineering, 13*, S125−S130.

Burt, R. K., Testori, A., Craig, R., Cohen, B., Suffit, R., & Barr, W. (2008). Hematopoietic stem cell transplantation for autoimmune diseases: What have we learned? *Journal of Autoimmunity, 30*, 116−120.

Cai, L., Friedman, N., & Xie, X. S. (2006). Stochastic protein expression in individual cells at the single molecule level. *Nature Cell Biology, 440*, 358−362.

Chen, C. Y., Wo, A. M., & Jong, D. S. (2012). A microfluidic concentration generator for dose-response assays on ion channel pharmacology. *Lab on a Chip, 12*, 794−801.

Chin, V. I., Taupin, P., Sanga, S., Scheel, J., Gage, F. H., & Bhatia, S. N. (2004). Microfabricated platform for studying stem cell fates. *Biotechnology and Bioengineering, 88*, 399−415.

Choi, S., Karp, J. M., & Karnik, R. (2012). Cell sorting by deterministic cell rolling. *Lab on a Chip, 12*, 1427−1430.

Chung, B. G., flanagan, L. A., Rhee, S. W., Schwartz, P. H., Lee, A. P., Monuki, E. S., et al. (2005). Human neural stem cell growth and differentiation in a gradient-generating microfluidic device. *Lab on a Chip, 5*, 401−406.

Chung, B. G., Park, J. W., Hu, J. S., Huang, C., Monuki, E. S., & Jeon, N. L. (2007). A hybrid microfluidic-vacuum device for direct interfacing with conventional cell culture methods. *BMC Biotechnology, 7*, 60.

Chung, S., Sudo, R., Mack, P. J., Wan, C. R., Vickerman, V., & Kamm, R. D. (2009). Cell migration into scaffolds under co-culture conditions in a microfluidic platform. *Lab on a Chip, 9*, 269−275.

Clewes, O., Narytnyk, A., Gillinder, K. R., Loughney, A. D., Murdoch, A. P., & Sieber-Blum, M. (2011). Human epidermal neural crest stem cells (hEPI-NCSC) – characterization and directed differentiation into osteocytes and melanocytes. *Stem Cell Reviews, 7*, 799–814.

Crews, N., Wittwer, C., & Gale, B. (2008). Continuous-flow thermal gradient PCR. *Biomedical Microdevices, 10*, 187–195.

Csete, M. (2010). Q&A: What can microfluidics do for stem-cell research? *Journal of Biology, 9*, 1.

Dahan, E., Bize, V., Lehnert, T., Horisberger, J. D., & Gijs, M. A. M. (2008). Rapid fluidic exchange microsystem for recording of fast ion channel kinetics in Xenopus oocytes. *Lab on a Chip, 8*, 1809–1818.

Davenport, R. J. (2005). What controls organ regeneration. *Science* (Vol. 309, p. 84).

Demello, A. J. (2006). Control and detection of chemical reactions in microfluidic systems. *Nature, 442*, 394–402.

Dhof, T. C. S. U., Wernig, M., Citri, A., Pang, Z. P., & Malenka, R. C. (2011). Comprehensive qPCR profiling of gene expression in single neuronal cells. *Nature Protocols, 7*, 1–10.

Dupin, E., & Coelho-Aguiar, J. M. (2012). Isolation and differentiation properties of neural crest stem cells. *Cytometry, 83*, 38–47.

El-Ali, J., Sorger, P. K., & Jensen, K. F. (2006). Cells on chips. *Nature, 442*, 403–411.

Ellison, D., Munden, A., & Levchenko, A. (2009). Computational model and microfluidic platform for the investigation of paracrine and autocrine signaling in mouse embryonic stem cells. *Molecular BioSystems, 5*, 1004.

Engler, A. J., Sen, S., Sweeney, H. L., & Discher, D. E. (2006). Matrix elasticity directs stem cell lineage specification. *Cell, 126*, 677–689.

Fatoyinbo, H. O., Hoettges, K. F., & Hughes, M. P. (2008). Rapid-on-chip determination of dielectric properties of biological cells using imaging techniques in a dielectrophoresis dot microsystem. *Electrophoresis, 29*, 3–10.

Fiedler, S., Shirley, S. G., Schnelle, T., & Fuhr, G. (1998). Dielectrophoretic sorting of particles and cells in a microsystem. *Analytical Chemistry, 70*, 1909–15.

Flaim, C. J., Chien, S., & Bhatia, S. N. (2005). An extracellular matrix microarray for probing cellular differentiation. *Nature Methods, 2*, 119–125.

Flaim, C. J., Teng, D., Chien, S., & Bhatia, S. N. (2008). Combinatorial signaling microenvironments for studying stem cell fate. *Stem Cells and Development, 17*, 29–40.

Flanagan, L. A., Lu, J., Wang, L., Marchenko, S. A., Jeon, N. L., Lee, A. P., et al. (2008). Unique dielectric properties distinguish stem cells and their differentiated progeny. *Stem Cells, 26*, 656–665.

Frenette, P. S., Subbarao, S., Mazo, I. B., von Andrian, U. H., & Wagner, D. D. (1998). Endothelial selectins and vascular cell adhesion molecule-1 promote hematopoietic progenitor homing to bone marrow. *Proceedings of the National Academy of Sciences of the U S A, 95*, 14423–14428.

Fu, A. Y., Spence, C., Scherer, A., Arnold, F. H., & Quake, S. R. (1999). A microfabricated fluorescence-activated cell sorter. *Nature Biotechnology, 17*, 1109–1111.

Fuhr, G., Müller, T., Schnelle, T., Hagedorn, R., Voigt, A., Fiedler, S., et al. (1994). Radiofrequency microtools for particle and liver cell manipulation. *Naturwissenschaften, 81*, 528–535.

Fukuda, J., Khademhosseini, A., Yeo, Y., Yang, X. Y., Yeh, J., Eng, G., et al. (2006). Micromolding of photo-crosslinkable chitosan hydrogel for spheroid microarray and co-cultures. *Biomaterials, 27*, 5259–5267.

Fung, W.-T., Beyzavi, A., Abgrall, P., Nguyen, N.-T., & Li, H.-Y. (2009). Microfluidic platform for controlling the differentiation of embryoid bodies. *Lab on a Chip, 9*, 2591.

Gagnon, Z. R. (2011). Cellular dielectrophoresis: Applications to the characterization, manipulation, separation and patterning of cells. *Electrophoresis, 32*, 2466–2487.

Gehling, U. M., Ergun, S., Schumacher, U., Wagener, C., Pantel, K., OTTE, M., et al. (2000). In vitro differentiation of endothelial cells from AC133-positive progenitor cells. *Blood, 95*, 3106–3112.

Glotzbach, J. P., Januszyk, M., Vial, I. N., Wong, V. W., Gelbard, A., Kalisky, T., et al. (2011). An information theoretic, microfluidic-based single cell analysis permits identification of subpopulations among putatively homogeneous stem cells. *PloS One, 6*, e21211.

Guilak, F., Cohen, D. M., Estes, B. T., Gimble, J. M., Liedtke, W., & Chen, C. S. (2009). Control of stem cell fate by physical interactions with the extracellular matrix. *Stem Cells, 5*, 17–26.

Guo, M. T., Rotem, A., Heyman, J. A., & Weitz, D. A. (2012). Droplet microfluidics for high-throughput biological assays. *Lab on a Chip, 12*, 2146.

Gupta, K., Kim, D.-H., Ellison, D., Smith, C., Kundu, A., Tuan, J., et al. (2010). Lab-on-a-chip devices as an emerging platform for stem cell biology. *Lab on a Chip, 10*, 2019.

Gurkan, U. A., Anand, T., Tas, H., Elkan, D., Akay, A., Keles, H. O., et al. (2011). Controlled viable release of selectively captured label-free cells in microchannels. *Lab on a Chip, 11*, 3979–3989.

Hoettges, K. F., Hübner, Y., Broche, L. M., Ogin, S. L., Kass, G. E. N., & Hughes, M. P. (2008). Dielectrophoresis-activated multiwell plate for label-free high-throughput drug assessment. *Analytical Chemistry, 80*, 2063–2068.

Holmes, D., Pettigrew, D., Reccius, C. H., Gwyer, J. D., van Berkel, C., Holloway, J., et al. (2009). Leukocyte analysis and differentiation using high speed microfluidic single cell impedance cytometry. *Lab on a Chip, 9*, 2881–2889.

Hosokawa, M., Hayata, T., Fukuda, Y., Arakaki, A., Yoshino, T., Tanaka, T., et al. (2010). Size-selective microcavity array for rapid and efficient detection of circulating tumor cells. *Analytical Chemistry, 82*, 6629–6635.

Hu, X. Y., Bessette, P. H., Qian, J. R., Meinhart, C. D., Daugherty, P. S., & Soh, H. T. (2005). Marker-specific sorting of rare cells using dielectrophoresis. *Proceedings of the National Academy of Sciences of the U S A, 102*, 15757–15761.

Huang, C. P., Lu, J., Seon, H., Lee, A. P., Flanagan, L. A., Kim, H.-Y., et al. (2009). Engineering microscale cellular niches for three-dimensional multicellular co-cultures. *Lab on a Chip, 9*, 1740–1748.

Huang, L. R., Cox, E. C., Austin, R. H., & Sturm, J. C. (2004). Continuous particle separation through deterministic lateral displacement. *Science, 304*, 987–990.

Huh, D., Matthews, B. D., Mammoto, A., Montoya-Zavala, M., Hsin, H. Y., & Ingber, D. E. (2010). Reconstituting organ-level lung functions on a chip. *Science, 328*, 1662–1668.

Hui, E. E., & Bhatia, S. N. (2007). Micromechanical control of cell-cell interactions. *Proceedings of the National Academy of Sciences of the U S A, 104*, 5722–5726.

Hur, S. C., Henderson-MacLennan, N. K., McCabe, E. R. B., & di Carlo, D. (2011). Deformability-based cell classification and enrichment using inertial microfluidics. *Lab on a Chip, 11*, 912–920.

Irimia, D., Geba, D. A., & Toner, M. (2006). Universal microfluidic gradient generator. *Analytical Chemistry, 78*, 3472–3477.

Jeon, N. L., Dertinger, S. K. W., Chiu, D. T., Choi, I. S., Stroock, A. D., & Whitesides, G. M. (2000). Generation of solution and surface gradients using microfluidic systems. *Langmuir, 16*, 8311–8316.

Jiang, Y., Jahagirdar, B. N., Reinhardt, R. L., Schwartz, R. E., Keene, C. D., Ortiz-Gonzalez, X. R., et al. (2002). Pluripotency of mesenchymal stem cells derived from adult marrow. *Nature, 418*, 41–49.

Karnoub, A. E., Dash, A. B., Vo, A. P., Sullivan, A., Brooks, M. W., Bell, G. W., et al. (2007). Mesenchymal stem cells within tumour stroma promote breast cancer metastasis. *Nature, 449*. 557-U4.

Karp, J. M., & Teol, G. S. L. (2009). Mesenchymal stem cell homing: The devil is in the details. *Cell Stem Cell, 4*, 206–216.

Karp, J. M., Yeh, J., Eng, G., Fukuda, J., Blumling, J., Suh, K. Y., et al. (2007). Controlling size, shape and homogeneity of embryoid bodies using poly(ethylene glycol) microwells. *Lab on a Chip, 7*, 786–794.

Keenan, T. M., Hsu, C. H., & Folch, A. (2006). Microfluidic 'jets' for generating steady-state gradients of soluble molecules on open surfaces. *Applied Physics Letters, 89*, 114103.

Khademhosseini, A., Ferreira, L., Blumling, J., 3rd, Yeh, J., Karp, J. M., Fukuda, J., et al. (2006). Co-culture of human embryonic stem cells with murine embryonic fibroblasts on microwell-patterned substrates. *Biomaterials, 27*, 5968–5977.

Khademhosseini, A., Yeh, J., Jon, S., Eng, G., Suh, K. Y., Burdick, J. A., et al. (2004). Molded polyethylene glycol microstructures for capturing cells within microfluidic channels. *Lab on a Chip, 4*, 425–430.

Kiermer, V. (2005). FACS-on-a-chip. *Nature Methods, 2*, 91.

Kim, S., Kim, H. J., & Jeon, N. L. (2010). Biological applications of microfluidic gradient devices. *Integrative Biology, 2*, 584–603.

Kim, U., Shu, C. W., Dane, K. Y., Daugherty, P. S., Wang, J. Y. J., & Soh, H. T. (2007). Selection of mammalian cells based on their cell-cycle phase using dielectrophoresis. *Proceedings of the National Academy of Sciences of the U S A, 104*, 20708–12.

Kobel, S. A., Burri, O., Griffa, A., Girotra, M., Seitz, A., & Lutolf, M. P. (2012). Automated analysis of single stem cells in microfluidic traps. *Lab on a Chip, 12*, 2843–2849.

Kopp, M. U., de Mello, A. J., & Manz, A. (1998). Chemical amplification. Continuous-flow PCR on a Chip. *Science, 280*, 1046–1048.

Kumachev, A., Greener, J., Tumarkin, E., Eiser, E., Zandstra, P. W., & Kumacheva, E. (2011). High-throughput generation of hydrogel microbeads with varying elasticity for cell encapsulation. *Biomaterials, 32*, 1477–1483.

Labeed, F., LU, J., Mulhall, H., Marchenko, S., Hoettges, K., Estrada, L., et al. (2011). Biophysical characteristics reveal neural stem cell differentiation potential. *PloS One, 6*, e25458.

Lanfer, B., Seib, F. P., Freudenberg, U., Stamov, D., Bley, T., Bornhäuser, M., et al. (2009). The growth and differentiation of mesenchymal stem and progenitor cells cultured on aligned collagen matrices. *Biomaterials, 30*, 5950–5958.

Lanza, R. P., Hayes, J. L., & Chick, W. L. (1996). Encapsulated cell technology. *Nature Biotechnology, 14*, 1107–1111.

Lecault, V., Vaninsberghe, M., Sekulovic, S., Knapp, D. J., Wohrer, S., Bowden, W., et al. (2011). High-throughput analysis of single hematopoietic stem cell proliferation in microfluidic cell culture arrays. *Nature Methods, 8*, 581–586.

Lee, C. H., Bose, S., van Vliet, K. J., Karp, J. M., & Karnik, R. (2011). Examining the lateral displacement of hl60 cells rolling on asymmetric p-selectin patterns. *Langmuir, 27*, 240–249.

Li, X., Valadez, A. V., Zuo, P., & Nie, Z. (2012). Microfluidic 3D cell culture: Potential application for tissue-based bioassays. *Bioanalysis, 4*(12), 1509–1525.

Lin, F., Nguyen, C. M. C., Wang, S. J., Saadi, W., Gross, S. P., & Jeon, N. L. (2005). Neutrophil migration in opposing chemoattractant gradients using microfluidic chemotaxis devices. *Annals of Biomedical Engineering, 33*, 475−482.

Liu, S., Dontu, G., & wicha, M. S. (2005). Mammary stem cells, self-renewal pathways, and carcinogenesis. *Breast Cancer Research: BCR, 7*, 86−95.

Lu, J., Barrios, C. A., Dickson, A. R., Nourse, J. L., Lee, A. P., & Flanagan, L. A. (2012). Advancing practical usage of microtechnology: A study of the functional consequences of dielectrophoresis on neural stem cells. *Integrative Biology, 4*, 1223−1226.

Mach, A. J., & di Carlo, D. (2010). Continuous scalable blood filtration device using inertial microfluidics. *Biotechnology and Bioengineering, 107*, 302−311.

Mach, A. J., Kim, J. H., Arshi, A., Hur, S. C., & di Carlo, D. (2011). Automated cellular sample preparation using a centrifuge-on-a-chip. *Lab on a Chip, 11*, 2827−2834.

Markey, A. L., Mohr, S., & Day, P. J. R. (2010). High-throughput droplet PCR. *Methods, 50*, 277−281.

Markx, G., & Davey, C. (1999). The dielectric properties of biological cells at radiofrequencies: Applications in biotechnology. *Enzyme and Microbial Technology, 25*, 161−171.

Martino, G., & Pluchino, S. (2006). The therapeutic potential of neural stem cells. *Nature Reviews Neuroscience, 7*, 395−406.

Mason, C., & Dunnill, P. (2008). A brief definition of regenerative medicine. *Regenerative Medicine, 3*, 1−5.

Mazo, I. B., Gutierrez-Ramos, J. C., Frenette, P. S., Hynes, R. O., Wagner, D. D., & von Andrian, U. H. (1998). Hematopoietic progenitor cell rolling in bone marrow microvessels: Parallel contributions by endothelial selectins and vascular cell adhesion molecule 1. *Journal of Experimental Medicine, 188*, 465−474.

Meyvantsson, I., & Beebe, D. J. (2008). Cell culture models in microfluidic systems. *Annual Review of Analytical Chemistry, 1*, 423−449.

Migliaccio, A. R., Whitsett, C., Papayannopoulou, T., & Sadelain, M. (2012). The potential of stem cells as an in vitro source of red blood cells for transfusion. *Cell Stem Cell, 10*, 115−119.

Mohamed, H., Murray, M., Turner, J. N., & Caggana, M. (2009). Isolation of tumor cells using size and deformation. *Journal of Chromatography, 1216*, 8289−8295.

Moon, H. S., Kwon, K., Kim, S. I., Han, H., Sohn, J., Lee, S., et al. (2011). Continuous separation of breast cancer cells from blood samples using multiorifice flow fractionation (MOFF) and dielectrophoresis (DEP). *Lab on a Chip, 11*, 1118−1125.

Moore, K. A., & Lemischka, I. R. (2006). Stem cells and their niches. *Science, 311*, 1880−1885.

Muller-Sieburg, C. E., Cho, R. H., Thoman, M., Adkins, B., & Sieburg, H. B. (2002). *Deterministic regulation of hematopoietic stem cell self-renewal and differentiation. Blood, 100*, 1302−1309.

Nagrath, S., Sequist, L. V., Maheswaran, S., Bell, D. W., Irimia, D., Ulkus, L., et al. (2007). Isolation of rare circulating tumour cells in cancer patients by microchip technology. *Nature, 450*, 1235−1239.

Nakatomi, H., Kuriu, T., Okabe, S., Yamamoto, S., Hatano, O., Kawahara, N., et al. (2002). Regeneration of hippocampal pyramidal neurons after ischemic brain injury by recruitment of endogenous neural progenitors. *Cell, 110*, 429−441.

Ng, E. S., D, R., Azzola, L., Stanley, E. G., & Elefanty, A. G. (2005). Forced aggregation of defined numbers of human embryonic stem cells into embryoid bodies fosters robust, reproducible hematopoietic differentiation. *Blood, 106*, 1601−1603.

Niu, X. Z., Gielen, F., Edel, J. B., & Demello, A. J. (2011). A microdroplet dilutor for high-throughput screening. *Nature Chemistry, 3*, 437−442.

Noebels, J. L., Avoli, M., Rogawski, M. A., Olsen, R. W., Delgado-Escueta, A. V., Naegele, J. R., et al. (2012). *Embryonic stem cell therapy for intractable epilepsy.* Bethesda (MD): National Center for Biotechnology Information (US).

Northrup, M. A., Ching, R. M., & Watson, A. R. T. (1993). DNA amplification with a microfabricated reaction chamber. In *Proceedings of the 7th international conference on solid state sensors and actuators, 1993 Yokohama, Japan* (pp. 924–926).

Notta, F., Doulatov, S., Laurenti, E., Poeppl, A., Jurisica, I., & Dick, J. E. (2011). Isolation of single human hematopoietic stem cells capable of long-term multilineage engraftment. *Science, 333*, 218–221.

Park, H. E., Kim, D., Koh, H. S., Cho, S., Sung, J.-S., & Kim, J. Y. (2011). Real-time monitoring of neural differentiation of human mesenchymal stem cells by electric cell-substrate impedance sensing. *Journal of Biomedicine and Biotechnology, 2011*, 1–8.

Park, J. Y., Hwang, C. M., Lee, S. H., & Lee, S. H. (2007). Gradient generation by an osmotic pump and the behavior of human mesenchymal stem cells under the fetal bovine serum concentration gradient. *Lab on a Chip, 7*, 1673–1680.

Park, J. Y., Kim, S.-K., Woo, D.-H., Lee, E.-J., Kim, J.-H., & Lee, S.-H. (2009). Differentiation of neural progenitor cells in a microfluidic chip-generated cytokine gradient. *Stem Cells, 27*, 2646–2654.

Patela, P., & Markxb, G. H. (2008). Dielectric measurement of cell death. *Enzyme and Microbial Technology, 43*, 463–470.

Pethig, R. (1996). Dielectrophoresis: Using inhomogeneous AC electrical fields to separate and manipulate cells. *Critical Reviews in Biotechnology, 16*, 331–348.

Pethig, R. (2010). Dielectrophoresis: Status of the theory, technology, and applications. *Biomicrofluidics, 4*, 022811.

Pethig, R., Lee, R., & Talary, M. (2004). Cell physiometry tools based on dielectrophoresis. *JALA, 9*, 324–330.

Phinney, D. G., & Prockop, D. J. (2007). Concise review: Mesenchymal stem/multipotent stromal cells: The state of transdifferentiation and modes of tissue repair — current views. *Stem Cells, 25*, 2896–2902.

Plouffe, B. D., Kniazeva, T., Mayer, J. E., Murthy, S. K., & Sales, V. L. (2009). Development of microfluidics as endothelial progenitor cell capture technology for cardiovascular tissue engineering and diagnostic medicine. *The FASEB Journal, 23*, 3309–3314.

Prieto, J. L., Lu, J., Nourse, J. L., Flanagan, L. A., & Lee, A. P. (2012). Frequency discretization in dielectrophoretic assisted cell sorting arrays to isolate neural cells. *Lab on a Chip, 12*, 2182–2189.

Qi, H., Huang, G., Han, Y. L., et al. (2016). In vitro spatially organizing the differentiation in individual multicellular stem cell aggregates. *Critical Reviews in Biotechnology, 36*(1), 20–31.

Reilly, G. C., & Engler, A. J. (2010). Intrinsic extracellular matrix properties regulate stem cell differentiation. *Journal of Biomechanics, 43*, 55–62.

Reitinger, S., Wissenwasser, J., Kapferer, W., Heer, R., & Lepperdinger, G. (2012). Electric impedance sensing in cell-substrates for rapid and selective multipotential differentiation capacity monitoring of human mesenchymal stem cells. *Biosensors and Bioelectronics, 34*, 63–69.

Roach, P., Parker, T., Gadegaard, N., & Alexander, M. R. (2010). Surface strategies for control of neuronal cell adhesion: A review. *Surface Science Reports, 65*, 145–173.

Roisen, F. J., Klueber, K. M., Lu, C. L., Hatcher, L. M., Dozier, A., Shields, C. B., et al. (2001). Adult human olfactory stem cells. *Brain Research, 890*, 11–22.

Roufosse, C. A., Direkze, N. C., Otto, W. R., & Wright, N. A. (2004). Circulating mesenchymal stem cells. *The International Journal of Biochemistry and Cell Biology, 36*, 585−597.
Scadden, D. T. (2006). The stem-cell niche as an entity of action. *Nature, 441*, 1075−1079.
Schaerli, Y., Wootton, R. C., Robinson, T., Stein, V., Dunsby, C., Neil, M. A. A., et al. (2009). Continuous-flow polymerase chain reaction of single-copy DNA in microfluidic microdroplets. *Analytical Chemistry, 81*, 302−306.
Schirhagl, R., Fuereder, I., Hall, E. W., Medeiros, B. C., & Zare, R. N. (2011). Microfluidic purification and analysis of hematopoietic stem cells from bone marrow. *Lab on a Chip, 11*, 3130−3135.
Schneegass, I., Brautigam, R., & Kohler, J. M. (2001). Miniaturized flow-through PCR with different template types in a silicon chip thermocycler. *Lab on a Chip, 1*, 42−49.
Schofield, R. (1978). The relationship between the spleen colony-forming cell and the haemopoietic stem cell. *Blood Cells, 4*, 7−25.
Serra, M., Brito, C., Correia, C., & Alves, P. M. (2012). Process engineering of human pluripotent stem cells for clinical application. *Trends in Biotechnology, 30*, 350−359.
Shamloo, A., Ma, N., Poo, M. M., Sohn, L. L., & Heilshorn, S. C. (2008). Endothelial cell polarization and chemotaxis in a microfluidic device. *Lab on a Chip, 8*, 1292−1299.
Sharma, S., Raju, R., Sui, S., & Hu, W.-S. (2011). Stem cell culture engineering − process scale up and beyond. *Biotechnology Journal, 6*, 1317−1329.
Shiba, Y., Fernandes, S., Zhu, W.-Z., Filice, D., Muskheli, V., Kim, J., et al. (2012). Human ES-cell-derived cardiomyocytes electrically couple and suppress arrhythmias in injured hearts. *Nature, 489*, 322−325.
Solanki, A., Shah, S., Memoli, K. A., Park, S. Y., Hong, S., & Lee, K.-B. (2010). Controlling differentiation of neural stem cells using extracellular matrix protein patterns. *Small, 6*, 2509−2513.
Solvas, X. C. I., & Demello, A. (2011). Droplet microfluidics: Recent developments and future applications. *Chemical Communications, 47*, 1936−1942.
Song, H., Chen, D. L., & Ismagilov, R. F. (2006). Reactions in droplets in microflulidic channels. *Angewandte Chemie International Edition, 45*, 7336−7356.
Song, H., Tice, J. D., & Ismagilov, R. F. (2003). A microfluidic system for controlling reaction networks in time. *Angewandte Chemie International Edition, 42*, 768−772.
Song, J. W., Cavnar, S. P., Walker, A. C., Luker, K. E., Gupta, M., Tung, Y.-C., et al. (2009). Microfluidic endothelium for studying the intravascular adhesion of metastatic breast cancer cells. *PloS One, 4*, e5756.
Stolberg, S., & McCloskey, K. E. (2009). Can shear stress direct stem cell fate? *Biotechnology Progress, 25*, 10−19.
Sun, K., Yamaguchi, A., Ishida, Y., Matsuo, S., & Misawa, H. (2002). A heater-integrated transparent microchannel chip for continuous-flow PCR. *Sensors and Actuators, A: Chemical, 84*, 283−289.
Sun, T., & Morgan, H. (2010). Single-cell microfluidic impedance cytometry: A review. *Microfluidics and Nanofluidics, 8*, 423−443.
Sykes, M., & Nikolic, B. (2005). Treatment of severe autoimmune disease by stem-cell transplantation. *Nature, 435*, 620−627.
Takahashi, K., & Yamanaka, S. (2006). Induction of pluripotent stem cells from mouse embryonic and adult fibroblast cultures by defined factors. *Cell, 126*, 663−676.
Talary, M. S., Mills, K. I., Hoy, T., Burnett, A. K., & Pethig, R. (1995). Dielectrophoretic separation and enrichment of Cd34+ cell subpopulation from bone-marrow and peripheral-blood stem-cells. *Medical, and Biological Engineering & Computing, 33*, 235−237.

Taly, V., Kelly, B. T., & Griffiths, A. D. (2007). Droplets as microreactors for high-throughput biology. *ChemBioChem, 8*, 263–272.

Tan, S. J., Yobas, L., Lee, G. Y. H., Ong, C. N., & Lim, C. T. (2009). Microdevice for the isolation and enumeration of cancer cells from blood. *Biomedical Microdevices, 11*, 883–892.

Tan, W. H., Suzuki, Y., Kasagi, N., Shikazono, N., Furukawa, K., & Ushida, T. (2005). A lamination micro mixer for mu-immunomagnetic cell sorter. *JSME International Journal Series C, 48*, 425–435.

Tewhey, R., Warner, J. B., Nakano, M., Libby, B., Medkova, M., David, P. H., et al. (2009). Microdroplet-based PCR enrichment for large-scale targeted sequencing. *Nature Biotechnology, 27*. 1025-U94.

Thomson, J. A., Itskovitz-ELDOR, J., Shapiro, S. S., Waknitz, M. A., Swiergiel, J. J., Marshall, V. S., et al. (1998). Embryonic stem cell lines derived from human blastocysts. *Science, 282*, 1145–1147.

Toh, Y.-C., Blagović, K., & Voldman, J. (2010). Advancing stem cell research with microtechnologies: Opportunities and challenges. *Integrative Biology, 2*, 305–325.

Toh, Y.-C., Blagovic, K., Yu, H., & Voldman, J. (2011). Spatially organized in vitro models instruct asymmetric stem cell differentiation. *Integrative Biology, 3*, 1179–1187.

Toh, Y.-C., & Voldman, J. (2011). Fluid shear stress primes mouse embryonic stem cells for differentiation in a self-renewing environment via heparan sulfate proteoglycans transduction. *The FASEB Journal, 25*, 1208–1217.

Toh, Y. C., Lim, T. C., Tai, D., Xiao, G. F., van Noort, D., & Yu, H. R. (2009). A microfluidic 3D hepatocyte chip for drug toxicity testing. *Lab on a Chip, 9*, 2026–2035.

Tumarkin, E., Tzadu, L., Csaszar, E., Seo, M., Zhang, H., Lee, A., et al. (2011). High-throughput combinatorial cell co-culture using microfluidics. *Integrative Biology, 3*, 653–662.

Underhill, G. H., & Bhatia, S. N. (2007). High-throughput analysis of signals regulating stem cell fate and function. *Current Opinion in Chemical Biology, 11*, 357–366.

Valastyan, S., & Weinberg, R. A. (2011). Tumor metastasis. *Molecular Insights and Evolving Paradigms Cell, 147*, 275–292.

van der Flier, L. G., & Clevers, H. (2009). Stem cells, self-renewal, and differentiation in the intestinal epithelium. *Annual Review of Physiology, 71*, 241–260.

van Midwoud, P. M., Verpoorte, E., & Groothuis, G. M. M. (2011). Microfluidic devices for in vitro studies on liver drug metabolism and toxicity. *Integrative Biology, 3*, 509–521.

Vanapalli, S. A., Duits, M. H. G., & Mugele, F. (2009). Microfluidics as a functional tool for cell mechanics. *Biomicrofluidics, 3*, 12006.

Vazin, T., & Schaffer, D. V. (2010). Engineering strategies to emulate the stem cell niche. *Trends in Biotechnology, 28*, 117–124.

Visvader, J. E., & Lindeman, G. J. (2012). Cancer stem cells: Current status and evolving complexities. *Cell Stem Cell, 10*, 717–728.

Vykoukal, D. M., Gascoyne, P. R. C., & Vykoukal, J. (2009). Dielectric characterization of complete mononuclear and polymorphonuclear blood cell subpopulations for label-free discrimination. *Integrative Biology, 1*, 477–484.

Vykoukal, J., Vykoukal, D. M., Freyberg, S., Alt, E. U., & Gascoyne, P. R. C. (2008). Enrichment of putative stem cells from adipose tissue using dielectrophoretic field-flow fractionation. *Lab on a Chip, 8*, 1386–1393.

Wan, J. (2012). Microfluidic-based synthesis of hydrogel particles for cell microencapsulation and cell-based drug delivery. *Polymers, 4*, 1084–1108.

Wang, M. M., TU, E., Raymond, D. E., Yang, J. M., Zhang, H., Hagen, N., et al. (2004). Microfluidic sorting of mammalian cells by optical force switching. *Nature Biotechnology, 23*, 83−87.

Wei, H. B., Chueh, B. H., Wu, H. L., Hall, E. W., Li, C. W., Schirhagl, R., et al. (2011). Particle sorting using a porous membrane in a microfluidic device. *Lab on a Chip, 11*, 238−245.

White, A. K., Vaninsberghe, M., Petriv, I., Hamidi, M., Sikorski, D., Marra, M. A., et al. (2011). High-throughput microfluidic single-cell RT-qPCR. *Proceedings of the National Academy of Sciences of the U S A, 108*, 13999−4004.

Wu, H.-W., Lin, C.-C., & Lee, G.-B. (2011). Stem cells in microfluidics. *Biomicrofluidics, 5*, 013401.

Wu, H. W., Lin, X. Z., Hwang, S. M., & Lee, G. B. (2009a). A microfluidic device for separation of amniotic fluid mesenchymal stem cells utilizing louver-array structures. *Biomedical Microdevices, 11*, 1297−1307.

Wu, Z. G., Willing, B., Bjerketorp, J., Jansson, J. K., & Hjort, K. (2009b). Soft inertial microfluidics for high throughput separation of bacteria from human blood cells. *Lab on a Chip, 9*, 1193−1199.

Xia, N., Hunt, T. P., Mayers, B. T., Alsberg, E., Whitesides, G. M., Westervelt, R. M., et al. (2006). Combined microfluidic-micromagnetic separation of living cells in continuous flow. *Biomedical Microdevices, 8*, 299−308.

Yamada, M., & Seki, M. (2005). Hydrodynamic filtration for on-chip particle concentration and classification utilizing microfluidics. *Lab on a Chip, 5*, 1233−1239.

Yim, E. K. F., Pang, S. W., & Leong, K. W. (2007). Synthetic nanostructures inducing differentiation of human mesenchymal stem cells into neuronal lineage. *Experimental Cell Research, 313*, 1820−1829.

Yung, C. W., Fiering, J., Mueller, A. J., & Ingber, D. E. (2009). Micromagnetic-microfluidic blood cleansing device. *Lab on a Chip, 9*, 1171−1177.

Zare, R. N., & Kim, S. (2010). Microfluidic platforms for single-cell analysis. *Annual Review of Biomedical Engineering, 12*, 187−201.

Zhang, J., Wei, X., Zeng, R., Xu, F., & Li, X. (2017). Stem cell culture and differentiation in microfluidic devices toward organ-on-a-chip. *Future Science OA, 3*(2), FSO187.

Zheng, S., Lin, H., Liu, J. Q., Balic, M., Datar, R., Cote, R. J., et al. (2007). Membrane microfilter device for selective capture, electrolysis and genomic analysis of human circulating tumor cells. *Journal of Chromatography, 1162*, 154−161.

Zhong, J. F., Chen, Y., Marcus, J. S., Scherer, A., Quake, S. R., Taylor, C. R., et al. (2007). A microfluidic processor for gene expression profiling of single human embryonic stem cells. *Lab on a Chip, 8*, 68−74.

Development of the immunoassay of antibodies and cytokines on nanobioarray chips

12

Samar Haroun, Jonathan Lee, Paul C.H. Li
Department of Chemistry, Simon Fraser University, Burnaby, BC, Canada

Questions:

1. Compare bioaffinity and covalent attachments for probe immobilizations in immunoassays.
2. Describe three detection methods employed for sensitive protein immunoassays.
3. Give an example each of the two types of proteins (e.g., antibody and cytokine) that are detected using immunoassays.

12.1 Introduction to immunoassays

Immunoassays have been utilized as a method of protein detection for biological samples. This method uses the immune reaction which takes place in between an antibody and an antigen. Antibodies are proteins secreted in the human body in order to identify and neutralize foreign objects invading the body. Antigens are markers on these objects that antibodies bind to in order to recognize the antigens. The introduction of immunoassays represented a significant leap in the ability to detect proteins, such as antibodies and cytokines secreted by human. Antibodies are utilized for the detection of diseases such as hepatitis and autoimmune disorders. Cytokines are involved in the studies of diseases such as Alzheimer's disease and cancer due to the gene regulation ability of the cytokines. As such, immunoassays have played important roles in protein detection and clinical diagnostics (Sutandy, Qian, Chen, & Zhu, 2013), see Table 12.1. Immunoassays have been classified as homogeneous and heterogeneous assays. In homogeneous assays, the probes and the samples will be mixed in the liquid phase; this method requires a separation step to detect the presence of the reaction products. In heterogeneous immunoassays, the samples in the liquid phase interact with the probes immobilized on a solid substrate, followed by a washing step to remove unbound samples. While both of these immunoassays are in practical use, heterogeneous assays are much more common due to the ease to wash away unbound samples from the solid substrate. Heterogeneous immunoassays usually take the form of the enzyme-linked immunosorbent assay (ELISA). The need of sample volumes in excess of 10 μL in

Table 12.1 Comparison of different commercial immunoassays based on the bioarray methods.

Product type	Product name	Company	Type of array	Protein content
Human protein	ProtoArray	Invitrogen	Functional	9000 human proteins
Kinase	Kinex	Kinexus Bioinformatics	Functional	200 human kinase proteins
Pathogen	Arrayit Pathogen Antigen Microarray	Arrayit Corporation	Functional	Essential proteins of different pathogens
Antibody for specific group of proteins	RayBio Human RTK Phosphorylation Antibody Array	RayBiotech, Inc	Analytical	Antibodies against 71 human kinases
	RayBio Human Cytokine Antibody Array	RayBiotech, Inc	Analytical	Antibodies against various human cytokines
	PlasmaScan 380 Antibody Microarray	Arrayit Corporation	Analytical	Antibodies for human plasma detection
	Cytokine Antibody Microarray	Full Moon BioSystems, Inc	Analytical	Antibodies against 77 human cytokines
	Kinase Antibody Microarray	Full Moon BioSystems, Inc	Analytical	Antibodies against 276 human kinases
Antibody for pathway detection	MAPK Pathway Phospho Antibody Array	Creative Bioarray	Analytical	185 antibodies against phospho-proteins in the MAPK pathways
	Signaling Explorer Antibody Microarray	Full Moon BioSystems, Inc	Analytical	1358 antibodies for multiple pathways

Table 12.1 Continued

Product type	Product name	Company	Type of array	Protein content
	Wnt Signaling Phospho Antibody Microarray	Full Moon BioSystems, Inc	Analytical	227 phospho-antibodies for cell growth, movement, and development pathways
Cell lysate	SomaPlex	Protein Biotechnologies	Reverse-phase	A variety of human cancer cell lysates

From Sutandy, F. X., Qian, J., Chen, C. S., & Zhu, H. (2013). Overview of protein microarrays. *Current protocols in protein science, 27*, 1−21. https://doi.org/10.1002/0471140864.ps2701s72.

ELISA poses a volume restriction to the detection of antibodies and cytokines. These proteins are found in low concentrations in low volumes in clinical samples. This makes the development of nanolitre volume liquid handling, and high detection sensitivity of low-volume, and low-concentration samples particularly important.

The miniaturization of the immunoassay technology came to light during the 1990s when development of DNA and protein microarrays began (Ekins, 1998). Furthermore, the need for simultaneous detection of a large number of analytes led to the development of multianalyte binding assays. Nanolitre volume liquid handling conducted in micron-sized channels provided a system in which minimal volume of liquid samples could be utilized while maintaining or even improving the sensitivity of the protein detection in these samples. The development of such technologies that can perform multianalyte detection in nanolitre volume of samples is called nanobioarray (NBA) chips which will be described in detail in subsequent sections.

12.2 Technologies

12.2.1 Microspot array

The most commonly developed immunoassay method is the spot array. It is a straightforward method where many probe spots are printed onto a chip substrate. Since the minimum volume of materials required for ELISA kits are limited to ∼ 10 μL, microspots that utilize liquid handling of nanoliters in microsized channels help to remove this limitation. Typically, the probe density is several thousand spots, and they are

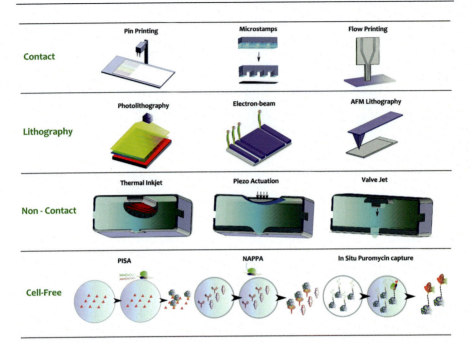

Figure 12.1 Summary of microspot array fabrication. (1) Contact pin printing; (2) Photolithography; (3) Thermal inkjet; (4) Cell-free protein in situ array.
From Romanov, V., Nikki Davidoff, S., Miles, A. R., Grainger, D. W., Galeabd, B. K., & Brooks, B. D. (2014). A critical comparison of protein microarray fabrication technologies. *Analyst, 139*, 1303−1326 with permission from Royal Society of Chemistry.

printed as a rectangular array within a single 1 cm × 1 cm square chip. This bioarray is then tested against a single sample, which is flowed on top of the chip. In this method, a large amount of data can be obtained from this test using a single sample.

There are three common methods utilized in microspotting the substrate: photolithography, mechanical microspotting, and inkjet printing (Schena et al., 1998; Romanov et al., 2014), see Fig. 12.1. These printing methods provide the ability to print multiple individualized spots on a single chip substrate.

Photolithography is used to pattern many spots accurately on the surface. This method is highly reproducible, with little variations in the microspot locations. This method does require a photomask for fabrication, which can be costly, as compared to other methods. This fabrication process is also time-consuming as each photomask must be designed and built before the chip fabrication can occur.

Mechanical microspotting utilizes a liquid droplet delivery mechanism with direct contact of spotting tips against the substrate to print the liquid from spots to spots. This method is straightforward and can be implemented in rapid prototyping. In addition, the microspotting procedure can be readily automated. Unlike the photolithography method, mechanical microspotting is not as precise, and so the high spot density cannot be achieved using photolithography. Nevertheless, this method remains a simple method of use in research labs.

Inkjet printing is a droplet delivery system using nozzles to transfer substances onto the substrate. This method allows for a spot density comparable to mechanical microspotting, while reducing the chip fabrication time as the inkjet liquid delivery method is contactless. The downside of this method is the robustness of the system. The delivery of the liquids is not always reliable and reproducible, due to clogging of the nozzle, which limits the use of this method.

12.2.2 Mosaic arrays

The mosaic array is a method that allows for multiple probes to react with multiple samples in immunoassays. Rather than having a single sample react with multiple probes, this method has several samples tested against multiple probes simultaneously.

In the mosaic array, the liquid flowed through polydimethylsiloxane (PDMS) channels sealed on top of the substrate (Bernard, Michel, & Delamarche, 2001; Dixit & Aguirre, 2014), see Fig. 12.2. This method is simple to use, and it utilizes micron-sized channels to define precisely and accurately the regions of the probes using nanoliters of reagents. This method requires the removal of the first chip and the assembly of a second chip before detection can occur. In other words, the channels in the chips must be intersecting in order to conduct the test in the manner of multiple probe and multiple sample.

In both methods of microspot and micromosaic arrays, a high spot density can be obtained. In the mosaic bioarray, the multiple probes will not only detect proteins in one sample but also detect multiple samples; whereas the microspot array will usually detect a single sample. However, the microspot array can be fabricated to generate

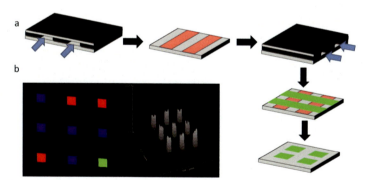

Figure 12.2 Methodology and results for developing micromosaic microarray. (a) Flow of biorecognition element of choice in the first direction using a network of parallel channels; immobilized strips of the biomolecule are created; secondary analyte solution is flown over the immobilized biomolecule strips, which creates second dimension lines; washing steps remove the undesired portions of the strip leaving spots of the size of channels; A 3X3 micromosaic illustration is shown in (b).
From Dixit, C. K., & Aguirre, G. R. (2014). Protein Microarrays with Novel Microfluidic Methods: Current Advances. *Microarrays (Basel Switzerland)*, 3, 180–202 with permission from Elsevier.

Table 12.2 Various microarray methods and their diagnostic applications.

Type of microarray	Method of development	Format	Density	Diagnostics application
DNA	Printing, in situ synthesis	Oligonucleotide, cDNA	Low-high	Respiratory, digestive tract infections
RNA	Printing	miRNA, total RNA	Low-high	Liver diseases, viral miRNA
Protein and peptide	Printing, stamping	Immunoassays, enzymatic assays, label-free	Moderate	Biomarker discovery, bacterial antigen
Carbohydrate	Stamping, drop-coating	Lectin assay	Moderate	Cell signaling. Biomarker discovery
Cellular	Droplet-coating	Immunoassays, protein assays, molecular assays	Low-moderate	Biomarker discovery, drug discovery, CTC identification

From Dixit, C. K., & Aguirre, G. R. (2014). Protein microarrays with novel microfluidic methods: Current advances. *Microarrays (Basel, Switzerland), 3*, 180−202. https://ds.doi.org./10.3390/microarrays3030180.

isolated detection regions. In this case, only one probe will detect each sample in each region. The microspot method is limited by the fact that each spot must have an individual probe and sample solution, whereas the micromosaic does not have this limitation. Recent advances show that a microspot array can be modified to alleviate this limitation by performing homogeneous-like immunoassays in which the probes are fixed on beads and remain in solutions for binding with samples in the same solution. This type of assay is commonly utilized in assays where a microwell is used to isolate the detection of samples at individual spots. Recent developments have shown increased stability of immobilized biomolecules, decreased assay times and cost, and instrument reduction with many disease detection applications, see Table 12.2 (Dixit & Aguirre, 2014).

12.3 Immobilization chemistry

In heterogeneous immunoassays, there are various methods of immobilizing the probes onto the surface (Kim & Kerr, 2013; Li & Chen, 2018; Liu & Yu, 2016; Rusmini, Zhong, & Feijen, 2007). Covalent attachment, adsorption, and bioaffinity attachment are the most common methods used, see Fig. 12.3 (Kim & Kerr, 2013).

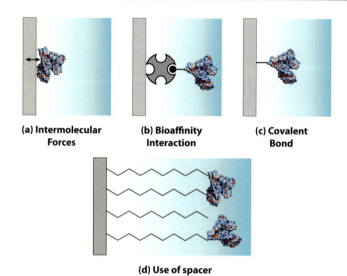

Figure 12.3 Common surface immobilization methods for heterogeneous assays. Schematic of immobilization mechanisms: (a) physisorption due to intermolecular forces, (b) bioaffinity interaction, and (c) covalent bond. The surface immobilization methods are often used in conjunction with (d) spacer for improved protein activity.
From Kim, D., & Herr, A. E. (2013). Protein immobilization techniques for microfluidic assays. *Biomicrofluidics 7*, 041501 with permission from AIP Publishing.

Adsorption is a simple method in which physisorption is commonly used to immobilize proteins onto a surface. This method can be achieved by adding proteins with high affinity to a particular substrate that is able to adsorb materials well. The drawback of this method is the occurrence of nonspecific binding. In addition, the weak binding force of physisorption means that desorption can easily occur through changes in reaction conditions, such as temperature, pH, and solvent composition. These drawbacks make this method rather limited in applications. While adsorption is a viable method in microspot arrays, it is not as ideal in micromosaic arrays.

In bioaffinity attachment, the most common method is through the use of biotinylated groups coupled to probes, which will attach to immobilized avidin analogs bound on a solid substrate. The high binding affinity of biotin to avidin groups and the ease of biotinylation of various probes make this a simple method for anchoring probes on solid substrates. In addition, the biotin-avidin link is very robust and is able to withstand many extreme conditions that may be encountered in a reaction (Moy, Florin, & Gaub, 1994). In order to avoid steric hindrance due to biotin on the active group of the probe, a carbon chain linker is usually used in between the biotin moiety and the probe. The drawback is that the probes must be biotinylated prior to being used which implies the requirement of an additional purification step.

Covalent attachment requires surface functionalization in order to attach the probes. Depending on the amino acids present in the protein or peptide probes, see Table 12.3 (Rushmini et al., 2007), there are several methods of surface functionalization, see Table 12.4 (Sutandy et al., 2013). Rusmini et al. (2007) lists two of these methods

Table 12.3 Comparison of immobilization techniques.

Side groups	Amino acids	Surfaces
$-NH_2$	Lys, hydroxyl-Lys	Carboxylic acid Active ester (NHS) Epoxy Aldehyde
$-SH$	Cys	Maleimide Pyridyl disulfide Vinyl sulfone
$-COOH$	Asp, Glu	Amine
$-OH$	Ser, Thr	Epoxy

From Rusmini, F., Zhong, Z. Y. & Feijen, J. (2007). Protein immobilization strategies for protein biochips. *Biomacromolecules, 8*, 1775−1789. With permission from American Chemical Society.

Table 12.4 Protein microarray fabrication common surfaces and their properties.

System	Surface	Properties
Covalent immobilization	Aldehyde, epoxy, NHS, carboxylic ester, etc.	Irreversible protein immobilization, good for covalent reactions, long immobilization
Adsorption	Polyvinylidene fluoride (PVDF), nitrocellulose membrane, polystyrene	High background signals in certain assays
Diffusion	Agarose/polyacrylamide gel, hydrogel	Good preservation of protein conformation, weak protein immobilization
Affinity capture	Ni^{2+}-NTA, streptavidin, glutathione	Possibility to control protein orientation
Metal	Gold, silver, steel, etc.	Conductive surface; compatible with SPR or mass spectrometry detection

From Sutandy, F. X., Qian, J., Chen, C. S., & Zhu, H. (2013). Overview of protein microarrays. *Current Protocols in Protein Science, 27*, 1−21. https://ds.doi.org/10.1002/0471140864.ps2701s72.

as: (1) N-hydroxysuccinimide (NHS) with 1-ethyl-3-(3-dimethylaminopropyl) carbodiimide (EDC) chemistry to couple with amino groups in proteins and (2) aldehyde chemistry to couple with amino groups in proteins. In the first method, EDC is used with NHS in various applications to create an amine-reactive NHS ester, which is easily attached to the amino groups of proteins through forming a stable amide bond. In the aldehyde method, glutaraldehyde (GA) may be used for the modification of the surface. Then, the aldehyde will interact with an amino group on the proteins. It is possible to modify the linker length to avoid steric hindrance and to improve the binding efficiency. However, the drawback of both methods is the requirement for a free primary amino group present in the protein molecules.

Although there still remain challenges with immobilization methods, site-selective attachment through nucleotide-binding sites, controlled protein orientation, and nonspecific adsorption allow for high protein loading. Multifunctional polymer coating and synthetic ligands-based site selective immobilization show promise for scale-up and automation purposes (Liu & Yu, 2016).

12.4 Detection methods

The common detection methods for immunoassays are based on tags that produce signals due to chemiluminescence, fluorescence, colorimetry, electrochemistry, and radioactivity (Pollard et al., 2007).

Chemiluminescent detection can be obtained by a horseradish peroxidase (HRP) tag, which is an enzyme that catalyzes chemiluminescent reaction of chemical substrates such as luminol. The HRP can be tagged onto the detection antibody which will be applied to the system. For instance, Langer, Niessner, and Seidel (2011) applied this method in an immunoassay for *Escherichia coli* (*E. coli*) detection, see Fig. 12.4. This method allows for a two orders of magnitude increase in detection ability as compared to the use of a fluorescent tag. The drawback of this method is the need of localization of the chemiluminescent reaction in the wells. The detection must also be completed rapidly upon the introduction of the substrate. In other words, this method of detection will be inaccurate if the substrate is not introduced to all detection regions or wells simultaneously. This method is excellent for high throughput detection, but light shielding from other wells (usually white) is required in order to prevent any residual light from bleeding into other wells, causing false positives.

Fluorescence can resolve the issues of the chemiluminescence by removing the need to introduce the HRP substrates as well as the need for reagent localization. In fluorescent detection, the tag is localized on the detection antibody, and no substrate is required for signal generation. For instance, Bilcharz et al. (2009) reported a fluorescence immunoassay method for cytokine detection. In terms of fluorescence, there is a variety of methods for the detection. The most direct method is attaching the fluorescent tag to the detection antibody. This method is the simplest and requires the least amount of time to detect. However, this method does not generate light as bright as chemiluminescence which has chemical amplification, and hence does not have as low detection limit as chemiluminescence. Nevertheless, fluorescent detection can be enhanced in many ways. One way is to multiply the number of fluorescent tags by adding a chain reaction or using a multiple tag antibody. Another way is by utilizing fluorescent beads for detection, and it is possible to increase the detection by two orders of magnitude. Fluorescence is a versatile method that can be utilized in a high throughput design, but light shielding from other wells (usually black) is required so that the light does not bleed from one spot to the next, thus causing false positives.

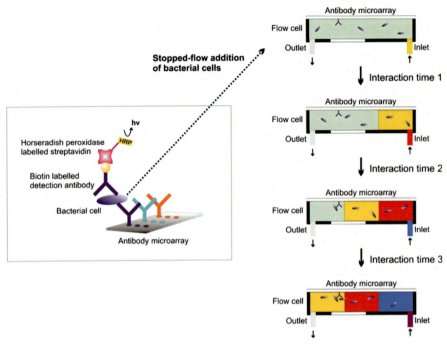

Figure 12.4 Detection of *E. coli* using chemiluminescence. A standard sandwich immunoassay is performed using the stop flow method. The biotin-conjugated polyclonal antibodies will first be coupled to the horseradish peroxidase (HRP) labeled streptavidin. HRP will then react with the chemiluminescent substrates. The various colored sections indicate the reagent volumes of 20 μL used in the various incubation steps. The results are shown in Fig. 12.7.
From Langer, V., Niessner, R. & Seidel, M. (2011). Stopped-flow microarray immunoassay for detection of viable *E. coli* by use of chemiluminescence flow-through microarrays. *Analytical and Bioanalytical Chemistry, 399*, 1041−1050. With permission from Springer-Verlag.

The third approach is colorimetric detection which can be achieved by a variety of methods. The simplest method is the introduction of a colorimetric substrate such as 3,3′,5,5′-tetramethylbenzidine that can be catalyzed by HRP to produce a colored compound. Another method for the colorimetric detection is immunogold silver staining (IGSS), see Fig. 12.5 (Yeh et al., 2009). This method uses silver or gold nanoparticles to aggregate against the gold-tagged detection protein (antibody or oligonucleotides) (Hayat, 1993; Holgate, Jackson, Cowen, & Bird, 1983). This method has a detection ability that is visible to the naked eye even at concentrations of 0.005 nM (Yeh et al., 2009). While normal colorimetric methods are not as sensitive as chemiluminescence or fluorescence, silver staining enhances the detection ability to a comparable level. In addition, the ease of this detection allows it to be viable for low cost detection equipment such as flat-bed scanners, when large and bulky instruments are unavailable.

Electrochemical detection utilizes the reduction and oxidation abilities of the materials for detection. For instance, Uliana, Peverari, Afonso, Cominetti, and Faria (2018) reported a method for detection of a cancer biomarker, see Fig. 12.6. The method requires electrodes (usually the working electrode in a three-electrode system) to be fabricated directly onto the device. This method is more sensitive than colorimetric

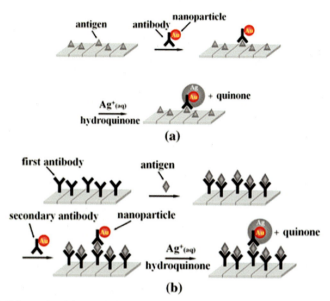

Figure 12.5 Schematic of the sandwich immunoassay using immunogold silver stain detection on a microspot bioarray. (a) The test used to evaluate the precipitation effects of the silver. (b) The actual method used to perform the ELISA (enzyme-linked immunosorbent assay)-type immunoassay. The results are shown in Fig. 12.8.
From Yeh, C. H., Hung, C. Y., Chang, T. C., Lin, H. P. & Un, Y. C. (2009). An immunoassay using antibody-gold nanoparticle conjugate, silver enhancement and flatbed scanner. *Microfluidics and Nanofluidics, 6,* 85–91. With permission from Springer Berlin/Heidelberg.

detection, and it does not require any transparent material. However, the detection is dependent on flow conditions within the channels, and the electrodes must be treated to prevent inaccurate results due to biofouling.

Radioactivity is another method that can be used for immunoassay detection. For instance, iodine-125 was used to label a protein for a radioactivity immunoassay (Mosley, Nguyen, Wu, & Kamei, 2016). In this method, the requirement for a transparent material can be bypassed as this method does not depend on optical detection methods. In addition, this method requires the radiolabeling of the protein, which allows for tracing of the protein. However, this method requires specialized equipment that reduces the compactness of this method. In addition, radioactive hazard is a concern that requires specialized safety training.

12.5 Applications

12.5.1 Antibody detection

Antibody detection has been utilized in a wide variety of applications. For instance, immunoassays have been applied in water analysis to detect pathogenic bacteria, such as *E. coli*. Conventional methods for detection of bacterial materials require

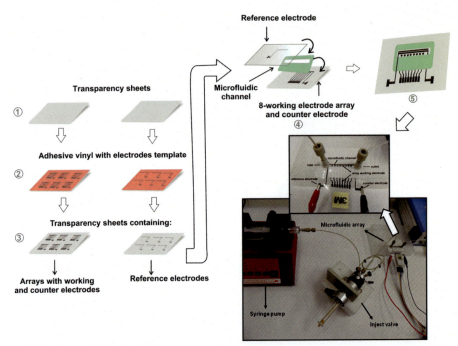

Figure 12.6 Construction of the microfluidic electrochemical device (μFED). Screen-printed electrodes: (1) transparency sheets, (2) transfer of vinyl masks to the transparency sheets and carbon ink screen-printing, followed by Ag|AgCl ink deposition on the reference electrode (RE); (3) vinyl mask removal. Assembly of the μFED: (4) sandwiching of the microfluidic channel between the polyester sheets, compressing the RE and working electrode (WE)/counter electrode (CE) sheets; (5) μFED ready for use, and image of the microfluidic setup. From Uliana, C. V., Peverari, C. R., Afonso, A. S., Cominetti, M. R., FAria, R. C. (2018). Fully disposable microfluidic electrochemical device for detection of estrogen receptor alpha breast cancer biomarker. *Biosensors and Bioelectronics, 99*, 156−162 with permission from Elsevier.

18−24 h to complete due to the required bacterial cultivation time. However, with the introduction of a stopped flow immunoassay system reported by Langer et al. (2011), the time required was reduced to 67 min (see Fig. 12.4). This method utilized the immobilization of polyclonal goat antibodies against *E. coli* cells utilizing 2000-Da diaminopolyethyleneglycol (DAPEG) to trap the cells. The detection was completed by the introduction of polyclonal detection antibodies conjugated with biotin, which would be coupled to streptavidin labeled with HRP. This will then react with chemiluminescent substrates to produce a signal. The detection limit obtained from this method, i.e., 4×10^5 cells/mL, is two orders of magnitude lower than a comparable conventional ELISA. In the stopped flow method, the standard microspot array has been modified to allow a solution to reach at, and react with, the microspots. The signal is enhanced when the flow rate of sample introduction is reduced (see Fig. 12.7). The benefit of this stop flow method is the ability to significantly enhance the signal compared to other methods which runs a sample continuously.

Development of the immunoassay of antibodies and cytokines on nanobioarray chips 501

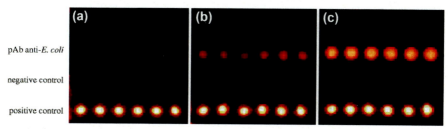

Figure 12.7 Chemiluminescent signals obtained from continuous flow at (a) 20 µL/s and (b) 0.5 µL/s, and from (c) stopped flow system for measurement of *E. coli* cells. In each image, the top row represent six spot replicates of pAb anti-*E. coli*, the middle of negative control and the bottom of positive control. The signals obtained from continuous flow are weaker than that using the stopped flow system The positive control was polyclonal antibody antiperoxidase and the negative control was spotting buffer. In each row, the interspot distance was 1100 µm. From Langer, V., Niessner, R. & Seidel, M. (2011). Stopped-flow microarray immunoassay for detection of viable *E. coli* by use of chemiluminescence flow-through microarrays. *Analytical and Bioanalytical Chemistry, 399*, 1041–1050. With permission from Springer-Verlag.

By using the immunoassay for detection of antibodies, we can specifically look for pathogenic cells, such as *E. coli* or *Staphylococcus aureus (S. aureus)* without killing them, as this will interfere with the ability to subsequently study these cells. In serum diagnostics, a multitude of proteins such as albumins, immunoglobulins (IgG), and regulatory proteins may be evaluated. In specific cases, the outcome of protein detection may just require a positive or negative result. IGSS is an excellent way to produce a rapid detection method that does not require expensive and bulky instruments and does generate fast results. This method was shown by Yeh, Hung, Chang, Lin, & Lin (2009) to detect protein A obtained from *S. aureus*, and IgGs obtained from human or goats (see Fig. 12.5). Over time, the signals gradually increase, resulting in the detection outcome of positive or negative result (see Fig. 12.8). In countries where expensive equipment is not readily available, these colorimetric immunoassays are economically viable.

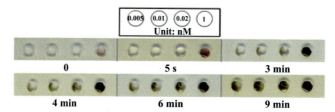

Figure 12.8 Images obtained from Immunogold silver staining (IGSS) results on a microspot array. Colorimetric changes were obtained from the immunoglobulin G-gold nanoparticles (IgG-AuNPs) conjugates once immersed in the silver enhancer solution from 0 s to 9 min. This demonstrated the IgG-AuNPs catalyzing the reduction of the silver ion solution to silver metal. From Yeh, C. H., Hung, C. Y., Chang, T. C., Lin, H. P. & Lin, Y. C. (2009). An immunoassay using antibody-gold nanoparticle conjugate, silver enhancement and flatbed scanner. *Microfluidics ond Nanofluidics, 6*, 85–91. With permission from Springer Berlin/Heidelberg.

In the paper by Yang, Janatova, Juenke, Mcmillin, and Andrade (2007), they demonstrated a microarray based on multiple wells to detect the antiepileptic drugs (AEDs), namely carbamazepine (CBZ), phenytoin (PHT), and valproic acid (VPA), simultaneously and quantitatively. The results of this competitive homogeneous immunoassay have a variation in results of less than 10%, as compared to values obtained from intra- and interassays, allowing for the method to be clinically viable.

Another system developed by Lee, Gulzar, Scott, and Li (2012) for the detection of antibodies involves the nanobioarray (NBA) chip method. This system is similar to the micromosaic approach but utilizes a spiral/radial chip configuration (see Fig. 12.9)

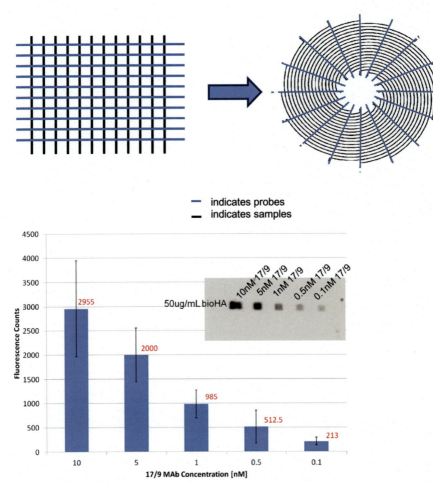

Figure 12.9 (a) The nanobioarray (NBA) chip (radial/spiral) as compared to the micromosaic chip (vertical/horizontal). (b) Results displaying the detection of monoclonal 17/9 antibodies dispensed into adjacent spiral channels intersecting with bioHA antigens immobilized along radial lines. Results were detected using a confocal fluorescence scanner.
With permission from the International Society for Optics and Photonics or SPIE.

rather than the horizontal/vertical chip configuration. This system utilizes the spiral channels to increase the residence time of the antibody—antigen reaction, thereby increasing the sensitivity of detection. This system utilizes a secondary antibody for fluorescence detection. The linear channel bioarray proposed by Bernard et al. (2001) was able to detect the antibodies to levels down to 0.5 nM. Utilizing the spiral NBA chip to detect monoclonal 17/9 antibodies (anti-influenza A clone 17/9), which bind to H3N2 hemagglutinin of the influenza virus A, 0.1 nM of the 17/9 Abs were detectable. A subsequent study by Sun et al. (2018) that used a secondary detection antibody allowed for detection of 0.01 nM of the same antibody.

12.5.2 Cytokine detection

Cytokines, e.g., interleukins, have been an area of interest as they are proteins that are important to human's immune response and are secreted by cells in diseases such as cancer, Alzheimer's disease as well as during organ transplant rejections. Although ELISA is the most common method to detect interleukins due to its high specificity, it is limited by long analysis time and its use of large sample size, high equipment cost and inflexibility in detecting various proteins simultaneously during a single experiment (Tonello et al., 2016). An immunoassay proposed by Zhou, Lu, Chen, and Sun (2010) utilizes a system which is designed for materials that are difficult to detect or that do not have a sandwich test kit for ELISA (see Fig. 12.10). The method proposed is called the specific analyte labeling and recapture assay. First, the antigen is bound to the capture antibody. Second, the bound antigen is labeled. Third, the labeled antigen is eluted. Fourth, the antigen is then recaptured utilizing the same capture antibody. This method allows for the use of a single detection antibody, rather than two antibodies—one for capture and one for detection. Moreover, the high specificity allows the same antigen to be recaptured. In this method, they trapped and detected various cytokines, the majority of which are interleukins (IL) such as: IL-1β, IL-4, IL-8, and IL-10; using their corresponding capture antibodies. Once the cytokines are trapped, they are then labeled with biotin. Finally, the antigens, which are released from the antibodies, are then recaptured using the same antibody. Poly-HRP streptavidin is then added for the detection of the antigens using the colorimetric substrate 2,2′-azinobis [3-ethylbenzothiazoline-6-sulfonic acid]-diammonium salt (ABTS). This system allows for multiple antigens to be detected from one sample. The sensitivity of this method allowed for detection of samples containing 0.01 ng/mL of cytokines.

In the study of Bilcharz et al. (2009) IL-6, IL-8 as well as other cytokines found in saliva of patients with pulmonary inflammatory diseases are detected. The cytokines in saliva have been detected through the use of microspheres in a homogeneous assay (see Fig. 12.11). The microspheres are surface-modified using aldehyde chemistry for immobilization of the corresponding monoclonal capture antibodies, such as anti-IL-8, on the surface. This method uses the sandwich detection method, in which the antigen is first captured and a biotinylated detection antibody is then incubated. Then, fluorescently labeled streptavidin is applied for detection. By utilizing fiber optics, each of these beads can be identified by their colors and intensities, allowing

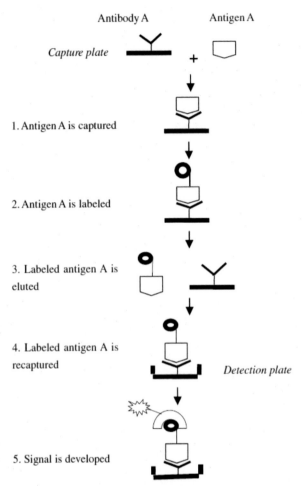

Figure 12.10 Cytokine Assay using Single Antibody. (1) Antigen A is captured on the surface utilizing an immobilized antibody A. (2) The captured antigen is then biotin labeled. (3) The labeled antigen is then eluted. (4) The eluted antigen is reintroduced into the system for recapture. (5) Streptavidin-HRP (horseradish peroxidase) is introduced to bind to the biotinylated antigen to develop a signal.
From Zhou, S. L., Lu, X. J., Chen, C. F. & Sun, D. X. (2010). An immunoassay method for quantitative detection of proteins using single antibodies. *Analytical Biochemistry, 400,* 213−218. With permission from Elsevier.

for a quantitative method for cytokine detection. This proof-of-concept experiment utilized the saliva samples obtained from patients to study the relationship between cytokines and pulmonary inflammatory diseases.

Another study by Gharibi, Haroun, Choy, and Li (2019) used an intersection bioarray approach to detect IL-2 ad IL-6, cytokines with diagnostic value that stimulate

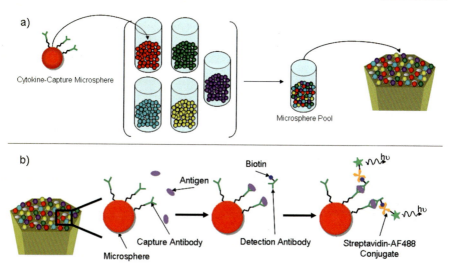

Figure 12.11 Microspheres for Cytokine Capture: (a) Capture antibodies are attached to the fluorescently encoded, amine functionalized microspheres. A mixture of various microspheres is loaded onto the fiber optic array. (b) The loaded microspheres are then incubated with the cytokines and then incubated with biotinylated antibodies.
From Blicharz, T. M., Siqueira, W. L., Helmerhorst, E. J., Oppenheim, F. G., Wexler, P. J., Little, F. F. & Walt, D. R. (2009). Fiber-optic microsphere-based antibody array for the analysis of inflammatory cytokines in saliva. *Analytical Chemistry, 81*, 2106–2114. With permission from American Chemical Society.

T-cells and play a role in acute phase protein production. Using direct immunoassays, they compared multiple immobilization surfaces of the capture antibody on a PDMS-glass microchip. They started with physical adsorption using poly-lysine (PLL), polystyrene (PS), and then covalent bonding by coupling primary amine groups on the aldehyde groups on the gluraraldehdye (GA) surface. For further optimization, they also modified the chip surface by introducing a protein G sublayer prior to antibody immobilization with a wash-out step to remove unbound molecules. For fluorescence detection, they used BioIgG first, followed by cyanine 5 labeled streptavidin (SA/Cy5). Optimized conditions were then applied to a sandwich bioarray method (see Fig. 12.12). In this study, Gharibi et al. were able to achieve a higher signal by immobilizing the antibodies on a GA surface compared to PS- and PLL-coated surfaces. Then by using a protein G sublayer prior to immobilization of antibodies, they were able to increase the fluorescent signal further. Through optimization, they were able to detect IL-6 concentrations as low as 3 ng/mL which translates to a detection level of 0.002 pg. These concentrations were comparable to those detected by Chikkaveeraiah, Mani, Patel, Gutkind, and Rusling (2011) using a microfluidic array that features nanostructured electrode and offline capture of antibodies as well as Kalpana, Thubashini and Sundharam (2014) in patients with recurrent aphthous stomatitis when using conventional ELISA kits.

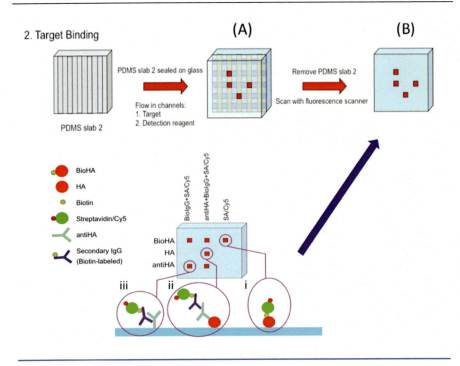

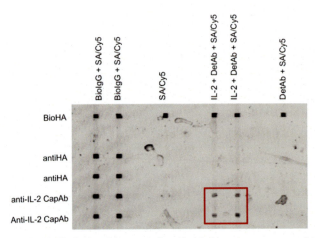

Figure 12.12 Scanned images of sandwich immunoassay on a chip for detection of human interleukin-2 (100 ng/mL). The glutaraldehyde surface was used for probe immobilization; IL-2 Incubation time was 60 min. Concentrations used for various reagents are provided in parentheses: BioHA (100 μg/mL), AntiHA (100 μg/mL), IL-2 capture antibody (500 μg/mL), IL-2 detection antibody (15 μg/mL), BioIgG (6 μg/mL), and SA/Cy5 (50 μg/mL). *Conadion Journal of Chemistry, 97*, 737−744.

12.6 Conclusion and future trends

This chapter describes the current developments in antibody detection based on the bioarray systems, which are initially developed for the nucleic acid detection (Sedighi & Li, 2014), and now the antibody bioarray systems show promise in multiplex detection of unpurified samples, low volume consumption, and fast reaction.

Further development with the bioarray method has shown improved detection signals and reduced equipment costs, making this a promising technique for future automation of diagnostic methods. Working toward automation will require confirming reproducibility especially with scaling up with large number of samples in a short amount of time. In terms of technology advances, there will be needs to improve the immunoassay systems for ease of automation. This will lead to much higher throughput and more reproducible results. While most of the instruments have automated operations, dispensing of the materials do not, which can lead to variations in detected signals. There still remain challenges to develop simple, versatile, stable, and cost-effective immobilization techniques for applications in high-performance bioanalytical devices. Site-selective attachment and controlled protein orientation with low nonspecific adsorption show great promise for biosensor/biochip fabrication. Another area that needs to be improved is the sensitivity of the instruments. It has been shown that the use of fluorescence detection results in lower detection limits in micro- or nanofluidic devices than in conventional methods like ELISA. To compete with chemiluminescence that offers better signal enhancement, a variety of methods such as fluorescence beads have also shown great promise in order to obtain better fluorescence signal. Finally, the ultimate goal is to improve upon this so that single molecule detection is possible. To achieve this goal, it will require system optimization as well as the development of novel detection methods involving the use of nanostructured materials.

Past applications were focused on samples that have ELISA kits developed. However, there are a wide variety of antibodies and cytokines that are not so easily captured. In addition to proteins that are difficult to analyze, many samples need to be purified before they can be analyzed. Furthermore, only a single aspect of these samples is currently analyzed. If instruments are able to completely characterize a sample, this will provide more information and improve our ability to understand the role of the antibodies and cytokines in a variety of physiological environments.

References

Bernard, A., Michel, B., & Delamarche, E. (2001). Micromosaic immunoassays. *Analytical Chemistry, 73*, 8–12. https://doi.org/10.1021/ac0008845

Blicharz, T. M., Siqueira, W. L., Helmerhorst, E. J., Oppenheim, F. G., Wexler, P. J., Little, F. F., et al. (2009). Fiber-optic microsphere-based antibody array for the analysis of inflammatory cytokines in saliva. *Analytical Chemistry, 81*, 2106–2114. https://doi.org/10.1021/ac802181

Chikkaveeraiah, B. V., Mani, V., Patel, V., Gutkind, J. S., & Rusling, J. F. (2011). Microfluidic electrochemical immunoarray for ultrasensitive detection of two cancer biomarker proteins in serum. *Biosensors and Bioelectronics, 26*, 4477−4483. https://doi.org/10.1016/j.bios.2011.05.005

Dixit, C. K., & Aguirre, G. R. (2014). Protein microarrays with novel microfluidic methods: Current advances. *Microarrays, 3*, 180−202. https://doi.org/10.3390/microarrays3030180

Ekins, R. P. (1998). Ligand assays: From electrophoresis to miniaturized microarrays. *Clinical Chemistry, 44*, 2015−2030. https://doi.org/10.1016/S0167-7799(99)01329-3

Gharibi, M., Haroun, S., Choy, J., & Li, P. C. H. (2019). A microfluidic antibody bioarray for fast detection of human interleukins in low sample volumes. *Canadian Journal of Chemistry, 97*, 737−744. https://doi.org/10.1139/cjc-2018-0506

Hayat, M. A. (1993). Immunogold-silver staining overview. *Journal of Histotechnology, 16*, 197−199. https://doi.org/10.1179/his.1993.16.3.197

Holgate, C. S., Jackson, P., Cowen, P. N., & Bird, C. C. (1983). Immunogold silver staining - new method of immunostaining with enhanced sensitivity. *Journal of Histochemistry and Cytochemistry, 31*, 938−944. https://doi.org/10.1177/31.7.6189883

Kalpana, R., Thubashini, M., & Sundharam, B. S. (2014). Detection of salivary interleukin-2 in recurrent aphthous stomatitis. *Journal of Oral and Maxillofacial Pathology, 18*, 361−364. https://doi.org/10.4103/0973-029X.151313

Kim, D., & Herr, A. E. (2013). Protein immobilization techniques for microfluidic assays. *Biomicrofluidics, 7*, 041501. https://doi.org/10.1063/1.4816934

Langer, V., Niessner, R., & Seidel, M. (2011). Stopped-flow microarray immunoassay for detection of viable *E. coli* by use of chemiluminescence flow-through microarrays. *Analytical and Bioanalytical Chemistry, 399*, 1041−1050. https://doi.org/10.1007/s00216-010-4414-0

Lee, J., Gulzar, N., Scott, J. K., & Li, P. C. H. (2012). A nanofluidic bioarray chip for fast and high-throughput detection of antibodies in biological fluids. In *SPIE 2012 global congress on nanomedicine, Incheon, South Korea, September 10−13, 2012, 8548* pp. 1−7). https://doi.org/10.1117/12.945970

Li, Z., & Chen, G.-Y. (2018). Current conjugation methods for immunosensors. *Nanomaterials, 8*(5), 278. https://doi.org/10.3390/nano8050278

Liu, Y., & Yu, J. (2016). Oriented immobilization of proteins on solid supports for use in biosensors and biochips: A review. *Microchim Acta, 183*, 1−19. https://doi.org/10.1007/s00604-015-1623-4

Mosley, G. L., Nguyen, P., Wu, B. M., & Kamei, D. T. (2016). Development of quantitative radioactive methodologies on paper to determine important lateral-flow immunoassay parameters. *Lab on a Chip, 16*, 2871−2881. https://doi.org/10.1039/C6LC00518G

Moy, V. T., Florin, E. L., & Gaub, H. E. (1994). Intermolecular forces and energies between ligands and receptors. *Science, 266*, 257−259. https://doi.org/10.1126/science.7939660

Pollard, H. B., Srivastava, M., Eidelman, O., Jozwik, C., Rothwell, S. W., Mueller, G. R., et al. (2007). Protein microarray platforms for clinical proteomics. *Proteomics - Clinical Applications, 1*, 934−952. https://doi.org/10.1002/prca.200700154

Rusmini, F., Zhong, Z. Y., & Feijen, J. (2007). Protein immobilization strategies for protein biochips. *Biomacromolecules, 8*, 1775−1789. https://doi.org/10.1021/bm061197b

Schena, M., Heller, R. A., Theriault, T. P., Konrad, K., Lachenmeier, E., & Davis, R. W. (1998). Microarrays: biotechnology's discovery platform for functional genomics. *Trends in Biotechnology, 16*, 301−306. https://doi.org/10.1016/S0167-7799(98)01219-0

Sedighi, A., & Li, P. C. H. (2014). Kras gene codon 12 mutation detection enabled by gold nanoparticles conducted in a nanobioarray chip. *Analytical Biochemistry, 448*, 58−64. https://doi.org/10.1016/j.ab.2013.11.019

Sun, Y., Gharibi, M., Lee, J., Li, P. C. H., Gulzar, N., Scott, J. K., et al. (2018). Rapid detection of antibody in biological fluids on a bioarray chip. *Analytical Letters.* https://doi.org/10.1080/00032719.2018.1500580

Sutandy, F. X., Qian, J., Chen, C. S., & Zhu, H. (2013). Overview of protein microarrays. *Current Protocols in Protein Science, 27*, 1−21. https://doi.org/10.1002/0471140864.ps2701s72

Tonello, S., Serpelloni, M., Lopomo, N. F., Sardini, E., Abate, G., & Uberti, D. L. (2016). Preliminary study of a low-cost point-of-care testing system using screen-printed biosensors: For early biomarkers detection related to Alzheimer disease. In *2016 IEEE international symposium on medical measurements and applications (MeMeA)* (pp. 1−6). https://doi.org/10.1109/MeMeA.2016.7533800

Uliana, C. V., Peverari, C. R., Afonso, A. S., Cominetti, M. R., & Faria, R. C. (2018). Fully disposable microfluidic electrochemical device for detection of estrogen receptor alpha breast cancer biomarker. *Biosensors and Bioelectronics, 99*, 156−162. https://doi.org/10.1016/j.bios.2017.07.043

Valentin Romanov, S., Davidoff, N., Miles, A. R., Grainger, D. W., Galeabd, B. K., & Brooks, B. D. (2014). A critical comparison of protein microarray fabrication technologies. *Analyst, 139*, 1303−1326.

Yang, X., Janatova, J., Juenke, J. M., Mcmillin, G. A., & Andrade, J. D. (2007). An ImmunoChip prototype for simultaneous detection of antiepileptic drugs using an enhanced one-step homogeneous immunoassay. *Analytical Biochemistry, 365*, 222−229. https://doi.org/10.1016/j.ab.2007.03.019

Yeh, C. H., Hung, C. Y., Chang, T. C., Lin, H. P., & Lin, Y. C. (2009). An immunoassay using antibody-gold nanoparticle conjugate, silver enhancement and flatbed scanner. *Microfluidics and Nanofluidics, 6*, 85−91. https://doi.org/10.1007/s10404-008-0298-0

Zhou, S. L., Lu, X. J., Chen, C. F., & Sun, D. X. (2010). An immunoassay method for quantitative detection of proteins using single antibodies. *Analytical Biochemistry, 400*, 213−218. https://doi.org/10.1016/j.ab.2010.01.038

Integrated microfluidic systems for genetic analysis

Siwat Jakaratanopas, Bin Zhuang, Wupeng Gan, Peng Liu
Department of Biomedical Engineering, Tsinghua University, School of Medicine, Haidian District, Beijing, China

Guided-reading questions

1. How do microfluidic systems benefit single-cell genetic analysis? What are some examples of technologies used for cell manipulation in microfluidic devices?
2. What are the different DNA extraction strategies utilized in microsystems for pathogen detection?
3. How do microbeads impact the development of integrated systems in various areas of genetic analysis?

13.1 Introduction

The completion of the human genome project (HGP) announced the start of the post-genome era (Lander et al., 2001; Venter et al., 2001). With the reference human genome sequence and ever-growing individual sequences established (Levy et al., 2007; Wang et al., 2008; Wheeler et al., 2008), researchers' attentions have been directed toward investigating the effects of DNA variations among individuals and their implications for diseases (Beckmann, Estivill, & Antonarakis, 2007; Buchanan & Scherer, 2008; Calvo et al., 2006; Fanciulli et al., 2007). Their completions also enabled the discoveries of genetic clues and evidence to better understand cellular behaviors (Blais & Dynlacht, 2005) and to develop more powerful genetic tools for application in forensics (Butler, 2006; Jobling & Gill, 2004), health care (Guttmacher, Porteous, & McInerney, 2007), food safety (Abee, van Schaik, & Siezen, 2004), and so on. These research interests have posed further challenges to current genetic analytical techniques. For example, to fully understand gene functions and the importance of genome structural variations (block substitutions, insertions, deletions, inversions, and duplications) to speciation, evolution, and diseases (Check, 2005; Ellegren, 2008; Zhao et al., 2004), numerous large-scale genomes need to be sequenced to obtain comparative information. A high-throughput and low-cost sequencing technology, which can generate accurate long-range read-lengths, is therefore of particular importance for many studies, such as the Cancer Genome Project. It is also known that subtle changes in gene expression are central for an organism to survive, and these changes can vary substantially among some type of cells under identical conditions (Acar, Mettetal, & van Oudenaarden, 2008; Choi, Cai, Frieda, & Xie, 2008). In addition, many biological processes, such as embryo development, and diseases such as cancer (Quintana et al., 2008), originate from a single cell. Therefore, a genetic and gene expression analysis platform, which can manipulate single cells efficiently and provide single-molecule sensitivity, will be greatly appreciated by researchers. Genetic analysis is poised to emerge from research laboratories and play an important role in our daily lives, such as in forensics and clinical diagnosis. Ideally, these applications require compact instruments that are fast, low-cost, easy to operate, and even portable for decentralized or point-of-care (POC) testing. Undoubtedly, all these challenges suggest that future genetic analytical techniques must require less cost and time, have high sensitivity and high throughput, and provide flexible platforms to meet various applicable situations.

Although conventional genetic analytical methods have advanced significantly through the application of robotics, there are several intrinsic limiting drawbacks.

(i) Sample loading: As the analytical targets are changing to single cells, the conventional serial dilution method for cell loading becomes ineffectual. Because the number of cells in each reaction follows the Poisson distribution, the variation of starting materials inevitably leads to irreproducible results.

(ii) Sample dilution: The liquid handling limitations of conventional analytical techniques are usually 5–10 µL, which not only consumes more expensive reagents, but also causes inevitable sample dilution. For example, to analyze a single gene (one DNA strand) in a cell, we conventionally put it into a working volume of 10 µL, which causes extreme dilution of this single template down to $<10^{-18}$ M. The most sensitive systems for DNA detection require concentrations in the femtomolar-picomolar range, which is already close to the maximum concentration of polymerase chain reaction (PCR) products practically generated from a single template in a 10 µL reaction.

(iii) Inefficient sample/product transport: During conventional genetic analysis, samples are transferred from one instrument to another several times, which can cause significant sample dilution and loss. For instance, in DNA capillary electrophoresis (CE) analysis, a sample of 1–2 µL is usually taken from 10 µL PCR products and later only ~2 nL of that sample is injected into the capillary for separation and detection (Butler, Buel, Crivellente, & McCord, 2004). This inefficient sample transfer compromises the sensitivity and quantitative capability of current analytical methods.

(iv) Contamination: Contamination issues become prominent when dealing with low-copy-number samples, since the contaminants can overwhelm real target signals. Current analytical processes that have multiple open sample transfer steps make contamination inevitable (Gill, Whitaker, Flaxman, Brown, & Buckleton, 2000). Nevertheless, the precipitous gap between the vast requirements of genetic analyses and the limited capabilities provided by current techniques will spur the improvement of existing tools and the innovation of new technologies.

13.2 Integrated microfluidic systems

Micrototal analysis systems (μTAS), or the so-called "lab-on-a-chip," have attracted increasing attention because of their ability to integrate multiple biochemical processes at pL-nL scale in a single device using microfabrication technology. The advantages of miniaturizing and integrating genetic analysis include high speed, less reagent consumption, and a reduction in size of instruments (Harrison et al., 1993; Manz, Graber, & Widmer, 1990, Manz et al., 1992). Moreover, microfabrication technology has the potential to overcome the hurdles associated with conventional techniques. Since the intrinsic length (μm) and volume scales (pL-nL) of microstructures in a device are close to those of single cells, efficient manipulation and loading of individual cells in a high-throughput manner becomes possible (Sims & Allbritton, 2007). The limited diffusion distances and concentrated reagents realized by performing assays in nanolitre-scale reactors could also substantially increase the sensitivity and speed of biochemical reactions (Jensen, 1998). By integrating the analytical process on a single device, efficient connections between each functional unit can be achieved, so that the loss and dilution of samples is minimized. Additionally, microfluidic automations can also eliminate the risks of sample mix-up and contamination, which are critical for high-sensitivity genetic analyses. Given all these inherent advantages, fully integrated microfluidic systems are a promising technology.

The development of integrated microdevices for genetic analyses has advanced rapidly. The early development of microfabricated genetic analysis devices focused on translating individual analytical steps into chip formats, such as DNA extraction, PCR, and microchannel capillary electrophoresis, to replace their counterparts in conventional genetic analyses. Current research work has centered on the development of fully integrated microsystems to provide complete solutions with enhanced performances to specific applications. Many review articles have been published, covering various aspects of microfluidic devices, including microfabrication, materials, device interface, fluidic control, and a wide range of applications (Fredrickson & Fan, 2004; Lagally & Mathies, 2004; Roman & Kennedy, 2007; West, Becker, Tombrink, & Manz, 2008). Therefore, this chapter focuses on the development of integrated genetic analyses that have significant impacts on DNA sequencing, gene expression analysis, pathogen/infectious disease detection, and forensic short tandem repeat (STR) typing.

13.3 Development of integrated microdevices

To develop fully integrated microsystems for gene expression and genetic analysis, several necessary chip elements must be strategically chosen, including device material, temperature control system for thermal cycling of reactions, microvalves for fluidic control, sample/product transport between analytical steps, and interface of microfluidic device to the macro world. We will briefly discuss these aspects as they closely relate to genetic analysis, but it is advisable to refer to other dedicated chapters on these aspects for more detailed information.

a. Device materials

The choice of device material is important for the development of integrated microsystems because the design, fabrication, and operation of the device are heavily dependent on the properties of the substrates used to manufacture them. Glass is a widely used substrate in integrated microfluidic devices for genetic analysis due to its beneficial advantages, including optical transparency for detection and mature surface chemistry manipulation (Blazej, Kumaresan, & Mathies, 2006; Ferrance et al., 2003; Lagally, Emrich, & Mathies, 2001; Waters et al., 1998). It is extensively used in CE applications because of its surface electroosmotic mobility and high thermoconductivity (Ren, Zhou, & Wu, 2013). Nevertheless, glass is brittle and has high fabrication cost with the heavy need for cleanroom facilities. Polymers including elastomers and plastics are later introduced, offering wide varieties of low-cost material alternatives suitable for different applications, making polymers the most commonly used microfluidic substrate. Polydimethylsiloxane (PDMS) is inarguably the most popular elastomeric substrate used worldwide due to its biocompatibility, ease of fabrication, optical transparency, and the ability to reversibly/irreversibly bond or conform to different substrate surfaces (McDonald et al., 2000; McDonald & Whitesides, 2002; Quake & Scherer, 2000). The main drawbacks of PDMS involve its inherent hydrophobicity, resulting in the adsorption of hydrophobic molecules onto the surface, and its gas permeability which can create undesirable solvent evaporation affecting assay performance (Kim & Herr, 2013; Mukhopadhyay, 2007; Ren et al., 2013). PDMS also swells in contact with organic solvents and is incompatible for applications involving these nonpolar solvents (Lee, Park, & Whitesides, 2003). Other polymer-based substrates include poly(methyl methacrylate) (PMMA), polycarbonate (PC), polystyrene (PS), polyethylene terephthalate (PET), and cyclic olefin copolymer (COC). Their distinctive characteristics are reviewed elsewhere (Becker & Gärtner, 2008). Recently, integrated paper-based devices containing on-chip nucleic acid extraction, amplification, and detection have been demonstrated, opening new possibilities for low-cost integrated microsystems in limited resource settings (Choi et al., 2016; Rodriguez et al., 2015; Tang et al., 2017).

b. Temperature control

Gene expression and genetic analyses usually include DNA or RNA amplification steps, which require rapid and accurate temperature control for thermally cycling reagents loaded in microreactors. To prevent the heat from affecting other chip elements and to reduce the thermal mass for rapid heating and cooling, the heating space should be precisely localized and minimized. Many temperature control methods, including contact and noncontact heating, have been successfully demonstrated on microdevices. Contact heating methods include external heaters attached to the chip surface, such as Peltier heaters (DuVall et al., 2016; Estes et al., 2012; Kopp, Mello, & Manz, 1998), and microfabricated thin film heaters made of Ti/Pt (Hsieh et al., 2008; Lagally et al., 2001), aluminum (Burns et al., 1996), chromium (Selva, Mary, & Jullien, 2010) or Indium Tin Oxide (ITO) (Fukuba, Yamamoto, Naganuma, & Fujii, 2004; Jha et al., 2012). Noncontact heating have been realized by means of infrared (IR) (Hettiarachchi, Kim, & Faris, 2012; Hühmer & Landers, 2000) and microwaves (Marchiarullo et al., 2013; Shaw et al., 2010). While these heating systems demonstrate comparable performances in laboratory settings, contact heating is generally more suitable for POC applications due to its inherently smaller size and no specialized equipment is needed.

c. Microfluidic control

Microvalves are essential parts for moving samples and products and preventing interference between each analytical step in a fully integrated microsystem (Oh & Ahn, 2006). Microvalves can be categorized into four different groups: actively mechanical, actively nonmechanical, passively mechanical, and passively nonmechanical. Table 13.1 lists several examples in each category that have been integrated into microdevices (Al-Faqheri et al., 2015; Baek, Yoon, Jeon, Seo, & Park, 2013; Chen et al., 2016; Cong et al., 2016; Feng & Chou, 2011; Feng, Zhou, Ye, & Xiong, 2003; Feng & Kim, 2004; Grover, Skelley, Liu, Lagally, & Mathies, 2003; Haefner, Koerbitz, Frank, Elstner, & Richter, 2018; Jadhav et al., 2015; Kistrup et al., 2014; Koh, Tan, Zhao, Ricco, & Fan, 2003; Li et al., 2004; Liu & Li, 2014; Nagai, Oguri, & Shibata, 2015; Oh, Han, Bhansali, & Ahn, 2002; Ouyang et al., 2013; Pappas & Holland, 2008; Park, Jung, Zhang, Lee, & Seo, 2012; Prakash & Kaler, 2007; Richter, Howitz, Kuckling, Kretschmer, & Arndt, 2004; Shaegh et al., 2018; Thio et al., 2011, 2013; Tice, Desai, Bassett, Apblett, & Kenis, 2014; Unger, Chou, Thorsen, Scherer, & Quake, 2000; Wang et al., 2015; Yang & Lin, 2009; Yobas, Huff, Lisy, & Durand, 2001; Yıldırım, Arıkan, & Külah, 2012; Zimmermann, Hunziker, & Delamarche, 2008). The following requirements should be taken into consideration when selecting microvalves: whether they are normally close or open mode, dead volume, power consumption, pressure resistance, and insensitivity to particle contamination. Generally speaking, actively mechanical microvalves have superior performance over other microvalves, hence are more commonly used in various microsystems. In addition, a micropump can be easily formed by connecting three active valves in serial on a microchip, emphasizing on its versatility (Grover et al., 2003; Quake & Scherer, 2000; Shaegh et al., 2018). Even though passive valves are not flexible and usually function-specific, they are gaining more attention due to its low-cost, simplicity, and ease of operation which can be effective and well-suited in some applications. For example, in an integrated PCR-CE microdevice, the interface between the viscous separation matrix and the PCR solution can act as a passive valve to restrain the PCR solution in the reactor during thermal cycling (Lagally et al., 2001). Park et al. utilized a narrow channel geometry and the hydrophobicity of PDMS to function as a passive capillary microvalve on an RNA purification rotary microsystem to prevent

Table 13.1 Microvalves for fluidic control on integrated devices.

Categories	Mechanism	References
Actively mechanical	Electromagnetic	(Liu and Li, 2014; Oh et al., 2002)
	Electrostatic	(Tice et al., 2014; Yobas et al., 2001; Yıldırım et al., 2012)
	Piezoelectric	(Chen et al., 2016; Li et al., 2004)
	Pneumatic	(Cong et al., 2016; Grover et al., 2003; Shaegh et al., 2018; Unger et al., 2000)
Actively nonmechanical	Hydrogel	(Haefner et al., 2018; Jadhav et al., 2015; Richter et al., 2004)
	Paraffin	(Baek et al., 2013; Feng and Chou, 2011; Yang and Lin, 2009)
	Biological	(Nagai et al., 2015; Pappas and Holland, 2008)
Passively mechanical	Check valves (flap, plug etc.)	(Al-Faqheri et al., 2015; Feng and Kim, 2004; Prakash and Kaler, 2007; Thio et al., 2011)
Passively nonmechanical	Hydrophobicity	(Feng et al., 2003; Ouyang et al., 2013; Wang et al., 2015)
	Capillary burst	(Kistrup et al., 2014; Park et al., 2012; Thio et al., 2013; Zimmermann et al., 2008)
	Gel valves	(Koh et al., 2003)

sample flow until adequate centrifugal force is applied to burst through capillary pressure (Park et al., 2012). These passive valves are incontrollable, nonresistant to high pressure, but are reliable in these situations.

d. Sample/product transport

The integration of the whole analytical process on a single device is more complex than simply combining several microfabricated units. Efficient and reproducible transport of the sample/product between function units is the key to a seamlessly integrated system and to fully demonstrate the advantages of sensitivity, reproducibility, and reliability. Examples of methods available for sample transportation within a device include: (1) sample moved by syringe pump (Easley et al., 2006; Hsieh, Ferguson, Eisenstein, Plaxco, & Soh, 2015), (2) sample driven by timing-controlled electric field (Liu, Toriello, & Mathies, 2006), (3) sample carried by transport vehicles, such as DNA captured and transported using magnetic beads (Beyor, Seo, Liu, & Mathies, 2008; Chang, Ding, Lin, Wang, & Lu, 2017; Liu, Li, Greenspoon, Scherer, & Mathies, 2011; Strohmeier et al., 2013; Ueberfeld, El-Difrawy, Ramdhanie, & Ehrlich, 2006), and (4) sample captured at the destination or captured then relocated downstream, such as filters (Gan et al., 2017; Khandurina, Jacobson, Waters, Foote, & Ramsey, 1999), capture gel (Blazej, Kumaresan, Cronier, & Mathies, 2007; Root, Agarwal, Kelso, & Barron, 2011), and solid phase extraction column (Long, Shen, Wu, Qin, & Lin, 2007). The pump and electric field methods are easy to implement but require precise timing and bulky instruments. Moreover, when there is a large volume mismatch between two structures, precious samples will be wasted or diluted. In contrast, the carrying and capture methods are more efficient and reliable, especially when volume mismatch exists in microdevices.

e. Macro-to-micro interface

Another aspect for successful microfluidic devices often overlooked during development is the connection between microfluidic device and off-chip components, also known as the macro-to-micro interface or world-to-chip interface. Reagents and samples are transferred from macroscopic environment in milliliters to microliters into microfluidic systems with nanoliter to picoliter reaction volume (Fredrickson & Fan, 2004). The volume mismatch between the device and outside world, therefore, is even more pronounced than the mismatch between microfluidic units; thus, a reliable interconnect is needed. Ideally, the interface must be easy to assemble, robust, leak-free, and chemically inert while having minimum dead volume that can potentially hinder assay efficiency and introduce contamination (Fredrickson & Fan, 2004; Tian & Finehout, 2009). Many fluid interface strategies have been explored, for instance on-chip reservoirs (Fang, Xu, & Fang, 2002; Lagally et al., 2001), integrated on-chip adaptors (Chen, Acharya, Gajraj, & Meiners, 2003), and removable modular adaptors (Nisisako, Ando, & Hatsuzawa, 2012; Nittis, Fortt, Legge, & de Mello, 2001; Yuen, 2016). The most widely used microfluidic interconnect to the macro world is the reservoir well which can be easily fabricated but require manual reagent loading before subsequent processes. Adaptors provide a more seamless connection, leading to a more streamlined operation and increased inlet density; however, most are device-specific with complex fabrication and assembly protocols (Fredrickson & Fan, 2004). Modular interconnects are gaining a lot of interests in recent years, with researches demonstrating interconnects with increased flexibility to tackle both module-to-module and world-to-chip connection challenges (Yuen, 2016) and the utilization of 3D printing technologies for rapid prototyping and highly customizable fluidic interconnects (Gong, Woolley, & Nordin, 2018; Paydar et al., 2014).

13.4 Applications of fully integrated systems in genetic analysis

a. DNA sequencing

As the demand for large-scale DNA sequencing grows, the National Institute of Health (NIH) in the United States continues to fund the development of new technologies to reduce the total cost of DNA sequencing from approximately $10 m to $1000 per genome (Blow, 2008), which will eventually make DNA sequencing a reliable and routine analytical procedure for biological researchers to explore complex biological processes, or even for physicians to tailor a personal treatment according to patients' genetic variations. To meet future expanding demands of DNA sequencing, extensive studies have been conducted to improve conventional Sanger sequencing and develop newer methods. Next-generation sequencing (NGS) technologies are evolving rapidly over the past decade and have been commercialized into many successful products providing massively parallel analysis with high throughput and low cost (Mardis, 2008; Shendure & Ji, 2008). Several published reviews provide a comprehensive introduction and analysis of their potential applications in the future (Goodwin, McPherson, & McCombie, 2016; Metzker, 2010; Shendure & Ji, 2008). In this section, the translation of Sanger sequencing onto microfluidic platforms and integrated Sanger sequencing microsystems will be highlighted, followed by achievements of microfluidics in improving NGS sample library preparation, including single-cell sequencing.

The first four-colour electrophoretic separation of Sanger sequencing products on a microfabricated glass CE chip was demonstrated by Woolley and Mathies (1995). Since then, numerous studies have been conducted to improve the data quality and read-length of chip-based DNA sequencing separations. By optimizing channel length and injector geometry (Liu, Shi, Ja, & Mathies, 1999), employing energy-transfer (ET) fluorescent reagents for fragment labeling (Berti, Medintz, Tom, & Mathies, 2001; Ju, Glazer, & Mathies, 1996; Kheterpal, Li, Speed, & Mathies, 1998) and utilizing novel separation matrixes and coating polymers (Chiesl et al., 2006; Doherty et al., 2004), DNA sequencings with >500 bp read-length and ~99% accuracy have been repeatedly demonstrated by many research groups (Backhouse et al., 2000; Liu et al., 1999; Schmalzing et al., 1998). Barron et al. developed a pDMA (Poly(N,N-dimethylacrylamide)) separation matrix and pHEA (poly(N-hydroxyethylacrylamide)) dynamic coating to achieve an ultrafast separation of 600 bases in just 6.5 min by microchip electrophoresis (Fredlake et al., 2008). To improve the sequencing throughput, a 768-lane DNA sequencing system, which alternatively runs two 394-lane plates, was also demonstrated by Aborn et al. (2005).

However, the potential of Sanger sequencing microdevice lies in the capability of integrating sample preparations with electrophoresis to achieve rapid and low-cost DNA sequencings. In 2006, Mathies et al. demonstrated a nanolitre-scale microfabricated bioprocessor, which integrates all three Sanger sequencing steps—thermal cycling, sample purification, and CE—into a four-inch hybrid glass PDMS wafer (Blazej et al., 2006). This fully integrated system contained a 250-nL reactor with microfabricated four-point resistance temperature sensors and an external thin film heater for rapid thermal cycling, PDMS micropumps, and valves for efficient sample transport from the reactor to the capture chamber, via a hole for transporting the samples from the top-layer to the bottom-layer channels. It has an affinity-capture chamber where Sanger sequencing fragments were captured by complimentary oligos for purification and concentration, and a 30-cm folded channel with taper turns for CE separation with a long-range single-base resolution. Complete DNA sequencing from 1 fmole of DNA template can be finished in under 30 min with a 556-base read-length and 99% accuracy, equivalent to those used in the initial human genome sequencing (Lander et al., 2001). For chip-based sequencing separation, Ueberfeld et al. developed a method for low-quantity DNA sample loading (Ueberfeld et al., 2006). DNA was reversibly captured onto paramagnetic microspheres, injected into a channel using a magnetized wire, and then released for separation. Although tenfold signal improvement was achieved, this method is not readily incorporated into an integrated microchip system. Later, a gel-based affinity DNA capture, concentration, and inline injection method integrated with on-chip CE was developed by Blazej et al. (2007). By replacing the conventional cross-injector with the new efficient, time-independent inline injector, 30 nL of sequencing sample produced from only 100 amol of human mitochondrial HVII template was near 100% immobilized in a capture gel and inline injected into a separation channel for electrophoresis. The successful development of these systems suggests that Sanger sequencing microsystem can potentially be used in clinical diagnosis, where a patient's short gene fragment can be quickly sequenced to aid diagnosis or personal treatments.

The advent of NGS provides a powerful tool for genome-wide analysis at an affordable price and gradually replaces the traditional Sanger sequencing method. As the technology continues to advance, sample preparation into template library ready for sequencing must not be overlooked in order to realize NGS full potential (Coupland, 2010). Microfluidics have made the automation of NGS library preparation possible, increasing the operation throughput while reducing reagent consumption of this normally labour-intensive, multi-step process. Kim et al. first demonstrated the use of digital microfluidic (DMF) as a central sample distribution hub between multiple external modules and to perform tasks required for NGS library preparation (Kim et al., 2011). Using external pump and electrowetting, the DMF interconnect enabled automated selective liquid fractioning from a continuous flow and droplet sorting into designated processing modules. With the precise droplet manipulation and AMPure XP magnetic beads, buffer exchange and washing procedures were shown on the central DMF platform, and the final average DNA recovery efficiency is 80% ± 4.8% in range of benchtop protocol. The group later extended this work into a fully integrated library preparation platform based on Nextera sample preparation protocol using bead-based assay for Illumina MiSeq system (Kim et al., 2013). DNA was extracted from a bacterial culture before loading onto the platform shown in Fig. 13.1 where all steps in

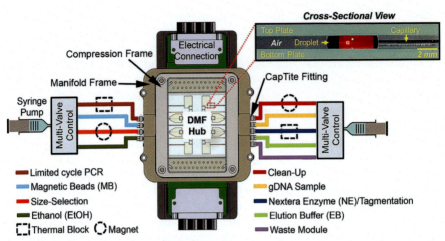

Figure 13.1 Integrated microsystem for preparing DNA libraries for sequencing showing the top view of an integrated system and the side view of the DMF (digital microfluidic)-capillary interface, featuring a central DMF hub for integrating multiple reagent and sample preparation modules (depicted in different colors), magnets, and thermal blocks coupled to module tubing for sample preparation, and multivalve syringe pumps for liquid handling.
Adapted from Kim et al. (2013).

Nextera workflow were implemented: DNA tagmentation, clean-up, PCR amplification, and size selection for off-chip sequencing. The system utilized the central DMF and syringe pumps for liquid manipulation similar to the previous work, but all sample preparation steps were performed on the peripheral modules, with some containing external magnets and heating blocks. Bacterial genome libraries prepared on this platform have >99% alignment to reference genomes with a good uniformity and data quality. For microsystem utilizing purification columns, Tan et al. reported an automated multicolumn chromatography chip that can process up to 16 different samples in parallel for library generation in Illumina MiSeq or Ion Torrent PGM systems (Tan et al., 2013). The device operated on a programmable integrated fluidic circuit (IFC) for liquid transport, valve actuation, and temperature control while the columns were formed with ChargeSwitch beads or carboxylated beads that can bind and release DNA effectively. Sequencing data prepared on the chip showed an alignment rate over 97% for both sequencing methods. Recently, Snider et al. leveraged magnetic bead motion controlled by an external magnet to navigate DNA-containing paramagnetic beads across the channel containing four aqueous buffers separated by immiscible oil for on-chip NGS library preparation (Snider, Nilsson, Dupal, Toloue, & Tripathi, 2019). The chip greatly simplified operation complexity from the absence of external pumps, valves, and electrode arrays while achieving >94% ± 1% accuracy to reference genome in 660 pg human gDNA. The benefits provided from these microfluidic advancements in automating library preparation will surely encourage a more efficient and widespread use of NGS in the future.

Single-cell genome sequencing has also seen improvements through the use of microfluidics regarding single-cell analyte preparation and library quality. Multiple displacement amplification (MDA) is a widely chosen whole genome amplification (WGA) method to generate adequate genomic DNA for sequencing from a scarce DNA source (i.e., single cell) (Rodrigue et al., 2009). However, MDA suffers from highly nonuniform amplification and one method to minimize this bias is the reduction of reaction volume via physically separated confinements in microfluidics (Marcy et al., 2007). Microfluidic MDA platforms can be categorized into two main formats: separation by fabricated microstructures or by droplet emulsion. Marcy et al. pioneered the first microfluidic single cell MDA which automatically isolate individual *E. coli* cells into nanoliter chambers for subsequent genome amplification (Marcy et al., 2007). The PDMS chip utilize several pneumatic valves for flow control, and on-chip single cell amplification was performed by traversing the solution across different amplification units representing each amplification protocols: cell lysis, DNA denaturation, neutralization, and MDA amplification. After amplification, samples were retrieved for off-chip quantitative polymerase chain reaction (qPCR) for amplification bias examination and for high-throughput pyrosequencing. PCR results were compared with 50 μL MDA control reactions, showing several undetected loci in 50 μL reactions, but all loci were detected in the 60 nL reactions, indicating reduction in bias and better representation for genome sequences. Fu et al. created an emulsion WGA performing single cell MDA in a large number of picoliter aqueous droplets immersed in oil (Fu et al., 2015). After cell lysing, genomic DNA were dehybridized and emulsified into 14 pL droplets containing one DNA fragment (∼10 kb) each on average via PDMS microfluidic cross junction. MDA reaction buffers were also incorporated into each droplet, and after amplification, the resulting DNA products were collected for qPCR and illumina sequencing. The method resulted in a more uniform coverage breadth with reduced amplification bias across the entire genome comparing to conventional MDA and multiple annealing and looping-based amplification cycles (MALBAC). Other recent researches utilized similar microfluidic platforms for massively parallel WGA (Hosokawa, Nishikawa, Kogawa, Takeyama, 2017; Sidore, Lan, Lim, & Abate, 2015; Wang, Fan, Behr, & Quake, 2012), and these microsystems would continue to facilitate advances in single-cell analysis.

b. Gene expression analysis

No cells are completely identical. Recent studies indicated that even genetically identical cells with seemingly identical cell histories and conditions can have significant differences regarding gene expression level (Cai, Friedman, & Xie, 2006; Choi et al., 2008; Raj, Peskin, Tranchina, Vargas, & Tyagi, 2006). Although gene expression is highly regulated for precise coordination within living organisms and is predicable on a general varying trend, the very low copy numbers of genes can cause random fluctuations of mRNA production in individual cells due to the thermal dynamic nature of biochemical reactions of only a few molecules, which cannot be averaged out by statistics of large numbers of reactants and lead to detectable differences in mRNA, protein, and eventually phenotype levels. Traditional analytical methods usually target cell contents extracted from 10^3 to 10^6 cells, the variations of which cannot be completely eliminated even by careful experimental design and control of cell conditions (Carlo & Lee, 2006). Therefore, the information obtained is the average response from a population of cells, which disguise the behaviors of individual cells and potentially give misleading information. Due to the difficulties of manipulating large number of tiny cells and detecting minute changes of low concentrations, conventional single-cell probing approaches usually suffer from intense manual operation, susceptibility to contamination, and extremely high cost. By combining microfabrication technology with these methods or translating the analyses into chip formats, significant improvements can be achieved due to the intrinsic small size and volume of microdevices, which are valuable for cell manipulation, sensitivity improvement, and system scale-up for high throughput operation. Here, we will illustrate several different microfabricated platforms for gene expression analysis by highlighting some impressive research results.

Fluorescence in-situ hybridization (FISH) is a powerful and widely used technique, which allows researchers to quantitatively probe single-copy mRNAs within individual living cells (Levsky, Shenoy, Pezo, & Singer, 2002; Raj et al., 2006). Microfluidic FISH platforms have actually been demonstrated in various approaches and applications. The analytical process normally include the incubation of fluorescence-labelled oligonucleotide probes with target cells followed by excess washes and visualization of cells using confocal fluorescence microscopy. One major hurdle of this method is the cell manipulation step, which can be dramatically improved by microfabrication technology. Matsunaga et al. developed a highly efficient single-cell entrapment system consisting of a microfabricated PET micromesh and PDMS microfluidic channels (Matsunaga et al., 2008). By applying negative pressure on the micromesh, 70%−80% of the introduced Raji Burkitt's lymphoma cells can be trapped and uniformly arranged in the microdevice. On-chip FISH assays including membrane permeabilization, hybridization, washing, and imaging were successfully performed to analyze β-actin mRNA expression in individual cells in a high-throughput manner. Riahi et al. reported a microfluidic device for single cell capture of circulating tumor cells (CTCs) capable of capturing 20−2000 cells with a high reproducibility for subsequent process (Riahi et al., 2014). The multilayer device contained around 56,320 capture chambers with individual pore channels, using cell size and deformability differences to trap single CTC inside each chamber while allowing smaller blood cells to pass through the pores into the outlet reservoir. The system reached 80% cell capture efficiency with minimal leukocyte contamination desirable for CTC detection, and it was later developed into an integrated, automated system commercialized as the Celsee PREP 400 system. Gogoi et al. utilized this label-free CTC capture system to perform DNA and mRNA FISH assays from blood samples of patients with metastatic breast, prostate, and colorectal cancers (Gogoi et al., 2016). The system can run four blood samples simultaneously and automatically dispense liquids into the inlet which are loaded into the chip via a vacuum pump. The system successfully performed both FISH assays, and the development of these systems hopefully would help open up more possibilities for FISH-based microfluidics outside of research laboratories.

Reverse transcription PCR (RT-PCR) plays a central role in gene expression analysis. Many efforts have been made to improve RT-PCR on sensitivity, automation, and throughput by miniaturizing and integrating the whole process on a microdevice. Additionally, since enclosed microsystems can effectively prevent mRNA from exposure to RNases, this reliability can be significantly improved. Chou et al. constructed a multilayer PDMS microsystem using the soft photolithography method, which is capable of performing single-cell lysis, affinity mRNA purification, and cDNA synthesis (Marcus, Anderson, & Quake, 2006a). Two key components implemented in this microsystem assured the success of on-chip quantitative mRNA analysis: enhanced reaction efficiency provided by nL-scale reactors and 100% sample transfer within the microdevice achieved using oligo(dT)-modified paramagnetic beads for mRNA capture. Meanwhile, the same authors also developed a microfluidic reactor array chip which consists of 8×9 (total 72) 450-pL reactors for RT-PCR. Taqman hydrolysis probe chemistry was employed to detect RNA templates with a limit of 34 copies, which are close to mRNA amounts usually obtained from single cells (Marcus, Anderson, & Quake, 2006b). Therefore, it is possible to develop a fully integrated system for gene expression analysis by combining the techniques described above. By using a similar device, Zhong et al. constructed an improved system for extracting total mRNAs from single human embryonic stem cells and synthesizing cDNA directly (Zhong et al., 2008). Bontoux et al. successfully integrated the single-cell trapping, total mRNA extraction, and RT-PCR into a microdevice using similar rotary reactors and PDMS microvalves developed by Bontoux et al. (2008); Chou, Unger, & Quake (2001). Both studies showed increased efficiency in extractions and reactions due to smaller volumes and integrated analytical processes. However, their dependence on off-chip amplification and detection limits their throughput and sensitivity.

The first giant leap forward was made by Toriello et al., describing a fully integrated PCR-CE microsystem with a single-cell sensitivity in measuring single-cell gene expression (Toriello et al., 2008). In this microdevice, single cells surface-modified with oligos can be captured via DNA hybridization by a size-limited gold pad modified with complimentary oligos and located in an RT-PCR reactor. Following cell lysis using dry ice, on-step RT-PCR was performed in this 200-nL reactor with a microfabricated RTD and a heater for 25 min. After amplification, a three-valve PDMS micropump was employed to move amplicons from the reactor to an oligo-modified capture gel matrix, where amplicons were captured, purified, and concentrated. By heating the chip over the DNA melting temperature, amplicons were released into a CE separation channel for a size-based separation. Single Jurkat cell analyses targeting GAPDH and 18S rRNA genes were successfully performed on the microdevice with a total analytical time of <75 min, and clearly revealed gene expression variations of GAPDH between eight individual cells compared with bulk measurement from 50 cells. This microsystem establishes the feasibility of performing single-cell gene expression analysis on an integrated device and provides a powerful tool for scientists to explore the stochastic nature of gene expression. Later, White et al. demonstrated a high-throughput integrated RT-qPCR device capable of performing 300 parallel single cell assays on the platform as shown in Fig. 13.2(a) (White et al., 2011). Steps including cell capture, cell lysis, reverse transcription, and qPCR were implemented

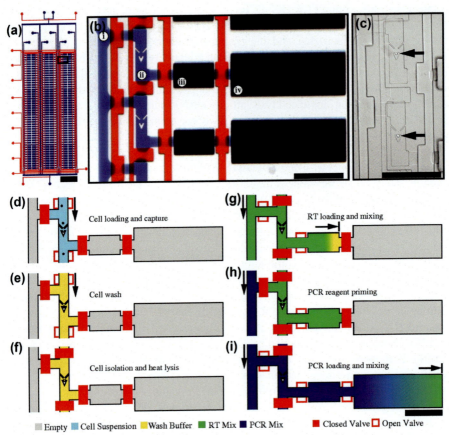

Figure 13.2 Microfluidic device for single-cell gene expression analysis. (a) Schematic of microfluidic device. The device features six sample input channels, each divided into 50 compound reaction chambers for a total of 300 RT-qPCRs (reverse transcription quantitative polymerase chain reactions) using approximately 20 μL of reagents. The *rectangular box* indicates the region depicted in (b). (b) Optical micrograph of array unit. For visualization, the fluid paths and control channels have been loaded with blue and red dyes, respectively. Each unit consists of (i) a reagent injection line, (ii) a 0.6-nL cell capture chamber with integrated cell traps, (iii) a 10-nL RT chamber, and (iv) a 50-nL PCR chamber. (c) Optical micrograph of 2 cell capture chambers with trapped single cells indicated by *black arrows*. Each trap includes upstream deflectors to direct cells into the capture region. (d) A single-cell suspension is injected into the device. (e) Cell traps isolate single cells from the fluid stream and permit washing of cells to remove extracellular RNA. (f) Actuation of pneumatic valves results in single-cell isolation prior to heat lysis. (g) Injection of reagent (green) for RT reaction (10 nL). (h) Reagent injection line is flushed with subsequent reagent (blue) for PCR. (i) Reagent for qPCR (blue) is combined with RT product in 50 nL qPCR chamber.
Adapted with permission from White et al. (2011).

using pneumatic valve actuation for liquid manipulation (Fig. 13.2(d−i)), along with a CCD camera mounted on a thermocycler plate for qPCR fluorescence detection. The reactor chambers were designed for sufficient dilution to avoid reaction inhibition from subpar cell lysate dilution at concentration beyond 10 cells/50 nL reaction. Moreover, RT-qPCR measurement noise became large with concentration below one copy/ 100 nL, and thus the optimized total reaction volume was 60.6 nL: 0.6-nL cell capture chamber, 10-nL RT chamber, and a 50-nL qPCR chamber (Fig. 13.2(b)). The system was applied to investigate single-cell miRNA expression in K562 cells with impressive results. In order to simplify instrumentation of integrated microsystem, Sun et al. reported the use of paramagnetic microbeads for mRNA capture and transport within the integrated RT-qPCR microfluidic chip (Sun et al., 2015). After cell lysis, microbeads containing oligo(dT)$_{25}$ residues were mixed with cell lysate to capture target mRNA templates, and these oligo(dT)$_{25}$ would also function as primers during reverse transcription. Two pneumatic valves were used to divert the flow while the beads can be transported within the device and retained by external magnet, reducing excessive use of microvalves thus simplifying the device complexity.

Another promising method to facilitate massively high-throughput single-cell mRNA analysis on a microsystem is the use of microemulsions. Single cells can be efficiently encapsulated into droplets that contain the necessary reagents for enzymatic amplifications (Edd et al., 2008; He et al., 2005; Kumaresan, Yang, Cronier, Blazej, & Mathies, 2008). The research by Mathies et al. showed that single-cell PCR can be performed within droplets (Kumaresan et al., 2008). Single-copy real-time reverse-transcription PCR was successfully demonstrated in isolated picolitre droplets (Beer et al., 2007, 2008). Advances regarding high-throughput mRNA profiling using droplets have been made in recent years. Macosko et al. developed the "Drop-Seq" technique for massively parallel analysis of mRNA expression in thousands of individual cells by partitioning single cells into droplets while remembering the cell's identity for each mRNA transcript (Macosko et al., 2015). A barcoding strategy was applied in synthesizing oligonucleotides on the beads such that each bead consists of the same set of "cell barcode" and "unique molecular identifier" (UMI) oligonucleotide regions that are different from other beads. Each bead is then coencapsulated with a single cell to capture its mRNA after cell lysis, which were collected for further off-chip reverse transcription, amplification, and sequencing. 44,808 mouse retinal cells were analyzed, showing 39 distinct populations and their differently expressed genes. We are excited to see higher degree of integration for these high-throughput, droplet-based microfluidics in realizing sample-in-answer-out capability in the future.

c. Pathogen/infectious disease detection

Another application that microchip technology can play an important role is in pathogen or infectious disease detection, where POC analysis is highly desirable (Ivnitski et al., 2003; Yeung, Lee, Cai, & Hsing, 2006). Routine standards for pathogen detection rely on culture plating and microscopy technologies, which are time-consuming and sometimes even not applicable since culture methods may be unknown. Ideally, new POC diagnostic devices should be fast, sensitive, accurate, cost-effective, and easy to use with minimal user intervention. Portability and disposability are also highly desirable especially for resource-limited settings or single-use devices. The benefits of microfluidics provide a potential solution to meet these criteria, and many integrated microfluidic systems have been created in recent years, demonstrating the capability of rapid, decentralized detection of various pathogens. In this section, advances in integrated microsystems and potential technologies based on nucleic acids for pathogen detection will be examined.

To replace culture-based methods, PCR-based detection technology has found a widespread-use for pathogen detection due to its speed, sensitivity (down to a single copy), as well as its capability of detecting minute amounts of targets from a huge nonpathogenic background. Real-time PCR is a potential method for rapid detection on a chip format because its combination of DNA amplification and detection on a single structure simplifies system design and operation. The first handheld real-time thermal cycler for bacterial detection was demonstrated by Higgins et al. (2003). This 1 kg in weight handheld advanced nucleic acid analyser (HANAA) can perform up to four real-time PCRs in about 30 min using a 12V battery pack. Later, the integration of real-time PCR with sample preparation on a single device was also explored (Cady, Stelick, Kunnavakkam, & Batt, 2005). A silicon microdevice, consisting of a serpentine microchannel filled with silica pillars for DNA purification and a chamber for real-time PCR amplification and detection, was packed with all the necessary electronics and optics into a suitcase-sized instrument for purposes of on-site analysis. As low as 10^4 *L. monocytogenes* cells could be detected in about 45 min using this system. Oblath et al. reported an integrated real-time PCR device utilizing monolithic aluminum oxide membrane (AOM) for on-chip DNA extraction (Oblath, Henley, Alarie, & Ramsey, 2013). The use of AOM eliminated subsequent washing steps required by other DNA extraction procedures. On-chip DNA extraction, amplification, and detection were demonstrated for identification of *Streptococcus mutans* in a saliva sample. These systems still required certain degree of user intervention like off-chip cell lysis or manual introduction of uncured PDMS into the outlet to seal the device in the later example, not yet achieving sample-in-answer-out capability.

Chip-based CE following DNA amplification can provide not only high sensitivity but also the capability of detecting multiple targets since additional information regarding amplicon sizes can be obtained through DNA separation. A portable system consisting of an integrated PCR-CE microdevice and a compact instrument for electrical control and laser-induced fluorescence detection has been developed by Lagally et al. (2004). The limit of detection of this system was determined as two to three bacterial cells using *E. coli* K12, and a complete run can be completed in 20 min. Analysis of both methicillin-sensitive and methicillin-resistant *S. aureus* directly from intact cells was also successfully performed on the microsystem. This integrated genetic analyser established the feasibility of on-site pathogen detection using electrophoresis as the final detection method. Prakash et al. integrated nine independent PCR chambers with one CE separation channel on a single chip for simultaneous amplification and sequential detection of respiratory pathogen *Bordetella Pertussis* (Prakash, De la Rosa, Fox, & Kaler, 2008). Nevertheless, these PCR-CE systems may suffer from low or even no PCR amplifications when processing crude samples containing PCR inhibitors due to the lack of integrated sample preparation step prior to PCR. Beyor et al. presented an integrated PCR-CE microdevice with cell preconcentration and purification on a single device (Beyor, Yi, Seo, & Mathies, 2009). *E. coli* cells are driven and captured on a fluidized immunomagnetic bead bed immobilized in microchannels. Cell-bead conjugates can be precisely transported and located into the PCR chamber using on-chip pumps and external magnets without delicate timing issues. An impressive sensitivity of 0.2 cfu/μL *E. coli* O157 cells in a 50 μL input volume was obtained on this integrated system.

To achieve sample-in-answer-out capability, Landers et al. developed an integrated microfluidic genetic analysis system (Fig. 13.3(a−c)), which can perform three major DNA processing steps: DNA extraction, PCR amplification, and electrophoretic separation (Easley et al., 2006). The entire analysis timeline, as shown in Fig. 13.3(d), is < 24 min, which is about 10 times less than conventional methods. DNA extraction from whole blood or nasal aspirate was performed in a microchannel packed with silica beads in under 10 min. The purified DNA samples together with a PCR mix were moved into a 550-nL PCR chamber, where rapid thermal cycling was conducted using a noncontact IR heating system in under 11 min. After that, PCR products and a sizing standard were pressure-injected into a separation channel for electrophoresis using an on-chip diaphragm pump. Although the detection limits of this system were not thoroughly investigated, the successful analyses of *Bacillus anthracis* (anthrax) in 750 nL of whole blood and of *Bordetella pertussis* in 1 μL of nasal aspirate from a patient clearly indicate the wide application of this integrated system for rapid and large-scale screening of disease outbreaks. Chen et al. demonstrated another sample-to-answer disposable microchip for the detection of pathogenic bacteria and HIV virus (Chen et al., 2010). The microchip is self-contained, with all the required buffers and dry PCR reagents stored in storage pouches and paraffin-passivated reaction chamber, respectively (Fig. 13.4(a) and (b)). The pouches were sealed with a removable aluminum tape while the paraffin film can be melted at 58°C before use. PCR-based procedure involved on-chip cell lysis, nucleic acid extraction using silica fiber matrix, nucleic acid purification, real-time PCR, or RT-PCR amplification depending on target molecule and fluorescence detection on an integrated lateral flow strip. A portable analyzer was used for fluid handling and thermocycling, and the system achieved a detection limit of 10^3 to 10^4 cells/mL for *B. Cereus* cells and 10^5 HIV virions/mL from saliva samples. More recently, Stumpf et al. reported the first fully automated, sample-to-answer centrifugal LabDisk with complete reagents prestorage for detecting respiratory pathogen (Stumpf et al., 2016). Liquid buffers were stored in aluminum stick-packs (van Oordt, Barb, Smetana, Zengerle, & von Stetten, 2013) which open from liquid pressure at certain rotation frequency, making sample loading the only manual liquid handling step. After initial sample introduction, the LabDisk was mounted on a prototype LabDisk player where lysis, bead-based nucleic acid

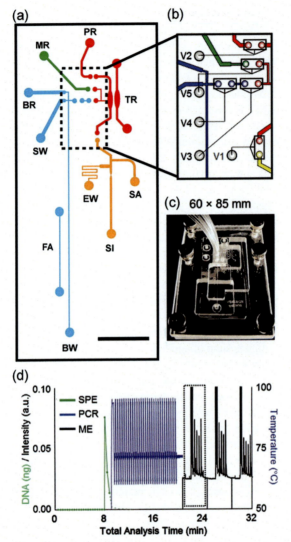

Figure 13.3 A fully integrated microfluidic genetic analysis system for pathogen detection. (a) Schematic of the microdevice. This device contains three domains for DNA extraction (yellow), polymerase chain reaction (PCR) amplification (red), and capillary electrophoresis (CE) separation (blue). All the reservoirs and structures are labeled as: sample inlet (SI), sidearm (SA), and extraction waste (EW) for DNA extraction; PCR reservoir (PR), marker reservoir (MR), sample waste (SW), and temperature reference (TR) chamber for PCR; buffer reservoir (BR), buffer waste (BW), and fluorescence alignment (FA) channel for electrophoresis. (b) Expanded view of the polydimethylsiloxane (PDMS) microvalves integrated on the chip for microfluidic control. V1 for the separation of PCR and DNA extraction domains. V2–V3–V4 forming a pump for sample pressure injection. V5–V3–V4 forming a pump for sizing ladder pressure injection. (c) A photograph of the chip assembly. (d) The timeline of the entire analysis performed on the microdevice. The *green line* is the DNA concentrations released from the solid-phase DNA extraction column as a function of time. The *blue line* is the temperature cycling profile for PCR. The *black line* is the three sequential separation traces.
Adapted with permission from Easley et al. (2006), Copyright (2006) National Academy of Sciences, U.S.A.

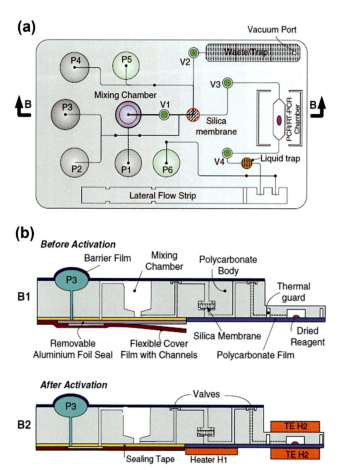

Figure 13.4 Schematic of the polycarbonate fluidic chip consisting of reagents storage pouches (P1–P6), on-chip diaphragm valves (V1–V4), a mixing chamber, a nucleic acid isolation chamber housing a silica membrane, a reverse transcription quantitative polymerase chain reactions (RT-PCR) chamber preloaded with dried reagents, an amplicon dilution trap, a waste chamber and liquid trap, and a lateral flow strip. (a) Top view; (b) cross sections of the cassette (indicated with the *arrows* B–B in (a) showing the cassette in storage state (B1) and operating (after activation) state (B2). Heaters H1 and H2 are components of the analyzer but not of the cassette. "TE" denotes the thermoelectric modules.
Reprinted from Chen et al. (2010) with permission of Springer Nature.

extraction, washing-elution, real-time RT-PCR were automatically executed. The device demonstrated the successful detection of influenza A H3N2 virus at 2.39×10^4 RNA copies per mL within 3.5 h. With further optimization and increase in multiplexing capabilities, the integrated PCR-based analyzers could potentially offer early diagnostics in POC testing.

An emerging technology recently applied in pathogen detection is digital PCR (dPCR) which offers absolute quantification of target nucleic acid without the need for standard curves by separating the sample into thousands of nanoliter-sized partitions. There are currently two commonly used microfluidic dPCR formats: microchamber dPCR (Ottesen, Hong, Quake, & Leadbetter, 2006) or droplet dPCR (Hindson et al., 2011). White et al. utilized microfluidic RT-dPCR to quantify an occult RNA virus GB Virus Type C (coinfected with HIV-1) in cell supernatant by using the 48.770 Digital Array microfluidic chip from Fluidigm (White, Quake, & Curr, 2012). The device can process up to 48 samples per chip with a total of 36,960 nL-sized chambers. Individual target molecules were physically confined within each chamber resulting in the presence or absence of target in the chambers, enabling digital counting of positive chambers after amplification and calculation of target concentration. Strain et al. demonstrated the first use of droplet dPCR in quantifying HIV DNA targets in human blood samples (Strain et al., 2013). Droplet generation was performed by Bio-Rad QX-100 system where sample containing PCR reaction mixture and oil containing surfactants were flown through a flow-focusing junction, generating monodisperse droplets at high throughput. Each reaction was confined within individual droplets with volume of 0.91 nL, and positive droplets were quantified. Both studies showed an increase in precision and sensitivity of dPCR over qPCR, desirable for detecting low copies of target nucleic acid in high background. Recently, Athamanolap et al. developed the first microfluidic platform capable of performing both multiple bacterial identification and antimicrobial susceptibility test on a single device from a polymicrobial sample (Athamanolap et al., 2019). Samples were separated into two parts: one was exposed to antibiotic of interest and one was not, and after off-chip preparation, both samples were separately loaded onto the nanoarray platform comprised of multiple 1 nL chamber array modules. On-chip dPCR utilizing universal primer was performed to amplify all isolated bacterial DNAs followed by high resolution melt (HRM) to obtain HRM profiles of individual wells for bacterial species quantification and identification via machine-learning algorithm. Difference in occupancy ratio of the bacteria in both modules represented whether it is a susceptible or resistant strain, and five different bacteria commonly found in urinary tract infection were correctly identified with 4 h total turnaround time. Despite the intrinsic benefits of dPCR, the integration of on-chip sample preparation presents a challenge and further development is needed to fully realize the potential of dPCR as a fully integrated POC system.

To overcome the requirements of precise and rapid temperature control for thermocycling in PCR-based systems, isothermal nucleic acid amplification methods offer promising alternatives for POC devices. Examples of commonly used isothermal technologies in pathogen detection include loop-mediated isothermal amplification (LAMP), recombinase polymerase amplification (RPA), nucleic acid sequence-based amplification (NASBA) and helicase-dependent amplification (HDA). Liu et al. reported a fully integrated disposable microfluidic cassette using LAMP for detecting HIV virus in oral fluids (Liu et al., 2011a). The cassette device consists of a single chamber containing Flinders Technology Associates (FTA) membrane for isolating target RNA and removal of inhibitors. Target capture, purification, LAMP amplification, and real-time fluorescence detection were performed in a single chamber, with the cassette mounted on a holder containing thin film heater, thermocouple, and mounted optical reader. A detection limit of <10 HIV particles was demonstrated. Kim et al. presented the use of RPA in a fully automated, integrated centrifugal microfluidic for the detection of *Salmonella enteritidis* (Kim, Park, Kim, & Cho, 2014). The major processing steps including DNA extraction, isothermal amplification, and detection were performed on chip. Sample enrichment was done using immunomagnetic bead separation before loading, and laser diode was applied for cell lysis, microvalve control, and noncontact heating during amplification. The whole procedure was done within 30 min with detection limits of 10 CFU/mL and 10^2 CFU/mL of *Salmonella* in phosphate-buffered saline (PBS) and milk, respectively. To reduce operation complexity and dependence on off-chip amplification instrument, Tang et al. demonstrated a sample-in-answer-out, paper-based microfluidic system performing the HDA-based method for nucleic acid testing (Tang et al., 2017). The battery-powered device consisted of three modules corresponding to the three major processing steps. DNA extraction buffers were stored in sponge-based reservoirs sealed with sealing rubbers, and amplification reagents were dry-stored. After the sample introduction, DNA extraction can be initiated with the press of a button where DNA was captured by Fusion 5 disk then simultaneously moved with HDA reagents to amplification module. Colorimetric signal was visible with the naked eye on a lateral flow strip, showing successful detection of *Salmonella typhimurium* with a detection limit of 10^2 CFU/mL within 1 h. Future advances in integration and cost reduction of these isothermal systems would make them powerful POC genetic analysis tools in resource-limited settings.

d. Short tandem repeat analysis

STR assays have become an indispensable and routine technique in forensic investigations due to their ability to produce highly distinctive profiles from minute amounts of DNA (Andersen et al., 1996; Butler, 2006; Chakraborty, Stivers, Su, Zhong, & Budowle, 1999; Jobling & Gill, 2004). The current STR typing process includes DNA extraction from collected evidences, DNA quantitation for sample characterization, multiplex PCR amplification using an STR typing kit, and amplicon separation and detection using a slab gel or capillary electrophoresis. Although the automation of the STR analytical process is underway using robotics (Butler et al., 2004; Greenspoon et al., 2006; Montpetit, Fitch, & O'Donnell, 2005), a mere displacement of manual operations with automated instruments can only provide a limited degree of improvement, as this process is still performed in μL-scale volume on several bulky instruments. The limited genotyping technologies and the rising number of DNA samples submitted for DNA testing have resulted in an escalating backlog of crime scene evidence pending examination in forensic laboratories worldwide. In addition to the huge demands for STR typing, forensic investigators are facing a unique challenge, in that forensic casework samples usually have lower amplification efficiency due to DNA degradation by exposure to environmental elements or natural contaminants, or low copy number DNA extracted from "touch evidence" (Butler, Shen, & McCord, 2003; Gill et al., 2000; Whitaker, Cotton, & Gill, 2001; Wickenheiser, 2002). Integrated microfluidic systems can substantially improve STR typing by miniaturization, potentially offering system portability for on-site analysis.

In the past few decades, impressive progress has been achieved in the translation of STR analysis procedure to microchip-based instruments. Ehrlich et al. demonstrated baseline resolved separations of single-locus STR samples in 30 s using a microfabricated CE microchip with a 2.6-cm-long separation channel (Schmalzing et al., 1997). Analyses of PCR samples containing four loci (CSF1PO, TPOX, THO1, and vWA) were completed in under 2 min. Mathies et al. presented a 96-channel microfabricated capillary array electrophoresis (μCAE) device coupled with a four-colour confocal fluorescence scanner for high-throughput STR typing (Yeung et al., 2006b). A prototype of the Berkeley μCAE device was successfully installed at the Virginia Department of Forensic Science for testing of routine forensic STR analyses (Greenspoon et al., 2008). Regarding amplification, Liu et al. constructed an integrated PCR-CE microdevice for forensic STR analysis, as well as a portable analysis instrument containing all the electronics and optics for chip operation and four-colour fluorescence detection (Liu et al., 2007). Multiplex amplification of amelogenin and three Y STR loci (DYS390, DYS393, DYS439) with 35 PCR cycles and CE separation were completed in 1.5 h with a detection limit of 20 copies of genomic DNA. To further explore the concept of performing rapid STR analyses outside of forensic laboratory, they conducted real-time DNA analyses at a mock crime scene (Liu et al., 2008). The crime scene was investigated following standard procedures, and three blood stain samples were extracted, amplified, and correctly typed at the scene. A DNA profile search against a mock CODIS database with a "convicted offender" sample was successfully conducted within 6 hours of arrival at the crime scene. The miniaturization of other "upstream" STR steps is also under investigation toward fully integrated microfluidic systems for automated STR analysis. For example, Bienvenue et al. developed a single-channel extraction device and method for on-chip sperm cell lysis and DNA purification, which has direct implications on forensic STR analysis (Bienvenue, Duncalf, Marchiarullo, Ferrance, & Landers, 2006). The purity and concentration of the DNA samples obtained from on-chip extraction were verified using conventional STR amplification and separation. Later, they reported another glass microdevice that integrated a silica bead column and a PCR chamber together for fast DNA extraction and STR amplification from whole blood samples (Bienvenue, Legendre, Ferrance, & Landers, 2010). The successful technology transfer and demonstration of on-site STR typing at a crime scene validates the feasibility of real-time human identification for crime scene investigation using microfluidics.

To improve the sensitivity of conventional STR analysis, post-PCR sample purification prior to CE has been employed (Smith & Ballantyne, 2007). Yeung et al. have developed an integrated STR sample cleanup and separation microdevice and method that employs a streptavidin capture gel chemistry coupled to a simple direct-injection geometry (Yeung, Liu, Del Bueno, Greenspoon, & Mathies, 2009). Compared to microchip CE experiments performed using a cross-injector under similar conditions, fluorescence intensity can be improved by 10−50 times for monoplex samples, and 14−19-fold for nine-plex STR products. The analyses of two artificial degraded DNA samples on the inline-injection CE microchip provided ∼33% and ∼71% more allelic markers, respectively, than those on the cross-injection chip. This enhanced sensitivity is highly valuable for low copy number and degraded DNA typing. Furthermore, the capture structure incorporated into the high-throughput μCAE has also been reported (Liu, Scherer, Greenspoon, Chiesl, & Mathies, 2011). The near 100% amplicon product transfer between processing steps provided by the capture, concentration, and inline injection method should significantly advance the STR typing on the sensitivity, robustness, and data quality for a variety of applications.

After the successful translation of benchtop STR processes onto a microfluidic format, several groups later demonstrated fully integrated microsystems for forensic STR typing. Hopwood et al. successfully developed an integrated microfluidic system that consists of a DNA extraction and amplification cartridge coupled with a CE microchip for rapid STR analysis from reference buccal samples (Hopwood et al., 2010). An aliquot of 150 μL of the sample lysate was introduced into the extraction and amplification cartridge. Using several electrochemical pumps and wax valves, the lysate was first mixed with ChargeSwitch magnetic beads for DNA extraction. Then, the purified DNA was loaded into a 10-μL PCR chamber where PowerPlex ESI 16 PCR mix was prepackaged. After amplification, amplicons along with preloaded sizing standards were injected into a separated CE chip via tubing for separation. During the overall analytical process, no manual operation was needed. Liu et al. developed a fully integrated μTAS that includes sequence-specific DNA template purification, PCR, post-PCR cleanup and capture inline injection, and CE (Liu et al., 2011b). While these systems demonstrated impressive performances, complicated operations need to be overcome before they can be practically applied in real forensic cases. Le Roux et al. reported a compact, integrated sample-in-answer-out microchip for STR typing from buccal swab or FTA paper (Le Roux et al., 2014). The system incorporated heat-activated enzyme for DNA preparation, removing the need for washing steps and additional reservoirs. PCR amplification utilized noncontact IR heating, and electrophoresis separation was carried out in a microchannel with an effective length of only 7 cm achievable by hydrophobically modified polyacrylamide polymer. An 18-plex STR profile was successfully generated in 2 h from buccal swab or FTA paper. To eliminate microvalve/pump, Kim et al. developed a slidable, valveless microsystem performing solid phase DNA extraction, PCR, and CE required for on-site STR typing (Kim et al., 2016). Each step can be independently performed, and sample transport between each compartment was easily done by simply sliding the topmost slidable chamber to different processing unit. The detection of amelogenin and mini Y STR loci was demonstrated from human whole blood within 60 min. Recently, Liu's group reported a fully integrated microsystem combining disposable plastic DNA extraction and amplification (DEA) chip with glass capillary array electrophoresis (CAE) chip for automated STR analysis as shown in Fig. 13.5(a) (Han et al., 2017). The system was built upon the group's previous work on a sample-to-answer microsystem for pharmacogenetic analysis where filter paper–based DNA extraction and "in situ" PCR were performed directly in the same chamber without elution, and a needle-shaped injection electrode was used for effective sample transfer to the CAE chip (Zhuang et al., 2016). Here, DEA chip was redesigned into a three-layered structure to reduce DNA polymerase

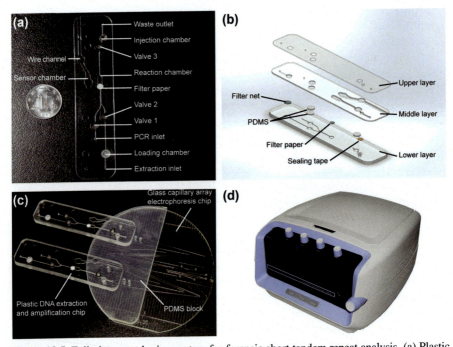

Figure 13.5 Fully integrated microsystem for forensic short tandem repeat analysis. (a) Plastic DNA extraction and amplification microchip. The extraction and polymerase chain reaction (PCR) unit contains an extraction inlet, a PCR inlet, a waste outlet, a loading chamber, a reaction chamber, an injection chamber, and three microvalves. (b) Exploded view of the DNA extraction and amplification (DEA) microchip structure. The microchip was formed by three poly(methyl methacrylate) (PMMA) layers sandwiched together with embedded polydimethylsiloxane (PDMS), nylon filter, and Fusion 5 filter. (c) Assembled microdevice containing two plastic DNA extraction and amplification chips and a glass capillary array electrophoresis chip. (d) Photograph of the compact instrument for microdevice control and detection. The instrument with dimensions of 48 × 35 × 35 cm contains a confocal optical system for detecting four different fluorescence signals, four high-voltage power supplies for electrophoresis, a fluidic control system, and all the electronics for system operation. Reproduced from Han et al. (2017) with permission of The Royal Society of Chemistry.

adsorption (Fig. 13.5(b)), and various PCR additive including bovine serum albumin (BSA), polyethylene glycol (PEG), and MgCl2 were optimized for an improved PCR efficiency. After the pretreatment of the CAE chip, samples were pipetted into the DEA which was sealed and assembled with the CAE chip (Fig. 13.5(c)) on a control and detection instrument that automatically carried out the remaining STR process (Fig. 13.5(d)). The generated STR profile correctly resolved all alleles from both oral swab and venous blood samples with a total analysis time of around 2 h. The implementation of the Fusion 5 filter paper in the reaction chamber for "in situ" PCR drastically simplified the DEA system while the reversible assembly of DEA and CAE chips offered the versatility in processing diverse forensic sample types as different DEA chip can be designed and easily swapped by the users. Building on the modular integration concept, the group later demonstrated the first modular-based, fully integrated microsystem with two different sample preparation modules (SPMs) for processing different forensic DNA samples (Gu et al., 2019). The first SPM module named "direct SPM" was used for direct PCR procedure of buccal swab sample and the "extraction SPM," with additional sample loading chamber and quartz filter paper, was for more challenging samples. The newly developed chitosan-modified quartz filter paper was utilized for DNA extraction, providing >90% DNA capture efficiency with a low PCR inhibition effect compared to other/unmodified filter papers. The system successfully generated full STR profile from 1 ng of buccal swab without DNA extraction in around 2 h and showcased that full STR profile can be automatically obtained from minute amount of blood (0.25 μL), highly diluted blood (0.5 μL blood in 1 mL buffer), and latent bloodstains (5 μL bloodstain on cloth washed with detergent). Even though several crude sample processing steps are still done off-chip, the modular strategy offered an increase in utility for fully integrated microsystems in tackling wider forensic samples for a more practical use in different applications.

13.5 Future of integrated microfluidic systems

Over the past 2 decades, microfluidic devices for genetic analysis have advanced rapidly. From early efforts in translating benchtop analytical steps into chip formats to successful demonstrations of fully integrated microsystems with superior performance over their conventional counterparts, microfluidic devices have proven themselves to be a promising powerful tool for the ever-growing field of genetic analysis. Although many companies have invested in developing and commercializing this new technology, the majority of the research and clinical societies are not fully embracing microfluidic solutions. This is because most microfluidic systems to date only function as one single conventional step in the overall multistep process or is only optimized for one specific application. Moreover, many still rely heavily on manual human intervention and the support from off-chip instruments in order to function properly, with different microsystems requiring different custom components. The lack of standardization, additional time, and capital investments needed to adopt microfluidic techniques limit its widespread use and still outweigh the advantages offered by microfluidics.

We believe fully integrated microfluidic systems, which contain all the necessary analytical steps and provide a complete solution to users, are the inevitable direction to look toward to in finding the "killer app" for microfluidics. Multiple researches have shown the potentials of these integrated systems in providing extraordinary advantages for genetic analysis while still harboring the same benefits offered by discrete microchips. Full automation of the whole analysis process can be realized with faster and better assay performance achievable even from minimally trained personnel. Future systems may be more self-contained with all reagents prestored on the device, robotics may play a bigger role for further automation, and standardized components in performing common chip functions may become more universal. As the field continue to mature, we will start to see more commercialized microsystems with higher degrees of integration, sensitivity, throughput, and versatility but for a lower cost per assay. We are certain that with a team effort from both academia and industry, the future of integrated microsystems looks bright.

References

Abee, T., van Schaik, W., & Siezen, R. J. (2004). Impact of genomics on microbial food safety. *Trends in Biotechnology, 22*, 653–660. https://doi.org/10.1016/j.tibtech.2004.10.007

Aborn, J. H., El-Difrawy, S. A., Novotny, M., Gismondi, E. A., Lam, R., Matsudaira, P., et al. (2005). A 768-lane microfabricated system for high-throughput DNA sequencing. *Lab on a Chip, 5*, 669–674. https://doi.org/10.1039/B501104C

Acar, M., Mettetal, J. T., & van Oudenaarden, A. (2008). Stochastic switching as a survival strategy in fluctuating environments. *Nature Genetics, 40*, 471–475. https://doi.org/10.1038/ng.110

Al-Faqheri, W., Ibrahim, F., Thio, T. H. G., Aeinehvand, M. M., Arof, H., & Madou, M. (2015). Development of novel passive check valves for the microfluidic CD platform. *Sensors and Actuators A: Physical, 222*, 245–254. https://doi.org/10.1016/j.sna.2014.12.018

Andersen, J. F., Greenhalgh, M. J., Butler, H. R., Kilpatrick, S. R., Piercy, R. C., Way, K. A., et al. (1996). Further validation of a multiplex STR system for use in routine forensic identity testing. *Forensic Science International, 78*, 47–64. https://doi.org/10.1016/0379-0738(95)01861-1

Athamanolap, P., Hsieh, K., O'Keefe, C. M., Zhang, Y., Yang, S., & Wang, T.-H. (2019). Nanoarray digital polymerase chain reaction with high-resolution melt for enabling broad bacteria identification and pheno–molecular antimicrobial susceptibility test. *Analytical Chemistry, 91*, 12784–12792. https://doi.org/10.1021/acs.analchem.9b02344

Backhouse, C., Caamano, M., Oaks, F., Nordman, E., Carrillo, A., Johnson, B., et al. (2000). DNA sequencing in a monolithic microchannel device. *Electrophoresis, 21*, 150–156. https://doi.org/10.1002/(sici)1522-2683(20000101)21:1<150::Aid-elps150>3.0.Co;2-5

Baek, S.-K., Yoon, Y.-K., Jeon, H.-S., Seo, S., & Park, J.-H. (2013). A wireless sequentially actuated microvalve system. *Journal of Micromechanics and Microengineering, 23*, 045006. https://doi.org/10.1088/0960-1317/23/4/045006

Becker, H., & Gärtner, C. (2008). Polymer microfabrication technologies for microfluidic systems. *Analytical and Bioanalytical Chemistry, 390*, 89−111. https://doi.org/10.1007/s00216-007-1692-2

Beckmann, J. S., Estivill, X., & Antonarakis, S. E. (2007). Copy number variants and genetic traits: Closer to the resolution of phenotypic to genotypic variability. *Nature Reviews Genetics, 8*, 639−646. https://doi.org/10.1038/nrg2149

Beer, N. R., Hindson, B. J., Wheeler, E. K., Hall, S. B., Rose, K. A., Kennedy, I. M., et al. (2007). On-chip, real-time, single-copy polymerase chain reaction in picoliter droplets. *Analytical Chemistry, 79*, 8471−8475. https://doi.org/10.1021/ac701809w

Beer, N. R., Wheeler, E. K., Lee-Houghton, L., Watkins, N., Nasarabadi, S., Hebert, N., et al. (2008). On-chip single-copy real-time reverse-transcription PCR in isolated picoliter droplets. *Analytical Chemistry, 80*, 1854−1858. https://doi.org/10.1021/ac800048k

Berti, L., Medintz, I. L., Tom, J., & Mathies, R. A. (2001). Energy-transfer cassette labeling for capillary array electrophoresis short tandem repeat DNA fragment sizing. *Bioconjugate Chemistry, 12*, 493−500. https://doi.org/10.1021/bc000155w

Beyor, N., Seo, T. S., Liu, P., & Mathies, R. A. (2008). Immunomagnetic bead-based cell concentration microdevice for dilute pathogen detection. *Biomedical Microdevices, 10*, 909. https://doi.org/10.1007/s10544-008-9206-3

Beyor, N., Yi, L., Seo, T. S., & Mathies, R. A. (2009). Integrated capture, concentration, polymerase chain reaction, and capillary electrophoretic analysis of pathogens on a chip. *Analytical Chemistry, 81*, 3523−3528. https://doi.org/10.1021/ac900060r

Bienvenue, J. M., Duncalf, N., Marchiarullo, D., Ferrance, J. P., & Landers, J. P. (2006). Microchip-based cell lysis and DNA extraction from sperm cells for application to forensic analysis. *Journal of Forensic Sciences, 51*, 266−273. https://doi.org/10.1111/j.1556-4029.2006.00054.x

Bienvenue, J. M., Legendre, L. A., Ferrance, J. P., & Landers, J. P. (2010). An integrated microfluidic device for DNA purification and PCR amplification of STR fragments. *Forensic Science International: Genetics, 4*, 178−186. https://doi.org/10.1016/j.fsigen.2009.02.010

Blais, A., & Dynlacht, B. D. (2005). Constructing transcriptional regulatory networks. *Genes and Development, 19*, 1499−1511.

Blazej, R. G., Kumaresan, P., Cronier, S. A., & Mathies, R. A. (2007). Inline injection microdevice for attomole-scale sanger DNA sequencing. *Analytical Chemistry, 79*, 4499−4506. https://doi.org/10.1021/ac070126f

Blazej, R. G., Kumaresan, P., & Mathies, R. A. (2006). Microfabricated bioprocessor for integrated nanoliter-scale Sanger DNA sequencing. *Proceedings of the National Academy of Sciences of the United States of America, 103*, 7240. https://doi.org/10.1073/pnas.0602476103

Blow, N. (2008). DNA sequencing: Generation next-next. *Nature Methods, 5*, 267−274. https://doi.org/10.1038/nmeth0308-267

Bontoux, N., Dauphinot, L., Vitalis, T., Studer, V., Chen, Y., Rossier, J., et al. (2008). Integrating whole transcriptome assays on a lab-on-a-chip for single cell gene profiling. *Lab on a Chip, 8*, 443−450. https://doi.org/10.1039/B716543A

Buchanan, J. A., & Scherer, S. W. (2008). Contemplating effects of genomic structural variation. *Genetics in Medicine, 10*, 639−647. https://doi.org/10.1097/GIM.0b013e318183f848

Burns, M. A., Mastrangelo, C. H., Sammarco, T. S., Man, F. P., Webster, J. R., Johnsons, B. N., et al. (1996). Microfabricated structures for integrated DNA analysis. *Proceedings of the National Academy of Sciences of the United States of America, 93*, 5556. https://doi.org/10.1073/pnas.93.11.5556

Butler, J. M. (2006). Genetics and genomics of core short tandem repeat loci used in human identity testing. *Journal of Forensic Sciences, 51*, 253–265. https://doi.org/10.1111/j.1556-4029.2006.00046.x

Butler, J. M., Buel, E., Crivellente, F., & McCord, B. R. (2004). Forensic DNA typing by capillary electrophoresis using the ABI Prism 310 and 3100 genetic analyzers for STR analysis. *Electrophoresis, 25*, 1397–1412. https://doi.org/10.1002/elps.200305822

Butler, J. M., Shen, Y., & McCord, B. R. (2003). The development of reduced size STR amplicons as tools for analysis of degraded DNA. *Journal of Forensic Sciences, 48*, 1054–1064.

Cady, N. C., Stelick, S., Kunnavakkam, M. V., & Batt, C. A. (2005). Real-time PCR detection of Listeria monocytogenes using an integrated microfluidics platform. *Sensors and Actuators B: Chemical, 107*, 332–341. https://doi.org/10.1016/j.snb.2004.10.022

Cai, L., Friedman, N., & Xie, X. S. (2006). Stochastic protein expression in individual cells at the single molecule level. *Nature, 440*, 358–362. https://doi.org/10.1038/nature04599

Calvo, S., Jain, M., Xie, X., Sheth, S. A., Chang, B., Goldberger, O. A., et al. (2006). Systematic identification of human mitochondrial disease genes through integrative genomics. *Nature Genetics, 38*, 576–582. https://doi.org/10.1038/ng1776

Carlo, D. D., & Lee, L. P. (2006). Dynamic single-cell analysis for quantitative biology. *Analytical Chemistry, 78*, 7918–7925. https://doi.org/10.1021/ac069490p

Chakraborty, R., Stivers, D. N., Su, B., Zhong, Y., & Budowle, B. (1999). The utility of short tandem repeat loci beyond human identification: Implications for development of new DNA typing systems. *Electrophoresis, 20*, 1682–1696. https://doi.org/10.1002/(SICI)1522-2683(19990101)20:8<1682::AID-ELPS1682>3.0.CO;2-Z

Chang, Y.-M., Ding, S.-T., Lin, E.-C., Wang, L., & Lu, Y.-W. (2017). A microfluidic chip for rapid single nucleotide polymorphism (SNP) genotyping using primer extension on microbeads. *Sensors and Actuators B: Chemical, 246*, 215–224. https://doi.org/10.1016/j.snb.2017.01.160

Check, E. (2005). Human genome: Patchwork people. *Nature, 437*, 1084–1086. https://doi.org/10.1038/4371084a

Chen, H., Acharya, D., Gajraj, A., & Meiners, J.-C. (2003). Robust interconnects and packaging for microfluidic elastomeric chips. *Analytical Chemistry, 75*, 5287–5291. https://doi.org/10.1021/ac034179i

Chen, S., Lu, S., Liu, Y., Wang, J., Tian, X., Liu, G., et al. (2016). A normally-closed piezoelectric micro-valve with flexible stopper. *AIP Advances, 6*, 045112. https://doi.org/10.1063/1.4947301

Chen, D., Mauk, M., Qiu, X., Liu, C., Kim, J., Ramprasad, S., et al. (2010). An integrated, self-contained microfluidic cassette for isolation, amplification, and detection of nucleic acids. *Biomedical Microdevices, 12*, 705–719. https://doi.org/10.1007/s10544-010-9423-4

Chiesl, T. N., Putz, K. W., Babu, M., Mathias, P., Shaikh, K. A., Goluch, E. D., et al. (2006). Self-associating block copolymer networks for microchip electrophoresis provide enhanced DNA separation via "inchworm" chain dynamics. *Analytical Chemistry, 78*, 4409–4415. https://doi.org/10.1021/ac060193u

Choi, P. J., Cai, L., Frieda, K., & Xie, X. S. (2008). A stochastic single-molecule event triggers phenotype switching of a bacterial cell. *Science, 322*, 442. https://doi.org/10.1126/science.1161427

Choi, J. R., Hu, J., Tang, R., Gong, Y., Feng, S., Ren, H., et al. (2016). An integrated paper-based sample-to-answer biosensor for nucleic acid testing at the point of care. *Lab on a Chip, 16*, 611−621. https://doi.org/10.1039/C5LC01388G

Chou, H. P., Unger, M. A., & Quake, S. R. (2001). A microfabricated rotary pump. *Biomedical Microdevices, 3*(4), 323−330. https://doi.org/10.1023/A:1012412916446

Cong, Y., Katipamula, S., Geng, T., Prost, S. A., Tang, K., & Kelly, R. T. (2016). Electrokinetic sample preconcentration and hydrodynamic sample injection for microchip electrophoresis using a pneumatic microvalve. *Electrophoresis, 37*, 455−462. https://doi.org/10.1002/elps.201500286

Coupland, P. (2010). Microfluidics for the upstream pipeline of DNA sequencing − a worthy application? *Lab on a Chip, 10*, 544−547. https://doi.org/10.1039/B917560A

Doherty, E. A. S., Kan, C.-W., Paegel, B. M., Yeung, S. H. I., Cao, S., Mathies, R. A., et al. (2004). Sparsely cross-linked "nanogel" matrixes as fluid, mechanically stabilized polymer networks for high-throughput microchannel DNA sequencing. *Analytical Chemistry, 76*, 5249−5256. https://doi.org/10.1021/ac049721x

DuVall, J. A., Le Roux, D., Tsuei, A.-C., Thompson, B. L., Birch, C., Li, J., et al. (2016). A rotationally-driven polyethylene terephthalate microdevice with integrated reagent mixing for multiplexed PCR amplification of DNA. *Analytical Methods, 8*, 7331−7340. https://doi.org/10.1039/C6AY01984F

Easley, C. J., Karlinsey, J. M., Bienvenue, J. M., Legendre, L. A., Roper, M. G., Feldman, S. H., et al. (2006). A fully integrated microfluidic genetic analysis system with sample-in−answer-out capability. *Proceedings of the National Academy of Sciences of the United States of America, 103*, 19272−19277. https://doi.org/10.1073/pnas.0604663103

Edd, J. F., Di Carlo, D., Humphry, K. J., Köster, S., Irimia, D., Weitz, D. A., et al. (2008). Controlled encapsulation of single-cells into monodisperse picolitre drops. *Lab on a Chip, 8*, 1262−1264. https://doi.org/10.1039/B805456H

Ellegren, H. (2008). Comparative genomics and the study of evolution by natural selection. *Molecular Ecology, 17*, 4586−4596. https://doi.org/10.1111/j.1365-294X.2008.03954.x

Estes, M. D., Yang, J., Duane, B., Smith, S., Brooks, C., Nordquist, A., et al. (2012). Optimization of multiplexed PCR on an integrated microfluidic forensic platform for rapid DNA analysis. *Analyst, 137*, 5510−5519. https://doi.org/10.1039/C2AN35768B

Fanciulli, M., Norsworthy, P. J., Petretto, E., Dong, R., Harper, L., Kamesh, L., et al. (2007). FCGR3B copy number variation is associated with susceptibility to systemic, but not organ-specific, autoimmunity. *Nature Genetics, 39*, 721−723. https://doi.org/10.1038/ng2046

Fang, Q., Xu, G.-M., & Fang, Z.-L. (2002). A high-throughput continuous sample introduction interface for microfluidic chip-based capillary electrophoresis systems. *Analytical Chemistry, 74*, 1223−1231. https://doi.org/10.1021/ac010925c

Feng, G.-H., & Chou, Y.-C. (2011). Fabrication and characterization of thermally driven fast turn-on microvalve with adjustable backpressure design. *Microelectronic Engineering, 88*, 187−194. https://doi.org/10.1016/j.mee.2010.10.011

Feng, G.-H., & Kim, E. S. (2004). Micropump based on PZT unimorph and one-way parylene valves. *Journal of Micromechanics and Microengineering, 14*, 429−435. https://doi.org/10.1088/0960-1317/14/4/001

Feng, Y., Zhou, Z., Ye, X., & Xiong, J. (2003). Passive valves based on hydrophobic microfluidics. *Sensors and Actuators A: Physical, 108*, 138–143. https://doi.org/10.1016/S0924-4247(03)00363-7

Ferrance, J. P., Wu, Q., Giordano, B., Hernandez, C., Kwok, Y., Snow, K., et al. (2003). Developments toward a complete micro-total analysis system for Duchenne muscular dystrophy diagnosis. *Analytica Chimica Acta, 500*, 223–236. https://doi.org/10.1016/j.aca.2003.08.067

Fredlake, C. P., Hert, D. G., Kan, C.-W., Chiesl, T. N., Root, B. E., Forster, R. E., et al. (2008). Ultrafast DNA sequencing on a microchip by a hybrid separation mechanism that gives 600 bases in 6.5 minutes. *Proceedings of the National Academy of Sciences of the United States of America, 105*, 476. https://doi.org/10.1073/pnas.0705093105

Fredrickson, C. K., & Fan, Z. H. (2004). Macro-to-micro interfaces for microfluidic devices. *Lab on a Chip, 4*, 526–533. https://doi.org/10.1039/B410720A

Fukuba, T., Yamamoto, T., Naganuma, T., & Fujii, T. (2004). Microfabricated flow-through device for DNA amplification—towards in situ gene analysis. *Chemical Engineering Journal, 101*, 151–156. https://doi.org/10.1016/j.cej.2003.11.016

Fu, Y., Li, C., Lu, S., Zhou, W., Tang, F., Xie, X. S., et al. (2015). Uniform and accurate single-cell sequencing based on emulsion whole-genome amplification. *Proceedings of the National Academy of Sciences of the United States of America, 112*, 11923. https://doi.org/10.1073/pnas.1513988112

Gan, W., Gu, Y., Han, J., Li, C.-X., Sun, J., & Liu, P. (2017). Chitosan-modified filter paper for nucleic acid extraction and "in situ PCR" on a thermoplastic microchip. *Analytical Chemistry, 89*, 3568–3575. https://doi.org/10.1021/acs.analchem.6b04882

Gill, P., Whitaker, J., Flaxman, C., Brown, N., & Buckleton, J. (2000). An investigation of the rigor of interpretation rules for STRs derived from less than 100 pg of DNA. *Forensic Science International, 112*, 17–40. https://doi.org/10.1016/S0379-0738(00)00158-4

Gogoi, P., Sepehri, S., Zhou, Y., Gorin, M. A., Paolillo, C., Capoluongo, E., et al. (2016). Development of an automated and sensitive microfluidic device for capturing and characterizing circulating tumor cells (CTCs) from clinical blood samples. *PLoS One, 11*, e0147400. https://doi.org/10.1371/journal.pone.0147400

Gong, H., Woolley, A. T., & Nordin, G. P. (2018). 3D printed high density, reversible, chip-to-chip microfluidic interconnects. *Lab on a Chip, 18*, 639–647. https://doi.org/10.1039/C7LC01113J

Goodwin, S., McPherson, J. D., & McCombie, W. R. (2016). Coming of age: Ten years of next-generation sequencing technologies. *Nature Reviews Genetics, 17*, 333–351. https://doi.org/10.1038/nrg.2016.49

Greenspoon, S. A., Sykes, K. L. V., Ban, J. D., Pollard, A., Baisden, M., Farr, M., et al. (2006). Automated PCR setup for forensic casework samples using the normalization wizard and PCR Setup robotic methods. *Forensic Science International, 164*, 240–248. https://doi.org/10.1016/j.forsciint.2006.02.027

Greenspoon, S. A., Yeung, S. H. I., Johnson, K. R., Chu, W. K., Rhee, H. N., McGuckian, A. B., et al. (2008). A forensic laboratory tests the Berkeley microfabricated capillary array electrophoresis device*. *Journal of Forensic Sciences, 53*, 828–837. https://doi.org/10.1111/j.1556-4029.2008.00750.x

Grover, W. H., Skelley, A. M., Liu, C. N., Lagally, E. T., & Mathies, R. A. (2003). Monolithic membrane valves and diaphragm pumps for practical large-scale integration into glass microfluidic devices. *Sensors and Actuators B: Chemical, 89*, 315–323. https://doi.org/10.1016/S0925-4005(02)00468-9

Guttmacher, A. E., Porteous, M. E., & McInerney, J. D. (2007). Educating health-care professionals about genetics and genomics. *Nature Reviews Genetics, 8*, 151−157. https://doi.org/10.1038/nrg2007

Gu, Y., Zhuang, B., Han, J., Li, Y., Song, X., Zhou, X., et al. (2019). Modular-based integrated microsystem with multiple sample preparation modules for automated forensic DNA typing from reference to challenging samples. *Analytical Chemistry, 91*, 7435−7443. https://doi.org/10.1021/acs.analchem.9b01560

Haefner, S., Koerbitz, R., Frank, P., Elstner, M., & Richter, A. (2018). High integration of microfluidic circuits based on hydrogel valves for MEMS control. *Advanced Materials Technologies, 3*, 1700108. https://doi.org/10.1002/admt.201700108

Han, J., Gan, W., Zhuang, B., Sun, J., Zhao, L., Ye, J., et al. (2017). A fully integrated microchip system for automated forensic short tandem repeat analysis. *Analyst, 142*, 2004−2012. https://doi.org/10.1039/C7AN00295E

Harrison, D. J., Fluri, K., Seiler, K., Fan, Z., Effenhauser, C. S., & Manz, A. (1993). Micromachining a miniaturized capillary electrophoresis-based chemical analysis system on a chip. *Science, 261*, 895. https://doi.org/10.1126/science.261.5123.895

He, M., Edgar, J. S., Jeffries, G. D. M., Lorenz, R. M., Shelby, J. P., & Chiu, D. T. (2005). Selective encapsulation of single cells and subcellular organelles into picoliter- and femtoliter-volume droplets. *Analytical Chemistry, 77*, 1539−1544. https://doi.org/10.1021/ac0480850

Hettiarachchi, K., Kim, H., & Faris, G. W. (2012). Optical manipulation and control of real-time PCR in cell encapsulating microdroplets by IR laser. *Microfluidics and Nanofluidics, 13*, 967−975. https://doi.org/10.1007/s10404-012-1016-5

Higgins, J. A., Nasarabadi, S., Karns, J. S., Shelton, D. R., Cooper, M., Gbakima, A., et al. (2003). A handheld real time thermal cycler for bacterial pathogen detection. *Biosensors and Bioelectronics, 18*, 1115−1123. https://doi.org/10.1016/S0956-5663(02)00252-X

Hindson, B. J., Ness, K. D., Masquelier, D. A., Belgrader, P., Heredia, N. J., Makarewicz, A. J., et al. (2011). High-throughput droplet digital PCR system for absolute quantitation of DNA copy number. *Analytical Chemistry, 83*, 8604−8610. https://doi.org/10.1021/ac202028g

Hopwood, A. J., Hurth, C., Yang, J., Cai, Z., Moran, N., Lee-Edghill, J. G., et al. (2010). Integrated microfluidic system for rapid forensic DNA analysis: Sample collection to DNA profile. *Analytical Chemistry, 82*, 6991−6999. https://doi.org/10.1021/ac101355r

Hosokawa, M., Nishikawa, Y., Kogawa, M., & Takeyama, H. (2017). Massively parallel whole genome amplification for single-cell sequencing using droplet microfluidics. *Scientific Reports, 7*, 5199. https://doi.org/10.1038/s41598-017-05436-4

Hsieh, K., Ferguson, B. S., Eisenstein, M., Plaxco, K. W., & Soh, H. T. (2015). Integrated electrochemical microsystems for genetic detection of pathogens at the point of care. *Accounts of Chemical Research, 48*, 911−920. https://doi.org/10.1021/ar500456w

Hsieh, T.-M., Luo, C.-H., Huang, F.-C., Wang, J.-H., Chien, L.-J., & Lee, G.-B. (2008). Enhancement of thermal uniformity for a microthermal cycler and its application for polymerase chain reaction. *Sensors and Actuators B: Chemical, 130*, 848−856. https://doi.org/10.1016/j.snb.2007.10.063

Hühmer, A. F. R., & Landers, J. P. (2000). Noncontact infrared-mediated thermocycling for effective polymerase chain reaction amplification of DNA in nanoliter volumes. *Analytical Chemistry, 72*, 5507−5512. https://doi.org/10.1021/ac000423j

Ivnitski, D., O'Neil, D. J., Gattuso, A., Schlicht, R., Calidonna, M., & Fisher, R. (2003). Nucleic acid approaches for detection and identification of biological warfare and infectious disease agents. *Biotechniques, 35*, 862−869. https://doi.org/10.2144/03354ss03

Jadhav, A. D., Yan, B., Luo, R. C., Wei, L., Zhen, X., Chen, C. H., et al. (2015). Photoresponsive microvalve for remote actuation and flow control in microfluidic devices. *Biomicrofluidics, 9*, 034114. https://doi.org/10.1063/1.4923257

Jensen, K. (1998). Smaller, faster chemistry. *Nature, 393*, 735–737. https://doi.org/10.1038/31590

Jha, S. K., Chand, R., Han, D., Jang, Y.-C., Ra, G.-S., Kim, J. S., et al. (2012). An integrated PCR microfluidic chip incorporating aseptic electrochemical cell lysis and capillary electrophoresis amperometric DNA detection for rapid and quantitative genetic analysis. *Lab on a Chip, 12*, 4455–4464. https://doi.org/10.1039/C2LC40727B

Jobling, M. A., & Gill, P. (2004). Encoded evidence: DNA in forensic analysis. *Nature Reviews Genetics, 5*, 739–751. https://doi.org/10.1038/nrg1455

Ju, J., Glazer, A. N., & Mathies, R. A. (1996). Energy transfer primers: A new fluorescence labeling paradigm for DNA sequencing and analysis. *Nature Medicine, 2*, 246–249. https://doi.org/10.1038/nm0296-246

Khandurina, J., Jacobson, S. C., Waters, L. C., Foote, R. S., & Ramsey, J. M. (1999). Microfabricated porous membrane structure for sample concentration and electrophoretic analysis. *Analytical Chemistry, 71*, 1815–1819. https://doi.org/10.1021/ac981161c

Kheterpal, I., Li, L., Speed, T. P., & Mathies, R. A. (1998). A three-wavelength labeling approach for DNA sequencing using energy transfer primers and capillary electrophoresis. *Electrophoresis, 19*, 1403–1414. https://doi.org/10.1002/elps.1150190835

Kim, H., Bartsch, M. S., Renzi, R. F., He, J., Van de Vreugde, J. L., Claudnic, M. R., et al. (2011). Automated digital microfluidic sample preparation for next-generation DNA sequencing. *Journal of the Association for Laboratory Automation, 16*, 405–414. https://doi.org/10.1016/j.jala.2011.07.001

Kim, D., & Herr, A. E. (2013). Protein immobilization techniques for microfluidic assays. *Biomicrofluidics, 7*, 041501. https://doi.org/10.1063/1.4816934

Kim, H., Jebrail, M. J., Sinha, A., Bent, Z. W., Solberg, O. D., Williams, K. P., et al. (2013). A microfluidic DNA library preparation platform for next-generation sequencing. *PLoS One, 8*, e68988. https://doi.org/10.1371/journal.pone.0068988

Kim, Y. T., Lee, D., Heo, H. Y., Sim, J. E., Woo, K. M., Kim, D. H., et al. (2016). Total integrated slidable and valveless solid phase extraction-polymerase chain reaction-capillary electrophoresis microdevice for mini Y chromosome short tandem repeat genotyping. *Biosensors and Bioelectronics, 78*, 489–496. https://doi.org/10.1016/j.bios.2015.11.079

Kim, T.-H., Park, J., Kim, C.-J., & Cho, Y.-K. (2014). Fully integrated lab-on-a-disc for nucleic acid analysis of food-borne pathogens. *Analytical Chemistry, 86*, 3841–3848. https://doi.org/10.1021/ac403971h

Kistrup, K., Poulsen, C. E., Østergaard, P. F., Haugshøj, K. B., Taboryski, R., Wolff, A., et al. (2014). Fabrication and modelling of injection moulded all-polymer capillary microvalves for passive microfluidic control. *Journal of Micromechanics and Microengineering, 24*, 125007. https://doi.org/10.1088/0960-1317/24/12/125007

Koh, C. G., Tan, W., Zhao, M.-Q., Ricco, A. J., & Fan, Z. H. (2003). Integrating polymerase chain reaction, valving, and electrophoresis in a plastic device for bacterial detection. *Analytical Chemistry, 75*, 4591–4598. https://doi.org/10.1021/ac0343836

Kopp, M. U., Mello, A. J. D., & Manz, A. (1998). Chemical amplification: Continuous-flow PCR on a chip. *Science, 280*, 1046. https://doi.org/10.1126/science.280.5366.1046

Kumaresan, P., Yang, C. J., Cronier, S. A., Blazej, R. G., & Mathies, R. A. (2008). High-throughput single copy DNA amplification and cell analysis in engineered nanoliter droplets. *Analytical Chemistry, 80*, 3522–3529. https://doi.org/10.1021/ac800327d

Lagally, E. T., Emrich, C. A., & Mathies, R. A. (2001). Fully integrated PCR-capillary electrophoresis microsystem for DNA analysis. *Lab on a Chip, 1*, 102−107. https://doi.org/10.1039/B109031N

Lagally, E. T., & Mathies, R. A. (2004). Integrated genetic analysis microsystems. *Journal of Physics D: Applied Physics, 37*, R245−R261. https://doi.org/10.1088/0022-3727/37/23/r01

Lagally, E. T., Scherer, J. R., Blazej, R. G., Toriello, N. M., Diep, B. A., Ramchandani, M., et al. (2004). Integrated portable genetic analysis microsystem for pathogen/infectious disease detection. *Analytical Chemistry, 76*, 3162−3170. https://doi.org/10.1021/ac035310p

Lander, E. S., Linton, L. M., Birren, B., Nusbaum, C., Zody, M. C., Baldwin, J., et al. (2001). Initial sequencing and analysis of the human genome. *Nature, 409*, 860−921. https://doi.org/10.1038/35057062

Le Roux, D., Root, B. E., Hickey, J. A., Scott, O. N., Tsuei, A., Li, J., et al. (2014). An integrated sample-in-answer-out microfluidic chip for rapid human identification by STR analysis. *Lab on a Chip, 14*, 4415−4425. https://doi.org/10.1039/C4LC00685B

Lee, J. N., Park, C., & Whitesides, G. M. (2003). Solvent compatibility of poly(dimethylsiloxane)-based microfluidic devices. *Analytical Chemistry, 75*, 6544−6554. https://doi.org/10.1021/ac0346712

Levsky, J. M., Shenoy, S. M., Pezo, R. C., & Singer, R. H. (2002). Single-cell gene expression profiling. *Science, 297*, 836. https://doi.org/10.1126/science.1072241

Levy, S., Sutton, G., Ng, P. C., Feuk, L., Halpern, A. L., Walenz, B. P., et al. (2007). The diploid genome sequence of an individual human. *PLoS Biology, 5*, 2113−2144. https://doi.org/10.1371/journal.pbio.0050254

Li, H. Q., Roberts, D. C., Steyn, J. L., Turner, K. T., Yaglioglu, O., Hagood, N. W., et al. (2004). Fabrication of a high frequency piezoelectric microvalve. *Sensors and Actuators A: Physical, 111*, 51−56. https://doi.org/10.1016/j.sna.2003.10.013

Liu, C., Geva, E., Mauk, M., Qiu, X., Abrams, W. R., Malamud, D., et al. (2011). An isothermal amplification reactor with an integrated isolation membrane for point-of-care detection of infectious diseases. *Analyst, 136*, 2069−2076. https://doi.org/10.1039/C1AN00007A

Liu, X., & Li, S. (2014). An electromagnetic microvalve for pneumatic control of microfluidic systems. *Journal of Laboratory Automation, 19*, 444−453. https://doi.org/10.1177/2211068214531760

Liu, P., Li, X., Greenspoon, S. A., Scherer, J. R., & Mathies, R. A. (2011). Integrated DNA purification, PCR, sample cleanup, and capillary electrophoresis microchip for forensic human identification. *Lab on a Chip, 11*, 1041−1048. https://doi.org/10.1039/C0LC00533A

Liu, P., Scherer, J. R., Greenspoon, S. A., Chiesl, T. N., & Mathies, R. A. (2011). Integrated sample cleanup and capillary array electrophoresis microchip for forensic short tandem repeat analysis. *Forensic Science International: Genetics, 5*, 484−492. https://doi.org/10.1016/j.fsigen.2010.10.009

Liu, P., Seo, T. S., Beyor, N., Shin, K.-J., Scherer, J. R., & Mathies, R. A. (2007). Integrated portable polymerase chain reaction-capillary electrophoresis microsystem for rapid forensic short tandem repeat typing. *Analytical Chemistry, 79*, 1881−1889. https://doi.org/10.1021/ac061961k

Liu, S., Shi, Y., Ja, W. W., & Mathies, R. A. (1999). Optimization of high-speed DNA sequencing on microfabricated capillary electrophoresis channels. *Analytical Chemistry, 71*, 566−573. https://doi.org/10.1021/ac980783v

Liu, C. N., Toriello, N. M., & Mathies, R. A. (2006). Multichannel PCR-CE microdevice for genetic analysis. *Analytical Chemistry, 78*, 5474−5479. https://doi.org/10.1021/ac060335k

Liu, P., Yeung, S. H. I., Crenshaw, K. A., Crouse, C. A., Scherer, J. R., & Mathies, R. A. (2008). Real-time forensic DNA analysis at a crime scene using a portable microchip analyzer. *Forensic Science International: Genetics, 2*, 301−309. https://doi.org/10.1016/j.fsigen.2008.03.009

Long, Z., Shen, Z., Wu, D., Qin, J., & Lin, B. (2007). Integrated multilayer microfluidic device with a nanoporous membrane interconnect for online coupling of solid-phase extraction to microchip electrophoresis. *Lab on a Chip, 7*, 1819−1824. https://doi.org/10.1039/B711741H

Macosko, E. Z., Basu, A., Satija, R., Nemesh, J., Shekhar, K., Goldman, M., et al. (2015). Highly parallel genome-wide expression profiling of individual cells using nanoliter droplets. *Cell, 161*, 1202−1214. https://doi.org/10.1016/j.cell.2015.05.002

Manz, A., Graber, N., & Widmer, H. M. (1990). Miniaturized total chemical analysis systems: A novel concept for chemical sensing. *Sensors and Actuators B: Chemical, 1*, 244−248. https://doi.org/10.1016/0925-4005(90)80209-I

Manz, A., Harrison, D. J., Verpoorte, E. M. J., Fettinger, J. C., Paulus, A., Lüdi, H., et al. (1992). Planar chips technology for miniaturization and integration of separation techniques into monitoring systems: Capillary electrophoresis on a chip. *Journal of Chromatography A, 593*, 253−258. https://doi.org/10.1016/0021-9673(92)80293-4

Marchiarullo, D. J., Sklavounos, A. H., Oh, K., Poe, B. L., Barker, N. S., & Landers, J. P. (2013). Low-power microwave-mediated heating for microchip-based PCR. *Lab on a Chip, 13*, 3417−3425. https://doi.org/10.1039/C3LC50461A

Marcus, J. S., Anderson, W. F., & Quake, S. R. (2006a). Microfluidic single-cell mRNA isolation and analysis. *Analytical Chemistry, 78*, 3084−3089. https://doi.org/10.1021/ac0519460

Marcus, J. S., Anderson, W. F., & Quake, S. R. (2006b). Parallel picoliter RT-PCR assays using microfluidics. *Analytical Chemistry, 78*, 956−958. https://doi.org/10.1021/ac0513865

Marcy, Y., Ishoey, T., Lasken, R. S., Stockwell, T. B., Walenz, B. P., Halpern, A. L., et al. (2007). Nanoliter reactors improve multiple displacement amplification of genomes from single cells. *PLoS Genetics, 3*, e155. https://doi.org/10.1371/journal.pgen.0030155

Mardis, E. R. (2008). Next-generation DNA sequencing methods. *Annual Review of Genomics and Human Genetics, 9*, 387−402. https://doi.org/10.1146/annurev.genom.9.081307.164359

Matsunaga, T., Hosokawa, M., Arakaki, A., Taguchi, T., Mori, T., Tanaka, T., et al. (2008). High-efficiency single-cell entrapment and fluorescence in situ hybridization analysis using a poly(dimethylsiloxane) microfluidic device integrated with a black poly(ethylene terephthalate) micromesh. *Analytical Chemistry, 80*, 5139−5145. https://doi.org/10.1021/ac800352j

McDonald, J. C., Duffy, D. C., Anderson, J. R., Chiu, D. T., Wu, H., Schueller, O. J., et al. (2000). Fabrication of microfluidic systems in poly(dimethylsiloxane). *Electrophoresis, 21*, 27−40. https://doi.org/10.1002/(sici)1522-2683(20000101)21:1<27::Aid-elps27>3.0.Co;2-c

McDonald, J. C., & Whitesides, G. M. (2002). Poly(dimethylsiloxane) as a material for fabricating microfluidic devices. *Accounts of Chemical Research, 35*, 491−499. https://doi.org/10.1021/ar010110q

Metzker, M. L. (2010). Sequencing technologies — the next generation. *Nature Reviews Genetics, 11*, 31–46. https://doi.org/10.1038/nrg2626

Montpetit, S. A., Fitch, I. T., & O'Donnell, P. T. (2005). A simple automated instrument for DNA extraction in forensic casework. *Journal of Forensic Sciences, 50*, 555–563.

Mukhopadhyay, R. (2007). When PDMS isn't the best. *Analytical Chemistry, 79*, 3248–3253. https://doi.org/10.1021/ac071903e

Nagai, M., Oguri, M., & Shibata, T. (2015). Characterization of light-controlled Volvox as movable microvalve element assembled in multilayer microfluidic device. *Japanese Journal of Applied Physics, 54*, 067001. https://doi.org/10.7567/jjap.54.067001

Nisisako, T., Ando, T., & Hatsuzawa, T. (2012). High-volume production of single and compound emulsions in a microfluidic parallelization arrangement coupled with coaxial annular world-to-chip interfaces. *Lab on a Chip, 12*, 3426–3435. https://doi.org/10.1039/C2LC40245A

Nittis, V., Fortt, R., Legge, C. H., & de Mello, A. J. (2001). A high-pressure interconnect for chemical microsystem applications. *Lab on a Chip, 1*, 148–152. https://doi.org/10.1039/B107836B

Oblath, E. A., Henley, W. H., Alarie, J. P., & Ramsey, J. M. (2013). A microfluidic chip integrating DNA extraction and real-time PCR for the detection of bacteria in saliva. *Lab on a Chip, 13*, 1325–1332. https://doi.org/10.1039/C3LC40961A

Oh, K. W., & Ahn, C. H. (2006). A review of microvalves. *Journal of Micromechanics and Microengineering, 16*, R13–R39. https://doi.org/10.1088/0960-1317/16/5/r01

Oh, K. W., Han, A., Bhansali, S., & Ahn, C. H. (2002). A low-temperature bonding technique using spin-on fluorocarbon polymers to assemble microsystems. *Journal of Micromechanics and Microengineering, 12*, 187–191. https://doi.org/10.1088/0960-1317/12/2/313

van Oordt, T., Barb, Y., Smetana, J., Zengerle, R., & von Stetten, F. (2013). Miniature stick-packaging — an industrial technology for pre-storage and release of reagents in lab-on-a-chip systems. *Lab on a Chip, 13*, 2888–2892. https://doi.org/10.1039/C3LC50404B

Ottesen, E. A., Hong, J. W., Quake, S. R., & Leadbetter, J. R. (2006). Microfluidic digital PCR enables multigene analysis of individual environmental bacteria. *Science, 314*, 1464. https://doi.org/10.1126/science.1131370

Ouyang, Y., Wang, S., Li, J., Riehl, P. S., Begley, M., & Landers, J. P. (2013). Rapid patterning of 'tunable' hydrophobic valves on disposable microchips by laser printer lithography. *Lab on a Chip, 13*, 1762–1771. https://doi.org/10.1039/C3LC41275J

Pappas, T. J., & Holland, L. A. (2008). Fluid steering in a microfluidic chip by means of thermally responsive phospholipids. *Sensors and Actuators B: Chemical, 128*, 427–434. https://doi.org/10.1016/j.snb.2007.06.031

Park, B. H., Jung, J. H., Zhang, H., Lee, N. Y., & Seo, T. S. (2012). A rotary microsystem for simple, rapid and automatic RNA purification. *Lab on a Chip, 12*, 3875–3881. https://doi.org/10.1039/C2LC40487G

Paydar, O. H., Paredes, C. N., Hwang, Y., Paz, J., Shah, N. B., & Candler, R. N. (2014). Characterization of 3D-printed microfluidic chip interconnects with integrated O-rings. *Sensors and Actuators A: Physical, 205*, 199–203. https://doi.org/10.1016/j.sna.2013.11.005

Prakash, A. R., De la Rosa, C., Fox, J. D., & Kaler, K. V. I. S. (2008). Identification of respiratory pathogen *Bordetella pertussis* using integrated microfluidic chip technology. *Microfluidics and Nanofluidics, 4*, 451–456. https://doi.org/10.1007/s10404-007-0195-y

Prakash, R., & Kaler, K. V. I. S. (2007). An integrated genetic analysis microfluidic platform with valves and a PCR chip reusability method to avoid contamination. *Microfluidics and Nanofluidics, 3*, 177−187. https://doi.org/10.1007/s10404-006-0114-7

Quake, S. R., & Scherer, A. (2000). From micro- to nanofabrication with soft materials. *Science, 290*, 1536. https://doi.org/10.1126/science.290.5496.1536

Quintana, E., Shackleton, M., Sabel, M. S., Fullen, D. R., Johnson, T. M., & Morrison, S. J. (2008). Efficient tumour formation by single human melanoma cells. *Nature, 456*, 593−598. https://doi.org/10.1038/nature07567

Raj, A., Peskin, C. S., Tranchina, D., Vargas, D. Y., & Tyagi, S. (2006). Stochastic mRNA synthesis in mammalian cells. *PLoS Biology, 4*, e309. https://doi.org/10.1371/journal.pbio.0040309

Ren, K., Zhou, J., & Wu, H. (2013). Materials for microfluidic chip fabrication. *Accounts of Chemical Research, 46*, 2396−2406. https://doi.org/10.1021/ar300314s

Riahi, R., Gogoi, P., Sepehri, S., Zhou, Y., Handique, K., Godsey, J., et al. (2014). A novel microchannel-based device to capture and analyze circulating tumor cells (CTCs) of breast cancer. *International Journal of Oncology, 44*, 1870−1878. https://doi.org/10.3892/ijo.2014.2353

Richter, A., Howitz, S., Kuckling, D., Kretschmer, K., & Arndt, K.-F. (2004). Automatically and electronically controllable hydrogel based valves and microvalves − design and operating performance. *Macromolecular Symposia, 210*, 447−456. https://doi.org/10.1002/masy.200450650

Rodrigue, S., Malmstrom, R. R., Berlin, A. M., Birren, B. W., Henn, M. R., & Chisholm, S. W. (2009). Whole genome amplification and de novo assembly of single bacterial cells. *PLoS One, 4*, e6864. https://doi.org/10.1371/journal.pone.0006864

Rodriguez, N. M., Linnes, J. C., Fan, A., Ellenson, C. K., Pollock, N. R., & Klapperich, C. M. (2015). Paper-based RNA extraction, in situ isothermal amplification, and lateral flow detection for low-cost, rapid diagnosis of influenza A (H1N1) from clinical specimens. *Analytical Chemistry, 87*, 7872−7879. https://doi.org/10.1021/acs.analchem.5b01594

Roman, G. T., & Kennedy, R. T. (2007). Fully integrated microfluidic separations systems for biochemical analysis. *Journal of Chromatography A, 1168*, 170−188. https://doi.org/10.1016/j.chroma.2007.06.010

Root, B. E., Agarwal, A. K., Kelso, D. M., & Barron, A. E. (2011). Purification of HIV RNA from serum using a polymer capture matrix in a microfluidic device. *Analytical Chemistry, 83*, 982−988. https://doi.org/10.1021/ac102736g

Schmalzing, D., Adourian, A., Koutny, L., Ziaugra, L., Matsudaira, P., & Ehrlich, D. (1998). DNA sequencing on microfabricated electrophoretic devices. *Analytical Chemistry, 70*, 2303−2310. https://doi.org/10.1021/ac971381a

Schmalzing, D., Koutny, L., Adourian, A., Belgrader, P., Matsudaira, P., & Ehrlich, D. (1997). DNA typing in thirty seconds with a microfabricated device. *Proceedings of the National Academy of Sciences of the United States of America, 94*, 10273−10278. https://doi.org/10.1073/pnas.94.19.10273

Selva, B., Mary, P., & Jullien, M.-C. (2010). Integration of a uniform and rapid heating source into microfluidic systems. *Microfluidics and Nanofluidics, 8*, 755−765. https://doi.org/10.1007/s10404-009-0505-7

Shaegh, S. A. M., Pourmand, A., Nabavinia, M., Avci, H., Tamayol, A., Mostafalu, P., et al. (2018). Rapid prototyping of whole-thermoplastic microfluidics with built-in microvalves using laser ablation and thermal fusion bonding. *Sensors and Actuators B: Chemical, 255*, 100−109. https://doi.org/10.1016/j.snb.2017.07.138

Shaw, K. J., Docker, P. T., Yelland, J. V., Dyer, C. E., Greenman, J., Greenway, G. M., et al. (2010). Rapid PCR amplification using a microfluidic device with integrated microwave heating and air impingement cooling. *Lab on a Chip, 10*, 1725−1728. https://doi.org/10.1039/C000357N

Shendure, J., & Ji, H. (2008). Next-generation DNA sequencing. *Nature Biotechnology, 26*, 1135−1145. https://doi.org/10.1038/nbt1486

Sidore, A. M., Lan, F., Lim, S. W., & Abate, A. R. (2015). Enhanced sequencing coverage with digital droplet multiple displacement amplification. *Nucleic Acids Research, 44*. https://doi.org/10.1093/nar/gkv1493. e66-e66.

Sims, C. E., & Allbritton, N. L. (2007). Analysis of single mammalian cells on-chip. *Lab on a Chip, 7*, 423−440. https://doi.org/10.1039/B615235J

Smith, P. J., & Ballantyne, J. (2007). Simplified low-copy-number DNA analysis by post-PCR purification. *Journal of Forensic Sciences, 52*, 820−829. https://doi.org/10.1111/j.1556-4029.2007.00470.x

Snider, A., Nilsson, M., Dupal, M., Toloue, M., & Tripathi, A. (2019). A microfluidics workflow for sample preparation for next-generation DNA sequencing. *Slas Technology: Translating Life Sciences Innovation, 24*, 196−208. https://doi.org/10.1177/2472630318796133

Strain, M. C., Lada, S. M., Luong, T., Rought, S. E., Gianella, S., Terry, V. H., et al. (2013). Highly precise measurement of HIV DNA by droplet digital PCR. *PLoS One, 8*, e55943. https://doi.org/10.1371/journal.pone.0055943

Strohmeier, O., Emperle, A., Roth, G., Mark, D., Zengerle, R., & von Stetten, F. (2013). Centrifugal gas-phase transition magnetophoresis (GTM) − a generic method for automation of magnetic bead based assays on the centrifugal microfluidic platform and application to DNA purification. *Lab on a Chip, 13*, 146−155. https://doi.org/10.1039/C2LC40866J

Stumpf, F., Schwemmer, F., Hutzenlaub, T., Baumann, D., Strohmeier, O., Dingemanns, G., et al. (2016). LabDisk with complete reagent prestorage for sample-to-answer nucleic acid based detection of respiratory pathogens verified with influenza A H3N2 virus. *Lab on a Chip, 16*, 199−207. https://doi.org/10.1039/C5LC00871A

Sun, H., Olsen, T., Zhu, J., Tao, J., Ponnaiya, B., Amundson, S. A., et al. (2015). A bead-based microfluidic approach to integrated single-cell gene expression analysis by quantitative RT-PCR. *RSC Advances, 5*, 4886−4893. https://doi.org/10.1039/C4RA13356K

Tang, R., Yang, H., Gong, Y., You, M., Liu, Z., Choi, J. R., et al. (2017). A fully disposable and integrated paper-based device for nucleic acid extraction, amplification and detection. *Lab on a Chip, 17*, 1270−1279. https://doi.org/10.1039/C6LC01586G

Tan, S. J., Phan, H., Gerry, B. M., Kuhn, A., Hong, L. Z., Min Ong, Y., et al. (2013). A microfluidic device for preparing next generation DNA sequencing libraries and for automating other laboratory protocols that require one or more column chromatography steps. *PLoS One, 8*, e64084. https://doi.org/10.1371/journal.pone.0064084

Thio, T., Nozari, A. A., Soin, N., Kahar, M. K. B. A., Dawal, S. Z. M., Samra, K. A., et al. (2011). Hybrid capillary-flap valve for vapor control in point-of-care microfluidic CD. In *Paper presented at the 5th Kuala Lumpur international conference on biomedical engineering 2011, Berlin, Heidelberg*.

Thio, T. H. G., Soroori, S., Ibrahim, F., Al-Faqheri, W., Soin, N., Kulinsky, L., et al. (2013). Theoretical development and critical analysis of burst frequency equations for passive valves on centrifugal microfluidic platforms. *Medical and Biological Engineering and Computing, 51*, 525−535. https://doi.org/10.1007/s11517-012-1020-7

Tian, W.-C., & Finehout, E. (2009). Interfacing microfluidic devices with the macro world abstract. In *Microfluidics for biological applications* (pp. 93–115). Boston, MA: Springer US.

Tice, J. D., Desai, A. V., Bassett, T. A., Apblett, C. A., & Kenis, P. J. A. (2014). Control of pressure-driven components in integrated microfluidic devices using an on-chip electrostatic microvalve. *RSC Advances, 4*, 51593–51602. https://doi.org/10.1039/C4RA10341F

Toriello, N. M., Douglas, E. S., Thaitrong, N., Hsiao, S. C., Francis, M. B., Bertozzi, C. R., et al. (2008). Integrated microfluidic bioprocessor for single-cell gene expression analysis. *Proceedings of the National Academy of Sciences of the United States of America, 105*, 20173. https://doi.org/10.1073/pnas.0806355106

Ueberfeld, J., El-Difrawy, S. A., Ramdhanie, K., & Ehrlich, D. J. (2006). Solid-support sample loading for DNA sequencing. *Analytical Chemistry, 78*, 3632–3637. https://doi.org/10.1021/ac052201x

Unger, M. A., Chou, H.-P., Thorsen, T., Scherer, A., & Quake, S. R. (2000). Monolithic microfabricated valves and pumps by multilayer soft lithography. *Science, 288*, 113. https://doi.org/10.1126/science.288.5463.113

Venter, J. C., Adams, M. D., Myers, E. W., Li, P. W., Mural, R. J., Sutton, G. G., et al. (2001). The sequence of the human genome. *Science, 291*, 1304. https://doi.org/10.1126/science.1058040

Wang, J., Fan, H. C., Behr, B., & Quake, S. R. (2012). Genome-wide single-cell analysis of recombination activity and de novo mutation rates in human sperm. *Cell, 150*, 402–412. https://doi.org/10.1016/j.cell.2012.06.030

Wang, S., Wang, T., Ge, P., Xue, P., Ye, S., Chen, H., et al. (2015). Controlling flow behavior of water in microfluidics with a chemically patterned anisotropic wetting surface. *Langmuir, 31*, 4032–4039. https://doi.org/10.1021/acs.langmuir.5b00328

Wang, J., Wang, W., Li, R., Li, Y., Tian, G., Goodman, L., et al. (2008). The diploid genome sequence of an Asian individual. *Nature, 456*, 60–65. https://doi.org/10.1038/nature07484

Waters, L. C., Jacobson, S. C., Kroutchinina, N., Khandurina, J., Foote, R. S., & Ramsey, J. M. (1998). Multiple sample PCR amplification and electrophoretic analysis on a microchip. *Analytical Chemistry, 70*, 5172–5176. https://doi.org/10.1021/ac980447e

West, J., Becker, M., Tombrink, S., & Manz, A. (2008). Micro total analysis systems: Latest achievements. *Analytical Chemistry, 80*, 4403–4419. https://doi.org/10.1021/ac800680j

Wheeler, D. A., Srinivasan, M., Egholm, M., Shen, Y., Chen, L., McGuire, A., et al. (2008). The complete genome of an individual by massively parallel DNA sequencing. *Nature, 452*, 872–876. https://doi.org/10.1038/nature06884

Whitaker, J. P., Cotton, E. A., & Gill, P. (2001). A comparison of the characteristics of profiles produced with the AMPFlSTR® SGM Plus™ multiplex system for both standard and low copy number (LCN) STR DNA analysis. *Forensic Science International, 123*, 215–223. https://doi.org/10.1016/S0379-0738(01)00557-6

White, R. A., Quake, S. R., & Curr, K. (2012). Digital PCR provides absolute quantitation of viral load for an occult RNA virus. *Journal of Virological Methods, 179*, 45–50. https://doi.org/10.1016/j.jviromet.2011.09.017

White, A. K., VanInsberghe, M., Petriv, O. I., Hamidi, M., Sikorski, D., Marra, M. A., et al. (2011). High-throughput microfluidic single-cell RT-qPCR. *Proceedings of the National Academy of Sciences of the United States of America, 108*, 13999–14004. https://doi.org/10.1073/pnas.1019446108

Wickenheiser, R. A. (2002). Trace DNA: A review, discussion of theory, and application of the transfer of trace quantities of DNA through skin contact. *Journal of Forensic Sciences, 47*, 442−450.

Woolley, A. T., & Mathies, R. A. (1995). Ultra-high-speed DNA sequencing using capillary electrophoresis chips. *Analytical Chemistry, 67*, 3676−3680. https://doi.org/10.1021/ac00116a010

Yang, B., & Lin, Q. (2009). A latchable phase-change microvalve with integrated heaters. *Journal of Microelectromechanical Systems, 18*, 860−867. https://doi.org/10.1109/JMEMS.2009.2024806

Yeung, S. H. I., Greenspoon, S. A., McGuckian, A., Crouse, C. A., Emrich, C. A., Ban, J., et al. (2006b). Rapid and high-throughput forensic short tandem repeat typing using a 96-lane microfabricated capillary array electrophoresis microdevice*. *Journal of Forensic Sciences, 51*, 740−747. https://doi.org/10.1111/j.1556-4029.2006.00153.x

Yeung, S.-W., Lee, T. M.-H., Cai, H., & Hsing, I.-M. (2006). A DNA biochip for on-the-spot multiplexed pathogen identification. *Nucleic Acids Research, 34*. https://doi.org/10.1093/nar/gkl702. e118-e118.

Yeung, S. H. I., Liu, P., Del Bueno, N., Greenspoon, S. A., & Mathies, R. A. (2009). Integrated sample Cleanup−Capillary electrophoresis microchip for high-performance short tandem repeat genetic analysis. *Analytical Chemistry, 81*, 210−217. https://doi.org/10.1021/ac8018685

Yobas, L., Huff, M. A., Lisy, F. J., & Durand, D. M. (2001). A novel bulk micromachined electrostatic microvalve with a curved-compliant structure applicable for a pneumatic tactile display. *Journal of Microelectromechanical Systems, 10*, 187−196. https://doi.org/10.1109/84.925734

Yuen, P. K. (2016). A reconfigurable stick-n-play modular microfluidic system using magnetic interconnects. *Lab on a Chip, 16*, 3700−3707. https://doi.org/10.1039/C6LC00741D

Yıldırım, E., Arıkan, M. A. S., & Külah, H. (2012). A normally closed electrostatic parylene microvalve for micro total analysis systems. *Sensors and Actuators A: Physical, 181*, 81−86. https://doi.org/10.1016/j.sna.2012.05.008

Zhao, S., Shetty, J., Hou, L., Delcher, A., Zhu, B., Osoegawa, K., et al. (2004). Human, mouse, and rat genome large-scale rearrangements: Stability versus speciation. *Genome Research, 14*, 1851−1860. https://doi.org/10.1101/gr.2663304

Zhong, J. F., Chen, Y., Marcus, J. S., Scherer, A., Quake, S. R., Taylor, C. R., et al. (2008). A microfluidic processor for gene expression profiling of single human embryonic stem cells. *Lab on a Chip, 8*, 68−74. https://doi.org/10.1039/B712116D

Zhuang, B., Han, J., Xiang, G., Gan, W., Wang, S., Wang, D., et al. (2016). A fully integrated and automated microsystem for rapid pharmacogenetic typing of multiple warfarin-related single-nucleotide polymorphisms. *Lab on a Chip, 16*, 86−95. https://doi.org/10.1039/C5LC01094B

Zimmermann, M., Hunziker, P., & Delamarche, E. (2008). Valves for autonomous capillary systems. *Microfluidics and Nanofluidics, 5*, 395−402. https://doi.org/10.1007/s10404-007-0256-2

Paper-based microfluidic devices for low-cost assays

Merwan Benhabib[1], XiuJun (James) Li[2]
[1]Telegraph Technologies, llc, San Francisco, CA, United States; [2]Department of Chemistry and Biochemistry, University of Texas at El Paso, El Paso, TX, United States

Guided-reading questions:

1. What techniques have been to fabricate paper-based devices, and what are their strengths and challenges?
2. What applications are paper-based devices currently tackling?
3. What issues does the field needs to focus on in the next decade to achieve broader applications?

14.1 Introduction

Lab-on-a-chip devices can provide the sensitivity, specificity, robustness, and rapidity needed for biomedical diagnostics. However, their cost and the skilled labor necessary to operate them make them difficult to access in resource-poor settings. To provide a low-cost, easy-to-use analytical tool, the Whitesides Group introduced paper-based microfluidic devices (μPADs) (Martinez et al., 2007). Paper is a cellulose fiber web with a high surface area, abundant, inexpensive, and compatible with biological samples, that has been extensively used since the early 20th century as a substrate for analytical and clinical chemistry (Clegg, 1950; Feigle, 1939; Helfferich, Giddings, & Keller, 1965). Nowadays, paper and paper like materials are one of the most prevalent substrates for point-of-care diagnostic (Von Lode, 2005). Immunochromatographic strips (ICS) are widely used as quantitative or semiquantitative tests in nonlaboratory settings (Abe et al., 2010). Additionally, paper is an ideal substrate for a disposable equipment-free testing solution because cellulose is biodegradable and can transport fluids by capillarity effect. μPAD's objective is to be a simple, portable, and mass-producible solution that combines all the benefits of microfluidics and paper. μPADs are an appealing diagnostic tool in home settings, for less-industrial countries, in remote or resource-poor locations, or during bioemergencies and first response accidents. They also can be of great use for environmental and food safety monitoring.

To circulate the fluids, μPADs rely on capillary action. It naturally occurs in the microscale channels, which are well-defined hydrophilic areas patterned on the hydrophobized sheet of paper (Li, Tian, & Shen, 2010a). When patterned with microstructures, paper becomes a platform where sample preparations and purifications, as well as multiple bioreactions can occur simultaneously without cross-contamination.

14.2 Fabrication techniques for paper-based microfluidic devices

There are two major patterning strategies: a one-step selective hydrophobization of certain areas of the device that leaves untouched the hydrophilic fluidic paths; and a two-step hydrophobization of the complete device followed by selective dehydrophobization of certain areas for fluidic flow. The dehydrophobization is achieved by etching away or dissolving the previously deposited hydrophobic agent to expose the underlying original hydrophilic paper. The straight forward, one step method, preserves the fluidic channels and detection zones, leaving their physicochemical properties unaltered (e.g., no paper color change, no residues). Hydrophobizing reagents used to fabricate µPADs can be classified in three categories depending on their function: physical filling of pores, deposition of a hydrophobizing agent, and chemical hydrophobization of the paper-fiber. This study will explore the different fabrication strategies in function of the category of hydrophobization reagent and patterning strategy used. But before, let us start first by reviewing the different types of paper suitable as substrate for the fabrication of microfluidic devices.

14.2.1 Paper-based materials used as substrates

A large variety of paper materials can be used as substrate for µPADs. The selection of the appropriate one depends on the field of application and the method of fabrication. Most researchers use cellulose paper, which is affordable, naturally hydrophilic, and allows for fast liquid penetration. Among the different kinds of cellulosic paper, Whatman filters are the most popular (Apilux et al., 2010; Fenton et al., 2008; Li et al., 2010b; Martinez et al., 2009). They are categorized in function of their porosity, particle retention, and flow rate. Whatman filter No. 1, their standard grade filter, allows for medium retention and flow rate. Although widely adopted due to its compatibility with many of the patterning techniques (Apilux et al., 2010; Carvalhal et al., 2010a; Ellerbee et al., 2009; Fenton et al., 2008; Hossain et al., 2009a; Martinez et al., 2008a, 2009, 2010; Songjaroen et al., 2011; Yu et al., 2011), Whatman No. 1 is not always ideal. For instance, Li et al. needed a filter paper with larger pores to balance the solvent-induced swelling of the cellulose fibers that happens with etch printing, and used a Whatman No 4 (Li et al., 2010b). Nie et al. required for their electrochemical detection (ECD) device a uniform structure to avoid the deformation of the screen-printed electrodes when wetted by fluids and used a chromatography paper (Nie et al., 2010a). The latter also has the advantage of lacking additives that could interfere with an electrochemical reaction (Wang et al., 2012a). Other groups reported using chemically modified cellulosic substrate usually blended with an inorganic filler, such as polyester. They are available commercially as ion exchange paper. They are nondegradable and present a smoother surface better suited for surface chemical modification or deposition (Arena et al., 2010; Nie et al., 2010a).

Another important type of paper substrate is the hydrophobic nitrocellulose (NC) membranes, which are smooth and with reasonably uniform pore size (0.45 µm) that allows for a more stable and reproducible liquid flow. They have been used for a long time for antigen immobilization (Hawkes, Niday, & Gordon, 1982) in, for instance, dot-immunobinding assays (Cheng et al., 2010) because they manifest a high degree of nonspecific binding toward biomolecules, making them suitable for immobilization of enzymes (Lu et al., 2009a, 2009b; Martinez et al., 2008a), proteins (Fenton et al., 2008), DNA (Cretich et al., 2010), and cell (Li, Ballerini, & Shen, 2012). Besides, pores in NC can perform purification based on size by filtrating impurities of larger diameter than the analyte which can mitigate interferences during the assay (Abe et al., 2010).

14.2.2 Techniques based on physical filling of pores with a hydrophobic polymer

14.2.2.1 Photolithography

The original method to pattern fluidics on paper is a two-step method derived from silicon lithographic techniques applied to chromatography paper substrate. This fabrication technique named Fast Lithographic Activation of Sheets (FLASH) and developed by Martinez et al. (2007, 2008, 2008b) is capable of creating features as small as 100 µm wide, and hydrophobic barriers to direct the flow as small as 200 µm wide. It requires an inkjet printer or copier machine, a UV light, and a hot plate. The patterning technique of a device, which takes less than 30 min, is described in Fig. 14.1. First, the sheet is impregnated with a hydrophobic polymer, photoresist (e.g., SU8); second, its front side gets covered with a transparent film and its backside with a black construction paper. Then, the microfluidic pattern gets printed on the transparent film, and the three components structure is exposed to UV. Finally, the backing and transparent films are removed, the sheet is baked, and the excess of photoresist gets removed during the development step with a mixture of isopropyl alcohol and acetone. The first device fabricated combined a glucose and protein tests (Martinez et al., 2007) with the reagents spotted in each detection regions and allowed to air-dry. The photoresist used, SU8, is the major cost driver of these devices at $0.93/m^2 of paper. It also requires over 20 min to cure and a plasma oxidation treatment to ensure full recovery of hydrophilicity. One can use less expensive alternative photoactive polymers, but most of them are very opaque making UV exposure through the full paper depth difficult (Klasner et al., 2010). Then, it becomes necessary to align and expose the backside of the device as well, adding more complexity to the process (Carrilho et al., 2009). Some novel polymer like Klasner's blend of polymers can be used to make devices in less than 3 min, without plasma oxidation and give similar minimum feature size. He reported features at 90 µm and barriers at 250 µm (Klasner et al., 2010). But, his method requires organic solvents, which can damage the flexibility

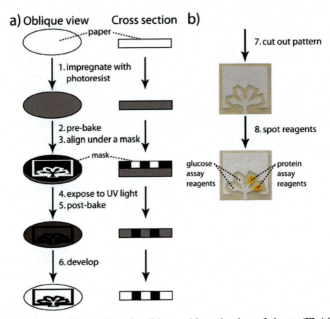

Figure 14.1 Schematic of the method fast lithographic activation of sheets (FLASH) for fabricating paper-based microfluidic devices. (a) Procedure for patterning paper with hydrophobic photoresist. (b) Derivatization of the device for assays.
Adapted with permission from Martinez, A. W., et al. (2008a). Simple telemedicine for developing regions: Camera phones and paper-based microfluidic devices for real-time, off-site diagnosis. *Analytical Chemistry, 80*(10), 3699–3707 Copyright © 2008 American Chemical Society.

of the paper and uses expensive brittle hydrophobic polymers (SU8 and PMMA) that makes the devices susceptible to folding and bending (Dungchai, Chailapakul, & Henry, 2011; Li et al., 2010; Songjaroen et al., 2011). It also involves many complicated, laborious, and time-consuming steps and requires clean rooms with sophisticated equipment and skilled labor, which are not ubiquitous across the world. However, this method is capable of creating small barriers and yields sharp resolution between hydrophobic and hydrophilic areas.

14.2.2.2 Plotting with an analog plotter

Another less complicated way to define hydrophobic patterns on paper than the multistep lithographic process is printing the hydrophobic polymer. Printing uses smaller volumes of readily available and less expensive polymers. It was first investigated by Bruzewicz et al., when they modified a plotter to print onto filter paper hydrophobic barriers made of a hexane solution of PDMS (polydimethylsiloxane), an inexpensive, nontoxic, and readily available polymer (Bruzewicz, Reches, & Whitesides, 2008). They created their own PDMS dispensing pens for the x, y plotter using PDMS and polyurethane and optimized their ink to ensure its rapid flow and its entire penetration through the sheet's thickness. It takes 1 h at 70°C for the elastomer to cure, during which PDMS spreads laterally reducing the printing resolution. Even though, the smallest feature and barrier were reported to be 1 mm, in practice, 2 to 4 mm wide channels are needed because patterned lines are hardly straight. Indeed, paper, a nonuniform porous substrate, does not permit a controllable penetration of PDMS (Li et al., 2008). Compared to FLASH devices, PDMS devices are flexible and bendable, making foldable devices (3D) (that can be folded without destruction of the channel) possible. They are also 50 times less expensive than at $0.02/m^2. Other elastomers like teflon, polystyrene, polypropylene, or polyisobutylene can be used as "ink" with a plotter, but PDMS is cheap and commonly used in microfluidics. Although this method does not damage the flexibility of the paper, it is time-consuming, requires modification of a hard to find plotter, and requires the special preparation of the elastomer diluted in hexane (Songjaroen et al., 2011).

14.2.3 Techniques based on soaking the paper with a hydrophobic chemical

14.2.3.1 Inkjet etching

Inspired by the FLASH method, Abe et al. used a two-step approach: impregnation of the paper with a polymer to fill the paper matrix with a hydrophobic layer, then patterning the microfluidic channels by finely dissolving the polymer with a solvent using a microdrop dispenser (such as an inkjet printer). Inkjets are commonly used in the manufacture of plastic electronics and polymer light emitting diodes. They are simpler and less expensive than the equipment required in photolithography. First, a filter paper is soaked in a 1.0 wt% solution of polystyrene in toluene for 2 h for complete hydrophobicity. Then, after letting it dry for 15 min at room temperature, the modified paper is patterned by inkjet printing toluene to locally dissolve the polymer and precisely reexpose hydrophilic areas that will constitute the fluidic paths. A 550 µm wide flow channel with a sensing area of 1.5 mm × 1.5 mm was printed on filter paper by inkjet etching for simultaneous determination of pH, total protein, and glucose (Abe, Suzuki, & Citterio, 2008). And a single apparatus (the inkjet printer) was used to dissolve the hydrophobic coating (patterning) and print the biochemical indicator inks (reagent deposition). Compared to a plotting system, an inkjet printer dispenses a precise volume of liquid in a reproducible and controlled manner, which permits not only the created hydrophilic–hydrophobic contrasts but also deposits the exact quantity of sensing reagents required, which makes this technique more cost-effective and less time-consuming (Abe et al., 2010). Even antibody immobilization on cellulosic surfaces by printing them as an ink was demonstrated (Abe et al., 2010). In addition, in contrast with lithography, inkjet printing is flexible (easy to change the design of the fluidic pattern), at lower cost, and adapted to mass manufacturing. However, photoresist-based fluidic channel can guide fluids with extremely low surface tension without any leaks because the polymer fills the paper pores. With polystyrene only, hydrophobic fluid can be transported (surface tension has to be higher than 35 mN/m) (Olkkonen, Lehtinen, & Erho, 2010). Another disadvantage of poly(styrene) is that it is time-consuming to coat the paper with it, about 2 h. And multiple printing runs are necessary to remove the coat, Abe et al. used 10 to 30 printing cycles for best results. This method also requires a customized potentially expensive inkjet printer (Dungchai et al., 2011).

14.2.3.2 Flexographic printing

Olkkonen used flexographic printing to pattern polystyrene boundaries onto chromatographic paper (Olkkonen et al., 2010). Although this technology can be used with many different hydrophobizing agents (such as alkyl ketene dimer (AKD), polymethylmethacrylate, or cross-linked polyvinyl alcohol), polystyrene was favored because it does not require heat treatment and it is biocompatible. With a 5% polystyrene ink and a single impression cycle, patterns of polystyrene are formed on the front side of the device and partially penetrate the paper thickness. To complete the waterproofing through all the paper thickness, a uniformed polystyrene layer is printed on the backside. This approach leads to devices that have shallow channels (about 50 μm), and thus requiring less sample volume. The minimum barrier and channel size made that way is 400 μm. This flexographic method is compatible with roll-to-roll mass production of fluidic devices using existing tools already present in printing houses. Fig. 14.2 shows a schematic of the process. The ink is first pipetted into an ink reservoir, and then gets transferred to the anilox roll which is covered with thousands of

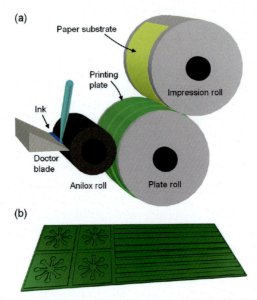

Figure 14.2 (a) Schematic illustration of the flexography unit used in the study. (b) Relief patterns in the printing plate define the hydrophobic regions to be formed into paper.
Adapted with permission from Olkkonen, J., Lehtinen, K., & Erho, T. (2010). Flexographically printed fluidic structures in paper. *Analytical Chemistry, 82*(24), 10246–10250 Copyright © 2010 American Chemical Society.

small volume cells. Each cell of anilox transfers its ink content onto the printing plate which contains the pattern. When printing, the anilox rotates four time to transfer the ink to the printing plate which in turn transfers it into the paper by pressing the paper against the impression roll as it rotates at 60 m/min. The ink penetration is promoted by pressure between the printing plate and the paper substrate. He reports 500 μm wide channels with 30 μm boundary roughness, in reproducible manner, and with negligible lateral ink spreading.

14.2.3.3 Wax printing

Wax is another hydrophobic plastic that inspired two groups Whitesides and Lin to use it as material for fluidic barrier on paper (Carrilho, Martinez, & Whitesides, 2009b; Lu et al., 2009a). It is malleable at ambient temperature, insoluble in water, easy to get anywhere in the world, inexpensive, sustainable, nontoxic, biodegradable, and with a relatively low viscosity when melted. In wax printing, first, a pattern of wax is deposited on a sheet of paper using a commercially available solid-ink printer in the case of large volume productions, or using a wax pen when doing only manual prototyping. The paper is then heated to melt the wax so that it diffuses through the entire thickness of the paper. The method is simple to learn, rapid ($\sim$5 min), and only requires two pieces of equipment—a solid-ink printer and a hot plate or oven. Compared to the previous fabrication methods, it relies on cheaper consumable and is more environmentally friendly. However, melted wax in paper spreads by capillarity in all directions, with the lateral component of that flow allowing the wax feature to change shape and size. This undesirable effect is amplified by the anisotropic character of paper fibers, being more horizontally than vertically aligned, and renders the patterns ill-defined and wider. Despite this lack of resolution, and because molten wax in paper behaves as a fluid in porous media, a simple relationship can predict the final width of the hydrophobic barrier and is used to take into account this phenomenon in the design. In fact, the spreading distance is constant for a given heating time and temperature. The features fabricated with this method are not as sharp as those generated by photolithography. By heating at 150°C for 120 s, Carrilho measured a spreading distance of 300 μm with a root mean square roughness of 57 μm. They produced a minimum barrier and channel widths of 850 and 560 μm, respectively (Carrilho et al., 2009). Nevertheless, with this procedure, they showed they can fabricate a 96-zone paper plate with sample distribution channels and a 384-zone microliter paper plate. To improve resolution, vacuum can be applied to drive the flow of molten wax into the paper thickness and minimize lateral spreading. Also, the wax pattern can be printed on both sides, reducing by two the required spreading distance. Additionally, the more uniform and smaller pores of the NC membranes enable to more controlled and precise wax patterns. Lu et al., report channels as thin as 300 μm and barriers of 60 μm on NC (Lu et al., 2009b). In one hand, wax has the advantage of not needing the use of solvents in the fabrication process. In the other, wax printed channels are not compatible with organic solvents since they react with it. That can be an advantage: one can remove interferences in a sample by washing them away with organic solvents (Leung et al., 2010).

14.2.3.4 Screen printing

Wax printing is a method that combines high-speed, simplicity, versatility, adaptability, and low-cost, and can accommodate large batch productions (Wang et al., 2012b). However, for most developing countries, wax printers are not a standard readily available tool and are expensive (Dungchai et al., 2011). To overcome this limitation, Dungchai et al. modified this method and introduced screen printing for wax (Dungchai et al., 2011). The technique consists in rubbing solid wax onto a paper filter through an ink-blocking stencil supported by a mesh. This mesh, made of porous fabric finely woven stretched over a frame, can transfer through material pressed against it, such as ink or wax. The loading of the wax is controlled by the size of the mesh and is fully blocked in the areas where the mesh has an impermeable coating. Then, similarly to wax printing, the device is put on a hot plate, and the wax is melted to form a hydrophobic barrier throughout the entire paper thickness. The wax penetration can be controlled by adjusting the temperature and the time of heating (the ideal condition was found to be 100°C for 60 s). A direct linear relationship exists between the width of the hydrophobic barrier deposited and the width of its design on the mask. The minimum designable channel and barrier widths are, on a whatman #1, 0.65 mm and 1.3 mm, respectively (Dungchai et al., 2011). Compared to using a wax printer, this technique is simpler and adequate for remote places where such complex equipment is unavailable. And as opposed to manually depositing wax with a pen, this technique is scalable and reproducible, as long as the force applied to the solid wax can be controlled.

14.2.3.5 Wax dipping

Because it is difficult to control the pressure on the wax with precision, screen printing suffers from poor reproducibility between batches which lead Songjaroen et al. to develop another wax-based fabrication method: wax dipping. This technique uses a mold that is pressed against the sheet of paper before the two are dipped for 1 s into melted wax at 120°C. After cooling, the sheet is peeled off and only has the areas protected by the mold remain without wax, as shown in Fig. 14.3 (Songjaroen et al., 2011). This 1-min method creates good resolution channels in a single dipping step. The relationship between the mask dimensions and the final hydrophilic dimensions is simple to derive. The smallest channel size rendered is 639 µm, similar to what is obtained with wax printing or wax screen-printing, but the reproducibility is better than the latter (%CV between 2% and 7%) when the temperature and the length of the dip in the bath of wax is perfectly controlled. The estimated total cost of a µPAD made by wax dipping is less than five cents.

14.2.4 Techniques based on the chemical modification of the paper surface

Certain reagents can change the wetting properties of the cellulose paper surface, and therefore be used to create hydrophilic—hydrophobic contrasts. This approach is simpler and more affordable than pore filling or deposition. AKD and alkenyl succinic

Paper-based microfluidic devices for low-cost assays 559

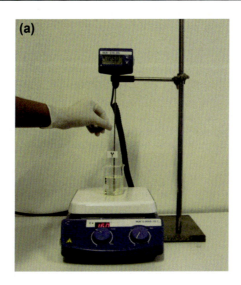

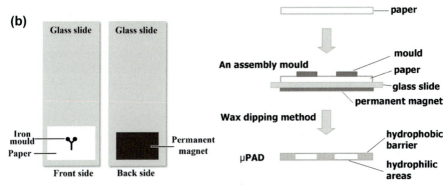

Figure 14.3 Fabrication process of the paper-based analytical device (PAD) using the wax dipping method: (a) simple wax dipping setup system and (b) procedure for patterning paper by wax dipping in top view (left) and lateral view (right).
Adapted with permission from Songjaroen, T., et al. (2011). Novel, simple and low-cost alternative method for fabrication of paper-based microfluidics by wax dipping. *Talanta, 85*(5), 2587–2593 Copyright © 2011 Elsevier B.V.

acid anhydrate (ASA) are commonly used for that purpose in paper sizing. They are very low cost patterning agents that impart hydrophobicity by esterification of the hydroxy group of the cellulose (Li et al., 2010a). Flexography, inkjet, and gravure are the most suitable methodologies to deposit sizing agents. After deposition, AKD and ASA require curing, typically in an oven at 100°C for 5 min. With this technique, the paper treated retains its original flexibility making packaging and handling easier. Moreover, the hydrophobic areas of the device show no visible mark or change of color, which is a critical characteristic for colorimetric-based assays.

14.2.4.1 Plasma oxidation etching

Li et al. are the first to have developed a two-steps process using a paper sizing reagent (Li et al., 2008, 2010a, 2010b). First, the paper is sized in AKD heptane solution and cured for 45 min at 100°C, making the treated paper strongly hydrophobic with contact angles greater than 110°. Then, sandwiched between two metal masks, the paper undergoes a plasma treatment that patterns hydrophilic area following the mask design. Although over-etching is common with plasma processes (the long mean free path of the energized electron causing bigger hydrophilic patterns than the mask), once the treatment duration and intensity are optimized, this process leads to very reproducible hydrophilic areas. The requirement for long curing times and a plasma oxidation tool (a sophisticated equipment not readily available) are the main production challenges to this technique. An additional drawback to this process is it creates hydrophilic areas that got exposed to solvents and polymers, which can be undesirable for certain assays (Songjaroen et al., 2011).

14.2.4.2 Inkjet printing

Inkjet printing relies on a digital inkjet printer to accurately deposit an AKD—heptane solution where the paper needs to be hydrophobic (Li et al., 2010). After printing, the device gets heated to allow curing, and, in a second step, the same printer can be used to deposit bioindicators in the sensing zones. This hydrophobic deposition requires only a single-side print to deposit the agent which then freely penetrates through the thickness of the sheet (and laterally). The use of heptane, a very volatile solvent, allows for the few picolitres printed solution to quickly evaporate and minimize lateral spread of the agent. This printing method is adapted to low-cost high-volume manufacturing. This process combines the advantage of PDMS printing (affordable devices which can withstand folding and bending) with the advanced patterning definition of photolithography. Finer wettable channels then 300 μm on Whatman paper (No. 4) have been reported. The estimated cost of a device with this method is a 1000 time lower than barrier-based PDMS devices. Digital inkjet printing is an easy and rapid fabrication process, with the pattern design solely requiring software changes to be modified. It is suitable for high-speed production of a large number of devices, with multiple devices printable on a single piece of paper with a single print-heat cycle (Li et al., 2010b). In addition, among all deposition processes, inkjet has the benefit of being a noncontact liquid deposition, which is highly desirable for printing biomolecules while minimizing cross-sample contamination and risk of substrate damage (Gauvreau & Laroche, 2005; Li et al., 2010a; Nagler, 2008).

However, an important limitation to the use of AKD and ASA is their nonresistance to the penetration of oil or low surface tension aqueous solution (typically solution with surface tension < 35 mN/m). To overcome that limitation, fluorocarbon-based sizing agents are used instead. Other alternatives such as thread-based device, that do not rely on hydrophobic barriers, have been successfully used to transport oil (Li et al., 2010a).

14.2.5 Other techniques
14.2.5.1 Laser printing and treatment
Laser printing is a one-step patterning method that starts with a hydrophobic paper substrate such as parchment, wax, or palette paper and uses CO_2 laser to pattern hydrophilic areas (Chitnis et al., 2011). The surfaces treated become more fibrous, and oxidized hydrophilic groups are formed. They can then trap chemicals but do not allow lateral diffusion of liquid. To achieve fluidic circulation, an additional coating of silica microparticles is needed. Therefore, after laser printing, an aqueous suspension of these particles is poured on top of the patterned paper, and after water evaporation and heavy shaking, they only remain in the hydrophilic areas. The high resolution and speed of this technique are its main advantages. By controlling the laser power and the scanning speed, it is possible to design features with little roughness and as small as 62 ± 1 μm.

14.2.5.2 Paper cutting and paper taping
The simplest method to fabricate paper-based devices is by cutting and taping. Fluidic flow in these kinds of devices is not bound in channels by hydrophobic barrier but by air instead. Cutting is rapid and only requires a cutting instrument such as a pair of scissors or, for complex patterns and mass-manufacturing, a laser cutter, or die cutter (Wang et al., 2012a). With this method, using tape is necessary to support any free-standing structures, which represents an extra step in the fabrication process.

Fenton et al. fabricated a NC lateral flow device that was shaped in two dimensions by a computer controlled knife on an XY plotter (Fenton et al., 2008). The resulting cut device was sandwiched between a vinyl and a polyester film to minimize evaporation, dehydration, and protect against external contamination. This technique is simple, direct, rapid, and suitable for mass manufacturing as well as prototyping, and can work with any type of cellulosic substrate. The smallest achievable features are in the millimeter range. And, with this technique, interpretational errors can be minimized by carving descriptive labels and instructions directly on the test strip.

Fabrication of 3D paper-based devices has been demonstrated using double-sided adhesive, as depicted on Fig. 14.4 (Martinez, Phillips, & Whitesides, 2008). Regular μPADs rely on 1D lateral flow wicking. 3D devices combine lateral and vertical wicking for an increased microfluidic capability, which opens the door to array-based analytical strategies commonly used in the pharmaceutical and drug discovery industries. Martinez used water-impermeable double-sided carpet tape and SU-8 photolithography patterning. Each individual layer of paper and tape were cut then stacked, alternating patterned paper and tape with via holes (60 μm thick and 800 μm in diameter). Via holes were punched through the tape and filled with a cellulose paste to create a vertical fluidic path. Finally, the reagents were spotted before device assembly. As an example of application, they demonstrated glucose test with control, four samples were tested for four analytes. The 3D device showed reliable and reproducible distribution of the sample to multiple detection zones in 1 min, making it easy to produce calibration curves. The estimated cost for a 3D device is

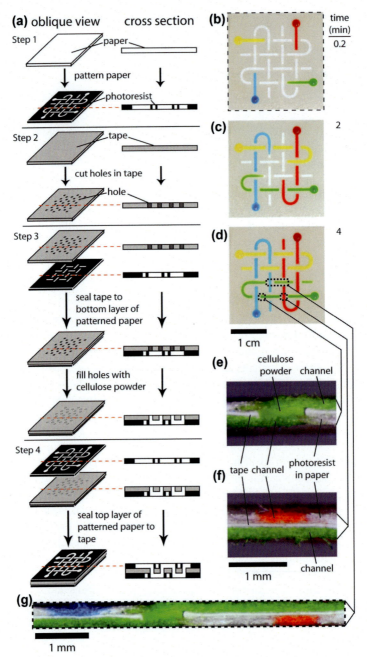

Figure 14.4 Preparation and demonstration of a 3D paper-based analytical device (PAD). (a) Fabrication. (b) Photograph of a basketweave system 10 s after adding red, yellow, green, and blue aqueous solutions of dyes to the sample reservoirs. The *dotted lines* indicate the edge of the device. (a and d) Photographs taken 2 (c) and 4 (d) min after adding the dyes. The streams of fluids crossed each other multiple times in different planes without mixing. The *dotted lines* in (d) show the positions of the cross sections shown in (e–g). (e) Cross section of the device showing a channel connecting the top and bottom layers of paper. (f) Cross section of the device

approximately US$30/m². Fig. 14.5 shows another technique utilizing wax as an adhesive to bond multiple layers to form a 3D chip (Gong et al., 2010). Patterns that will form fluidic channels were cut out from the substrate, and then the substrate was soaked in melted wax and sandwiched between glass or polymer sheets. And, using vacuum, the wax is pumped out from the channel. This bonding process is durable, compatible with cell culture, reversible, and provides a good seal. Origami methods have also been used for 3D building of paper-based devices, as shown on Fig. 14.6 (Liu & Crooks, 2011).

14.3 Detection and read-out technologies

In order to obtain a complete analytical instrument, an adequate transduction strategy needs to be chosen. That is done in function of the type of analytes and sample matrices handled, as well as the desired concentration ranges and accuracies. In addition, read-out strategies need to comply with the overall goals associated with paper devices: simplicity, mass manufacturability, and lower cost. Optical and electrochemical methods are generally the most simple, compact, low-power, and low-cost analytical techniques. They are, therefore, the best suited for paper-based assays. To date, the majority of the analytical assays for paper-based devices that have been reported rely on one or a combination of these detection techniques: colorimetry, electrochemistry, conductivity, chemiluminescence (CL), or electrochemiluminescence (ECL) (Sanjay et al., 2015). Let us explore each one.

14.3.1 Colorimetric detection

Colorimetric assays are reactions that lead to a change of color due to an enzymatic or chemical interaction between spotted reagents and the analyte. μPADs are well-suited for colorimetric biochemical assays; already most commercially available paper strip tests use color changes to qualitatively detect analytes (Dungchai et al., 2010). Colorimetric assays are ideal for simple semiquantitative answers, or when a yes/no answer is needed. When μPADs were first introduced, they successfully were applied to the colorimetric detection of glucose and protein, at levels that are clinically relevant

◄

showing the three layers of the device with orthogonal channels in the top and bottom layers of paper. (g) Cross section of the device showing the layers and the distribution of fluid (and colors) in each layer of the device shown in (d). The *dotted lines* indicate the edges of the cross section. Adapted with permission from Martinez, A. W., Phillips, S. T., & Whitesides, G. M. (2008). Three-dimensional microfluidic devices fabricated in layered paper and tape. *Proceedings of the National Academy of Sciences of the United States of America, 105*(50), 19606−19611. Copyright © 2008 National Academy of Sciences, USA.

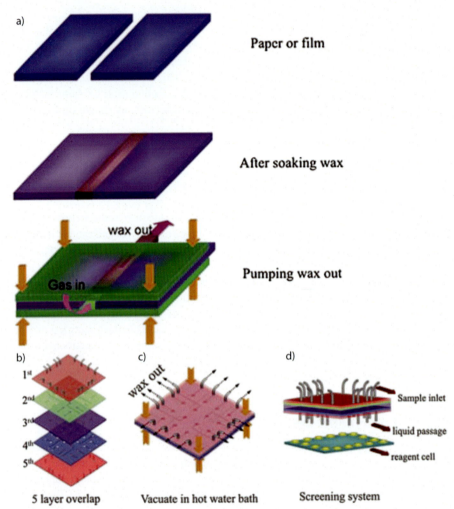

Figure 14.5 (a) After laser or scalpel cutting, the paper or film absorbed wax at the wax's melting point. After cooling, the film or paper was sandwiched between two glass slides and immersed in a hot-water bath. The gas was introduced from the inlet to the outlet through which the wax in the channel was pushed. (b) Five layers were overlapped and aligned. All of the layers were wetted by melt wax before being overlapped. (c) Layers were pressed together by four clamps at four corners (*yellow arrows*). (d) Structure of bacterial screening system comprised an upper screening chamber and a lower reagent cell. The liquid passage was a glass capillary which allowed the movement of liquid by capillary action.
Adapted with permission from Gong, X., et al. (2010). Wax-bonding 3D microfluidic chips. *Lab on a Chip, 10*(19), 2622−2627. Copyright © 2010 Royal Society of Chemistry.

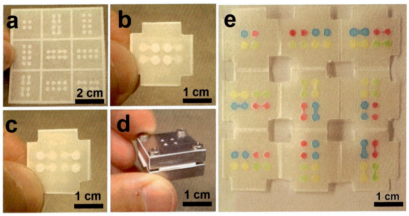

Figure 14.6 (a) Chromatography paper (100 μm thick) having photolithographically patterned channels, reservoirs, and a folding frame. All channels were 900 μm wide, and the reservoirs were 2.5 mm in diameter. (b) Top layer of the folded paper revealing four inlet reservoirs in the center of the device. The four flanking circular features are present within the 3-D structure of the device but are visible due to the transparency of the paper. Four corners of the folded paper were cut, so it could be clamped in the aluminum housing shown in (d). (c) Bottom layer of the folded paper. (d) The aluminum housing used to support the 3-D paper microfluidic system. The four holes drilled in the top of the housing are used for injecting solutions. (e) An unfolded, nine-layer paper microfluidic device after injecting four 1.0 mM, aqueous, colored solutions (rhodamine 6G, red; erioglaucine, blue; tatrazine, yellow; and a mixture of erioglaucine and tatrazine, 1:10, green) through the four injection ports in the aluminum clamp. The colored solutions passed through their designated channels and reservoirs without mixing. Adapted with permission from Liu, H., & Crooks, R. M. (2011). Three-dimensional paper microfluidic devices assembled using the principles of origami. *Journal of the American Chemical Society, 133*(44), 17564–17566. Copyright © 2011 American Chemical Society.

(Martinez et al., 2007). The testing of glucose was done by reacting the sample with potassium iodine mixed with horseradish peroxidase and glucose oxidase, which leads to the detection zone changing color from clear to brown proportionally to the glucose concentration. In a similar fashion, using citrate buffer with tetrabromophenol, a change of color from blue to yellow is obtained in function of protein concentration. These two examples are well-established colorimetric chemistries routinely used in laboratory for urine analyses. In the case of paper devices, the chemicals and enzymes involved in the colorimetric assay are usually spotted at the last step of fabrication and left to dry in the detection zones before final packaging. Similar glucose and protein tests were tried on devices patterned with different method: PDMS plotting (Bruzewicz et al., 2008), wax printing (Lu et al., 2009a), wax dipping (Songjaroen et al., 2011), inkjet printing of the device as well as the reagents (Abe et al., 2008). Other colorimetric tests published include: glucose using glucose oxidase with phenol red (Olkkonen et al., 2010) or bromocresol green (Songjaroen et al., 2011) as colored indicators; pH with bromothymol blue (Abe et al., 2008; Bruzewicz et al., 2008); nitrite test based on the Griess reaction principle (Klasner et al., 2010; Li et al., 2010);

uric acid test based on a bicinchoninate chelate method (Dungchai et al., 2010); protein test (Wang et al., 2010); lactate test (Dungchai et al., 2010); ketones test using the first spatially separated online double chemical derivatization (Klasner et al., 2010); total iron test ion using 1,10-phenanthroline (Dungchai et al., 2011); and IgG immunosensing pathogen detection (Abe et al., 2010). For these assays, a linear response over the range of interest is generally observed. And this dynamic range is limited by the amount of reagent and sample present, with most reactions stopping when the sample has completely evaporated and/or the channels have dried out. Therefore, colorimetric reactions need to be faster than the rate of evaporation. Keeping the device incubated in a humidity chamber reduces evaporation and improves the dynamic range (Klasner et al., 2010).

Visually comparing the color intensity of a reaction spot by naked eye is challenging. It represents a major hindrance to making this technology quantitative. Many factors including visual perception of color, lighting, and difference of color between a dry printed color on a label and the color on the reacted wetted paper can influence the reading (Dungchai et al., 2009).

In an attempt to quantify results more accurately, multiple researchers have digitalized the resulting color. They used a handheld optical colorimeter that measures the transmission of light through paper (Ellerbee et al., 2009), cell phone cameras (Martinez et al., 2008a; Xu et al., 2019), and scanners (Apilux et al., 2010; Klasner et al., 2010). The widespread existence of cell phone communication infrastructures and the omnipresence of camera-embedded phones and smartphones make this digital exchange affordable. It also allows for a better deployment of resources by enabling the monitoring to be done by untrained personnel.

In 2014, an android smartphone application was developed to process images of a paper-based device for measuring nitrite concentration and pH of water samples (Fig. 14.7). This work demonstrates the ability to detect multiple analytes on one device and to obtain immediate results in the field (Lopez-Ruiz et al., 2014). In this

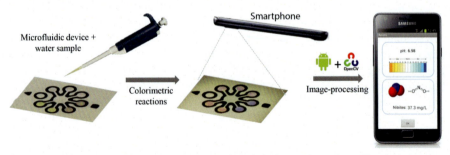

Figure 14.7 Scheme showing use of the paper-based device to determine pH and nitrite concentration with analysis by smartphone.
Adapted with permission from Lopez-Ruiz, N., et al. (2014). Smartphone-based simultaneous pH and nitrite colorimetric determination for paper microfluidic devices. *Analytical Chemistry*, 86(19), 9554–9562. Copyright © 2014 American Chemical Society.

device, Griess reagents immobilized on the paper reacted with nitrite to produce a color change from colorless to pink, allowing quantification. The pH was measured by a color change in two pH indicators stored on the paper, phenol red, and chlorophenol red. The device only required one drop of water sample, and after 15 min, the analytes have reacted with the stored reagents. The android application ensures that camera placement is consistent for each sample by aligning marks on the device and uses the camera flash for consistency in lighting. The change in the hue and saturation coordinates of the hue-saturation-value (HSV) color space combined with a custom algorithm give a final readout. The μPAD and android application obtained comparable results to a standard potentiometric method for pH determination; however, it was less accurate for nitrite analysis. Despite these limitations, the work demonstrates the development of a smartphone application that provides consistent, objective analysis of colorimetric data in the field.

Even with digitization, however, experimental conditions such as lighting, sensitivity of the color measurement device, and background color of the paper substrate that can change with time and in between batches remain sources of interpretation errors. These reading mistakes can be minimized if, as Li et al. proposed, an internal calibration standard is run in parallel to the sample using the same device under the same conditions (Li et al., 2010b). He used inkjet printing of AKD to pattern a six branch device to analyze for nitrite ion and uric acid, and a low-cost desktop scanner for the image digitalization. He spotted the unknown solution in one of the detection zone and five dilutions from a standard in the rest and then introduced the indicator reagents in the central inlet zone, as described on Fig. 14.8. He obtained an increase in reliability and accuracy approaching that of conventional UV-Vis spectrophotometry. Similarly, Wang et al. developed a tree-shape design, depicted on Fig. 14.9, that is convenient for multiplexed assays and can integrate a self-calibration curve to eliminate systematic errors (Wang et al., 2010). The paper-based device enables a uniform flow of water from its stem to the multiple branches where each single analysis takes place. After the assay is completed, the operator can easily compare the color of the unknown with the standards. Another strategy to improve accuracy and help visual reading can be achieved by using multiple indicators for the same analyte that will generate different colors and react at different levels of analyte concentrations (Dungchai et al., 2010). This approach, used by Dungchai et al., can be accomplished by spotting an oxidase enzyme that produces hydrogen peroxide proportionally to the analyte's concentration and spotting indicators that react at different levels of concentration of hydrogen peroxidase. This method was used to develop a nine branch device for simultaneous analytical measurement of glucose, lactate, and uric acid in clinically relevant ranges and demonstrated a significant improvement in reading accuracy (Dungchai et al., 2010).

Among colorimetric indicators, gold and silver nanoparticles (NPs) with their strong extinction coefficient are superior. Their absorption spectra have the unique property of depending on their size; therefore, any reaction that can cause these NPs to aggregate or dissociate leads to an observable change of color (Prasad et al., 2020). Zhao et al. leveraged these properties and demonstrated that DNA cross-linked gold NPs can be used for adenosine biosensing on paper devices. The paper

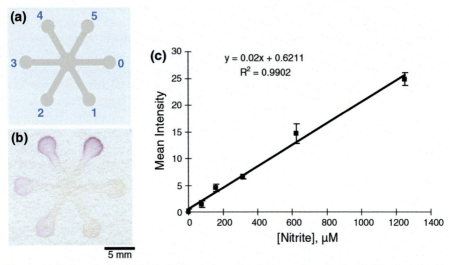

Figure 14.8 Quantitative biological/chemical assay using paper-based microfluidic devices. (a) The assay design: NO$_2$—standard solutions (0.5 lL) with different concentration from 0 to 1250 lmol/L were deposited into detection zone 0 to zone 5 in sequence; (b) NO$_2$—indicator solution was added into the device from central inlet zone and caused different color changes in different detection zones; (c) Calibration curve created by color density measurement using Adobe Photoshop of the scanned images of the tests. Error bars were obtained from six repeated measurements.
Adapted with permission from Li, X., Tian, J., & Shen, W. (2010a). Progress in patterned paper sizing for fabrication of paper-based microfluidic sensors. *Cellulose, 17*(3), 649–659. Copyright © Springer Science + Business Media B.V. 2010.

substrate served as a protection from nonspecific stimuli making the aggregated gold NPs stable for weeks and able to be stored without loss of performance (Zhao et al., 2008). The NPs would only dissociate (thus change color) upon addition of the target. Sensitive detection of adenosine and endonuclease was performed, and with the use of DNA aptamers, the assay can be generalized to many targets. Colorimetric assays based on the aggregation (as oppose to dissociation) of NPs have also been successfully demonstrated. For instance, to produce a copper detector, silver NPs were functionalized with homocysteine (Hcy) and dithiothreitol (DTT) and spotted on a paper-based device. Upon addition of copper, which induced their aggregation through amino-carboxyl binding, they showed a change of color with a limit of detection (LOD) as low as 7.8 nM (Ratnarathorn et al., 2012).

Many groups have addressed the pitfalls listed above by integrating new sensing motifs on μPADs. For example, an aptamer-based fluorescent μPAD capable of multiplexed screening of cancer cells was developed in 2016 (Liang et al., 2016). This paper device presented on Fig. 14.10 is coated with graphene oxide and quantum dots (QDs) that are functionalized with DNA aptamers. The aptamers not only target specific lines of cancer cells but also bind to graphene through π-π stacking, effectively quenching

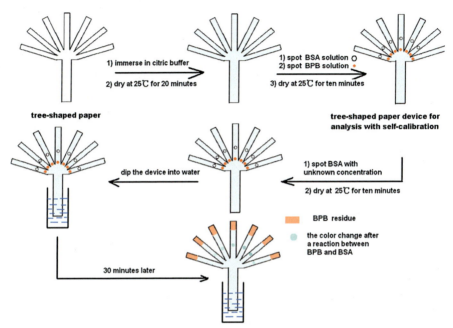

Figure 14.9 Diagram of the procedure for tree-shaped device with self-calibration for detection. Adapted with permission from Wang, W., Wu, W. Y., & Zhu, J. J. (2010). Tree-shaped paper strip for semiquantitative colorimetric detection of protein with self-calibration. *Journal of Chromatography A, 1217*(24), 3896–3899. Copyright © 2010 Elsevier B.V.

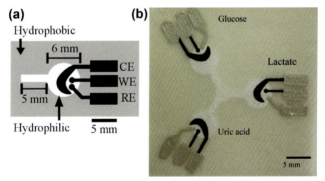

Figure 14.10 Schematic representation of the fabrication process of the multiplexed microfluidic paper-based analytical device (μPAD) and quantum dot(QD)–coated silica beads developed by Liang et al. (a) μPAD consists of three negative control areas that are not connected to the sample inlet and three sample wells each containing a different QD/aptamer pair. (b) Functionalization of silica nanoparticles with QDs and aptamers.
Adapted with permission from Liang, L., et al. (2016). Aptamer-based fluorescent and visual biosensor for multiplexed monitoring of cancer cells in microfluidic paper-based analytical devices. *Sensors and Actuators B: Chemical, 229*, 347–354. Copyright © 2016 Elsevier B.V.

the fluorescence of the QDs. When the aptamers bind to their respective cancer cells, the QDs are unquenched and fluoresced. Each cell line is represented by a different color QD, so the color of the fluorescence indicates the cell type detected. The device can be used with the naked eye for qualitative testing but can also be used with a fluorescence detector for sensitive quantitative measurements with low detection limits. Sensitivity was enhanced by coating mesoporous silica NPs with the QDs. The NPs have a large surface-area-to-volume ratio, which increased the number of QDs available for binding with cells on the surface of the device, compared with QDs adsorbed on paper alone. This work is an example of µPAD research focused on improving sensitivity and LODs, and multiplexed testing. Although, LODs on paper can be improved over traditional colorimetric detection through techniques like fluorescence, another method often used to lower detection limits is electrochemistry.

14.3.2 Electrochemical detection

ECD as opposed to colorimetric assays is generally capable of precise quantification of the analyte's concentration. As presented in the various examples below, this detection strategy may still require some form of chemical amplification, such as enzyme or metal ion—based enhancements, to further lower detection limits to clinically relevant levels (Scida et al., 2014). These procedures of enhancement often require expensive reagents, multiple steps for the end user, and a complex device fabrication. They are, therefore, not quite adapted to paper-based devices. ECD is a redox-based method that relies on a three electrode system: the working, the counter, and the reference electrodes. On paper-based devices, these electrodes can be screen printed with a conductive ink at a low cost. Commonly, a carbon ink is used for the working, and counter electrodes and a silver/silver chloride ink for the reference electrode and the pads (Apilux et al., 2010; Dungchai et al., 2009). Fig. 14.11 shows screen-printed electrodes; they have the advantage to be disposable and easy to functionalize by chemical derivatization. Although ECD on paper requires external equipment, the latter remains minimal, consumes little power, and can be miniaturized (Dungchai et al., 2009). The first microfluidic paper-based electrochemical device (µPED) was introduced by Dungchai et al. with the simultaneous quantification of glucose, lactate, and uric acid in biological samples (Dungchai et al., 2009). After being printed, the electrodes were chemically modified with Prussian Blue to improve their selectivity toward hydrogen peroxide, then they were spotted with the appropriate oxidase enzymes, which catalyzed the oxidation of their substrate (the analyte) while reducing oxygen to hydrogen peroxide. When a sample drop is deposited at the center of the paper, it flows to the reaction sites where chronoamperometry is performed using the optimal potential for hydrogen peroxide production. Low detection limits within the range of clinical relevance were obtained with performances comparable to the ones from traditional diagnostic tools (Dungchai et al., 2011). Nie et al. also demonstrated glucose testing using chronoamperometry and showed a LOD five times lower than traditional glucometers and twice lower than colorimetric assays (Nie et al., 2010a). They also fabricated a paper-based device with four electrodes to be used with commercial handheld glucometer (Nie et al., 2010b). Additionally, they demonstrated ECD's good

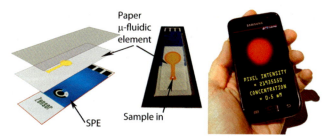

Figure 14.11 (a) Basic design of the electrochemical detection cell for paper-based microfluidic devices. *CE*, counter electrode; *RE*, reference electrode; *WE*, working electrode. (b) Picture of three electrode paper-based microfluidic devices. The hydrophilic area at the center of the device wicks sample into the three separate test zones where independent enzyme reactions occur. The silver electrodes and contact pads are made from Ag/AgCl paste with the black electrode portions being the Prussian Blue modified carbon electrodes. The device size is 4 cm × 4 cm.
Adapted with permission from Dungchai, W., Chailapakul, O., & Henry, C. S. (2009). Electrochemical detection for paper-based microfluidics. *Analytical Chemistry, 81*(14), 5821–5826. Copyright © 2009 American Chemical Society.

selectivity by specifically quantify Pb(II) at ppb-levels concentrations in solutions containing Zn(II) and Pb(II) using anodic stripping voltammetry.

When electrodes are fabricated directly onto paper, they have most of their surface occupied by cellulose fibers, and as a result, their sensitivity is lowered. Recently, to overcome this limitation, Crooks et al. presented hollow-channel μPADs (Renault et al., 2013, 2014; Scida et al., 2014) which incorporated microwire electrodes. These devices, called ePADs, are capable of performing bulk solution electrochemistry under flow conditions. They have faster flow rates (therefore shorter analysis times) and have electrodes amenable to surface modification external to the device, and that could better resist harsher pretreatments without damaging and/or contaminating the paper substrate.

ECD can readily be combined with a separation step for improved sensing. Carvalhal et al. separated via chromatography and then analyzed by chronoamperometry a mixture of uric and ascorbic acid on a paper-based device (Carvalhal et al., 2010b). The separation, which efficiency depends on the thickness, the length, and the quality of the paper, happened during travel of the sample thought the paper column.

A hurdle for the common methods used in ECD, amperometric, and coulometric is their need for external bulky electrochemical detectors. An alternative method requiring only a simple reader is the electrical conductivity measurement (Steffens et al., 2009). Another one is the monitoring of streaming potentials, as described by Leung et al. Their group showed that these potentials are sensitive to the presence of charged polymers adsorbed on the surface of the paper. So, they proposed derivatizing the cellulosic channel to bind the target and detecting the binding events by measuring the changes in streaming potential (Apilux et al., 2010; Leung et al., 2010). Electrochemical Impedance Spectroscopy (EIS) is another detection method that can detect binding events, the ones that occur on a transducer surface. It was used on an ePAD by the Henry Group (Adkins, Noviana, & Henry, 2016). They derivatized gold microwire electrodes through surface assembled monolayer (SAM) chemistry which inferred a bioaffinity to the analyte through a stepwise bioconjugation process. Each binding event produced an increase in the measured impedance, and using flow-based PAD, they increased the mass transfer of species to the electrode surface and showed they can detect the West Nile Virus (WNV) at limits comparable to those achieved with enzyme-linked immunosorbent assay (ELISA). To overcome another hindrance from ECD, the inability to detect certain analytes and/or to prevent the overlapping response of contaminants with the analyte of interest, a strategy of dual electrochemical and colorimetric assays on a single device can be adopted. Apilux et al. used that option to simultaneously screen for Au(III) and Fe(III), which have reduction currents that overlap (Apilux et al., 2010). They detected Au(III) using square wave voltammetry in aqua regia buffer, and Fe(III) using a phenanthroline-based colorimetric assay. More recently, a device with dual detection system was developed for the quantification of heavy metals (Rattanarat et al., 2014). Fe^{3+}, Ni^{2+}, Cr^{6+}, and Cu^{2+} were quantified using a colorimetric method (with as dyes and in order, dimethylglyoxime, phenanthroline, 1,5 diphenylcarbazide, and with a mixture of bathocuproine and polyethylene glycol), and Pb^{2+} and Cd^{2+} were using square-wave anodic stripping voltammetry. With the adequate pick of electrode material and detection potential, μPEDs represent a solution that combines simplicity, moderate cost, portability, and speed with the required accuracy, sensitivity, and selectivity.

14.3.3 Chemiluminescent and electrochemiluminescent detections

CL is simple, highly sensitive, and can be performed in the dark, thus independently of any ambient light. Yu et al. designed a μPADs for the simultaneous analysis of glucose and uric acid relying on the CL reaction between rhodamine derivatives and hydrogen peroxide (Yu et al., 2011). The hydrogen was generated by the two oxidase enzymes immobilized on separate channels.

ECL detection corresponds to a CL reaction in which luminescence is established and controlled by the application of an electrical potential. This method inherits of the advantages from CL, such as emission of light independently of the ambient light, with an improved selectivity and an increased dynamic range due to the better control of the reaction through electrochemistry (Delaney et al., 2011; Ge et al., 2012; Yan et al., 2012). And like ECD, ECL is highly sensitivite and permits a good control over timing and spatial location of the reaction (Delaney et al., 2011). Fig. 14.12 shows the first ECL-based sensing paper-based device by Delaney et al. (2011). They used screen printed electrodes and chronoamperometry to induce ECL between a biological compound, nicotinamide adenine dinucleotide, and an ECL reagent, tris(bipyridine)ruthenium(II), which yields an orange luminescence. Using a phone camera as a photo sensor, they successfully obtained calibration curves with detection limits lower than colorimetric assays. Additionally, they showed that the mass transport was unaffected by the fibrous substrate.

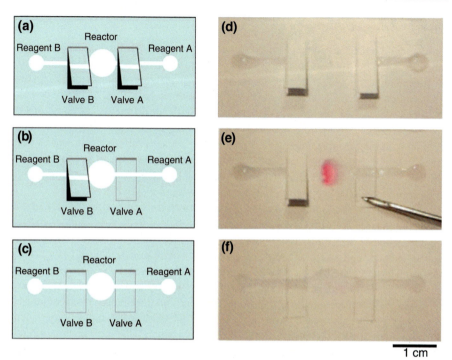

Figure 14.12 Electrochemiluminescence (ECL) detection of a sample solution (2-(dibutylamino)-ethanol (DBAE)). The device was filled with a 10 mM Ru(bpy)$_3^{2+}$ solution before drying, and was then aligned and fixed onto the face of the screen-printed electrode (SPE) by laminating with transparent plastic. A drop of sample was introduced through a small aperture in the plastic at the base of the channel. After the detection zone being fully wetted, a potential of 1.25 V was applied and the resulting emission was captured and analyzed. Adapted with permission from Delaney, J. L., et al. (2011). Electrogenerated chemiluminescence detection in paper-based microfluidic sensors. *Analytical Chemistry, 83*(4), 1300–1306. Copyright © 2011 American Chemical Society.

14.4 Application of paper-based microfluidic devices

Made of readily available material, small, lightweight, easy to stack, store, and transport, paper-based microfluidics have the potential to be a privileged analytical platform for a wide range of applications. We will explore three major areas: medical diagnostics, environmental monitoring, and food quality assessment. Relying on the different detection techniques described earlier, μPADs can provide qualitative and/or quantitative (sometimes semiquantitative) results for the detection of a single or multiple analytes. They exist under two major formats: the on-demand devices, which are empty generic platforms that require the user to introduce detection reagents into the device prior to testing; and the ready-to-use devices, which are complete devices with reactive sensing reagents already integrated in the detection zones. We will discuss examples in these two categories and look at their strengths and challenges which constitute important considerations in future developments and improvements in the field.

14.4.1 On-demand μPADs

On-demand devices are general-purpose tools with only the desired microfluidic features for handling fluids. They are generic platforms that can be utilized for common biological or chemical assays, such as quantifying an analyte concentration or creating a calibration curve. Li et al. presented an example of such devices, a star shape platform that allows a single drop of indicator react with six different concentrations of nitrate (Li et al., 2010a). Another example is Bruzewicz's design which has an inlet channel splitting into five equally sized channels leading to different test zones where the user can pipette different reagents for parallel testing. He used an open inlet channel with no border, which allows a simple dipping of the inlet edge of the device to draw some sample in and start the assays (Bruzewicz et al., 2008).

To perform more complex and reliable measurements while having the ease of use of conventional lateral flow tests, on-demand devices need to include sample processing capabilities. Two-dimensional fluidic networks on paper can enable these sophisticated features and render multiple steps assays possible. The Yager Group, after doing quantitative studies on flow in fluidic networks, has showed several methods for controlling fluid transport (Kauffman et al., 2010; Fu et al., 2010a, 2011). Like by playing with the geometry of the fluidic network and introducing dissolvable barriers, they enable automated sequential delivery of fluid and sample pretreatment before analysis (Fu et al., 2010b; Lutz et al., 2011). In general, the introduction of functional elements to actively control fluid movements is critical to the development of improved assay execution on paper. Li et al. developed a simple element, shown on Fig. 14.13, that functions as a switch (Li et al., 2010a). A reactor has been made using two switches that control the access of two liquid reactants from their dosing sites (A1, A2) to the reactor site B (Li et al., 2010). Other circuit elements have been fabricated such as a fluidic timer based on paraffin wax (Noh & Phillips, 2010a, 2010b), an "on" button for connecting and disconnecting the fluidic flow (Martinez et al., 2010), a filter that separates plasma from whole blood (Yang et al., 2012). Additional works on adapting common microfluidic techniques to paper-based devices include hydrodynamic focusing, sized-based extraction of molecules, micromixing, and dilution (Osborn et al., 2010; Rezk et al., 2012).

14.4.2 The ready-to-use μPADs

We define ready-to-use devices as devices that already incorporate the reagents needed in a particular detection chemistry meant for a specific analyte. They correspond to most of the published works and are designed to respond to the needs of a given field. Table 1 presents a compilation of most of the reported analytes and the methods used for their detection, in function of the field of application: health diagnostics, biochemical analysis, environmental monitoring, food quality control, and forensic.

In health diagnostics, μPADs find an application as low-cost, disposable, and easy to fabricate testing devices that, if quantitative enough, can be used to directly establish a diagnostic. And when only semiquantitative or semiqualitative, they represent a fast and inexpensive initial screening tool that can indicate if a more expensive and labor-

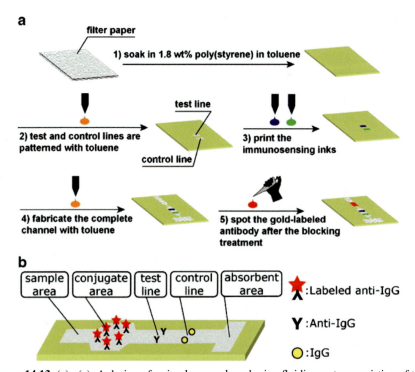

Figure 14.13 (a)–(c): A design of a simple paper-based microfluidic reactor consisting of two sample dosing sites, two valves and one central reaction site; (d)–(f) A paper-based microfluidic reactor based on this design was tested using acid–base neutralization reaction; ((d) Phenolphthalein indicator solution was deposited onto the central reaction zone. NaOH and HCl solutions were added into reagent zones A and B, respectively; (e) NaOH solution was introduced into the reaction zone to trigger color change; (f) HCl solution was introduced later into the reaction zone via valve B to neutralize NaOH in the reaction zone).
Adapted with permission from Li, X., Tian, J., Shen, W. (2010a). Progress in patterned paper sizing for fabrication of paper-based microfluidic sensors. *Cellulose, 17*(3), 649–659. Copyright © Springer Science + Business Media B.V. 2010.

intensive examination is required. To be of clinical use, μPADs (such as the ones reported in Table 1) have to be capable of analyzing samples from body fluid such as urine, saliva, sputum, or blood. Additionally, to be the most representative of the patient's health condition, they are usually designed for simultaneous detection of multiple analytes using a single sample drop. Examples include the simultaneous detection in urine of glucose and protein (Martinez et al., 2007, 2008a) or in saliva of nitrite and uric acid, which are potential biomarkers for monitoring hemodialysis (Li et al., 2010a).

Besides, nowadays, a large range of commercially available health testing tools are based on immunorecognition assays. Some example include the urine test for pregnancy or blood test for hepatitis C. Usually, with these immunotest strips, the analyte flows by capillarity effect to spotted antibodies and subsequently bound to them leading to a color appearance at the test line (Dungchai et al., 2010). They are extremely sensitive, reliable, and fast. By using these existing immune-based assays and the powerful platform that is microfluidics, paper-based devices open up new possibilities for clinical testing (Fenton et al., 2008). For instance, Khan demonstrated a paper-based device for blood typing using a three arms prototype, where each arm was treated with a different solution of antibody (A, B, and O) (Khan et al., 2010). After a drop of whole blood was spotted at the center of the device, it flowed to the different arms, and when the red cells, carried with the blood, encountered their specific antibodies they agglutinated causing a visible chromatographic mark on that arm. This paper-based diagnostics, at a cost of only a few cents, can promote health in the developing world by rapidly providing the blood test result necessary to many chirurgical procedures. Other work relying on antigenic binding include the electroluminescent detection-based method for diagnostic of carcinoembryonic antigen from real serum sample (Yan et al., 2012), and the CL detection of four cancer biomarkers (Ge et al., 2012). Another major immunologic test adapted to paper-fluidics is the ELISA, which combines antibodies and enzymes to provide specificity and sensitivity (Abe et al., 2010; Cheng et al., 2010; Martinez, 2011; Wang et al., 2009, 2012b). Fig. 14.14 from Abe et al. shows the fabrication process of a paper-based device using immunosensing inks and gold-labeled antibodies. They demonstrate that the antibodies get successfully adsorbed on the cellulose and get released from their immobilization site only upon sample application. Likewise, Wang et al. wax-printed a device combining the specific ELISA method with the sensitive CL detection and showed quantitative clinical testing of three tumor markers (Wang et al., 2012b). In parallel, to satisfy the need for high throughput, low cost, and low volume ELISA assays, Cheng et al. printed paper-based microarray plates (Cheng et al., 2010). They represent an affordable equivalent to the conventional 96-microzone plate, onto which researchers demonstrated quantitative detection of HIV-1. All these testing devices used in conjunction with the modern communication tools such as camera phone are powerful telemedicine and general health monitoring tools. μPADs have the potential to be useful in food quality control as well, where inspections from production to packaging are required, and where monitoring the lifetime of products once on the shelves is critical. They have been used to assess various analytes, from amine vapors in fish to mycotoxins in cereals, and more frequently bacteria such as *Escherichia coli* and *Salmonella* (Adkins et al., 2017; Srisa-Art et al., 2018; Yao et al., 2018). Adkins et al., for instance, used two types of μPADs to indirectly detect *E. coli* and *Enterococcus*. Enzymes released by these bacteria were reacted with substrates that produced p-nitrophenol (PNP), o-nitrophenol (ONP), and p-aminophenol (PAP). The PNP, ONP, and PAP were detected colorimetrically with a spot test and electrochemically with an ePAD, and good in-laboratory calibration curves were obtained. The major disadvantage of these bacterial tests, however, remains the requirement to enrich real samples by growing the bacteria to generate detectable concentrations. Unfortunately, the 4–24 h preenrichment process required seven steps prior to quantification, increasing both the analysis time and complexity of the assay. Srisa-Art et al. reported a colorimetric spot test and distance-based μPAD for quantifying salmonella

Paper-based microfluidic devices for low-cost assays 577

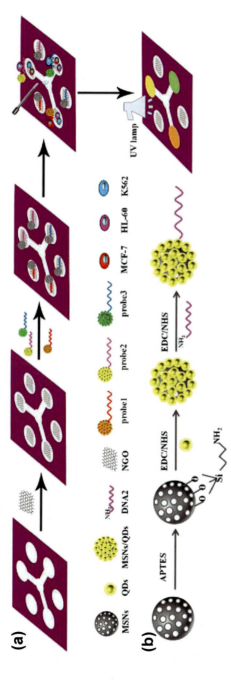

Figure 14.14 (a) Fabrication process of the inkjet-printed microfluidic immunosensing strip. Patterning of the test/control lines (step 2), dispensing of the immunosensing inks onto the test/control lines (step 3), and patterning of the entire channel and remaining areas (step 4) are performed on the same inkjet printing apparatus (the *pen symbol* indicates the use of the inkjet printer). A gold-labeled antibody is spotted onto the conjugate area by a micropipette. (b) Schematic representation of the finalized strip featuring a microfluidic channel consisting of a sample inlet area, a conjugate area, a sensing area containing a test line and a control line, and an absorbent area.
Adapted with permission from Abe, K., et al. (2010) Inkjet-printed paperfluidic immuno-chemical sensing device. *Analytical and Bioanalytical Chemistry*, 398(2), 885–893. Copyright © Springer Science + Business Media B.V. 2010.

(Srisa-Art et al., 2018). They added of a "chemometer" strip to measure the length of the color band and help with quantification without the need for an external instrument.

Park et al. used delayed flow and channel partition formation on a NC membrane to achieve a simple, single-step device for on-site detection of *Salmonella*. Two types of antibody-conjugated gold nanoparticles (AuNPs) are used for each pathogen being detected, and three gold enhancer components, used to amplify the colorimetric signals, are preloaded and dried on the NC membrane. This one-step operation device uses a compressed dipstick with dehydrated reagents to carry out a multistep reaction scheme: The device is dipped into a sample solution, and the analyte reacts with the antibody conjugated AuNPs, and the immunocomplexes are then captured by antibodies at the test line for colorimetric signals. This device was able to detect *E. coli* and *Salmonella* with comparable detection limits to current USDA standards for these bacteria, ($\sim$ 100 CFU/mL) but faced a high standard deviation in signal intensity, and therefore, more work to increase precision is needed.

Other examples include the work of Nie et al. on an electrochemical μPADs that used a commercial glucometer to measure on-site the concentration of ethanol in food products (Nie et al., 2010b), and the one by Hossain et al. on the detection of acetylcholinesterase (AChE) inhibitors, including organophosphate pesticides in foods and beverages (Hossain et al., 2009b). Their colorimetric assay relied on a printed sol–gel silica ink that entrapped AChE and a chromogenic substrate on the paper-based device. They reported excellent detection limits and successful detections in milk and apple juice, demonstrating its applicability for on the field rapid trace testing. The articles discussed above are just a few of the many published in which researchers are attempting to develop more efficient means of food monitoring in resource-limited areas to prevent foodborne illnesses.

Lastly, a major field of application for testing is the environmental and water monitoring, where extremely low-cost, real-time, and on-site detection tests are highly needed. The major categories of contaminants sought for are heavy metals, chemical and agricultural pollutants as well as toxins and pathogens. For ionic metals, a good example of μPAD is the one from Apilux et al. on the monitoring of gold refining waste. They designed a dual electrochemical/colorimetric μPAD for detecting both Au(III) and Fe(III) on the same device (Apilux et al., 2010). Iron needed to be measured calorimetrically since it interferes with the ECD of gold. Additional harmful ions include lead and zinc for which Nie et al. designed a rapid and cost-effective μPAD based on anodic stripping voltammetry (Nie et al., 2010a). Another device with dual colorimetry/electrochemistry capabilities was demonstrated for the measure of multiple heavy metals (Fe^{3+}, Ni^{2+}, Cr^{6+}, Cu^{2+}, Pb^{2+}, and Cd^{2+}) with a 0.01 μg uncertainty for the analytes relying on colorimetry and 0.01 ng for the ones relying on electrochemistry (Rattanarat et al., 2014). Agricultural runoffs carrying pesticides and insecticide also constitute a threat to human health and the environment. Hossain et al. tested bioactive paper sensors sensitive to organophosphates, which are a class of chemicals widely used in agriculture (Hossain et al., 2009a). Regarding the probing of biohazards, and toxins in particular, Wang et al. developed a simple but high-performance fibrous-based biosensor faster than traditional ELISA. They impregnated a paper-based device with antibody-coated single-walled carbon nanotubes, which electrical conductivity depended on the concentration in the toxins the spotted antibodies are sensitive to (Wang et al., 2009). They demonstrated the effectiveness of their platform by detecting, at levels lower than the World Health Organization standard, microcystin, a lethal toxin that travels to the liver, binds covalently to protein phosphatases, and disrupts cellular control processes.

14.5 Current limitations and future perspectives in paper-based microfluidics

Microfluidic paper devices have the potential to be widely adopted analytical tools. Their low cost, portability, disposability, limited waste, simplicity, speed, lower consumption of reagents and sample, ease of fabrication, and use make them very attractive (Auroux et al., 2002; Coltro et al., 2010; Li et al., 2012; Liana et al., 2012; Reyes et al., 2002). Their downsized reaction zones compared to dipstick tests makes them appealing for the analysis of scarce and hard-to-get samples (Abe et al., 2008). However, to become a standard tool, they still need to overcome multiple limitations and match the performance of conventional analytical techniques. Some are impediments related to the substrate's nature, others originate from fabrication and detection hurdles.

A large volume of the sample gets lost during transport across a μPAD. In fact, at least half of it is retained within the paper matrix or evaporates in the air before reaching the detection zones, resulting in less concentrated, thus harder to detect, analytes (Li et al., 2012b). These losses are particularly undesirable when quantities of samples are limited. To improve sample delivery and avoid evaporation, groups have proposed various methods to enclose devices (Schilling et al., 2012). Fully enclosing devices have the additional benefits of protecting channels from outside contamination, improving storage of reagents, and easing its handling and transport. Prior to Schilling et al., others reported using double-sided tape to enclose 3D devices, but the adhesion of the protective tape becomes poor when the device gets wet and diffusion of adhesive in paper over time can be an issue. Back-side protection was proposed as well, using polyester-backed NC (Fenton et al., 2008) or flexographic printing of a polyester layer (Olkkonen et al., 2010). In addition, for the performance of separations on the paper device, a closed system enables a better control over eluent's vapor pressure, thus decreasing separation times and improving separation efficiencies (Carvalhal et al., 2010a, 2010b). To mitigate sample retention, other groups have suggested using nonporous V-groove channels on polymer instead of cellulose (Tian et al., 2010), or thread-based microfluidic system, where sewed threads through a supporting substrate such as a polymer film are used to channel fluids (Li et al., 2010c; Reches et al., 2010). These threaded devices have higher wet strength compared with the paper-based ones. Recently, the Li group pioneered a new type of paper hybrid devices, paper/polymer hybrid microfluidic devices, to combine the benefits of both paper and polymer substrates (Dou et al., 2014; Sanjay et al., 2016; Zuo et al., 2013).

To make lab-on-paper and low-cost diagnostic tool, its fabrication needs to be compatible with high-speed, high-volume manufacturing without compromising quality. It is critical to ensure that channels extend through the full thickness of the paper and hold the fluid properly. Because paper fibers are intertwined in a planar fashion and layered on top of each other (making hydrophobic wicking anisotropic), it is challenging for single-step fabrication processes to pattern thin and well-defined channels (Li et al., 2010a). As for the two-steps method, a common issue is the interference of the sample with some residues of hydrophobic reagent that would not have been completely removed from the channel (Dungchai et al., 2011). Furthermore, all patterning strategies relying on hydrophobic agents cannot build hydrophobic barriers strong enough to withstand samples of low surface tension, such as biological samples with surfactant. To have effective transport of any kind of liquid, it is best to pattern by blocking cellulosic pores. But, this strategy uses extensive amounts of material. Another challenge that can be solved with novel fabrication designs are the difficulty in multiplex analysis and in high integration of multiple analytical procedures on a single device, which are important features to ensure quantitative analyses (Wang et al., 2012b). 3D structures described previously are a tentative to achieve this goal. The future will see more of these intricate devices and novel techniques to route fluids, separate analytes, and wash, all while avoiding fluidic cross-talks.

μPADs need to detect very low concentrations of biomarkers and contaminants to be relevant. Commonly, food and drinking water levels of contamination are in the ppb- to ppt-range, and currently typical colorimetric-based devices are limited to ppm. Research to enhance sensitivity and selectivity has already started with the development of AuNPs-based detection and biorecognition on paper (Zhao et al., 2008a, 2008b). In addition, any detection strategy needs to be compatible with transport and room temperature long-time storage. Understanding biomolecules immobilization and their stability is complex, and comprehensive optimizations still need to be conducted. Finally, to stay appealing, any detection strategy on μPADs needs to preserve their portability and their low power consumption. An innovation by Thom et al., consisting in galvanic cells patterned within the paper device, represents an attractive approach toward self-powered analytical assays (Thom et al., 2012).

Since its introduction, paper has shown tremendous potential as a substrate material for sensing devices. Although many applications have been reported, paper-based microfluidics is still at an early stage. Any commercial success will depend on μPADs being mass producible at a low-cost, with an acceptable shelf life in resource-limited areas, capable of reliable and easy-to-interpret results, and capable of measuring a suite of analytes. Additionally, commercial adoption will be slow for μPADs applications that require complicated or expensive external equipment. Therefore, in the coming years, we foresee the development to focus on improving manufacturability, sensitivity, and detection limits, developing new techniques for long-term and stable storage of reagents on paper in uncontrolled conditions, and fabricating devices capable of multiplexed testing. We also expect the field to move toward applications that require regular measurements, such as human health preventative screenings and environmental assessment.

References

Abe, K., et al. (2010). Inkjet-printed paperfluidic immuno-chemical sensing device. *Analytical and Bioanalytical Chemistry, 398*(2), 885−893.

Abe, K., Suzuki, K., & Citterio, D. (2008). Inkjet-printed microfluidic multianalyte chemical sensing paper. *Analytical Chemistry, 80*(18), 6928−6934.

Adkins, J. A., et al. (2017). Colorimetric and electrochemical bacteria detection using printed paper- and transparency-based analytic devices. *Analytical Chemistry, 89*(6), 3613−3621.

Adkins, J. A., Noviana, E., & Henry, C. S. (2016). Development of a quasi-steady flow electrochemical paper-based analytical device. *Analytical Chemistry, 88*(21), 10639−10647.

Apilux, A., et al. (2010). Lab-on-paper with dual electrochemical/colorimetric detection for simultaneous determination of gold and iron. *Analytical Chemistry, 82*(5), 1727−1732.

Arena, A., et al. (2010). Flexible ethanol sensors on glossy paper substrates operating at room temperature. *Sensors and Actuators B: Chemical, 145*(1), 488−494.

Auroux, P. A., et al. (2002). Micro total analysis systems. 2. Analytical standard operations and applications. *Analytical Chemistry, 74*(12), 2637−2652.

Bruzewicz, D. A., Reches, M., & Whitesides, G. M. (2008). Low-cost printing of poly(dimethylsiloxane) barriers to define microchannels in paper. *Analytical Chemistry, 80*(9), 3387−3392.

Carrilho, E., et al. (2009). Paper microzone plates. *Analytical Chemistry, 81*(15), 5990−5998.

Carrilho, E., Martinez, A. W., & Whitesides, G. M. (2009). Understanding wax printing: A simple micropatterning process for paper-based microfluidics. *Analytical Chemistry, 81*(16), 7091−7095.

Carvalhal, R. F., Carrilho, E., & Kubota, L. T. (2010a). The potential and application of microfluidic paper-based separation devices. *Bioanalysis, 2*(10), 1663−1665.

Carvalhal, R. F., et al. (2010b). Electrochemical detection in a paper-based separation device. *Analytical Chemistry, 82*(3), 1162−1165.

Cheng, C. M., et al. (2010). Paper-based ELISA. *Angewandte Chemie International Edition, 49*(28), 4771−4774.

Chitnis, G., et al. (2011). Laser-treated hydrophobic paper: An inexpensive microfluidic platform. *Lab on a Chip, 11*(6), 1161−1165.

Clegg, D. L. (1950). Paper chromatography. *Analytical Chemistry, 22*(1), 48−59.

Coltro, W. K. T., et al. (2010). Toner and paper-based fabrication techniques for microfluidic applications. *Electrophoresis, 31*(15), 2487−2498.

Cretich, M., et al. (2010). Coating of nitrocellulose for colorimetric DNA microarrays. *Analytical Biochemistry, 397*(1), 84−88.

Delaney, J. L., et al. (2011). Electrogenerated chemiluminescence detection in paper-based microfluidic sensors. *Analytical Chemistry, 83*(4), 1300−1306.

Dou, M., et al. (2014). A versatile PDMS/paper hybrid microfluidic platform for sensitive infectious disease diagnosis. *86*(15), 7978−7986.

Dungchai, W., Chailapakul, O., & Henry, C. S. (2009). Electrochemical detection for paper-based microfluidics. *Analytical Chemistry, 81*(14), 5821−5826.

Dungchai, W., Chailapakul, O., & Henry, C. S. (2010). Use of multiple colorimetric indicators for paper-based microfluidic devices. *Analytica Chimica Acta, 674*(2), 227−233.

Dungchai, W., Chailapakul, O., & Henry, C. S. (2011). A low-cost, simple, and rapid fabrication method for paper-based microfluidics using wax screen-printing. *Analyst, 136*(1), 77−82.

Ellerbee, A. K., et al. (2009). Quantifying colorimetric assays in paper-based microfluidic devices by measuring the transmission of light through paper. *Analytical Chemistry, 81*(20), 8447–8452.

Feigle, F. (1939). In A. Freidsohn (Ed.), *Qualitative analysis by spot tests*.

Fenton, E. M., et al. (2008). Multiplex lateral-flow test strips fabricated by two-dimensional shaping. *ACS Applied Materials and Interfaces, 1*(1), 124–129.

Fu, E., et al. (2010a). Controlled reagent transport in disposable 2D paper networks. *Lab on a Chip, 10*(7), 918–920.

Fu, E., et al. (2010b). Chemical signal amplification in two-dimensional paper networks. *Sensors and Actuators B: Chemical, 149*(1), 325–328.

Fu, E., et al. (2011). Transport in two-dimensional paper networks. *Microfluidics and Nanofluidics, 10*(1), 29–35.

Gauvreau, V., & Laroche, G. (2005). Micropattern printing of adhesion, spreading, and migration peptides on poly (tetrafluoroethylene) films to promote endothelialization. *Bioconjugate Chemistry, 16*(5), 1088–1097.

Ge, L., et al. (2012). Three-dimensional paper-based electrochemiluminescence immunodevice for multiplexed measurement of biomarkers and point-of-care testing. *Biomaterials, 33*(4), 1024–1031.

Gong, X., et al. (2010). Wax-bonding 3D microfluidic chips. *Lab on a Chip, 10*(19), 2622–2627.

Hawkes, R., Niday, E., & Gordon, J. (1982). A dot-immunobinding assay for monoclonal and other antibodies. *Analytical Biochemistry, 119*(1), 142–147.

Helfferich, F., Giddings, J., & Keller, R. (1965). *Advances in chromatography* (Vol. 1). New York: Marcel Dekker.

Hossain, S. M. Z., et al. (2009a). Development of a bioactive paper sensor for detection of neurotoxins using piezoelectric inkjet printing of sol–gel-derived bioinks. *Analytical Chemistry, 81*(13), 5474–5483.

Hossain, S. M. Z., et al. (2009b). Reagentless bidirectional lateral flow bioactive paper sensors for detection of pesticides in beverage and food samples. *Analytical Chemistry, 81*(21), 9055–9064.

Kauffman, P., et al. (2010). Visualization and measurement of flow in two-dimensional paper networks. *Lab on a Chip, 10*(19), 2614–2617.

Khan, M. S., et al. (2010). Paper diagnostic for instantaneous blood typing. *Analytical Chemistry, 82*(10), 4158–4164.

Klasner, S. A., et al. (2010). Paper-based microfluidic devices for analysis of clinically relevant analytes present in urine and saliva. *Analytical and Bioanalytical Chemistry, 397*(5), 1821–1829.

Leung, V., et al. (2010). Streaming potential sensing in paper-based microfluidic channels. *Colloids and Surfaces A: Physicochemical and Engineering Aspects, 364*(1), 16–18.

Liang, L., et al. (2016). Aptamer-based fluorescent and visual biosensor for multiplexed monitoring of cancer cells in microfluidic paper-based analytical devices. *Sensors and Actuators B: Chemical, 229*, 347–354.

Li, X., Ballerini, D. R., & Shen, W. (2012). A perspective on paper-based microfluidics: Current status and future trends. *Biomicrofluidics, 6*(1), 011301-011301-13.

Li, X., et al. (2008). Paper-based microfluidic devices by plasma treatment. *Analytical Chemistry, 80*(23), 9131–9134.

Li, X., et al. (2010). Fabrication of paper-based microfluidic sensors by printing. *Colloids and Surfaces B: Biointerfaces, 76*(2), 564–570.

Li, X., Tian, J., & Shen, W. (2010a). Progress in patterned paper sizing for fabrication of paper-based microfluidic sensors. *Cellulose, 17*(3), 649–659.

Li, X., Tian, J., & Shen, W. (2010b). Quantitative biomarker assay with microfluidic paper-based analytical devices. *Analytical and Bioanalytical Chemistry, 396*(1), 495–501.

Li, X., Tian, I., & Shen, W. (2010c). Thread as a versatile material for low-cost microfluidic diagnostics. *ACS Applied Materials & Interfaces, 2*(1), 1–6.

Liana, D. D., et al. (2012). Recent advances in paper-based sensors. *Sensors, 12*(9), 11505–11526.

Liu, H., & Crooks, R. M. (2011). Three-dimensional paper microfluidic devices assembled using the principles of origami. *Journal of the American Chemical Society, 133*(44), 17564–17566.

Lopez-Ruiz, N., et al. (2014). Smartphone-based simultaneous pH and nitrite colorimetric determination for paper microfluidic devices. *Analytical Chemistry, 86*(19), 9554–9562.

Lu, Y., et al. (2009a). Rapid prototyping of paper-based microfluidics with wax for low-cost, portable bioassay. *Electrophoresis, 30*(9), 1497–1500.

Lu, Y., et al. (2009b). Fabrication and characterization of paper-based microfluidics prepared in nitrocellulose membrane by wax printing. *Analytical Chemistry, 82*(1), 329–335.

Lutz, B. R., et al. (2011). Two-dimensional paper networks: Programmable fluidic disconnects for multi-step processes in shaped paper. *Lab on a Chip, 11*(24), 4274–4278.

Martinez, A. W. (2011). Microfluidic paper-based analytical devices: From POCKET to paper-based ELISA. *Bioanalysis, 3*(23), 2589–2592.

Martinez, A. W., et al. (2007). Patterned paper as a platform for inexpensive, low-volume, portable bioassays. *Angewandte Chemie International Edition, 46*(8), 1318–1320.

Martinez, A. W., et al. (2008a). Simple telemedicine for developing regions: Camera phones and paper-based microfluidic devices for real-time, off-site diagnosis. *Analytical Chemistry, 80*(10), 3699–3707.

Martinez, A. W., et al. (2008b). FLASH: A rapid method for prototyping paper-based microfluidic devices. *Lab on a Chip, 8*(12), 2146–2150.

Martinez, A. W., et al. (2009). Diagnostics for the developing world: Microfluidic paper-based analytical devices. *Analytical Chemistry, 82*(1), 3–10.

Martinez, A. W., et al. (2010). Programmable diagnostic devices made from paper and tape. *Lab on a Chip, 10*(19), 2499–2504.

Martinez, A. W., Phillips, S. T., & Whitesides, G. M. (2008). Three-dimensional microfluidic devices fabricated in layered paper and tape. *Proceedings of the National Academy of Sciences of the United States of America, 105*(50), 19606–19611.

Nagler, R. M. (2008). Saliva analysis for monitoring dialysis and renal function. *Clinical Chemistry, 54*(9), 1415–1417.

Nie, Z., et al. (2010a). Electrochemical sensing in paper-based microfluidic devices. *Lab on a Chip, 10*(4), 477–483.

Nie, Z., et al. (2010b). Integration of paper-based microfluidic devices with commercial electrochemical readers. *Lab on a Chip, 10*(22), 3163–3169.

Noh, H., & Phillips, S. T. (2010a). Fluidic timers for time-dependent, point-of-care assays on paper. *Analytical Chemistry, 82*(19), 8071–8078.

Noh, H., & Phillips, S. T. (2010b). Metering the capillary-driven flow of fluids in paper-based microfluidic devices. *Analytical Chemistry, 82*(10), 4181–4187.

Olkkonen, J., Lehtinen, K., & Erho, T. (2010). Flexographically printed fluidic structures in paper. *Analytical Chemistry, 82*(24), 10246–10250.

Osborn, J. L., et al. (2010). Microfluidics without pumps: Reinventing the T-sensor and H-filter in paper networks. *Lab on a Chip, 10*(20), 2659–2665.

Prasad, K. S., et al. (2020). New method to amplify colorimetric signals of paper-based nanobiosensors for simple & sensitive pancreatic cancer biomarker detection. *Analyst*.

Ratnarathorn, N., et al. (2012). Simple silver nanoparticle colorimetric sensing for copper by paper-based devices. *Talanta, 99*, 552–557.

Rattanarat, P., et al. (2014). Multilayer paper-based device for colorimetric and electrochemical quantification of metals. *Analytical Chemistry, 86*(7), 3555–3562.

Reches, M., et al. (2010). Thread as a matrix for biomedical assays. *ACS Applied Materials & Interfaces, 2*(6), 1722–1728.

Renault, C., et al. (2013). Hollow-channel paper analytical devices. *Analytical Chemistry, 85*(16), 7976–7979.

Renault, C., et al. (2014). Three-dimensional wax patterning of paper fluidic devices. *Langmuir, 30*(23), 7030–7036.

Reyes, D. R., et al. (2002). Micro total analysis systems. 1. Introduction, theory, and technology. *Analytical Chemistry, 74*(12), 2623–2636.

Rezk, A. R., et al. (2012). Uniform mixing in paper-based microfluidic systems using surface acoustic waves. *Lab on a Chip, 12*(4), 773–779.

Sanjay, S. T., et al. (2015). Biomarker detection for disease diagnosis using cost-effective microfluidic platforms. *Analyst, 140*(21), 7062–7081.

Sanjay, S. T., et al. (2016). A paper/polymer hybrid microfluidic microplate for rapid quantitative detection of multiple disease biomarkers. *Scientific Reports, 6*, 30474.

Schilling, K. M., et al. (2012). Fully enclosed microfluidic paper-based analytical devices. *Lab on a Chip, 84*(3), 1579–1585.

Scida, K., et al. (2014). Simple, sensitive, and quantitative electrochemical detection method for paper analytical devices. *Analytical Chemistry, 86*(13), 6501–6507.

Songjaroen, T., et al. (2011). Novel, simple and low-cost alternative method for fabrication of paper-based microfluidics by wax dipping. *Talanta, 85*(5), 2587–2593.

Srisa-Art, M., et al. (2018). Highly sensitive detection of *Salmonella typhimurium* using a colorimetric paper-based analytical device coupled with immunomagnetic separation. *Analytical Chemistry, 90*(1), 1035–1043.

Steffens, C., et al. (2009). Low-cost sensors developed on paper by line patterning with graphite and polyaniline coating with supercritical CO_2. *Synthetic Metals, 159*(21), 2329–2332.

Thom, N. K., et al. (2012). "Fluidic batteries" as low-cost sources of power in paper-based microfluidic devices. *Lab on a Chip*.

Tian, J., et al. (2010). Capillary driven low-cost V-groove microfluidic device with high sample transport efficiency. *Lab on a Chip, 10*(17), 2258–2264.

Von Lode, P. (2005). Point-of-care immunotesting: Approaching the analytical performance of central laboratory methods. *Clinical Biochemistry, 38*(7), 591–606.

Wang, L., et al. (2009). Simple, rapid, sensitive, and versatile SWNT– paper sensor for environmental toxin detection competitive with ELISA. *Nano Letters, 9*(12), 4147–4152.

Wang, P., et al. (2012a). Paper-based three-dimensional electrochemical immunodevice based on multi-walled carbon nanotubes functionalized paper for sensitive point-of-care testing. *Biosensors and Bioelectronics, 32*(1), 238–243.

Wang, S., et al. (2012b). Paper-based chemiluminescence ELISA: Lab-on-paper based on chitosan modified paper device and wax-screen-printing. *Biosensors and Bioelectronics, 31*(1), 212–218.

Wang, W., Wu, W. Y., & Zhu, J. J. (2010). Tree-shaped paper strip for semiquantitative colorimetric detection of protein with self-calibration. *Journal of Chromatography A, 1217*(24), 3896–3899.

Xu, X., et al. (2019). A smartphone-based on-site nucleic acid testing platform at point-of-care settings. *40*(6), 914–921.

Yan, J., et al. (2012). Paper-based electrochemiluminescent 3D immunodevice for lab-on-paper, specific, and sensitive point-of-care testing. *Chemistry, 18*(16), 4938–4945.

Yang, X., et al. (2012). Integrated separation of blood plasma from whole blood for microfluidic paper-based analytical devices. *Lab on a Chip, 12*(2), 274–280.

Yao, L., et al. (2018). A microfluidic impedance biosensor based on immunomagnetic separation and urease catalysis for continuous-flow detection of *E. coli* O157:H7. *Sensors and Actuators B: Chemical, 259*, 1013–1021.

Yu, J., et al. (2011). Microfluidic paper-based chemiluminescence biosensor for simultaneous determination of glucose and uric acid. *Lab on a Chip, 11*(7), 1286–1291.

Zhao, W., et al. (2008). Paper-based bioassays using gold nanoparticle colorimetric probes. *Analytical Chemistry, 80*(22), 8431–8437.

Zuo, P., et al. (2013). A PDMS/paper/glass hybrid microfluidic biochip integrated with aptamer-functionalized graphene oxide nano-biosensors for one-step multiplexed pathogen detection. *13*(19), 3921–3928.

Microfluidic devices for viral detection

Wenfu Zheng[1], Jiashu Sun[1], Xingyu Jiang[2]
[1]CAS Key Laboratory for Biomedical Effects of Nanomaterials and Nanosafety, CAS Center for Excellence in Nanoscience, National Center for NanoScience and Technology, Beijing, P.R. China; [2]Department of Biomedical Engineering, Southern University of Science and Technology, Shenzhen, Guangdong, P.R. China

Guiding questions:

1. How to detect virus by microfluidic immunoassay?
2. How to detect nucleic acids of virus by microfluidics?
3. How to detect virus by microfluidic flow cytometry?

15.1 Introduction

Infectious diseases result from pathogenic microorganisms, such as bacteria, viruses, parasites, and fungi (Fauci & Morens, 2012). The outbreak of infectious diseases severely threatens public health and greatly increases the risk of morbidity and mortality, especially in developing countries (Leke, 2010; Pang & Peeling, 2007). Viral infectious diseases, including human immunodeficiency virus (HIV), hepatitis B, hepatitis C, are the major causes of death in the world (Leke, 2010). In recent years, the emergence of new viruses such as Ebola virus, MERS-CoV, SARS-CoV, and COVID-2019 has brought enormous threaten to human health worldwide (Cui, Li, & Shi, 2019; Towner et al., 2008; Zhu et al., 2020). Rapid and effective diagnostic technologies are crucial for identifying viruses and pathogens, providing appropriate treatment, and preventing the outbreak of infection (Dong, Liu, Mou, Deng, & Jiang, 2019; Sun, Xianyu, & Jiang, 2014; Yang, Liu, & Jiang, 2019). Gold-standard techniques for detection of viral infectious disease include tissue culture, enzyme-linked immunosorbent assay (ELISA), and polymerase chain reaction (PCR) (Foudeh, Didar, Veres, & Tabrizian, 2012; Mackay, 2004). Although these diagnostic approaches are commonly adopted in the developed world, they are still labor intensive, time consuming, and typically associated with high equipment and reagent expenses (Yang & Rothman, 2004). For example, diagnosis of HIV involves an enzyme immunoassay combined with a Western blot (Branson, 2007). These tests are not suitable to be performed outside the laboratory, or without trained personnel (Sturenburg & Junker, 2009). For detection of very low density infections, PCR remains the most effective tool, but is limited in low-resource settings because of their high cost, long analysis time, and the influence of contamination (Drakeley & Reyburn, 2009). Despite the fact that diagnostic methods are well established in the developed world, these approaches are generally not affordable or feasible in resource-poor settings where modern healthcare infrastructure is not available (Yager, Domingo, & Gerdes, 2008). Cost-effective, portable, disposable, and point-of-care (POC) diagnostic approaches are needed in order to enhance the health-related quality of life in worldwide populations. Microfluidic technologies, with increased sensitivity and decreased cost, hold great promise to develop effective diagnostic tools to overcome the hurdles imposed by conventional methods (Chin, Linder, & Sia, 2012; Gervais, de Rooij, & Delamarche, 2011; Govindarajan, Ramachandran, Vigil, Yager, & Bohringer, 2012). These technologies provide many benefits, including compactness, portability, disposability, and integration of multiple functions. The small dimension of microfluidic channels inherently reduces reagent consumption, decreases reaction time, and provides the ability to analyze low volume samples (Bange, Halsall, & Heineman, 2005; Beebe, Mensing, & Walker, 2002; Melin & Quake, 2007; Sia & Whitesides, 2003). Microfluidic technologies can automate various steps of assays, including sample preparation, reaction, transportation, and analysis, inside a single chip (Melin & Quake, 2007). This enclosed, integrated, and automated format of microfluidics significantly avoids cross-contamination and enables multiplexed detection of pathogens. In addition, mass production of disposable microfluidic devices for viral detection can be implemented by using low-cost plastic fabrication and screen-printing techniques (Dong, Li, Zhang, Cao, & Gan, 2007; Liu, Cady, & Batt, 2007). Currently, microfluidic systems are becoming essential and revolutionary tools for POC viral diagnostics (Kelly & Woolley, 2005; Sun et al., 2014; Zhang et al., 2012).

15.2 Microfluidic technologies used for viral detection

This section introduces a variety of promising microfluidic technologies used for viral detection. These technologies hold great potential for addressing issues raised by conventional methods including immunological detection, nucleic acid amplification, and flow cytometry.

15.2.1 Microfluidic immunoassay

Immunological detection is one of the most powerful clinical tools for viral diagnostics because of its relative simplicity (Jiang, Ng, Stroock, Dertinger, & Whitesides, 2003; Wang et al., 2002). Immunoassays rely on high-affinity antibody—antigen interaction to test either the antigen or the antibody (Wu, 2006). Among a diverse set of immunoassays, ELISA is the most widely used one, involving enzyme-conjugated antibodies and the enzyme's substrate to detect antigens of interest indicated by a color change (Fig. 15.1) (Borkowsky et al., 1987). Because of the high sensitivity and selectivity of antigen—antibody binding, ELISA has been commonly adopted for diagnosis of infectious diseases (Cordes & Ryan, 1995; Misiani et al., 1992). However, ELISA often requires labor-intensive procedures, long assay times, and expensive reagents, making

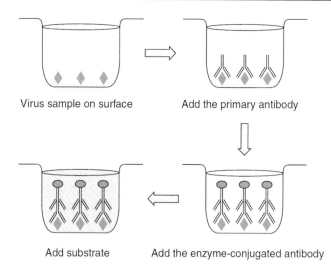

Figure 15.1 Schematic of enzyme-linked immunosorbent assay (ELISA). Briefly, the virus sample (pathogenic antigen) is immobilized on a solid substrate. The substrate is then incubated with the serum, which contains the corresponding antibody (the primary antibody). A second, enzyme-conjugated antibody is added to bind the primary antibody, followed by adding a substrate for this enzyme. The substrate changes color upon reaction with the enzyme.

this technology poorly suited for low-resource settings (Qu, Liu, Liu, Wang, & Jiang, 2011; Yang, Niu, et al., 2008). Another commonly used immunological method for viral detection is the Western blot (protein immunoblot) that uses gel electrophoresis to separate proteins, followed by subsequent blotting to identify proteins. The Western blot is a widely accepted HIV diagnostic assay, but requires cumbersome manual protocols during assays (He et al., 2015; Pan, Chen, & Jiang, 2010; Song et al., 2012).

Microfluidic immunoassay can address many of these issues raised by conventional immunological detection. To perform a microfluidic immunoassay, a microfluidic network (µFN) is designed to pattern different antigens on the substrate, followed by blocking the unpatterned areas with bovine serum albumin (BSA) to prevent nonspecific binding of proteins. The next step is to introduce a sample solution containing specific antibodies to bind with antigens using a second µFN. As the immunobinding occurs along micrometer-wide intersecting lines, a mosaic of signals from crossreacted zones can be read using a fluorescence microscope (Fig. 15.2) (Bernard, Michel, & Delamarche, 2001). This miniaturized format of microfluidic assays only uses a small amount of reagent such as antibodies and enzymes that are often hundreds of dollars per milligram, thus dramatically reducing the cost of each test. Moreover, microfluidic techniques allow the integration and automation of immunoassay procedures such as sample preparation, reagent delivery, and multiple incubation and washing steps. Because of the rapid transportation inside the microchannels, the time required for each incubation step can be dramatically reduced from 1 h to 5 min (Rossier & Girault, 2001).

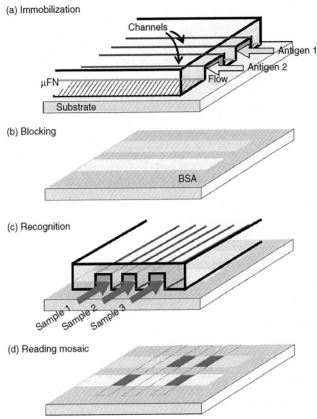

Figure 15.2 Schematic of microfluidic immunoassay. (a) A microfluidic network (μFN) to pattern different antigens on the substrate. (b) Block unpatterned area with bovine serum albumin (BSA) to prevent nonspecific binding of proteins. (c) Introduce antibodies to bind with antigens using a second μFN. (d) Read the binding mosaic pattern.
Reprinted with permission from Bernard et al. (2001), copyright 2001 American Chemical Society.

We developed a microfluidic immunoassay device consisting of a microdilutor network (μDN) and an antigen-coated polycarbonate (PC) membrane. The μDN dilutes the serum sample by one half each time the sample flows through a branch (Fig. 15.3(a)) (Jiang et al., 2003). To induce local mixing inside each branch in which laminar flow is dominated at small Reynolds number, chaotic advective mixers are designed on the channel surface, each of which includes four cycles of herringbone patterns (Jiang et al., 2005). For diagnosis of HIV infection, a piece of PC membrane was first coated by antigens by microfluidics, and placed between the μDN and a flat polydimethylsiloxane (PDMS). The sample of serum containing anti-gp120 and anti-gp41 is introduced from the left inlet, and the buffer containing 5% BSA is injected from the right inlet. As the sample flows orthogonally across the antigen-coated

Microfluidic devices for viral detection 591

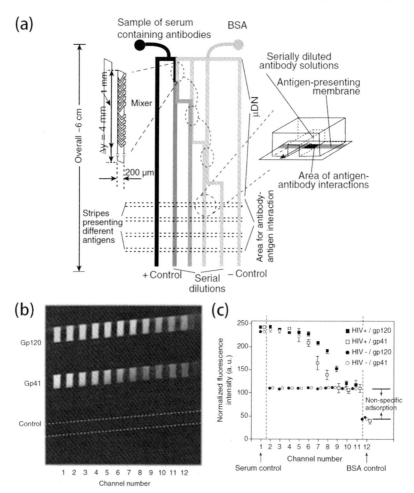

Figure 15.3 The microfluidic immunoassay device for detecting HIV infection. (a) Schematic of the microdilutor network (μDN). (b) Immunofluorescence image of anti-gp120 and anti-gp41 interaction with the membrane-bound antigens. (c) Plots of the normalized fluorescence intensity versus the channel number.
Reprinted with permission from Jiang et al. (2003), copyright 2003 American Chemical Society.

membrane, the antibodies in the serum bind to the immobilized antigens, observed as a fluorescent micromosaic pattern (Fig. 15.3(b)). To generate a calibration curve for quantification of analytes, the solution of human immunoglobulin Gs (IgGs) with known concentrations is flowed through the μDN, followed by plotting the fluorescent intensities of micromosaic versus the channel number. Based on this calibration curve, the absolute concentrations of anti-gp120 and anti-gp41 in serum can be determined (Fig. 15.3(c)). A similar design is adopted for quantitative analysis of multiple HIV samples simultaneously inside a single chip (Song et al., 2012). These microfluidic immunoassay devices are promising for sensitive and effective POC viral diagnostics.

In addition, microfluidic devices can be designed to perform parallel, quantitative assays of multiple viral samples in one test. Researchers reported a silicon microchip with immobilized antibodies for microfluidic enzyme immunoassays using chemiluminescence detection. They evaluated different immobilization protocols and buffer selection to reach the best assay stability and sensitivity (Yakovleva et al., 2002). A microfluidic diagnostic system consisting of several reaction wells, micropneumatic valves, peristaltic micropumps, and an automatic platform was reported. The micropneumatic valves were used to separate analytes and reagents, while the spider-web peristaltic micropumps were employed to drive the fluids into the microchannels. After the analytes and reagents gradually entered the reaction/detection area, fluorescence signals caused by antibody–antigen interaction were detected by a fluorescent reader so as to detect the diseases. This integrated microfluidic system allowed fast diagnosis of hepatitis C virus and syphilis in an automated and efficient format (Fig. 15.4) (Wang & Lee, 2005).

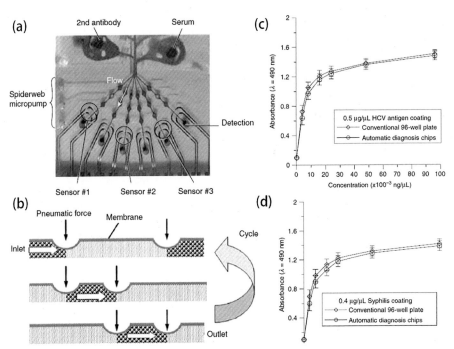

Figure 15.4 Microfluidic diagnostic system. (a) An automated microfluidic system consisting of micropneumatic valves and peristaltic micropumps for fast immunoassays. (b) Schematic diagram of the working principle of peristaltic micropumps. Results of detecting hepatitis C virus (c) and syphilis (d) by using the microfluidic chip.
Reprinted with permission from Wang and Lee (2005), copyright 2005 Elsevier.

We applied electrospun nanofibrous membranes as the solid substrates to detect HIV-specific antibodies from human serum samples (Yang et al., 2008). These nanofibers with large specific surface areas could increase the adsorption of proteins, thus improving the sensitivity and signal-to-noise ratio of microfluidic immunoassays (Fig. 15.5). Moreover, fabrication of these nanofibrous membranes was simple and cost-effective, which could be easily incorporated with existing microchannel designs.

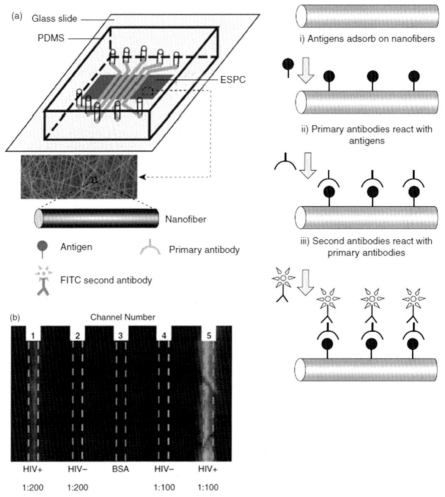

Figure 15.5 Electrospun nanofibrous membranes as the solid substrates to detect HIV-specific antibodies from human serum samples. (a) A microfluidic device for HIV immunoassays with the electrospun polycarbonate fibrous membrane (ESPC) as the solid substrate. ESPC substrate with the large specific surface areas can increase antigen adsorption. (b) Results of the assays using different samples of patient serum to detect anti-gp41 at lower concentrations. Reprinted with permission from Yang et al. (2008), copyright 2008 WILEY-VCH.

This membrane-based microfluidic assay was well-suited for resource-poor settings. We further designed a fluorescent microfluidic immunoassay for rapid, multiple HIV sample screening and confirmation through removing the blocking step (Song et al., 2012). This method could significantly improve the assay speed while keeping the limit of detection comparable to conventional ELISA, which made it an excellent candidate for a quick HIV test for both screening and confirmation. The detection of inflammatory factors generated in human body is crucial for diagnosis of virus infection. However, the concentrations of these inflammatory factors range broadly from the pg/mL level to µg/mL level in serum samples. To realize simultaneous and multiplexed assays of these biomarkers, we used click chemistry to assemble horseradish peroxidase (HRP) in a controlled fashion to generate enzyme assemblies as probes for multiplexed bioassays. The assays were carried in a lab-on-a-chip format, with a limit of detection of 0.47 pg/mL for interleukin-6, 2.6 pg/mL for procalcitonin, and 40 ng/mL for C-reactive protein. This technique can serve as a POC platform for viral infection diagnostics (Xianyu et al., 2018).

We developed a microfluidic Western blot by combining a microfluidic immunoassay with conventional protein blotting, which was termed as µWB (Pan et al., 2010). This µWB consisted of five steps: (1) using sodium dodecyl sulfate polyacrylamide gel electrophoresis (SDS-PAGE) to separate proteins in cell lysates according to their molecular weights; (2) transferring proteins from the polyacrylamide gel to a polyvinylidene fluoride (PVDF) membrane by an electrotransfer system; (3) placing a µFN on the blotted membrane with the channels perpendicular to the protein bands; (4) detecting multiple proteins simultaneously on the PVDF membrane by incubating different primary antibodies in parallel microfluidic channels; and (5) peeling off the µFN and incubating the whole PVDF membrane in fluorescent dye–labeled secondary antibody solution. This microfluidic system could analyze multiple proteins simultaneously consuming only microliters of antibodies and indicated a new avenue for POC diagnosis of viral infection. To make the µWB compatible with the commonly used multilane blotting in biolabs, we updated the microfluidics into parallel and serpentine microfluidic channels, thus achieving the identification of multiple targets in multiple samples simultaneously. Moreover, the adjacent blotting bands inside the parallel microchannels could be easily distinguished, which is difficult to achieve in conventional blotting assay (He et al., 2015). Following the concept of µWB, researchers applied an automated microfluidic Western blot to detect purified HIV proteins gp120 and p24 from human sera with the increased protein blotting efficiency and reduced reagent consumption (Hughes & Herr, 2012; Kim, Karns, Tia, He, & Herr, 2012). This microfluidic system also decreased the overall assay time to 10–60 min, enabled multiplexed analyte detection, lowered the detection limit to 50 pM, and realized quantitation over a wide dynamic range. These improvements were attributed to unique microscale conditions. Apart from protein–protein interaction, aptamers could be utilized to detect virus due to their advantages such as high stability and durability, low cost, and ease of chemical synthesis. By combining aptamer and microfluidics, researchers realized automatic and accurate detection of H1N1 virus, which achieved a detection limit of 0.032 hemagglutination units (Tseng, Wang, Chang, & Lee, 2016).

15.2.2 Microfluidic nucleic acid detection

15.2.2.1 Microfluidic nucleic acid amplification

Over the past decades, nucleic acid amplification methods have evolved as the cornerstone of clinical assessment and prevention of infectious diseases (Fang, Liu, Kong, & Jiang, 2010; Yager et al., 2008). Advantages of nucleic acid amplification-based diagnostic assays include the increased detection sensitivity that can theoretically amplify a single copy (at least 10^6 higher than lateral flow immunoassays), the improved specificity to differentiate pathogen strains, and the faster diagnostic time than tissue culture (Mackay, 2004). Strategies for nucleic acid amplification can be simply classified as nonisothermal amplification (e.g., PCR) and isothermal amplification (such as loop-mediated isothermal amplification (LAMP), nucleic acid sequence-based amplification (NASBA), and nicking enzyme amplification reaction (NEAR)) (McCalla & Tripathi, 2011). PCR relies on thermal cycling consisting of repeated temperature changes to realize deoxyribonucleic acid (DNA) denaturation, annealing, and extension. PCR testing can rapidly and accurately screen hepatitis C virus, hepatitis B virus, HIV-1, and HIV-2 in blood samples (Peeters et al., 1992; Roth, Weber, & Seifried, 1999). Isothermal amplification technologies use a constant temperature rather than thermal cycling, thus performing assays in a simple and effective manner (Notomi et al., 2000). Isothermal amplification assays have been developed for detecting circulating HIV-1 virus in blood, malaria, and tuberculosis (Iwamoto, Sonobe, & Hayashi, 2003; Kievits et al., 1991; Poon et al., 2006). As microfluidic technology carries many advantages, such as disposable, low cost, reduced cross-contamination and biohazard risks, on-chip nucleic acid amplification is expected to have great impact on viral diagnostics.

A real-time microfluidic-based PCR system consisting of six individual thermal cycling modules was developed (Cho et al., 2006). In comparison with conventional PCR machines, which require 25 μL of reaction mixtures and 2—3 h reaction time, the on-chip PCR systems consumes only 1 μL of reaction mixtures and amplifies DNA within 20 min. This on-chip PCR system was used to conduct large-scale clinical screening of the hepatitis B virus infection, the results of which showed a sensitivity of 94% and specificity of 93%. Another popular format of microfluidic-based PCR for viral diagnostics is the droplet emulsion PCR system, which relies on the integration of microfluidic PCR and discrete water-in-oil droplets as the reaction chambers generated by flow focusing or electric field (Park, Zhang, Lin, Wang, & Yang, 2011). Each of millions of aqueous droplets containing PCR mixtures is protected by immiscible oil, enabling the large-scale and high-throughput amplification and screening of the nucleic acid of viruses with decreased risk of cross-containment. Researchers reported the use of a droplet emulsion PCR system for pathogenic cell detection in a high background of normal cells with the detection limit of $1/10^5$ (Fig. 15.6) (Zeng, Novak, Shuga, Smith, & Mathies, 2010).

To simplify the sample processing of PCR, researchers reported a POC apparatus for hepatitis virus detection. They developed an automated sample-to-answer disc based on a double rotation axes centrifugal microfluidic system. The release of

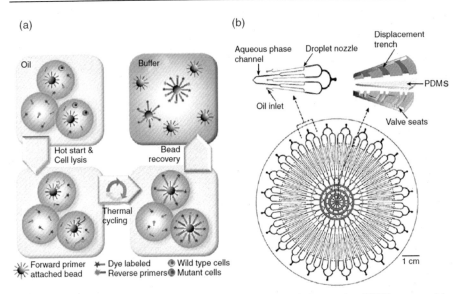

Figure 15.6 Schematic of the droplet emulsion polymerase chain reaction (PCR) system. (a) Statistically dilute beads and templates are encapsulated into uniform nanoliter volume droplets for PCR amplification. (b) Layout of the integrated microfluidic chip composed of a single ring pump and 96 droplet generators for droplet-based PCR system.
Reprinted with permission from Zeng et al. (2010), copyright 2010 American Chemical Society.

prestored reagents, the separation of serum from whole blood, the extraction of DNA from the virus, and real-time PCR were automatically conducted on the disk. The whole detection process could be finished within 48 min with a sample concentration down to 100 copies/mL (Fig. 15.7) (Li, Miao, Li, Sun, & Peng, 2019). Based on a centrifugal disk, researchers performed real-time reverse transcription polymerase chain reaction (RT-PCR) to detect influenza A H3N2 virus with sample concentrations down to 2.39×10^4 viral ribonucleic acid (RNA) copies per mL (Stumpf et al., 2016).

Compared with PCR systems, isothermal amplification strategies can eliminate the thermal cycling steps, thus simplifying both the chip design and the instrument configuration. Researchers demonstrated a microfluidic real-time NASBA system for diagnosis of human papillomavirus (HPV) (Gulliksen et al., 2004). NASBA is an isothermal, transcription-based amplification technique specifically designed for amplification of RNA that requires two primers and three enzymes to proceed (McCalla & Tripathi, 2011). The microfluidic NASBA chip was made by bonding the etched silicon wafer with glass to form a 10- or 50-nL reaction chamber and fluid delivery channels. The reaction mixture was preheated at 65°C before loading into the chamber, which was placed above a heater at a temperature around 41°C. Real-time NASBA process inside the microfluidic chip was monitored by using fluorescent

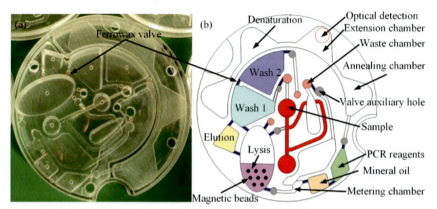

Figure 15.7 Photograph of the disc (a) and schematic of the microfluidic layout (b) for sample-to-result HBV DNA detection from whole blood. The whole blood is pipetted into the sample chamber while DNA extraction reagents are prestored in the washing 1 chamber, washing 2 chambers, and the eluate chamber, which are connected to the DNA extraction chamber wherein the magnetic beads and lysis buffer are prestored. The microfluidic channels and ferrowax valves are used for controlling the movement of the liquid. Primers and probes are prestored in the polymerase chain reaction (PCR) reagent chamber. The annealing, extension, and denaturation chamber are applied to RT (reverse transcription)-PCR.
Reprinted with permission from Li et al. (2019), copyright 2019 American Chemical Society.

molecular beacon probes and an external optical detection system. This proof-of-concept system successfully amplified and detected HPV positive control (1 μM) and single stranded deoxyribonucleic acid (ssDNA) (0.1 μM) in nanoliter volumes. A microfluidic device that integrated the functions of RNA purification and NASBA was developed (Dimov et al., 2008). This integrated microfluidic device had two functional domains: a silica bead-bed chamber for RNA purification and a NASBA chamber for real-time amplification and detection (Fig. 15.8). Cell lysate samples first passed over the silicon beads that were used to capture and purify RNA. The genetic material was washed off the beads and delivered into the NASBA channel, followed by heating at 65°C before adding enzymes. An adjacent no-template negative control was included on the same chip for direct comparison. On-chip amplification was monitored in real time using molecular beacon fluorescent probe technology. This microfluidic NASBA system enabled 10 times faster (<3 min) and 10 times less volume (2 μL) than conventional reactions.

Another intensively developed isothermal amplification technology is LAMP, which bypasses thermal cycling by using a set of specially designed primers and a DNA polymerase for strand displacement (Notomi et al., 2000). We developed a microfluidic system (μLAMP) for virus detection. This system had an octopus-like configuration containing 10 microchambers, each of which was connected to the corresponding thin microchannel via a dimension gradient bridge (Fang, Chen, Yu, Jiang, & Kong, 2011). The microchambers were precoated with specific LAMP probe sets,

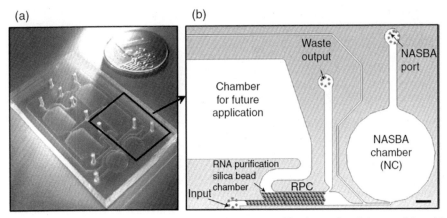

Figure 15.8 Schematic of microfluidic device for RNA purification and real-time nucleic acid sequence-based amplification NASBA of *E. coli* bacteria. (a) Photograph of microfluidic architecture that is mirrored to allow a NASBA reaction and a negative control in the same chip. (b) Layout of the single device incorporating RNA purification chamber and real-time NASBA chamber.
Reprinted with permission from Dimov et al. (2008), copyright 2008 The Royal Society of Chemistry.

and the separate microchannels were used to forbid the cross-talk of probes among different microchambers. This microfluidic system was applied to simultaneously differentiate three types of human influenza in a single chip, with the detection limit of less than 10 copies/μL in 2 μL quantities of sample within 0.5 h. Identification of eight important swine viruses was also performed using the octopus-like μLAMP system. We also integrated LAMP with a multichannel microfluidic system (μLAMP) for parallel detection of the pseudorabies virus (PRV) with high sensitivity and specificity (Fig. 15.9(a)) (Fang et al., 2010). The μLAMP allows the direct analysis of a sample of 0.4 μL of interested DNA in less than 1 h with the detection limit of 10 fg/μL. The readout of μLAMP could be either by the naked eye or via absorbance measured by an optic sensor (Fig. 15.9(b)). The μLAMP system with a parallel, multiple, high-throughput, and integrated format has a huge potential to facilitate the realization of POC viral diagnostics.

Researchers designed a microfluidic LAMP cassette equipped with an integrated Flinders Technology Associates (FTA) membrane for on-chip HIV-1 detection (Liu et al., 2011). As the saliva sample flowed through the cassette, the nucleic acids were captured and concentrated by the FTA membrane, which were directly used as templates for real-time LAMP monitored by a fluorescent reader. The FTA-based LAMP device had a simple chip design with a detection limit of less than 10 HIV particles. Researchers also developed a microfluidic-based real-time fluorescence LAMP device using cyclic olefin polymer microchips and a monochromatic charge-coupled

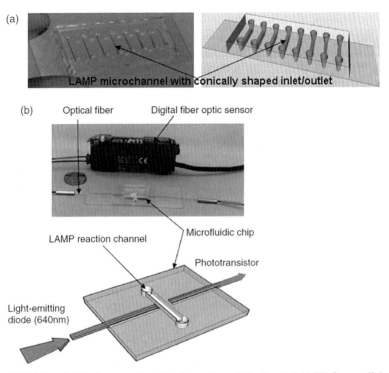

Figure 15.9 Microfluidic loop-mediated isothermal amplification (μLAMP) for parallel detection of pseudorabies virus (PRV). (a) Photograph and schematic of the eight-channel μLAMP chip for amplification and detection of PRV. (b) Photograph and schematic of the quantitative analysis unit. (c) Dynamic curves (upper) and standard curve (lower) of the real-time absorbance detection of μLAMP method.
Reprinted with permission from Fang et al. (2010), copyright 2010 American Chemical Society.

device (CCD) camera. This microfluidic LAMP assay was used to rapidly and sensitively detect waterborne pathogens within 20 min (Ahmad et al., 2011). These microfluidic nucleic acid amplification and detection systems hold great significance for rapid diagnosis of viral infections. To make the assay easier for conducting in resource-poor settings, we used capillaries as a reactor to carry out LAMP (cLAMP). The reagents for LAMP, sealed by segments of water droplets to prevent contamination, were heated by a pocket warmer, and the results were displayed as fluorescent signal excited by a handheld flashlight. Two target RNA segments of HIV could be simultaneously detected on the cLAMP system with a sensitivity of two copies of standard plasmid (Zhang, Zhange, Sun et al., 2014). Furthermore, the cLAMP system was integrated with a piece of FTA membrane for capturing and concentrating nucleic acids, which were directly used as templates for real-time LAMP assay. This device was capable of doing sample-to-answer screening of single nucleotide polymorphisms

(SNPs) of target genes (Zhang, Zhange, Wang, et al., 2014). Furthermore, we developed a micropipette tip-based nucleic acid detection strategy. A small piece of FTA card was embedded in a pipette tip for extracting and trapping DNA/RNA from raw samples. The induction of raw sample, washing buffer, and LAMP reagents in sequence and subsequently sealing the two sides of the tip make the pipette a minireactor for nucleic acid amplification. Equipped with a mini-heater and a handheld UV flashlight, the LAMP reaction could be conducted and the results could be read out (visualize by fluorescence). The limit of detection of this method was two copies of plasmid containing Ebola nucleic acid fragments (Lu et al., 2016).

Another isothermal amplification strategy is rolling circle amplification (RCA). By carrying RCA in microfluidics with a dumbbell-shaped padlock probe, amplified DNA could form hydrogels, which can block microchannel flow of a dyed liquid to indicate the presence of positive DNA samples with the naked eye (Lee et al., 2015). However, this process took 2 h to completely block channel flow. To accelerate the reaction process, researchers tethered primer on thousands of microbeads packed in a microfluidic channel. When a targeted viral DNA meets the corresponding particular template, the DNAs will rapidly amplify into a dumbbell shape through the RCA process. Due to the large surface area of the microbeads, the amplified DNA could rapidly (within 15 min) form hydrogel to block the flow path. By staining the hydrogel, the target pathogens could be determined with the naked eyes (Fig. 15.10). On a multichannel chip, simultaneous phenotyping of Ebola, Middle East respiratory syndrome (MERS), Dengue, Zika virus could be performed (Na, Nam, Lee, & Shin, 2018).

15.2.2.2 Amplification-free nucleic acid detection on microfluidics

Amplification-free nucleic acid detection, which only needs to capture target nucleic acids and read out their signals, does not require an amplification process that needs specialized training and facilities and can provide a rapid and simple diagnostic test. Plasmonic sensing (Stockman, 2015), electrochemical detection (Henihan et al., 2016), and advanced microscopy (Tao et al., 2015) can achieve amplification-free nucleic acid detection. Antiresonant reflecting optical waveguide (ARROW) is a technique that can create femtoliter excitation volumes on a chip to effectively excite and detect individual labeled target nucleic acid molecules. Researchers developed a viral detection technique based on ARROW and a sample preparation multiplexer (SPM) on a microfluidic chip. Metered air bubbles were generated on the chip to stir up magnetic beads carrying capture probes to realize effect target nucleic acid capture. All the sample processing procedures including target capture, wash, and release were performed automatically on the chip without manual intervention. By using this platform, a detection limit of 0.021 pfu/mL of Ebola virus RNA was achieved (Du et al., 2017).

15.2.3 Microfluidic flow cytometry

Flow cytometry has been routinely used for rapidly counting and differentiating cells based on their biophysical properties and plays significant roles in clinical estimation

Microfluidic devices for viral detection 601

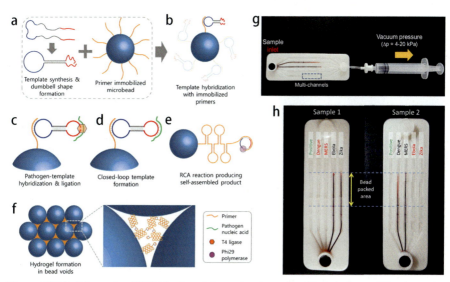

Figure 15.10 Schematic of DNA hydrogel formation through rolling circle amplification using agarose-based microbeads. (a) The templates are self-assembled to form an asymmetric dumbbell shape. And the primers are immobilized on the microbeads. (b) The templates are hybridized with primers immobilized on microbeads surface. (c) When the template on the microbead hybridized with a target pathogen, (d) the template can be ligated to form a closed-loop template. (e) Rolling circle amplification (RCA) products are elongated by Phi29 polymerase. (f) The dumbbell-shaped long DNAs are aggregated with neighbor DNAs and form a DNA gel in bead voids. (g) Photograph of the experimental apparatus. (h) The results of multiple detection of sample 1 (Dengue and MERS) and sample 2 (Ebola and Zika) using microchip.
Reprinted with permission from Na et al. (2018), copyright 2018 Elsevier.

of viral infections such as HIV and hepatitis B virus (Cheng et al., 2007; Stoop et al., 2005). Over the last two decades, substantial improvements and refinements to this established technique have been made using microfluidic approaches. Microfluidic flow cytometry has competitive advantages including downscaling sizes, automated process, high-throughput, and accurate measurements, making the technology ideal for POC viral diagnostics such as influenza, baculovirus (BV), and dengue virus (Ferris, McCabe, Doan, & Rowlen, 2002; Stoffel, Kathy, & Rowlen, 2005; Yang, Lien, Huang, Lei, & Lee, 2008). There are several components for design and construction of the microfluidic flow cytometer: (1) a miniaturized fluidics system combined with hydrodynamic focusing, acoustophoresis, or dielectrophoresis to rapidly align biological samples inside the microfluidic channel; (2) an integrated optical or/and electrical detection system to interrogate particles/cells based on their physicochemical characteristics when they flow through the detection zone of the microfluidic chip; and (3) an on-chip post-processing system to sort, differentiate, and recover samples. Researchers constructed a microfluidic flow cytometer for rapid detection of single viruses (Ferris et al., 2002). They used an argon ion laser operating at 488-nm emission combined with a photomultiplier tube (PMT)−based optical system to produce a diffraction-limited spot size of ∼0.5 μm and a probe volume of ∼8 fL, and successfully detected and enumerated fluorescently stained viruses including adenovirus-5, respiratory syncytial virus, and influenza. Stoffel et al. constructed a dual-channel microfluidic flow cytometer to detect unpurified BV samples. They used a two-dye staining method, targeting both the protein capsid and genome of BV, and developed an algorithm to identify simultaneous events on the DNA and protein channels (Stoffel et al., 2005). A magnetic bead−based microfluidic flow cytometer was developed for fast viral detection (Yang et al., 2008). The antibody-conjugated magnetic beads were first used to capture target viruses, followed by using another dye-labeled antivirus antibody to mark the bead-bound virus for the subsequent optical detection. This system integrated multiple modules into a single chip such as sample incubation, delivery, focusing, sorting, and collecting, allowing automatic detection of the dengue virus with the detection limit of 10^3 PFU/mL (Fig. 15.11). Plaque-forming units (PFUs) are a measure of the quantity of viruses

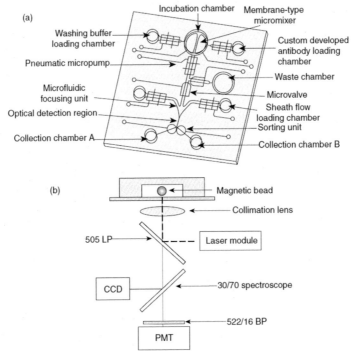

Figure 15.11 Magnetic bead−based microfluidic flow cytometer for fast viral detection. (a) Schematic of the magnetic bead−based microfluidic flow cytometer for fast viral detection. This system integrated multiple modules into a single chip such as sample incubation, delivery, focusing, sorting, and collecting. (b) Schematic of the optical detection system. Reprinted with permission from Yang et al. (2008), copyright 2008 Elsevier.

that are capable of lysing host cells and forming a plaque. A microfluidic contactless impedance cytometer containing a disposable biochip was reported. This chip can be inserted onto a printed circuit board (PCB) with reusable electrodes that can dramatically reduce the manufacturing costs of microfluidic cytometers. This microfluidic approach has potential for counting clusters of differentiation 4 (CD4) cells in blood samples from HIV patients in resource-poor settings (Emaminejad, Javanmard, Dutton, & Davis, 2012). These stated microfluidic flow cytometers can overcome the size and cost constraints of conventional flow cytometry, providing a new way for rapid, automated, and cost-effective viral diagnosis.

15.3 Examples of applications

This section provides three examples of microfluidic technologies for viral detection. These tools may advance conventional diagnostic techniques in terms of high throughput, integration, and automation.

15.3.1 Barcoded microchip for immunoassay

The use of a barcode scanner and smartphone application to read out the barcode results of multiplexed assays was pioneered by our group. We developed a barcoded microchip for protein detection. Barcodes can store and organize a large amount of data by arranging dark bars and light spaces with different widths. Varying the different combinations of bars and spaces can represent different information. The barcoded microchip contained several sets of microchannels with different widths (Fig. 15.12). The presence of positive immunoassay in the microchannel can be reflected as HRP-catalyzed colorimetric reaction, which displays a dark-blue color thus changing the width of the dark lines. By contrast, a negative immunoassay will not cause any color change. A barcoded microchip can simultaneously perform tens of immunoassays (encode) and display all the results by a portable barcode reader or a smartphone (decode). Simultaneous detection of three HIV proteins (anti-gp41 antibody, anti-gp120 antibody, and anti-gp36 antibody) from six human serum samples was realized on the chip (Zhang et al., 2015). To realize mass-manufacturing of barcoded analytical devices, we utilized an inkjet printer and an XYZ dispensing platform to generate codes on papers and designed a new group of barcodes which possess 16 times higher coding capacity than the standard Codabar code. The detection of HBV antibody, HCV antigen, and HIV antigen be completed within 10 min on this device (Yang, Javanmard, Dutton, & Davis, 2017; Yang, Zhang, Yang, et al., 2017).

Barcode microfluidic chips show their potential in immunoassays; however, the operations concerning sample introduction, incubation, and washing in the microfluidic channels are not easy for nonprofessionals. We developed an efficient mass

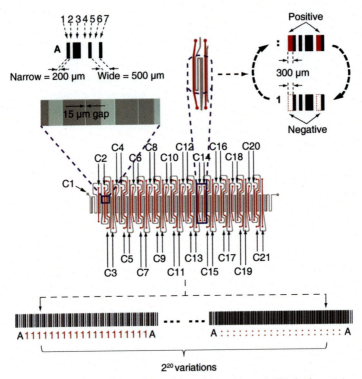

Figure 15.12 Design of microfluidic barcodes. The gray channel, C1, is the constant region displayed as dark bars after bioassays. The red channels, C2–C21, are variable regions filled with samples/solutions which could be either bars or spaces, depending on the positive ":" or negative "1" results of the assays. The magnified inset shows a part of the master with a small gap between the variable region and the constant region.
Reprinted with permission from Zhang et al. (2015), copyright 2015 American Chemical Society.

manufacturing method to fabricate paper-based barcode chips for multiplexed immunoassays. Codabar code and the constant thickness of papers were utilized to perform immunoassays. Three sheets of paper could form a wide module while one sheet of paper formed a narrow module or an intercharacter space. Gold nanoparticles (AuNPs) were used to generate colorimetric signals (red) in the test regions. The positive immunoassay could generate wide modules, changing the characters of "1" to ":"; otherwise, the negative immunoassay will not change the width of the bars and will not lead to the change of the characters (Fig. 15.13(a)). The barcode assay system consists of two parts: the paper-based barcode chips and the lateral flow test strips (Fig. 15.13(b)). The lateral flow test strip was used to load and transfer the target samples to the test regions while the paper-based barcode chip can immobilize capture probes, conduct immunoassays, and support the readout of the barcode results. After the completion of the immunoreaction, the barcode results of multiplex biomarkers were directly deciphered by a barcode scanner (Fig. 15.13(c)). Sandwich immunoassay was performed

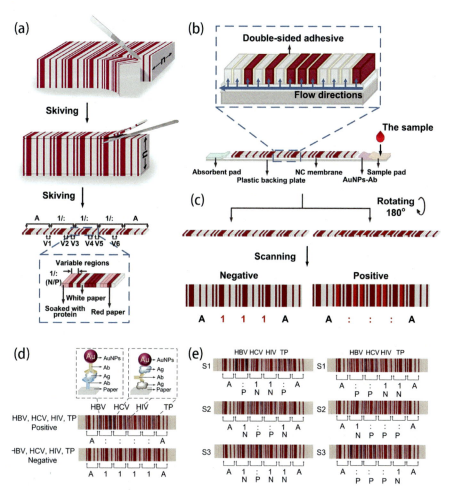

Figure 15.13 Paper-based barcode assay for virus detection. (a) Fabrication of paper-based chips by gluing the white papers, the red papers, and the papers soaked with capture probes together according to the Codabar rules and skived the combined papers into a small size. V1 and V2, V3 and V4, and V5 and V6 are variable regions used for target 1, target 2, and target 3. N, negative; P, positive. (b) Assay system on the chip. (c) Readout of the results. In an indirect or sandwich assay, when the targets are all positive, the result is read as "A:::A"; otherwise, the result is read as "A111A."(d) Positive and negative results of the simultaneous detection of HBV surface antigen and human anti-HCV, HIV-1, and TP antibodies. (e) Detection of six samples from patients infected by HBV, HCV, HIV-1, and TP.
Reprinted with permission from Yang, Zhang, Yang, et al. (2017), copyright 2017 American Association for the Advancement of Science.

on the barcode chip to detect HBV surface antigen and HCV, HIV-1, and *Treponema pallidum* (TP) antibodies from patient's blood (Fig. 15.13(d) and (e)). The results were read out by a barcode scanner connected to a computer, which were consistent with the results detected by ELISA. This paper-based barcode assay system provides a tool for highly efficient, accurate, and objective diagnoses (Yang, Zhang, Zheng et al., 2017; Yang, Zhang, Yang, et al., 2017).

15.3.2 CRISPR-Cas13a-based virus detection on a microchip

In recent years, clustered regularly interspaced short palindromic repeats (CRISPR) bacterial adaptive immune system has been adopted as a group of novel tools for infectious disease detection. 2 CRISPR-Cas types, CRISPR-Cas12, and CRISPR-Cas13 have been utilized as novel platforms for detection of DNA and RNA, respectively (Hatoum-Aslan, 2018). Cas13a can be reprogrammed with CRISPR RNAs (crRNAs) to provide a platform for specific virus (e.g., Zika and Dengue viruses) RNA sensing at a single base level (Gootenberg et al., 2017). The binding of Cas13a-cRNA to target RNA can induce a conformational change to activate Cas13a to cleavage nonspecific RNA. Cas13a can cleave about 10^4 nonspecific RNA when cleaving a target RNA (Fig. 15.14(a)). To improve the detection sensitivity

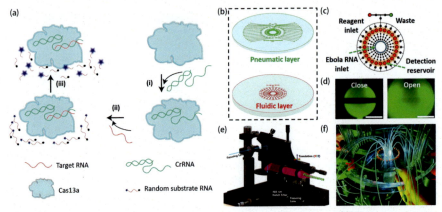

Figure 15.14 (a) Schematic of CRISPR-Cas13a-based sensing mechanism: (i) purified Cas13a binds with CRISPR RNA. (ii) The Cas13a-CRISPR RNA complex hybridizes with Ebola target RNA. (iii) The Cas13a-CRISPR RNA-Ebola RNA complex cleaves random RNA strands and releases fluorophores into the solution. (b) Design of the automated CRISPR microfluidic chip for Ebola virus detection. (c) Blow up of design of the fluidic layer. Ebola target RNA is pumped into the detection reservoir and reacted with Cas13a–crRNA. (d) Open (left) and closed (right) states of a microvalve. (e) Design of a benchtop fluorometer system integrated with a microfluidic device for in situ virus sensing. (f) Photograph of chip and detection system.
Reprinted with permission from Qin et al. (2019), copyright 2019 American Chemical Society.

without amplifying target RNA, researchers developed an automated and multiplexing microfluidic chip which can mix and hybridize virus nucleic acid. The microfluidic chip was mounted on a custom designed benchtop fluorometer for in situ and low volume (~10 μL) virus detection (Fig. 15.14(b−f)). On this device, Ebola virus could be detected with a detection limit of ~20 pfu/mL (5.45×10^7 copies/mL) within 5 min (Qin et al., 2019).

15.3.3 Microfluidic flow cytometer for monitoring HIV infection

The important clinical parameters in managing HIV-infected subjects are the absolute number and percentage of $CD4^+$ T lymphocytes (Hulgan et al., 2007). A microfluidic flow cytometer was developed to enable simultaneously counting the number and the percentage of $CD4^+$ T lymphocytes based on resistive pulse sensing and fluorescence detection (Wang et al., 2008). The microfluidic chip used for cell analysis consists of a three-terminal PDMS microfluidic circuit bonded to a glass substrate. The horizontal fluidic circuit is composed of two large microchannels sandwiching a small sensing channel of 16 μm × 30 μm in cross-section and 150 μm in length. A vertical microchannel connects the sensing channel to the gate of a metal−oxide−semiconductor field-effect transistor (MOSFET), which amplifies the voltage pulses caused by the translocation of cells through the small sensing channel. Meanwhile, an optical fiber is arranged close to the sensing channel for detecting fluorescently labeled cells (Fig. 15.15). In the experiment, lymphocytes are obtained from healthy donors, in which $CD4^+$ T cells are fluorescently labeled by immunostaining. The mixture of stained $CD4^+$ T and other unstained lymphocytes is introduced into the microchannel by electroosmosis. When a cell passes through the sensing channel, it will displace a volume of electrolyte equivalent to its own volume, resulting in a transient resistance change. This resistance change is proportional to the cell size, which is amplified ten-fold by a MOSFET (Sun, Stowers, Boczko, & Li, 2010). The so-called MOSFET-based resistive pulse sensing can count and size the cells passing through the aperture, whether the cells are fluorescently labeled or not. The characterization run shows that the diameter of lymphocytes ranges from 5.33 to 7.53 μm, consistent with the results from the commercial flow cytometer. To determine the percentage of fluorescently labeled $CD4^+$ T lymphocytes, an optical fluorescence system is integrated with the MOSFET-based resistive pulse sensing. When the stained cells pass through the sensing channel, the fluorescence signals are detected by the optical fiber and converted to electrical signals. As a 50% stained cell suspension flows through the sensing channel, both MOSFET drain current and fluorescence signal are recorded (Fig. 15.15). MOSFET signals indicate the total number of the cells passing through the sensing aperture, whereas the fluorescence signals show the translocation events of fluorescently labeled cells. The measured percentage of the stained cells is 48.7%, indicating a comparable accuracy with the result of 46.1% from commercial flow cytometer. This microfluidic flow cytometer is small, cost effective, easy to operate, and comparably accurate and may eventually be used to monitor HIV progression in infected patients.

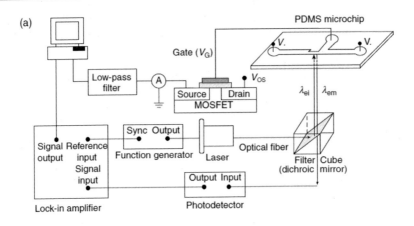

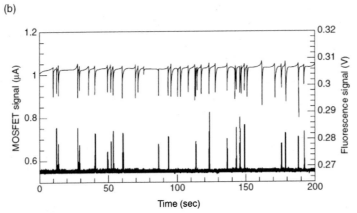

Figure 15.15 Microfluidic flow cytometer for detection of lymphocytes. (a) Schematic of measurement setup of the microfluidic flow cytometer. This system consists of a microchip, a MOSFET (metal−oxide−semiconductor field-effect transistor)-based resistive pulse sensor and a fluorescence detector. (b) Detection of a 50% stained cell suspension. The upper plot and left axis indicate the MOSFET signals indicating the total number of the cells passing through the sensing aperture; the lower plot and right axis indicate the fluorescent signals showing the translocation events of fluorescently labeled $CD4^+$ T lymphocytes cells.
Reprinted with permission from Wang et al. (2008), copyright 2008 The Royal Society of Chemistry.

The detection of virus in patient's blood faces challenges of high background. To solve this problem, researchers developed a spiral inertial microfluidics that can separate blood cells from viral particles and free nucleic acids (Fig. 15.16). By using this device, they collected plasma samples with excellent recovery of viral (cytomegalovirus) nucleic acids, highlighting the potential of this device in processing clinical samples for viral genome sequencing (Choi et al., 2018).

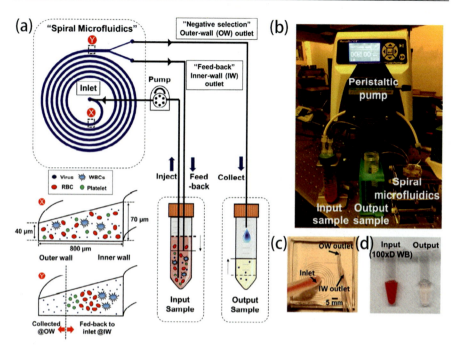

Figure 15.16 Spiral microfluidic device for separating blood cell and viral particles. (a) Schematic of the spiral microfluidic device for separating blood cell and viral particles. (b) Photograph of experimental setup (c) Magnified view of spiral microfluidic device (d) Comparison between input (100 times diluted whole blood) and microfluidics-treated samples. Reprinted with permission from Choi et al. (2018), copyright 2018 American Chemical Society.

15.4 Conclusion and future trends

Low-cost, high-efficient, POC, and automated assays for viral diagnosis are the pressing need for global health improvement. Microfluidic technologies have shown great potential to advance conventional diagnostic techniques in terms of high throughput, integration, and automation. This chapter reviews microfluidic methods for viral detection including microfluidic immunoassay, microfluidic nucleic acid detection, and microfluidic flow cytometry. Several samples of microfluidic devices used for selective and sensitive viral detection are presented.

Despite the promising success of microfluidics for the detection of viral infection, most devices are proof-of-concept prototypes. One challenge of commercializing microfluidic-based viral detection tools is batch fabrication of multifunctional microchips. The multilayer chips containing on-chip pumps, valves, mixers, or heaters for biological assays are usually assembled one by one by trained personnel. Another challenge is the design and construction of miniaturized and an automated fluid-control system equipped with microfluidic devices. The control system, which can precisely manipulate micro- to nanoliter volumes of fluid, is necessary to ensure the stability and performance of microfluidic assays. Integration of detection system for signal readout and measurement is also a challenge because the detection area of a microchip is relatively small. Further efforts in developing microfluidic viral diagnostic tools also include user-friendly software for data acquisition and analysis, and remote data collection with the ultimate goal of publicly available assays.

Acknowledgments

W. Z., J. S and X. J. acknowledge financial support from the National Key R&D Program of China (2018YFA0902600, 2017YFA0205901), the National Natural Science Foundation of China (21535001, 81730051, 21761142006, and 81673039) and the Chinese Academy of Sciences (QYZDJ-SSW-SLH039, 121D11KYSB20170026, XDA16020902); Tencent Foundation through the XPLORER PRIZE for financial support. W. Z., J. S and X. J. gratefully acknowledge Elsevier, American Chemical Society, The Royal Society of Chemistry, American Association for the Advancement of Science, and Wiley-VCH for their permission to reprint materials from publications.

References

Ahmad, F., Seyrig, G., Tourlousse, D. M., Stedtfeld, R. D., Tiedje, J. M., & Hashsham, S. A. (2011). A CCD-based fluorescence imaging system for real-time loop-mediated isothermal amplification-based rapid and sensitive detection of waterborne pathogens on microchips. *Biomedical Microdevices, 13*, 929−937.

Bange, A., Halsall, H. B., & Heineman, W. R. (2005). Microfluidic immunosensor systems. *Biosensors and Bioelectronics, 20*, 2488−2503.

Beebe, D. J., Mensing, G. A., & Walker, G. M. (2002). Physics and applications of microfluidics in biology. *Annual Review of Biomedical Engineering, 4*, 261−286.

Bernard, A., Michel, B., & Delamarche, E. (2001). Micromosaic immunoassays. *Analytical Chemistry, 73*, 8−12.

Borkowsky, W., Krasinski, K., Paul, D., Moore, T., Bebenroth, D., & Chandwani, S. (1987). Human-immunodeficiency-virus infections in infants negative for anti-Hiv by enzyme-linked immunoassay. *Lancet*, 1168−1171.

Branson, B. M. (2007). State of the art for diagnosis of HIV infection. *Clinical Infectious Diseases, 45*, S221−S225.

Cheng, X. H., Irimia, D., Dixon, M., Sekine, K., Demirci, U., Zamir, L., et al. (2007). A microfluidic device for practical label-free CD4+T cell counting of HIV-infected subjects. *Lab on a Chip, 7*, 170−178.

Chin, C. D., Linder, V., & Sia, S. K. (2012). Commercialization of microfluidic point-of-care diagnostic devices. *Lab on a Chip, 12*, 2118−2134.

Choi, K., Ryu, H., Siddle, K. J., Piantadosi, A., Freimark, L., Park, D. J., et al. (2018). Negative selection by spiral inertial microfluidics improves viral recovery and sequencing from blood. *Analytical Chemistry, 90*, 4657−4662.

Cho, Y. K., Kim, J., Lee, Y., Kim, Y. A., Namkoong, K., Lim, H., et al. (2006). Clinical evaluation of micro-scale chip-based PCR system for rapid detection of hepatitis B virus. *Biosensors and Bioelectronics, 21*, 2161−2169.

Cordes, R. J., & Ryan, M. E. (1995). Pitfalls in HIV testing - application and limitations of current tests. *Postgraduate Medical Journal, 98*, 177- 177−180, 185−186, 189.

Cui, J., Li, F., & Shi, Z. L. (2019). Origin and evolution of pathogenic coronaviruses. *Nature Reviews Microbiology, 17*, 181−192.

Dimov, I. K., Garcia-Cordero, J. L., O'Grady, J., Poulsen, C. R., Viguier, C., Kent, L., et al. (2008). Integrated microfluidic tmRNA purification and real-time NASBA device for molecular diagnostics. *Lab on a Chip, 8*, 2071−2078.

Dong, R., Liu, Y., Mou, L., Deng, J., & Jiang, X. (2019). Microfluidics-based biomaterials and biodevices. *Advanced Materials, 31*, e1805033.

Dong, H., Li, C. M., Zhang, Y. F., Cao, X. D., & Gan, Y. (2007). Screen-printed microfluidic device for electrochemical immunoassay. *Lab on a Chip, 7*, 1752−1758.

Drakeley, C., & Reyburn, H. (2009). Out with the old, in with the new: The utility of rapid diagnostic tests for malaria diagnosis in Africa. *Transactions of the Royal Society of Tropical Medicine and Hygiene, 103*, 333−337.

Du, K., Cai, H., Park, M., Wall, T. A., Stott, M. A., Alfson, K. J., et al. (2017). Multiplexed efficient on-chip sample preparation and sensitive amplification-free detection of Ebola virus. *Biosensors and Bioelectronics, 91*, 489−496.

Emaminejad, S., Javanmard, M., Dutton, R. W., & Davis, R. W. (2012). Microfluidic diagnostic tool for the developing world: Contactless impedance flow cytometry. *Lab on a Chip, 12*, 4499−4507.

Fang, X. E., Chen, H., Yu, S. N., Jiang, X. Y., & Kong, J. L. (2011). Predicting viruses accurately by a multiplex microfluidic loop-mediated isothermal amplification chip. *Analytical Chemistry, 83*, 690−695.

Fang, X. E., Liu, Y. Y., Kong, J. L., & Jiang, X. Y. (2010). Loop-mediated isothermal amplification integrated on microfluidic chips for point-of-care quantitative detection of pathogens. *Analytical Chemistry, 82*, 3002−3006.

Fauci, A. S., & Morens, D. M. (2012). 200 NEJM anniversary article the perpetual challenge of infectious diseases. *New England Journal of Medicine, 366*, 454−461.

Ferris, M. M., McCabe, M. O., Doan, L. G., & Rowlen, K. L. (2002). Rapid enumeration of respiratory viruses. *Analytical Chemistry, 74*, 1849−1856.

Foudeh, A. M., Didar, T. F., Veres, T., & Tabrizian, M. (2012). Microfluidic designs and techniques using lab-on-a-chip devices for pathogen detection for point-of-care diagnostics. *Lab on a Chip, 12*, 3249−3266.

Gervais, L., de Rooij, N., & Delamarche, E. (2011). Microfluidic chips for point-of-care immunodiagnostics. *Advanced Materials, 23*, H151−H176.

Gootenberg, J. S., Abudayyeh, O. O., Lee, J. W., Essletzbichler, P., Dy, A. J., Joung, J., et al. (2017). Nucleic acid detection with CRISPR-Cas13a/C2c2. *Science, 356*, 438−442.

Govindarajan, A. V., Ramachandran, S., Vigil, G. D., Yager, P., & Bohringer, K. F. (2012). A low cost point-of-care viscous sample preparation device for molecular diagnosis in the developing world; an example of microfluidic origami. *Lab on a Chip, 12*, 174−181.

Gulliksen, A., Solli, L., Karlsen, F., Rogne, H., Hovig, E., Nordstrom, T., et al. (2004). Real-time nucleic acid sequence-based amplification in nanoliter volumes. *Analytical Chemistry, 76*, 9−14.

Hatoum-Aslan, A. (2018). CRISPR methods for nucleic acid detection herald the future of molecular diagnostics. *Clinical Chemistry, 64*, 1681−1683.

Henihan, G., Schulze, H., Corrigan, D. K., Giraud, G., Terry, J. G., Hardie, A., et al. (2016). Label- and amplification-free electrochemical detection of bacterial ribosomal RNA. *Biosensors and Bioelectronics, 81*, 487−494.

He, S., Zhang, Y., Wang, P., Xu, X., Zhu, K., Pan, W., et al. (2015). Multiplexed microfluidic blotting of proteins and nucleic acids by parallel, serpentine microchannels. *Lab on a Chip, 15*, 105−112.

Hulgan, T., Shepherd, B. E., Raffanti, S. P., Fusco, J. S., Beckerman, R., Barkanic, G., et al. (2007). Absolute count and percentage of CD4(+) lymphocytes are independent predictors of disease progression in HIV-infected persons initiating highly active antiretroviral therapy. *The Journal of Infectious Diseases, 195*, 425−431.

Hughes, A. J., & Herr, A. E. (2012). Microfluidic Western blotting. *Proceedings of the National Academy of Sciences of the United States of America, 109*, 21450−21455.

Iwamoto, T., Sonobe, T., & Hayashi, K. (2003). Loop-mediated isothermal amplification for direct detection of *Mycobacterium tuberculosis* complex, M-avium, and M-intracellulare in sputum samples. *Journal of Clinical Microbiology, 41*, 2616−2622.

Jiang, X. Y., Ng, J. M. K., Stroock, A. D., Dertinger, S. K. W., & Whitesides, G. M. (2003). A miniaturized, parallel, serially diluted immunoassay for analyzing multiple antigens. *Journal of the American Chemical Society, 125*, 5294−5295.

Jiang, X. Y., Xu, Q. B., Dertinger, S. K. W., Stroock, A. D., Fu, T. M., & Whitesides, G. M. (2005). A general method for patterning gradients of biomolecules on surfaces using microfluidic networks. *Analytical Chemistry, 77*, 2338−2347.

Kelly, R. T., & Woolley, A. T. (2005). Microfluidic systems for integrated, high-throughput DNA analysis. *Analytical Chemistry, 77*, 96a−102a.

Kievits, T., Vangemen, B., Vanstrijp, D., Schukkink, R., Dircks, M., Adriaanse, H., et al. (1991). Nasba isothermal enzymatic in vitro nucleic-acid amplification optimized for the diagnosis of Hiv-1 infection. *Journal of Virological Methods, 35*, 273−286.

Kim, D., Karns, K., Tia, S. Q., He, M., & Herr, A. E. (2012). Electrostatic protein immobilization using charged polyacrylamide gels and cationic detergent microfluidic Western blotting. *Analytical Chemistry, 84*, 2533−2540.

Lee, H. Y., Jeong, H., Jung, I. Y., Jang, B., Seo, Y. C., Lee, H., et al. (2015). DhITACT: DNA hydrogel formation by isothermal amplification of complementary target in fluidic channels. *Advanced Materials, 27*, 3513−3517.

Leke, R. G. F. (2010). Global health governance-the response to infectious diseases. *Lancet, 376*, 1200−1201.

Li, L., Miao, B., Li, Z., Sun, Z., & Peng, N. (2019). Sample-to-answer hepatitis B virus DNA detection from whole blood on a centrifugal microfluidic platform with double rotation axes. *ACS Sensors, 4*, 2738−2745.

Liu, Y. X., Cady, N. C., & Batt, C. A. (2007). A plastic microchip for nucleic acid purification. *Biomedical Microdevices, 9*, 769−776.

Liu, C. C., Geva, E., Mauk, M., Qiu, X. B., Abrams, W. R., Malamud, D., ... Bau, H. H. (2011). An isothermal amplification reactor with an integrated isolation membrane for point-of-care detection of infectious diseases. *Analyst, 136*, 2069−2076.

Lu, W., Wang, J., Wu, Q., Sun, J., Chen, Y., Zhang, L., et al. (2016). High-throughput sample-to-answer detection of DNA/RNA in crude samples within functionalized micro-pipette tips. *Biosensors and Bioelectronics, 75*, 28−33.

Mackay, I. M. (2004). Real-time PCR in the microbiology laboratory. *Clinical Microbiology and Infections, 10*, 190−212.
McCalla, S. E., & Tripathi, A. (2011). Microfluidic reactors for diagnostics applications. *Annual Review of Biomedical Engineering, 13*, 321−343.
Melin, J., & Quake, S. R. (2007). Microfluidic large-scale integration: The evolution of design rules for biological automation. *Annual Review of Biophysics and Biomolecular Structure, 36*, 213−231.
Misiani, R., Bellavita, P., Fenili, D., Borelli, G., Marchesi, D., Massazza, M., et al. (1992). Hepatitis-C virus-infection in patients with essential mixed cryoglobulinemia. *Annals of Internal Medicine, 117*, 573−577.
Na, W., Nam, D., Lee, H., & Shin, S. (2018). Rapid molecular diagnosis of infectious viruses in microfluidics using DNA hydrogel formation. *Biosensors and Bioelectronics, 108*, 9−13.
Notomi, T., Okayama, H., Masubuchi, H., Yonekawa, T., Watanabe, K., Amino, N., et al. (2000). Loop-mediated isothermal amplification of DNA. *Nucleic Acids Research, 28*, E63.
Pan, W. Y., Chen, W., & Jiang, X. Y. (2010). Microfluidic western blot. *Analytical Chemistry, 82*, 3974−3976.
Pang, T., & Peeling, R. W. (2007). Diagnostic tests for infectious diseases in the developing world: Two sides of the coin. *Transactions of the Royal Society of Tropical Medicine and Hygiene, 101*, 856−857.
Park, S., Zhang, Y., Lin, S., Wang, T. H., & Yang, S. (2011). Advances in microfluidic PCR for point-of-care infectious disease diagnostics. *Biotechnology Advances, 29*, 830−839.
Peeters, M., Gershydamet, G. M., Fransen, K., Koffi, K., Coulibaly, M., Delaporte, E., et al. (1992). Virological and polymerase chain-reaction studies of Hiv-1 Hiv-2 dual infection in cote-divoire. *Lancet, 340*, 339−340.
Poon, L. L. M., Wong, B. W. Y., Ma, E. H. T., Chan, K. H., Chow, L. M. C., Abeyewickreme, W., et al. (2006). Sensitive and inexpensive molecular test for falciparum malaria: Detecting *Plasmodium falciparum* DNA directly from heat-treated blood by loop-mediated isothermal amplification. *Clinical Chemistry, 52*, 303−306.
Qin, P., Park, M., Alfson, K. J., Tamhankar, M., Carrion, R., Patterson, J. L., et al. (2019). Rapid and fully microfluidic ebola virus detection with CRISPR-Cas13a. *ACS Sensors, 4*, 1048−1054.
Qu, W. S., Liu, Y. Y., Liu, D. B., Wang, Z., & Jiang, X. Y. (2011). Copper-mediated amplification allows readout of immunoassays by the naked eye. *Angewandte Chemie International Edition, 50*, 3442−3445.
Rossier, J. S., & Girault, H. H. (2001). Enzyme linked immunosorbent assay on a microchip with electrochemical detection. *Lab on a Chip, 1*, 153−157.
Roth, W. K., Weber, M., & Seifried, E. (1999). Feasibility and efficacy of routine PCR screening of blood donations for hepatitis C virus, hepatitis B virus, and HIV-1 in a blood-bank setting. *Lancet, 353*, 359−363.
Sia, S. K., & Whitesides, G. M. (2003). Microfluidic devices fabricated in poly(dimethylsiloxane) for biological studies. *Electrophoresis, 24*, 3563−3576.
Song, L. S., Zhang, Y., Wang, W. J., Ma, L. Y., Liu, Y., Hao, Y. L., et al. (2012). Microfluidic assay without blocking for rapid HIV screening and confirmation. *Biomedical Microdevices, 14*, 631−640.
Stockman, M. I. (2015). Applied optics. Nanoplasmonic sensing and detection. *Science, 348*, 287−288.

Stoffel, C. L., Kathy, R. F., & Rowlen, K. L. (2005). Design and characterization of a compact dual channel virus counter. *Cytometry, Part A, 65a*, 140−147.

Stoop, J. N., van der Molen, R. G., Baan, C. C., van der Laan, L. J. W., Kuipers, E. J., Kusters, J. G., et al. (2005). Regulatory T cells contribute to the impaired immune response in patients with chronic hepatitis B virus infection. *Hepatology, 41*, 771−778.

Stumpf, F., Schwemmer, F., Hutzenlaub, T., Baumann, D., Strohmeier, O., Dingemanns, G., et al. (2016). LabDisk with complete reagent prestorage for sample-to-answer nucleic acid based detection of respiratory pathogens verified with influenza A H3N2 virus. *Lab on a Chip, 16*, 199−207.

Sturenburg, E., & Junker, R. (2009). Point-of-Care testing in microbiology the advantages and disadvantages of immunochromatographic test strips. *Deutsches Arzteblatt International, 106*, 48−54.

Sun, J. S., Stowers, C. C., Boczko, E. M., & Li, D. Y. (2010). Measurement of the volume growth rate of single budding yeast with the MOSFET-based microfluidic Coulter counter. *Lab on a Chip, 10*, 2986−2993.

Sun, J., Xianyu, Y., & Jiang, X. (2014). Point-of-care biochemical assays using gold nanoparticle-implemented microfluidics. *Chemical Society Reviews, 43*, 6239−6253.

Tao, Y., Rotem, A., Zhang, H., Chang, C. B., Basu, A., Kolawole, A. O., et al. (2015). Rapid, targeted and culture-free viral infectivity assay in drop-based microfluidics. *Lab on a Chip, 15*, 3934−3940.

Towner, J. S., Sealy, T. K., Khristova, M. L., Albarino, C. G., Conlan, S., Reeder, S. A., et al. (2008). Newly discovered ebola virus associated with hemorrhagic fever outbreak in Uganda. *PLoS Pathogens, 4*, e1000212.

Tseng, Y. T., Wang, C. H., Chang, C. P., & Lee, G. B. (2016). Integrated microfluidic system for rapid detection of influenza H1N1 virus using a sandwich-based aptamer assay. *Biosensors and Bioelectronics, 82*, 105−111.

Wang, D., Coscoy, L., Zylberberg, M., Avila, P. C., Boushey, H. A., Ganem, D., et al. (2002). Microarray-based detection and genotyping of viral pathogens. *Proceedings of the National Academy of Sciences of the United States of America, 99*, 15687−15692.

Wang, Y. N., Kang, Y. J., Xu, D. Y., Chon, C. H., Barnett, L., Kalams, S. A., et al. (2008). On-chip counting the number and the percentage of CD4+T lymphocytes. *Lab on a Chip, 8*, 309−315.

Wang, C. H., & Lee, G. B. (2005). Automatic bio-sampling chips integrated with micro-pumps and micro-valves for disease detection. *Biosensors and Bioelectronics, 21*, 419−425.

Wu, A. H. B. (2006). A selected history and future of immunoassay development and applications in clinical chemistry. *Clinica Chimica Acta, 369*, 119−124.

Xianyu, Y., Wu, J., Chen, Y., Zheng, W., Xie, M., & Jiang, X. (2018). Controllable assembly of enzymes for multiplexed lab-on-a-chip bioassays with a tunable detection range. *Angewandte Chemie International Edition, 57*, 7503−7507.

Yager, P., Domingo, G. J., & Gerdes, J. (2008). Point-of-care diagnostics for global health. *Annual Review of Biomedical Engineering, 10*, 107−144.

Yakovleva, J., Davidsson, R., Lobanova, A., Bengtsson, M., Eremin, S. A., Laurell, T., et al. (2002). Microfluidic enzyme immunoassay using silicon microchip with immobilized antibodies and chemiluminescence detection. *Analytical Chemistry, 74*, 2994−3004.

Yang, S. Y., Lien, K. Y., Huang, K. J., Lei, H. Y., & Lee, G. B. (2008). Micro flow cytometry utilizing a magnetic bead-based immunoassay for rapid virus detection. *Biosensors and Bioelectronics, 24*, 855−862.

Yang, M., Liu, Y., & Jiang, X. (2019). Barcoded point-of-care bioassays. *Chemical Society Reviews, 48*, 850−884.

Yang, D. Y., Niu, X., Liu, Y. Y., Wang, Y., Gu, X., Song, L. S., et al. (2008). Electrospun nanofibrous membranes: A novel solid substrate for microfluidic immunoassays for HIV. *Advanced Materials, 20*, 4770−4775.

Yang, S., & Rothman, R. E. (2004). PCR-based diagnostics for infectious diseases: Uses, limitations, and future applications in acute-care settings. *The Lancet Infectious Diseases, 4*, 337−348.

Yang, M. Z., Zhang, W., Yang, J. C., Hu, B., Cao, F. J., Zheng, W. S., et al. (2017b). Skiving stacked sheets of paper into test paper for rapid and multiplexed assay. *Science Advances, 3*, eaao4862.

Yang, M., Zhang, W., Zheng, W., Cao, F., & Jiang, X. (2017a). Inkjet-printed barcodes for a rapid and multiplexed paper-based assay compatible with mobile devices. *Lab on a Chip, 17*, 3874−3882.

Zeng, Y., Novak, R., Shuga, J., Smith, M. T., & Mathies, R. A. (2010). High performance single cell genetic analysis using microfluidic emulsion generator arrays. *Analytical Chemistry, 82*, 3183−3190.

Zhang, Y., Sun, J., Zou, Y., Chen, W., Zhang, W., Xi, J. J., et al. (2015). Barcoded microchips for biomolecular assays. *Analytical Chemistry, 87*, 900−906.

Zhang, Y., Tang, Y. F., Hsieh, Y. H., Hsu, C. Y., Xi, J. Z., Lin, K. J., et al. (2012). Towards a high-throughput label-free detection system combining localized-surface plasmon resonance and microfluidics. *Lab on a Chip, 12*, 3012−3015.

Zhang, Y., Zhang, L., Sun, J., Liu, Y., Ma, X., Cui, S., et al. (2014). Point-of-care multiplexed assays of nucleic acids using microcapillary-based loop-mediated isothermal amplification. *Analytical Chemistry, 86*, 7057−7062.

Zhang, L., Zhang, Y., Wang, C., Feng, Q., Fan, F., Zhang, G., et al. (2014). Integrated microcapillary for sample-to-answer nucleic acid pretreatment, amplification, and detection. *Analytical Chemistry, 86*, 10461−10466.

Zhu, N., Zhang, D., Wang, W., Li, X., Yang, B., Song, J., et al. (2020). A novel coronavirus from patients with pneumonia in China, 2019. *New England Journal of Medicine, 382*, 727−733.

Microfluidic applications on pancreatic islets and β-cells study for human islet transplant

Yuan Xing[1], Pu Zhang[2], Yi He[1], Xiaoyu Yu[1], Sharon Lu[1], Farid Ghamsari[1], Sarah Innis[1], Joshua E. Mendoza-Elias[3], Melur K. Ramasubramanian[2], Yong Wang[1], José Oberholzer[1]

[1]Department of Surgery, University of Virginia, Charlottesville, VA, United States; [2]Department of Mechanical and Aerospace Engineering, University of Virginia, Charlottesville, VA, United States; [3]Department of Surgery, San Joaquin General Hospital, French Camp, CA, United States

Guided-reading questions:

1. How to develop a microfluidic system for in vitro islet multifunction assessments with a high spatiotemporal resolution as it could not only be useful in islet physiology study but may also predict the outcome of transplant?
2. How to utilize microfluidic techniques to fabricate islet hydrogel capsules to prevent immune-rejection and prolong islet grafts survival after transplantation?
3. How does the microfluidic technology benefits stem cell study to further solve problems in human islets transplantation?

16.1 Introduction

Since the introduction of the Edmonton Protocol in 2000, islet transplantation has emerged as a promising therapy for Type I diabetes mellitus (T1DM) and currently is the only therapy that can achieve glycemic control without the need for exogenous insulin (Alejandro, Barton, Hering, Wease, & Collaborative Islet Transplant Registry, 2008; Gangemi et al., 2008; Qi et al., 2014; Ricordi et al., 2016; Ryan et al., 2005). Transplanting islet cells for treating T1DM has several advantages over transplanting a whole pancreas since it involves only a minor surgical procedure with much lower morbidity and mortality and has a significantly lower cost. Although insulin replacement therapy via either injection or pumps has proven to be an effective therapy for controlling blood glucose levels and minimizing hypoglycemic episodes, the risk of hypoglycemia remains, as well as diabetes-related complications such as metabolic syndrome, cardiovascular renal disease, and retinopathy. The potential advantage of islet transplantation over insulin therapy is that the transplanted islets can maintain normal blood glucose levels under a wide range of physiological conditions without producing excess insulin that may result in hypoglycemic episodes (Alejandro et al., 2008; Gangemi et al., 2008; Qi et al., 2014; Ricordi et al., 2016; Ryan et al., 2005).

To date, islet transplantation has shown variable success in demonstrating both short- and long-term insulin independence (Alejandro et al., 2008; Bellin et al., 2008; Gangemi et al., 2008; Ryan et al., 2005), and much of this variability is associated with the factors relating to both organ donor and recipient. As a cell therapy, islet transplantation is a multistep process involving pancreas organ procurement and preservation, tissue digestion and dissociation, islet purification, cell culture, islet transplantation via the hepatic portal vein, and graft maintenance by nonsteroidal immunosuppressant regimens. Successful islet transplantation is dictated by the cumulative success of each aforementioned step.

16.1.1 Insulin secretory pathway: how glucose sensing and metabolic coupling translates to insulin kinetics?

A pancreatic islet is a cluster of 1000–2000 cells, which can range in size between 50 and 500 μm in diameter. Islets are composed of at least five different cell types: α-cells, secreting glucagon; β-cells, producing insulin and amylin; δ-cells, secreting somatostatin; PP cells, secreting pancreatic polypeptide; and ε-cells, secreting ghrelin. In diabetes research, we are primarily concerned with β-cells as they secrete insulin and compose 65%–80% of human islet mass. As seen in Fig. 16.1, β-cell insulin secretion is governed by cellular electrical activity, metabolic events, and ion signaling, which display complex biphasic and pulsatile kinetic profiles (Luciani, Misler, & Polonsky, 2006; Porksen et al., 2002). The first phase of the biphasic profile corresponds to a prompt, marked increase in the insulin secretory rate that is transient (4–8 min). In the absence of glucose, this profile decreases back to baseline. With continuous glucose stimulation, a secondary phase consisting of a gradual increase is observed (Henquin, Nenquin, Stiernet, & Ahren, 2006; Komjati, Bratusch-Marrain, & Waldhausl, 1986). Glucose-induced insulin secretion is a dynamic process that is tightly regulated. In short, glucose enters β-cells via GLUT2 facilitated transport; subsequent glycolysis generates pyruvate, entering the tricarboxylic acid cycle (TCA cycle) in the mitochondria. Newly produced NADH then enters the electron transport chain (ETC) to undergo oxidative phosphorylation, generating an electrical potential gradient across the mitochondrial membrane. Mitochondrial hyperpolarization then leads to ATP generation and the closure of ATP-sensitive K^+ (K_{ATP}) channels. This initiates plasma membrane depolarization and an increase in intracellular calcium concentration ($[Ca^{2+}]_i$) through a rapid influx of calcium ions via voltage-dependent calcium channels (VDCCs). In this way, glucose induces an increase in $[Ca^{2+}]_i$, which triggers the fusion of insulin granules to the cell plasma membrane resulting in the exocytosis of insulin, C-peptide, and proinsulin (Babenko, Aguilar-Bryan, & Bryan, 1998; Henquin, Schmeer, Nenquin, & Meissner, 1985; Roe et al., 1996; Warnotte, Gilon, Nenquin, & Henquin, 1994). Alternate pathways of glucose-stimulated insulin secretion (GSIS), independent of either K_{ATP} channels or $[Ca^{2+}]_i$, have been described

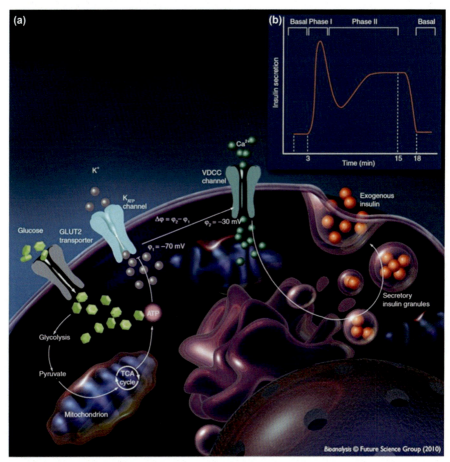

Figure 16.1 Insulin secretory pathway and kinetic profile. (a) Ionic control of secretion. (b) Biphasic insulin secretory kinetics (Wang et al., 2013).
Reprinted with permission from Future Science Ltd

(Gembal, Gilon, & Henquin, 1992; Straub & Sharp, 2002) but play a smaller role in insulin secretion. Some evidence demonstrates that glucose-induced $[Ca^{2+}]_i$ is associated with calcium concentration inside the mitochondria (Kennedy et al., 1996; Maechler, Kennedy, Wang, & Wollheim, 1998). The rise in intramitochondrial calcium, together with the aforementioned coupling messengers/factors, evokes insulin secretion independent from K_{ATP} channels or amplifies the K_{ATP}-dependent pathway (Kennedy et al., 1996; Maechler et al., 1998). However, it has been confirmed that the K_{ATP} and the $[Ca^{2+}]_i$-mediated pathway remains the primary mechanism of GSIS. Although only composing 1%−2% of pancreas mass, islets receive 2%−10% of pancreatic blood perfusion (Svensson, Sandler, & Jansson, 1994).

In addition to the mitochondria's well-established role in the insulin secretory pathway, mitochondrial energetics and calcium signaling are also essential for β-cell viability. Mitochondria actively mediate and regulate a variety of effector mechanisms involving cell life and death. Intracellular calcium acts as a secondary messenger in a variety of cells and tightly regulates many cellular functions within subcellular microdomains. In addition, the level and pattern of $[Ca^{2+}]_i$ modulate cell viability and influence both apoptotic and necrotic pathways (Duchen, 2000). In the search for a more reliable and β-cell-specific potency assay, several approaches to measuring mitochondrial integrity and calcium influx have been tested as an alternative assay, in the form of a single parameter or combined with other parameters for islet viability and potency.

For example, the static measurement of mitochondrial membrane potentials for islet viability using tetramethylrhodamine ethyl ester (TMRE) has been investigated in conjunction with either Newport Green (NP) (Ichii et al., 2005) or FluoZin-3 (Jayaraman, 2008), suggesting that β-cell mitochondrial integrity is critically important and has predictive value for transplant outcomes when compared to the gold standard immunodeficient nude mouse model; this has been confirmed by other researchers (Iglesias et al., 2008). While these results are promising, the aforementioned assessments of mitochondrial integrity measure a static value of β-cell energetic status with only retrospective values, since these assays may take days to conduct and cannot predict islet graft function at the time of transplant. Moreover, as the enzymatic dissociation of the islets is involved, the assays' methodology is often questioned for the introduction of artifacts, such as selective damage and loss of the β-cell population. Furthermore, most of these assays require more sophisticated laboratory setups, such as fluorescence-activated cell sorting (FACS), confocal microscope, and laser scanning cytometry.

Although individual assays that quantify either mitochondrial energetics or $[Ca^{2+}]_i$ have been used extensively to study β-cell stimulus-secretion coupling, they have never been combined with islet perifusion for human islet potency and viability studies. In this chapter, we will discuss a microfluidic-based islet perifusion apparatus with the integration of multichannel fluorescence imaging for changes in mitochondrial electrical potentials ($\Delta\Psi_M$) and $[Ca^{2+}]_i$ and off-chip insulin analysis for human islet function assessment.

16.1.2 Obstacles toward clinical use of the islet products

The U.S. Food and Drug Administration (FDA) defines the islet product as a biological drug; therefore, isolated human islets for transplant need to be prepared under FDA-approved guidance before islet transplant can be approved as a clinical therapy. Despite the application and standardization of current good manufacturing practices (cGMPs) in the islet isolation process, lot-to-lot variability still cannot be avoided. To reduce the risk of transplanting low-quality islets, appropriate product release tests are needed. While tests for identity, sterility, and purity are well established, so far, no reliable assessment of islet potency is available prior to transplant. This continues to be one of the key hurdles associated with uncontrollable clinical outcomes.

In addition, while islet cells have potential applications to functional treatments of T1DM, it may also be critical in addressing challenges with immunoisolation and immunoprotection in patients. Encapsulation of islet cells using biocompatible materials holds significant promise as a means to eliminate the need for immunosuppression. There are many approaches to protecting the islets from the host immune system, including conformal coating, macro- or microencapsulation, and bioscaffold. Microcapsules offer the advantage of a larger surface-to-volume ratio, allowing for faster nutrient and O_2 transport (Fig. 16.2). Various types, including sizes and composition, of microcapsules have been developed with promising advancements. Recent studies have demonstrated that encapsulated islets effectively reverse diabetes in small animal models. However, large animal (nonhuman primate) studies and clinical studies showed very limited success. One of the major obstacles to clinical application is the death of large portions of encapsulated islet cells due to severe hypoxia (deprivation of O_2) associated with larger capsule sizes (>500 μm). O_2 diffusion limitation in the capsule material, alginate, is only 200 μm. Furthermore, islets have a much higher metabolic requirement, especially in response to glucose and insulin secretion. The transplant site applied in animals and humans is in the intraperitoneal (IP) cavity due to volume requirements. However, the PoO_2 is much lower in IP than in the pancreas (~28 mmHg vs. ~44 mmHg). Therefore, capsule diameter is important to ensure sufficient O_2 transport, as well as proper insulin delivery.

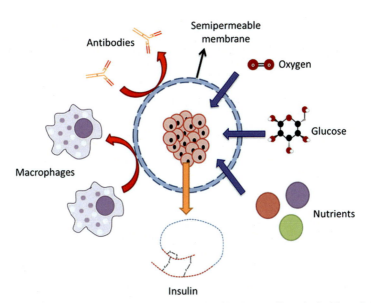

Figure 16.2 Principle of islet microencapsulation (Paredes Juarez, Spasojevic, Faas, & de Vos, 2014).
Reprinted with permission from Frontiers.

16.1.3 Standard assays currently used to determine islet potency

The existing standard assays for islet function and viability include static GSIS for potency and inclusive and exclusive dyes to stain membrane integrity for viability. Both of these assays have no predictive values and do not correlate well with clinical transplant outcomes (Armann, Hanson, Hatch, Steffen, & Fernandez, 2007; Papas, Pisania, Wu, Weir, & Colton, 2007b; Papas, Suszynski, & Colton, 2009; Street et al., 2004; Sweet et al., 2008). Therefore, clinicians are more dependent on morphology and islet cell mass, IEq (Islet Equivalent, a volumetric quantification of islet mass), to determine the suitability of a given islet preparation. The static GSIS only measures "bulk" insulin release from an islet product under extreme conditions (exposure to 16.7 mM glucose for 60 min) and fails to observe and quantify the dynamic nature of β-cell insulin secretory kinetics. In addition, insulin secretion data alone does not provide any useful information on the key stimulus coupling factors that control and regulate insulin secretion and, therefore, may be a source of false positives and false negatives in islet function and viability tests. For example, mild stress during the islet isolation process can lead to temporary insulin degranulation and leakage caused by cell membrane damage, even though the islets are still viable. Therefore, a low GSIS may not indicate irreversible loss of function, as temporarily impaired islet cells may recover once transplanted into a recipient. Likewise, a high GSIS result may be caused by insulin degranulation stemming from membrane damage.

In contrast to both GSIS and IEq assessments, an in vivo potency assay conducted by transplanting human islets into the kidney capsule of immunodeficient nude mice correlates extremely well with clinical transplant outcomes and is currently the "gold standard" for evaluating islet potency. However, this in vivo analysis takes several weeks to complete and, therefore, only provides a retrospective indication of islet function, which renders this assay impractical as a pretransplant assessment in the time-critical clinical setting (Bertuzzi & Ricordi, 2007; London, Thirdborough, Swift, Bell, & James, 1991; Ricordi, Lakey, & Hering, 2001; Ricordi, Scharp, & Lacy, 1988).

To address this problem, a variety of in vitro tests have been investigated in order to assess islet potency and viability prior to islet release for transplant, including: the measurement of the oxygen consumption rate (OCR) (Papas et al., 2007; Sweet & Gilbert, 2006; Sweet et al., 2008; Wang, Upshaw, Strong, Robertson, & Reems, 2005); the quantification of reactive oxygen species (ROS) (Armann et al., 2007); and ADP/ATP ratios (Goto, Holgersson, Kumagai-Braesch, & Korsgren, 2006; Kim et al., 2009). Apart from providing less predictive data and being of more retrospective usefulness, these assays also have multiple limitations. Most OCR and ROS assays are conducted in a static manner under a single static parameter. Additionally, OCR and ROS assays lack β-cell specificity, as an islet is composed of at least five different cell types, with β-cells contributing only 65%−80% of a human islet cell mass. Even with a weighted analysis of OCR and ROS for each individual cell group, this information may be confounded and artifactual. Recently, new research evidences chemical and ion communication among β-cells, or between β-cells and α-cells, being important for regulation of insulin secretion (Spigelman, Dai, & MacDonald, 2010). In addition, gap junctional complexes between adjacent islet cells are also needed to facilitate intraislet cell—cell communications and coordinate hormonal (Carvalho et al., 2012). Therefore, the ADP/ATP assay is often challenged for its accuracy since islet dissociation is involved.

16.1.4 Current methods for islet encapsulation

Emulsification and extrusion are the most popular dispersion steps currently employed in islet encapsulation (Schwarz, 2000). The emulsification method utilizes a polydimethylsiloxane (PDMS) membrane and neutralized collagen solution to fabricate cell-containing gel modules. The membrane is formed by spinning PDMS on an SU-8 molded Si wafer which contains an array of holes in a variety of shapes. The process of emulsification is performed by incubating gel modules in a 37°C environment for 1 h. The cell-containing gel modules' dimensions can be controlled from diameters from 40 to 1000 μm and heights from 100 to 1000 μm (McGuigan, Bruzewicz, Glavan, Butte, & Whitesides, 2008). This method requires a high cell density collagen solution to meet transplantation needs. The cell volume pregel module is inconsistent.

The current extrusion method utilizes a needle and air to form a droplet. The process starts with suspending islets in a polymer solution. This solution is pumped into the chamber and starts flowing out through the internal nozzle. The air flowing through the outer nozzle then shears off the polymer solution and forms droplets which are collected in a barium chloride bath where hydrogel microcapsules crosslink to form microcapsules as shown in Fig. 16.3. The microcapsules produced by this technique are consistently larger (>500 μm) and, therefore, not optimal for transplantation (Schwarz, 2000). Furthermore, they produce >50% empty capsules which lead to increased transplant volume and can provoke severe host immunoreaction.

16.2 Microfluidic technologies: the emergence of microfluidics applied to islet transplantation

Under normal in vivo conditions, islets experience a dynamically changing microenvironment where insulin is secreted in a biphasic oscillatory pattern in response to blood glucose levels which is oscillatory. Therefore, an imperative emerges to have a perfusion setup that can better mimic the native microenvironment islets are exposed to through the precise control of physiologically relevant parameters. In order to better understand β-cell physiology and pathophysiology, a series of perifusion devices have been developed in the past few decades with the capability to regulate perifusate temperature, pH, and the ability to switch between various streams of stimuli (Hoshi & Shreeve, 1973; Lacy, Knudson, Williams, Richards, & Midgley, 1976; Lacy, Walker, & Fink, 1972; Weaver, McDaniel, Naber, Barry, & Lacy, 1978). However, these

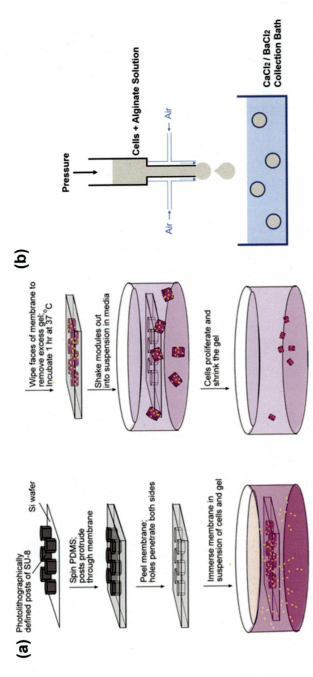

Figure 16.3 Schematic representation of the extrusion and emulsification method The figure depicts the principle of emulsification (a) (McGuigan et al., 2008) and the extrusion cell encapsulation (b). Reprinted from PLOS.

devices have several limitations including difficult operation, limited flow control, inadequate mimicking of the in vivo microenvironment, and a lack of integration with conventional analysis techniques.

In recent years, microfluidic technology has emerged as a valuable tool for studying pancreatic islets mainly due to its higher efficiency and configurable versatility. Microfluidic devices allow for the minimal consumption of reagents and analytes, as well as the leveraging of microscale phenomena such as laminar flow, capillary flow, electroosmotically driven flow, electrokinetically driven flow, microdroplet formation (Liu, Goodhouse, Jeon, & Enquist, 2008; Mosadegh et al., 2007; Taylor, Rhee, & Jeon, 2006), and rapid diffusion (Oppegard, Nam, Carr, Skaalure, & Eddington, 2009). Microfluidics allows the development and application of new experimental modalities and techniques currently not possible with conventional macroscale tools. Additionally, multiple tasks and/or analytical tools can be integrated to improve experimental throughput (Craighead, 2006; El-Ali, Sorger, & Jensen, 2006). In regard to microfluidic devices for islet transplantation, several advantages of the microscale are utilized such as: (i) islet immobilization; (ii) creation, maintenance, and optimization of culture microenvironments; (iii) continuous live-cell imaging of β-cell physiological function with the ability to resolve the rapid secretory and metabolic waveforms intrinsic to β-cells; (iv) integration with single or multiple analytical tools; and (v) mass production of islet products (e.g., islet capsule) for cell therapy of diabetes.

16.2.1 Islet immobilization: design considerations and strategies for live cell imaging

One of the greatest technical challenges in applying microfluidics to islets is the immobilization of islets owing to their unique cellular composition and 3-D cytoarchitecture, which must be preserved. One approach to immobilizing islets uses a PDMS plug or wall in order to position an islet into a microchannel, as shown in Fig. 16.4a (Dishinger, Reid, & Kennedy, 2009; Rocheleau & Piston, 2008; Rocheleau et al., 2004). In this method, the advantage lies in being able to predictably place and locate islets; however, a potential disadvantage is an introduction of mechanical stresses, which can cause islet damage and insulin leakage. As an alternative islet trapping method shown in Fig. 16.4b, others have designed an array of circular microwells (pockets) (Adewola et al., 2010; Mohammed et al., 2009). The bottom layer of the device achieves this immobilization with an array of circular wells (500 μm in diameter and 150 μm in depth), which allows the islets to fall, then passively sit and react to medium, without undue mechanical stress and shear forces. More than one islet can be analyzed simultaneously, increasing analytical throughput. However, this device pools the secreted products together, which can be either an advantage or a disadvantage, depending on the intended application.

In order to achieve single-islet and real-time imaging in some cases, the microfluidics must be further designed to enable a precise analysis of an individual cell in a

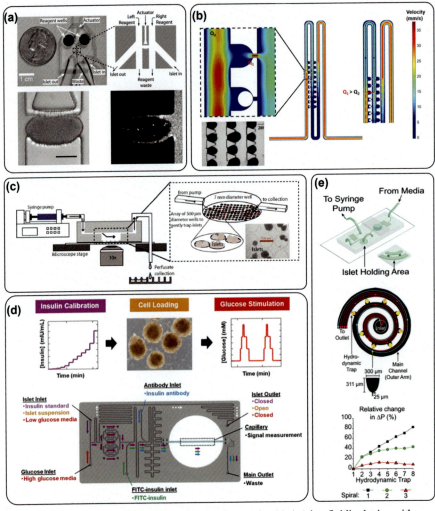

Figure 16.4 Microfluidic devices for islet function study. (a) A microfluidic device with a single-islet piston-like trap to assess glucose-induced intracellular oscillations of calcium in pancreatic islets (Rocheleau, Walker, Head, McGuinness, & Piston, 2004). (b) The flow dynamics in a microfluidic islet perifusion array (IPA). Computer simulation is generated with COMSOL Multiphysics 5.3. Islets image is captured under microscope to show trapped islets in the array. Scale bars are 200 μm (Nourmohammadzadeh et al., 2016; Xing et al., 2016). (c) A microfluidic islet perifusion chamber (IPC) device for multiparametric islet function assessment through imaging and ELISA (Mohammed, Wang, Harvat, Oberholzer, & Eddington, 2009). (d) The "Islet-on-a-Chip" design utilizes hydrodynamic trapping, fluorescent imaging, and on-chip continuous insulin measurement to study islet physiology (Glieberman et al., 2019). (e) A microfluidic device to enhance viral transduction of pancreatic islets. Schematic showing a section of a microfluidic device where islets are held in a series of hydrodynamic traps connected by bypass channels. The curve shows simulated pressure drop (ΔP) across islets to guide the design (Silva et al., 2016).
Reproduced with permission from PNAS, Springer Nature, Royal Society of Chemistry.

specific location, such as an array, with minimal shear force and cell stress. A hydrodynamic trapping approach is first described in 2008 by Tan and Takeuchi. Since then, many researchers have been applying this method to immobilize pancreatic islets for imaging (Glieberman et al., 2019; Mohammed et al., 2009; Silva et al., 2016; Xing et al., 2016) (see Fig. 16.4). In brief, the islets are trapped based on the flow resistant difference between the U-cup and the loop channel. When flow carries an islet to the junction between the U-cup (trapping area) and the loop channel, an islet will be trapped in the U-cup due to less resistance. The trapped islet results in increased resistance in the U-cup, and the flow is then redirected into the loop channel. This flow carries subsequent islets toward the next empty U-cup, iterating the trapping downstream throughout the device. Flow dynamic simulation is shown in Fig. 16.4c and indicates that the trapping area has lower flow resistance and higher flow velocity (Q1) than the loop channel (Q2), which results in particle movement into the trapping area when the U-cup is empty (Xing et al., 2016).

16.2.2 Fluid control: creation, maintenance, and optimization of culture microenvironments

A stable and flexible fluid control system is necessary for β-cell applications in microfluidics. Flow driven by pressure, in either a continuous or stepwise manner, is the standard method that has been proven adequate for many islet applications (Adewola et al., 2010; Chen et al., 2008; Dishinger et al., 2009). However, one potential obstacle is pressure oscillations at low flow rates and when starting or stopping as observed in syringe pumps. In response to this problem, reciprocating and continuous flow micropumps have been implemented (Zhang & Roper, 2009). Electroosmotic flow also plays an important role in the manipulation of liquid flow in microfluidic applications since electroosmotic velocities can be independent of channel size, which is beneficial when applied to small microchannels. Additionally, droplets have also been used in β-cell study using a syringe or vacuum (Chen et al., 2008; Zhang & Roper, 2009). As demonstrated by the Piston group using vacuum-driven flow, they were able to generate a passive method for microfluidic droplet sampling method that was used to quantify β-cell zinc secretion (zinc and insulin are cosecreted) with significantly improved spatiotemporal resolution (average droplet volume was 470 ± 9 pL under a flow rate of 0.100 μL/min) (Easley, Rocheleau, Head, & Piston, 2009). Furthermore, please read other dedicated chapters of this book to find more detailed microfluidic droplet technique.

Another microfluidic device employing droplet-based fluid flow was the chemistrode developed by the Ismagilov Group (Chen et al., 2008). In contrast to traditional path clamp electrode setups, which can be used to directly measure β-cell electrical activity, this method's strength lies in its ability to manipulate and record molecular signals with a high spatial and temporal resolution, requiring 50 ms for stimuli pulse and 1.5 s for secreted insulin sampling. This system has a maximum temporal resolution of 50 ns, with the ability to measure insulin secretion from a single islet at a frequency of 0.67 Hz. This high level of resolution is achieved by droplets that are continuously encapsulated and separated from an islet.

The generation of chemical gradients into microfluidic setups is needed to generate dynamically changing microenvironments that will help elucidate the mechanisms underlying β-cell secretory kinetics. In order to generate these gradients, the Roper Group has integrated two diaphragm pumps with off-chip valves that generate a chemical gradient in sine and triangle waveforms (Zhang & Roper, 2009). As another solution to this problem, our group currently employs an integrated on-chip inlet staggered herringbone chaotic mixer with computer-controlled syringes to generate preprogrammed glucose stimulation (Adewola et al., 2010; Lee et al., 2012; Mohammed et al., 2009).

16.2.3 Detection: live-cell imaging of islets and β-cells

Highly coordinated spatiotemporal changes in $[Ca^{2+}]_i$ regulate many β-cell cellular processes including GSIS and, therefore, require real-time detection of electrical, biochemical, and ion signaling activities. Thus, $[Ca^{2+}]_i$ may be a direct indicator of insulin secretory kinetics. One of the most critical limiting factors for studying calcium signaling using microfluidics is the spatiotemporal resolution. To address this problem, the use of fluorescent calcium indicator dyes such as Fura-2 AM or Fluo-4 AM (family of EGTA analogs) has been well-characterized to have high selectivity and sensitivity in conventional and microfluidic imaging applications. In contrast, the temporal resolution of calcium signaling remains a function of each microfluidic device's flow dynamics and can also be controlled by medium delivery methods, valves, and device geometry.

Another method that may be used as an assay for insulin secretion is the detection of zinc ions. In β-cells, zinc is complexed with insulin to form a 2-Zn-hexameric crystal. When insulin is secreted, along with c-peptide, zinc is also cosecreted into plasma. The Piston Group has utilized this feature of β-cells and has developed a droplet-based device with a sampling drop volume of approximately 0.47 nL (Easley et al., 2009). Their single islet studies demonstrated a high temporal resolution that allowed the detection of two zinc oscillatory frequencies: fast ($\sim$20–40 s) and slow ($\sim$5–10 min). Concurrently, zinc oscillatory waveforms were shown to closely coincide with intraislet calcium oscillations and secreted insulin patterns. Insulin quantification was determined off-chip using either enzyme-linked immunosorbent assay (ELISA) or radioimmunoassay (RIA). In a similar concept, the Kennedy Group developed a 15-channel microfluidic device capable of perifusing individual islets and then mixing perifusate with FITC-insulin and antiinsulin antibody to perform a competitive immunoassay (Dishinger et al., 2009). Performed in real-time, this system is capable of detecting insulin secretion at a resolution of 10 s. The ability to rapidly quantify temporally resolved insulin secretion at the single islet level will have significant applications in islet research.

In the pursuit of developing a reliable islet potency test to address a clinical need and overcome the limitations of current tests, we developed and characterized a three-layer microfluidic platform (Adewola et al., 2010; Mohammed et al., 2009) that combines the measurement of mitochondrial potential changes ($\Delta\Psi_{Mito}$), calcium influx ($[Ca^{2+}]_i$), and dynamic insulin kinetics into a single and real-time assay.

16.2.4 Biomanufacturing: islets microencapsulation

Microfluidic technology provides the technological advancement needed for future cell-based therapy for T1DM, including xenotransplantation to alleviate the islet supply constraints. Compared to needle and air jet encapsulation methods, microfluidics has the following advantages: the ability to manipulate small liquid volumes so that each capsule can be produced under control, an ease of automation, a multiplexing capability to scale production, and a high-throughput quality control. Furthermore, microfluidic technology also provides unique advantages in generating uniformly shaped capsules of desired size ranges that can be scaled to produce large volumes of encapsulations needed for clinical applications. A well-controlled process for the successful production of encapsulated islets with tight capsule specifications in size, shape, and porosity in volumes needed for transplant in humans is not currently available.

There are three major gelation mechanisms that have been widely employed within islets microencapsulation. Thermally sensitive gels (e.g., gelatin) are formed through a temperature change. Photoresistive (e.g., poly(ethylene glycol (PEG))) and ion-based (e.g., alginate) crosslinking materials are solidified by light (e.g., UV) and a divalent ion (e.g., Ca^{2+}), respectively (Kang, Park, Ju, Jeong, & Lee, 2014). The cell viability was observed to be significantly lower when the gelation process was exposed to a temperature change or UV light. Thus, the ion-based gelation method is viewed as the best approach for islet encapsulation.

In 2014, Headen demonstrated a microfluidic-based flow-focusing cell microencapsulation system for generating size-controlled hydrogels. Three independent flows of (1) mineral oil containing SPAN80 (a surfactant), (2) a crosslinker phase containing mineral oil and SPAN80 with an emulsion of aqueous dithiothreitol solution, and (3) PEG-4MAL macromer in aqueous physiological buffer were pumped into the microfluidic chip using syringe pumps (Headen et al., 2014). As the macromer phase approached the flow-focusing nozzle, a coflowing continuous phase of oil shielded the macromer from contact with the crosslinker-laden oil phase (Fig. 16.5a).

Microfiber, as shown in Fig. 16.5b, is another approach utilizing microfluidic-devices to encapsulate islets. Microfibers are easy to handle, whereas beads are not easily handled and sheets are delicate and difficult to implant due to size (Jun et al., 2013). Microfiber fabrication employs the coaxial flow principal similar to the one used in the extrusion method. Instead of using air to shear off hydrogels, the coaxial flow channel is filled with a calcium chloride solution to introduce calcium-dependent crosslinking at the cylindrical outlet channel, by which formed alginate microfiber. The diameter of

630 Microfluidic Devices for Biomedical Applications

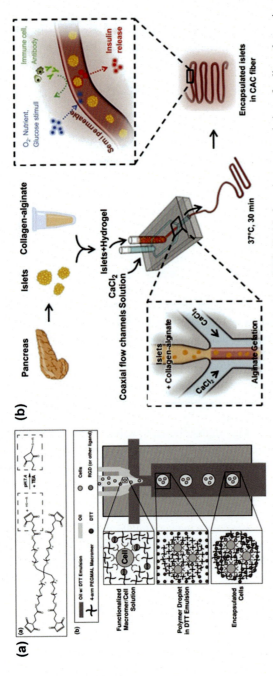

Figure 16.5 Schematic representation of the extrusion and emulsification method. (a) PEG-4MAL for microencapsulation of cells and proteins in a flow-focusing microfluidic chip using a cytocompatible crosslinking reaction. (a) PEG-4MAL macromer consists of a 4-arm branched polyethylene glycol (PEG) backbone modified with a maleimide group terminating each arm. At physiological pH, free thiol-containing molecules undergo a Michael-type addition reaction with maleimides, forming a covalent bond to macromer. This reaction is facilitated by nucleophilic buffers such as triethanolamine (TEA) and can be used to either functionalize the macromer or crosslink macromer into a hydrogel network. (b) A microfluidic device with flow focusing geometry is utilized to produce microgels (Headen, Aubry, Lu, & Garcia, 2014). (b) Schematic illustration of microfiber encapsulation. Collagen-alginate composite solution containing islets was used as a sample fluid, and calcium chloride solution was introduced into a sheath fluid. The two solutions were mixed at the cylindrical outlet channel, inducing Ca^{2+}-dependent crosslinking of coaxially focused alginate to form the microfiber (Jun et al., 2013).
Reprinted with permission from John Wiley and Sons and Elsevier.

the microfiber is strongly dependent on the flow rate ratio of the islets-suspended alginate solution and coaxial CaCl$_2$ solution. To secure cell viability, the outlet nozzle diameter must be larger than 250 μm to accommodate islets size.

16.2.5 Stem cell applications

Islet transplantation can serve as an effective intervention for restoring normoglycemia, but the demand for islets far outstrips the supply. Considering the unlimited potential of human pluripotent stem cells (hPSCs) for self-renewal, the generation of functional β cells from hPSCs has emerged as an attractive alternative. However, recent reports describe β and β-like cell formation from hPSCs, and these cells possess limited functionality. The fate of stem cells is highly regulated by the microenvironment (Morrison & Spradling, 2008). The microenvironment promotes stem cell maintenance and controls the differentiation of stem cells to achieve homeostasis. To direct the stem cell differentiation, it is crucial to know the role of various biochemical cues (e.g., growth factors, glucose, oxygen, etc. (Aguiari et al., 2008; Ivanovic, 2009)) in the decision-making process of stem cells. By controlling the fluidic properties like convection, diffusion, and reaction, microfluidics can tune the microenvironment around stem cells in a variety of ways beyond setting a concentration of chemicals (Fig. 16.6). By combing with different structures on the substrate, microfluidics can also tune the composition of the local population and cell—cell interactions, and, thus, provide a handy platform to probe various important biological processes like differentiation and evolution in more biological relevant conditions than conventional tissue culture dishes (Zhang & Austin, 2012).

Given the importance of islet cytoarchitecture for endocrine function, culture systems can be designed to recapitulate elements of the intricate 3D structure of the developing islet. Besides some traditional methods, like hanging drops, round bottom multiwell plates, and stirring cell culture, microfluidic technology has also been used to generate cell aggregates with controlled sizes due to its advanced fluid control. Multiple studies have reported improved function of reaggregated pseudoislets, either in vitro or in vivo after transplantation. There is also evidence that beta cells reaggregated with endothelial progenitor cells demonstrate improved GSIS compared to pseudoislets composed only of beta cells (Penko et al., 2011).

Furthermore, microfluidics offers a revolutionary way to perform high-throughput screening with many advantages like much lower amounts of starting cells, precise control of inoculation number, and dynamic adjustment of culture conditions. A fully automated cell culture screening system based on a microfluidic chip has been used to create arbitrary culture media formulations in 96 independent culture chambers (Gomez-Sjoberg, Leyrat, Pirone, Chen, & Quake, 2007). The device was able to change the condition of each culture chamber separately by using combinations of valves. As a proof of principles, the researchers inoculated the human primary

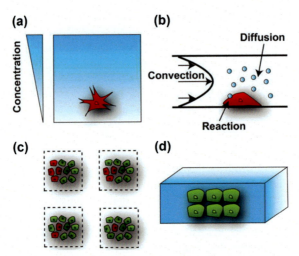

Figure 16.6 Illustrations, some key ideas of how microfluidics is used to analyze stem cells. (a) A concentration gradient of chemicals (e.g., growth factors, drugs) can be established in microfluidics devices by combining convection and diffusion, depending on the desired gradient profile. This is to mimic the heterogeneous environment in natural stem-cell niches. (b) By changing the geometry of devices or driving pressures, the flow and diffusion profile can be fine-tuned. This can be used to investigate the role of different signaling pathways on stem cell differentiation in a dynamic fashion. (c) The substrate of microfluidics devices can be patterned to study the effect of cell–cell interaction within same or different types of cells (e.g., if stem cell differentiation can be stimulated or suppressed by the presence of other cells nearby and how). (d) 3D microfluidics devices can be made from extracellular matrix, where stem cells are cultured in the more in vivo–like environment (Zhang & Austin, 2012).
Reprinted with permission from Springer Nature.

mesenchymal stem cells (hMSCs) to each chamber with feedback control to achieve the desired inoculation number and monitored the effect of osteogenic stimulation on differentiation and proliferation of hMSCs over weeks (Gomez-Sjoberg et al., 2007). Another example is using the microfluidic perifusion-based devices from Oberholzer's research group to test insulin secretory signals of pseudoislets derived from stem cells (Nair et al., 2019; Sui et al., 2018). Applying the microfluidic technology, dynamic detection could provide researchers with more information to guide the development of functional artificial islets derived from stem cells.

16.3 Design and validation of microfluidic devices for islet study and transplantation

Microfluidic-based techniques begin with the design, fabrication, and application of a specific device for the manipulation of fluids at the microscale level. Typically, micro means one of the following features: small volume (often in the scale of nL, pL, and fL), small size (submillimeter), low energy consumption, or the use of some physical phenomenon within the microdomain, such as surface area to volume ratio, laminar flow, or diffusion dominant transport. Several materials can be used for fabrication, including silicon, metal, glass, and polymers. In this chapter, we are discussing microfluidic design using devices from Oberholzer Lab and Ramasubramanian Lab as examples. Since all microfluidic devices here are composed of either PDMS or sometimes combined with glass components, only the design and fabrication of these devices will be briefly described.

16.3.1 Polydimethylsiloxane devices

Due to the ease of prototyping, stiffness, and high aspect ratio, SU8 photoresist has become the standard method for PDMS micromolding in microfluidic fabrication (Weibel, Diluzio, & Whitesides, 2007). The basic steps of soft photolithography have been described previously (Nourmohammadzadeh et al., 2016). Currently, soft photolithography manufacture is carried out in a cleanroom facility to prevent contamination with dust; however, given the application, they may be carried out in a conventional chemical hood. For the devices described in this chapter, the PDMS fabrication workflow begins with the design of a photomask using transparency printing, SU-8 master-mold fabrication, followed by PDMS curing, and ends with PDMS-glass bonding. Detailed fabrication protocol of PDMS devices using soft photolithography can be found in section 16.5.1 at the end of this chapter.

16.3.2 Design and validation of microfluidic devices for islet and β-cell perifusion and imaging

Microfluidics offers a practical solution to the ongoing clinical need to rapidly assess islet function. Parallel microchannels enable multiple experiments to be performed simultaneously and the imaging of cells within the microchannels, which is currently not possible with existing commercially available dynamic perfusion platforms. Additionally, microfluidic delivery of stimulatory solutions reduces the mechanical perturbation reducing stress to the islets. To successfully deploy a device at multiple transplantation centers, the device must be simple, robust, user-friendly, and provide quick, reproducible results that are predictive of transplant outcomes; a device failure during a characterization process may lead to discarding potentially lifesaving donor tissue.

The first-generation microfluidic device developed by Dr. José Oberholzer's research group is an islet perifusion chamber (IPC) device (Adewola et al., 2010; Mohammed et al., 2009). As shown in Fig. 16.4b, the IPC device is composed of three layers: the top layer, 500 μm in height, comprising inlet and outlet channels 2 mm wide (5 mm at fanned ends); the middle layer, composing a spacer layer; the bottom layer, 150 μm in height, containing microwells for islet immobilization. The microwells are 500 μm in diameter and 100 μm apart. In each perifusion chamber, the array of tiny circular wells can help to gently immobilize the islets without shielding them from the perfusion fluids to maximize the amount of islet surface area exposed to flow. This device allows researchers to simultaneously quantify the mitochondrial potential, $[Ca^{2+}]_i$, and the biphasic response of islets in response to dynamic glucose stimulation to provide a complete assessment of islet function.

However, challenges remain when using an IPC device, such as the inability to satisfactorily assess the heterogeneous property of individual islets, especially when testing a large number of islets simultaneously, as data are often averaged from islet populations. Examination of heterogeneous properties at the individual islet level often provides more detailed physiological or pathophysiological information than averaging-based population methodologies. To achieve the individual islet imaging, Oberholzer's team developed an islet perifusion array (IPA) device, which utilizes the hydrodynamic trapping principle to immobilize individual islets (Nourmohammadzadeh et al., 2016). As shown in Fig. 16.7a, the IPA device is a two-layer PDMS device. The top layer consists of an inlet, an outlet, and an array of U-shaped circular traps (300 μm in diameter, 250 μm in depth, and with a 50 μm opening) for islet immobilization. The bottom layer is a clear glass slide to ease the imaging process. During the loading of islets, islets are brought to the U-shaped traps following the fluid flow and pressure drop. Once a trap is occupied, islets will run into the next one due to the blockage of the opening until all traps are fulfilled. Applying this design, up to 300 islets can be trapped successfully in a single run for imaging.

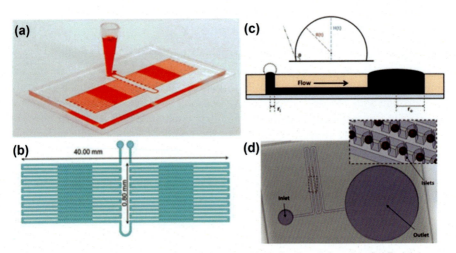

Figure 16.7 Microfluidic islet perifusion array. (a) Photo image of the microfluidic islet perifusion array (IPA) device. (b) Schematic of the IPA device (Nourmohammadzadeh et al., 2016). (c) Working principle of the surface tension driven flow delivery. (d) Schematic of the pumpless islet perifusion array (p-IPA) device integrated with islet array (Xing et al., 2016). Reprinted with permission from Springer Nature.

Furthermore, Xing et al. reported an improvement of the IPA device, surface tension—driven passive pumping system, shown in Fig. 16.7b (Xing et al., 2016). Traditionally, microfluidic devices use external energy sources, such as a syringe pump, for the steady delivery of fluids. External pumps are often bulky and operationally burdensome, which results in limitations to microfluidic biochips that can hinder the adaptability and use in wider applications in the field of diabetes research and treatment. For example, like most of the microfluidic devices, these systems need macroscale pumps and other accessory components to facilitate flow delivery and perifusate collection, and, thus, create a complexity of the operation and reduce the spatiotemporal resolution of measured hormones and physiological activities. In the novel design of pumpless islet perifusion array (p-IPA) device, while keeping the hydrodynamic trapping array structure, the pumpless flow delivery is achieved based on surface tension difference caused by different diameters of the inlet and the outlet ($R_{out} >> R_{in}$). For a 20-islet array chip with R_{out}: $R_{in} = 5:1$, it would only take less than 10 μL and 2.5 s for complete flow exchanges in the device, ultimately providing opportunities for a faster fluid delivery, more efficient stimulation to islets, and less solution consumption with improved spatiotemporal resolution of the parameters measured.

In Fig. 16.8, the curves show $[Ca^{2+}]_i$ fluorescent measurements of isolated rodent islets and human islets in the stimulation of glucose and KCl during perifusion using IPC and p-IPA devices, respectively (Xing et al., 2016). In Fig. 16.8a and c, the $[Ca^{2+}]_i$ of isolated rodent islets shows a 140% peak value and increase up to 170% in response to 14 mM glucose. Similarly, as shown in Fig. 16.8b and d, human islets from the same isolation show a 30% increase in 25 mM glucose, a 60% increase in 30 mM KCl solution using an IPC device, a 37% increase in 25 mM glucose, and then about an 80% increase in 30 mM KCl solution using a p-IPA device. For both experiments, the increased $[Ca^{2+}]_i$ occurred within 5 min postglucose stimulation and showed a typical biphasic profile that is a very important signature of islet calcium signaling for stimulation and regulation of efficient insulin secretion. More importantly, it is worth noting that the p-IPA device design has improved the precision of islet calcium signaling by not only increasing the detecting sensitivity but also effectively detecting subtle changes such as phase zero, which is often not detectable in previously designed IPC device.

16.3.3 Design and validation of microfluidic devices for islet microencapsulation

A microfluidic approach utilizing coaxial air flow to scaling up islet encapsulation was introduced by Ramasubramanian and Opara's research group (Tendulkar et al., 2012). The schematic diagram of the system is shown in Fig. 16.9a. The microfluidic device is designed using SolidWorks (Dassault Systemes Solidworks Corp., MA, USA) and 3D printed by using DSM Somos ProtoTherm 12120 polymer (3D Systems Corporation, South Carolina, USA) due to its high-resolution structuring

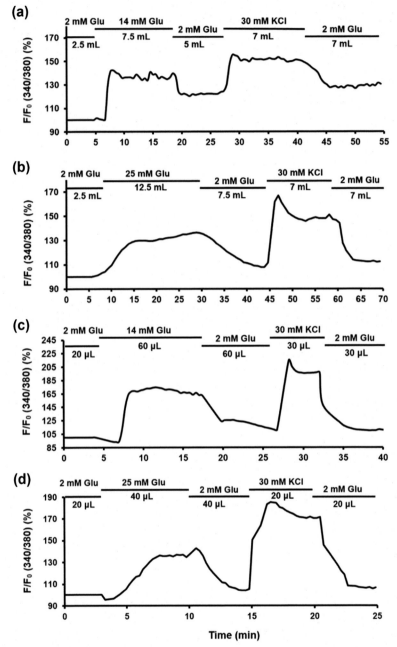

Figure 16.8 Microfluidic perifusion of rodent and human islets. (a) Representative trace of rodent islet calcium signaling in response to 14 mM glucose and 30 mM KCl using an islet perifusion chamber (IPC) device. (b) Representative trace of human islet calcium signaling in response to 25 mM glucose and 30 mM KCl using an IPC device. (c) Representative trace of rodent islet calcium signaling in response to 14 mM glucose and 30 mM KCl using a pumpless islet perifusion array (p-IPA) device. (d) Representative trace of human islet calcium signaling in response to 25 mM glucose and 30 mM KCl using a p-IPA device. N = 50–60 islets from three independent islet samples for each experiment (Xing et al., 2016).
Reprinted with permission from Springer Nature.

Microfluidic applications on pancreatic islets and β-cells study 637

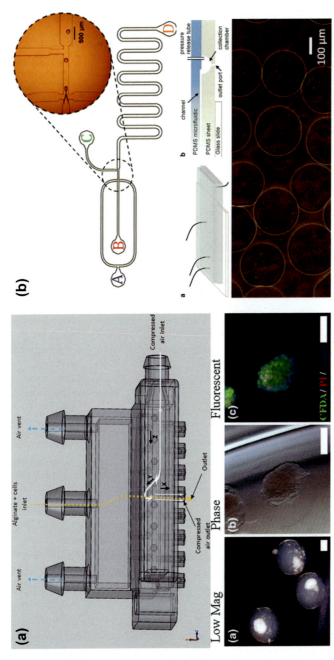

Figure 16.9 Schematic representation of the extrusion and emulsification method. (a) Shows the flow of alginate-cell mixture and compressed air through the microfluidic device. Encapsulation of rat pancreatic islets with microfluidic device. (a) Islets seen within the alginate capsules; (b) parallel phase contrast and (c) fluorescently labeled pancreatic islets for live and dead cells, Scale bars 0–200 μm (Tendulkar et al., 2012). (b) Microfluidic template design with the ports labeled: *(inlet port A)* light mineral oil with 3% (V/V) Span80; *(inlet port B)* 1.5% (w/v) alginate + 100 mM Ca-EDTA (1:1); *(inlet port C)* 1% (v/v) acetic acid + mineral oil; *(outlet port D)* collection port. 2. Final design integration. (a) 3D view with tubes connected. (b) Cross section of polydimethylsiloxane (PDMS) device with three layers: PDMS channel mold, PDMS sheet, and glass slide. (c) Uniformly sized alginate beads formed under the following conditions (Sharma, Hunckler, Ramasubramanian, Opara, & Katuri, 2017). Reprinted with permission from Springer Nature.

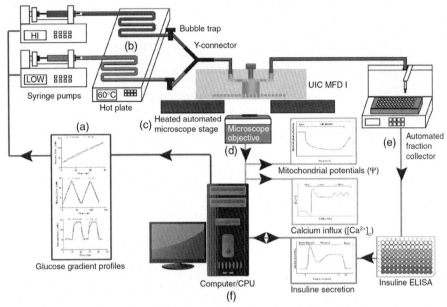

Figure 16.10 Microfluidic-based multimodal islet perifusion system and experimental setup. (a) A computer governs a syringe system and generates a preprogrammed temporal glucose gradient while maintaining constant total flow. (b) The incoming media is heated on a hot plate to be brought up to near physiological temperatures (37°C ± 3°C) and then passed through a bubble trap and Y-connector. (c) As the perifusing media enters the microdevice, the perifusion chamber temperature is maintained by a heating stage. (d) $[Ca^{2+}]_i$ and ϕ_{Mito} are recorded. (e) Perifusate leaving the device outlet is collected by a fraction collector and quantified off-chip by ELISA. (f) All physiological responsive data of $[Ca^{2+}]_i$, ϕ_{Mito}, and insulin are compiled (Wang et al., 2013).
Reprinted with permission from Elsevier.

capability (more applications of 3D-printed microfluidic devices will be discussed in Chapter 17). The microfluidic device consists of a 3D air supply and a multinozzle outlet for microcapsule generation. It has one alginate inlet and one compressed air inlet. The outlet has eight nozzles, each 380 μm in inner diameter, which produce hydrogel microspheres ranging from 500 to 700 μm in diameter. These nozzles are concentrically surrounded by air nozzles with a 2 mm inner diameter. There are two tubes connected at the top to allow the air to escape as the alginate solution fills the chamber. A variable flow pump is used to pump the alginate solution, and tubing is used to connect in-house air supply to the air channel and peristaltic/syringe pump to the alginate chamber. The flow rate of air is controlled via a pressure regulator. As shown in Fig. 16.9a, rat pancreatic islets were successfully encapsulated using this 3D microfluidic device. Pancreatic islets can be observed within the capsules as white spheroids approximately 100–200 μm in size. The pancreatic islets can stay viable in capsules as shown in Fig. 16.9a, where live cells are green and necrotic (dead) cells are red.

To achieve a better uniformity of capsule size and shape, Ramasubramanian and Opara's research group designed and fabricated an internal gelation microfluidic device. As shown in Fig. 16.9b, the islets-suspended droplets which contain calcium ethylenediaminetetraacetate (Ca-EDTA) are formed via a flow-focusing junction and carried through the acetic acid injected carrier fluid (Sharma et al., 2017). The calcium ions are released from a Ca-EDTA alginate mixed solution internally after the decline of the pH by injection of acetic acid. Alginate-calcium ion cross-linking is initiated immediately after the T-junction where the mineral oil with acetic acid is added to the horizontal channel. To accommodate islet microencapsulation, the channels' diameter within the microfluidic device must be large enough to let islet pallets pass through without clogging. Thus, a channel diameter of around 300–500 µm is recommended. An extension channel of 500 µm in diameter was added after the T-junction in order to secure the internal gelation processing time before the collection. Uniformly sized alginate beads with a diameter of 250 ± 20 µm are collected in the $CaCl_2$ solution and washed with Tween solution, as shown in Fig. 16.9b.

16.4 Protocol: materials

The following section outlines all the materials and equipment used in experiments with microfluidic devices from Oberholzer Lab. Section 16.4.1 covers microfluidic device fabrication. Section 16.4.2 covers islet isolation and culture. Section 16.4.3 covers simultaneous islet perifusion and fluorescence imaging. Section 16.4.4 covers islet on-chip microencapsulation.

16.4.1 Microfluidic device fabrication

16.4.1.1 Reagents and tools

- Photomask (CAD/Art service)
- Polydimethylsiloxane (PDMS) (Dow Corning)
- Photoresist SU-8–2150 (Microchem)
- SU-8 photoresist developer (Microchem)
- Silicon wafer (Silicon Sense, 4" dummy wafers)
- Acetone (Sigma-Aldrich)
- Methanol (Sigma-Aldrich)
- Isopropanol (Sigma-Aldrich)
- N_2 compressed gas (Airgas)
- Mixing spatula (Sigma-Aldrich)
- Tweezers (TDI Switzerland)
- Weighing boats (Sigma-Aldrich)
- 3M scotch tape (Office Depot)
- Razor blade/Scalpel (Office Depot)
- Gauge no. 11 stainless Luer needles as hole-punch (Grainger)
- Gauge no. 0 hole puncher (Cole-Parmer)
- Circular 3" 2.0 kg weights (custom machined)

16.4.1.2 Equipment

- Digital balance (Mettler Toledo Inc.)
- Spinner (Laurell Technologies, WS-400B 6NPP/LITE)
- 3 Hot plates (PMC Dataplate, 730) (for curing PDMS, replaceable with oven)
- UV-Lamp (EXFO-OmniCure, S1000)
- Digital profiler (Starrett, F2730−0) (for confirming photoresist thickness)
- Vacuum desiccator for degassing PDMS (Cole-Parmer)
- Plasma torch (Electro-Technic Products, Inc.)

16.4.2 Mouse islet isolation and culture

16.4.2.1 Reagents

- Collagenase P (Roche)
- RPMI 1640 (Mediatech) (see REAGENT SETUP)
- Fetal bovine serum (FBS) (Clontech)
- Streptomycin/Penicillin (Gibco)
- 1.018 kg m^{-3} Ficoll (Mediatech)
- 1.096 kg m^{-3} Ficoll (Mediatech)
- 1.069 kg m^{-3} Ficoll (Mediatech)
- 1.037 kg m^{-3} Ficoll (Mediatech)
- 1× HBSS (Mediatech)
- Isoflurane (Baxter)

16.4.2.2 Equipment and materials

- C57/B6 mice (Jackson Laboratory)
- Biosafety hood (NUAIR)
- Water bath with temperature control (Precision)
- Centrifuge (Beckman, J6-MI, maximum RPM 6000)
- Incubator (Thermo Electron, Thermo Series II)
- Inverted microscope (Leica, S6F)
- 35 × 10 mm Petri dish (Becton-Dickson)
- Surgical tools (Straight and curved forceps, 4 $\frac{1}{2}$ " iris scissors, 3 $\frac{1}{2}$ " hemostat clamp)
- 5 mL Syringe (Becton-Dickinson)
- 30g $\frac{1}{2}$ " needle (Becton-Dickinson)
- Isoflurane vaporizer (Viking Medical, model: ISOV-2)

16.4.2.3 Cell culture media

RPMI 1640 culture medium: supplemented with 10% of FBS (vol/vol) and 100 unit mL^{-1} of penicillin and 100 μg mL^{-1} of streptomycin.

16.4.3 Simultaneous islet perifusion and fluorescence imaging

16.4.3.1 Reagents

- Krebs-Ringer bicarbonate buffer (KRB) (see REAGENT SETUP)
- Sodium chloride, NaCl (Sigma-Aldrich)
- Sodium bicarbonate, NaHCO$_3$ (Sigma-Aldrich)
- Potassium chloride, KCl (Sigma-Aldrich)
- Monopotassium phosphate, KH$_2$PO$_4$ (Sigma-Aldrich)
- Calcium chloride dihydrate, CaCl$_2$ •2H$_2$O (Sigma-Aldrich)
- Magnesium sulfate heptahydrate, MgSO$_4$• 7H$_2$O (Sigma-Aldrich)
- HEPES (Mediatech)
- Insulin ELISA kit (Mercodia)
- D-Glucose (Sigma-Aldrich)
- Fura-2 AM (Invitrogen) (see REAGENT SETUP)
- Rhodamine 123 (Rh 123) (Sigma-Aldrich) (see REAGENT SETUP)
- Dimethyl sulfoxide (DMSO) (Fisher)
- Bovine serum albumin (BSA) (Sigma-Aldrich)
- Ethanol (Decon Laboratories)
- 0.22 μm Vacuum filter (Millipore)

16.4.3.2 Cell culture media

- KRB (mM): NaCl (129), NaHCO$_3$ (5.0), KCl (4.7), KH$_2$PO$_4$ (1.2), CaCl$_2$ •2H$_2$O (1.0), MgSO$_4$ •H$_2$O (1.2), HEPES (10), pH 7.35−7.40.
- *CRITICAL: Sterilize the working solution by filtration with a 0.22 μm vacuum filter. Adjust the buffer pH with KOH to prevent potential precipitation and store for no more than 1 week at 4°C.
- KRB stock solutions should be stored for no more than 1 month at 4°C.
- Preparation of Fura-2 AM stock solution: Add 100 μL DMSO to each tube (50 μg) so that the final concentration is 2 mM. Store at −20°C in the dark.
- Preparation of Rh 123 stock solution: Dissolve Rh 123 in 100% ethanol (vol/vol) at a concentration of 1 mg mL^{-1}. Store at −20°C in the dark.

16.4.3.3 Equipment and materials

- Microfluidic device (see PROCEDURE)
- Syringe pumps (Harvard Apparatus, Model 22)
- Digital hot plates (Dataplate, PMC 720 series)
- Thermometer (Omega Engineering, Inc, model HH-25TC)
- 60 mL Luer lock syringes (Becton-Dickinson)
- Fraction collector (Gibson, FC-203B)
- Epifluorescence microscopy setup (see Equipment setup)
- Leica DMI 4000B fluorescence microscope (see Equipment setup)
- Xenon light source
- Excitation and emission filter wheels (Chroma Technology)
- Lambda DG-4 wavelength switcher (Ludl Electronic Ltd.)

- Fura-2/FITC polychronic beam splitter and double band emission filter (Chroma Technology)
- High-speed and high-resolution charge-coupled device (Retiga-SRV, Fast 1394, QImaging)
- Imaging acquisition and analysis (SimplePCI, Hamamatsu Corp)
- LabVIEW 8.0 (National Instruments)
- 30" Silicone tubing (Cole Palmer 1/16 × 1/8")
- 1.5 mL Eppendorf tube (Fisher Scientific)
- Y-connectors (1/16" and 4 mm) (Cole Palmer)
- Syringe connectors (female Luer plug 1/16") (Cole Palmer)
- Straight connectors (1/16") (Cole Palmer)
- Elbow connector (1/16") (Cole Palmer)
- In-line bubble trap (Alltech Association)

16.4.3.4 Equipment and experimental setup (see Fig. 16.10)

The setup consists of a Leica DMI 4000B fluorescence microscope equipped with 10× and 20× objectives and a 1.4-megapixel CCD camera (12-bit digital output and IEEE 1394 USB interface). Dual wavelength Fura-2 is excited at 340 and 380 nm, and the increases in $[Ca^{2+}]_i$ are expressed as a ratio of F340/F380 (%). Rh123 is a lipophilic cation that partitions selectively into the negatively charged mitochondrial membrane. Mitochondrial energization causes hyperpolarization of the mitochondrial membrane resulting in the uptake of Rh123 into the mitochondria and fluorescence quenching expressed as F/F_0 (%). Rh123 is excited at 495 nm. Excitation wavelengths are controlled by means of corresponding excitation filters (Chroma Technology) mounted in a Lambda DG-4 wavelength switcher. Emission of Fura-2 (510 nm ± 10) and Rh123 fluorescence (530 nm ± 10) is filtered using a Fura-2/FITC polychronic beam splitter and a double band emission filter (Chroma Technology. Part number: 73.100bs). SimplePCI software (Hamamatsu Corp.) is used for image acquisition.

16.4.4 Islet on-chip microencapsulation

16.4.4.1 Reagents

- Aquapel (Aquapel Inc.)
- Ethanol (Sigma-Aldrich)
- Sodium citrate dihydrate (Sigma-Aldrich)
- Light mineral oil (Sigma-Aldrich)
- Alginate (Novamatrix)
- Calcium chloride (Sigma-Aldrich)
- Sodium-EDTA (Mallinckrodt)
- Span80 surfactant (Sigma-Aldrich)
- Acetic acid (Sigma-Aldrich)
- N_2 compressed gas (Airgas)

16.4.4.2 Equipment and materials

- HEPA filtered custom cleanroom or standard biosafety hood.
- Syringe pumps (Fusion 200, Chemyx Inc.)
- Syringes and needles (Dickinson)
- Polyethylene tubing (Intramedic polyethylene tubing, PE 60)

16.5 Protocol: procedures

The following section provides three protocols from Oberholzer Lab including device fabrication, mouse islet isolation, islet on-chip fluorescence imaging, and islet on-chip microencapsulation.

16.5.1 PDMS device fabrication and mouse islet isolation

16.5.1.1 Design of the photomask for the SU-8 negative master

Masks are designed using CAD programs that can generate vector-based graphic files and convert them into raster formats such as encapsulated PostScript (EPS) files. Photomasks then are printed at a resolution higher than that of the minimum feature size. In designing a photomask, at least three alignment markers should be included to facilitate photomask alignment during SU-8 master-mold fabrication if the design includes more than three layers.

16.5.1.2 Fabrication of the SU-8 negative master: timing 4 h

The following describes the fabrication of an SU-8 master with a 500 μm height using SU-8−2150 as an example. For other thicknesses, the parameters such as spin speed and exposure time can be found in the MicroChem manufacturer's references. Fabrication should be done in an HEPA filtered environment; this could be a cleanroom or in a biosafety hood to minimize particle contaminants. All manufacturing steps are intended for room temperature (25°C) unless otherwise indicated by hot plate temperatures. See Fig. 16.11a for a diagram of a typical PDMS workflow.

- 1| **Critical step:** Ensure that all working surfaces/tables are level, as tilted hot plates can cause flow of the photoresist and alter the heights of the microchannels.
- 2| Substrate pretreatment: Rinse a 3" (75 mm) Si wafer sequentially for 30 s with acetone, methanol, and isopropanol, followed by DI water. Dry with a stream of compressed N_2 gas. Perform a dehydration bake of the cleaned wafer on the hot plate at 120°C for 10 min to improve the adhesion of the photoresist to the wafer.
- 3| Expose the wafer to oxygen plasma for 30 s at a power of 100 W (Terra Universal) to oxidize any remaining organic residue.
- 4| Spin coat: Warm-up spinner before use by testing the spin program to ensure correct spin speeds. Spinner Program for SU-8−2150: 500 rpm, spread for 10 s and 1000 rpm, for 30 s to yield a thickness of 500 μm. Cover 25% of Si wafer surface with SU-8 photoresist and execute the spin program.

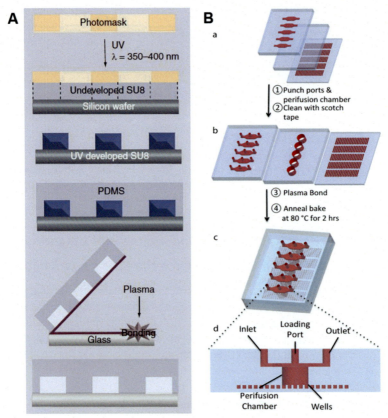

Figure 16.11 Polydimethylsiloxane (PDMS)-based microfluidic device fabrication. (a) Workflow of PDMS-based microfluidic device by photolithography. (b) Final assembly of islet perifusion chamber (IPC) device. (a) 3 layers are microfabricated using soft photolithography, as shown in Fig. 16.1, and prepared by punching appropriate ports and chambers. (b) Bonding surfaces are cleaned with scotch tape. (c) Bonding surfaces are plasma treated, bonded, and then followed by pressured contact on a hot plate while anneal baking. Each completed device is composed of five perifusion systems used in parallel with an automated stage or individually. (d) Cross-sectional view of a perifusion system. The completed device and device components shown here are proportional to the original device. For clarity, channels are indicated in red. Microwells in the bottom layer, not bounded by the perifusion chamber, are not connected to perifusion network. This microwell array is maintained for simplicity for the novice fabricator (Wang et al., 2013).
Reprinted with permission from Future Science Ltd and Elsevier.

- **Caution:** If the temperature in the cleanroom is ±2°C of room temperature, then adjust spin speed by 150 rpm ± 2°C inversely as to resist viscosity decreases with an increase in temperature.
- 5| Soft bake (preexposure bake): After spinning is complete, keep the coated wafer level and transfer it to hot plates in the following sequence: (i) 65°C for 10 min; (ii) 95°C for 120 min; (iii) 65°C for 1 min.

- **Critical step:** After these steps, turn off the hot plate and allow the coated wafer to cool down to room temperature.
- 6| Mask exposure: Take the high-resolution transparent mask (containing microfeatures and alignment markings) and overlay it on top of the SU-8 coated wafer. Expose the wafer to UV light (365 nm filtered Omnicure S1000) with an energy of 600 mJ cm^{-2}. If delamination occurs later in the development step, increase the UW irradiation dosage.
- **Caution:** Make sure to use UV safety goggles when the lamp shutter is open.
- 7| Postexposure bake: After exposing the SU-8, transfer the wafer back to the hot plate for further baking in the following sequence: (i) 65°C for 5 min; (ii) 95°C for 30 min; (iii) 65°C for 1 min.
- **Critical step:** After these steps, turn off the hot plate and allow the coated wafer to cool down to room temperature.
- 8| Develop master: Working under a hood, pour 200 mL of MicroChem SU-8 developer into a 500 mL flat beaker. Transfer the wafer into the developer and bathe for 30 min. Agitate the wafers throughout this duration to ensure adequate development of high aspect ratio features.
- **Caution:** SU-8 developer is a toxic volatile chemical. Work under a hood and a well-ventilated area with appropriate protective gear.
- 9| Rinse wafer with isopropanol to confirm development completion.
- **Critical step:** If the wafer is milky-white, then the SU-8 is not completely developed; return to the developer for an additional 20 s.
- 10| When development is complete, rinse thoroughly with isopropanol to wash away unexposed SU-8. Then, rinse with DI water and blow dry with compressed N_2 gas. Use a digital profiler to confirm the design specifications of microfeature heights.

PAUSE POINT: Developed master molds can be stored in a Petri dish sealed with parafilm (to prevent the entry of dust).

16.5.1.3 PDMS casting: timing 3 h

Here, we use the islets perifusion device, comprised of three molded PDMS layers, as an example.

- 11| Mixing PDMS: For a 3" wafer, weigh out 35 g of PDMS elastomer base and curing agent (Sylgard 184) at a 10:1 ratio into a weighing boat and mix thoroughly for 5 min.
- **Critical step:** If PDMS is NOT mixed thoroughly, or the catalyst is inadequate, the PDMS will not cure completely and the master-mold will be unusable.
- 12| Place the master-mold into a Petri dish, then slowly pour the mixed PDMS over the master-mold.
- 13| Degassing PDMS: Place the Petri dish that holds the master-mold into a dedicated PDMS-only vacuum desiccator. Seal and engage the desiccator for 30 min. Bubbles will be seen to move to the surface. Periodically vent the chamber (e.g., bleeder valve) to release the chamber pressure. After removal from the chamber, use a pipette bulb to expel remaining bubbles. At this point, also make PDMS plugs by filling some 1/16" straight connectors with PDMS and curing (step 14).
- 14| PDMS curing: Place the Petri dish on an 85°C hot plate for 2 h. When fully cured, the PDMS will become solid.

- **PAUSE POINT:** Casted PDMS molds can be stored in a Petri dish sealed with parafilm (to prevent the entry of dust).
- 15| PDMS mold release: Cut out the casted PDMS molds, using a scalpel or razor blade. Use tweezers to carefully and slowly peel PDMS away from the mold. Place the PDMS mold on a sheet of transparency film (microchannels facing downward) for preparation of bonding or storage.
- **PAUSE POINT:** Multiple PDMS molds can be made and stored at this point.
- **Critical step:** When cutting out cured PDMS, make sure to avoid touching the photoresist pattern or breaking the silicon wafer. If not, the master will become unusable and a new one must be produced.

16.5.1.4 Bonding of multilayer microfluidic device: timing 3 h

After molding and cutting of the three PDMS layers, assemble the device by chemical bonding using plasma-treated surface activation, in the following procedures (see Fig. 16.11b).

- 16| Prepare the top layer microchanneled PDMS by using a gauge 11 ($\sim$2 mm diameter) needle punch to carefully punch three holes for each perifusion network: 1 inlet, 1 outlet, 1 loading port. Make sure to remove the punch cores with tweezers before bonding.
- 17| Prepare the middle layer PDMS spacer by using a gauge 0 ($\sim$7 mm diameter) hole-punch to carefully punch one hole to make the perifusion chamber. Remove the cores.
- 18| Using Tape, clean and remove any dust and debris from the area to be bonded. Then, activate the bonding surfaces with the oxygen plasma torch. Alternating between the two surfaces, treat each bonding surface with plasma for 30 s for a total of three times on each bonding surface.
- **Critical step:** Do not touch or bend the activated surface, as this can prevent the device from bonding completely.
- 19| Then, align the bonding surfaces and apply pressure to the bonding area. Make sure to remove any air bubbles. Place the bonded device on an 85°C hot plate pressed with a 2.0 kg weight for 2 h.
- **Critical step:** The bonding process is irreversible. Make sure that the alignment is correct and that there is no debris or bubbles, as this will introduce leaks into the device and encourage delamination.
- 20| To make sure the device is bonded and sealed correctly, pump DI water with a 1 mL syringe to check for leaks. Alternatively, air can be pumped with a pipette with the device submerged in DI water.

16.5.1.5 Mouse pancreatic islet isolation

- 1| Enzyme preparation: Prepare Collagenase P solution at a concentration of a 0.375 mg mL^{-1} in hank's balanced salt solution (HBSS) for 5 mL per mouse pancreas and keep on ice.
- **Caution:** Optimal collagenase concentration is different for each strain of mouse.
- **Critical step:** Keep the collagenase enzyme on ice to prevent enzyme degradation.

- 2| Euthanize mice with compressed CO_2 and 3% isoflurane followed by cervical dislocation to ensure no discomfort to the animals. Disinfect the mouse by spraying it with 70% ethanol (vol/vol).
- **Caution:** Follow national and institutional guidelines for animal handling.
- 3| Make a V-incision starting at the genital area and move the bowel to the left side of the open mouse and clearly expose the common bile duct.
- 4| Clamp the ampulla on the surface of the duodenum using a hemostat.
- 5| Pancreas distension: Distend (in! ate) the pancreas through the bile duct with a 30-gauge needle and 5 mL syringe containing 2 mL of cold collagenase solution, starting at the gallbladder.
- 6| Digestion: Remove the distended pancreas and place it in a 15 mL tube containing 2 mL of the collagenase solution.
- 7| Place in 37°C water bath and incubate for 12 min.
- 8| Shake for 5 s, then add 10 mL of cold HBSS to stop digestion when 80% of the pancreas falls apart.
- **Critical step:** Do not shake too much. Otherwise, the islets will be overdigested and fragmented.
- 9| Centrifuge the digested tissue at 284 g (1000 rpm in a Beckman J6-MI) for 30 s at 4°C and discard the supernatant.
- 10| Resuspend the pellet with 14 mL of cold HBSS and centrifuge with the previous setting. Discard supernatant as completely as possible.
- **Critical step:** Remaining HBSS might cause a change in the Ficoll density (steps 11–13).
- 11| Discontinuous gradient purification: Add 5 mL of 1.108 kg m -3 Ficoll and vortex vigorously.
- 12| Layer 2 mL of Ficoll solutions in descending density gradients: 1.096, 1.069, and 1.037 kg m^{-3}.
- **Critical step:** Work quickly. Long-term exposure of Ficoll to islets is toxic.
- 13| Centrifuge at 640 g (1800 rpm in a Beckman J6-MI) for 15 min at 4°C, with brake off.
- 14| Pick islets from the interface between density layers 1.069 and 1.096 using a plastic transfer pipette and place in a 50 mL conical tube containing 25 mL of cold HBSS.
- 15| Wash: Wash two times with cold HBSS (repeating step 9).
- 16| Culture: Resuspend the islet pellet in 10 mL RPMI-1640 containing 10% FBS (vol/vol), 100 IU mL^{-1} penicillin, 100 μg mL^{-1} streptomycin, and 20 mM HEPES. Transfer it into a Petri dish and place it in a humidified incubator (37°C, 5% CO_2).

16.5.2 *Simultaneous islet perifusion and fluorescence imaging*

16.5.2.1 *Device preconditioning (see Fig. 16.12)*

- 1| Debubbling and vacuum loading of the microfluidic device: PDMS is a hydrophobic material that makes it difficult for aqueous solutions to coat the device and also is a source of bubbles. Therefore, we recommend this five-step process: (i) immerse the microfluidic device in a vessel and flush with 100% EtOH for 10 min; (ii) place ethanol-treated device in vacuum desiccator (Fisher Scientific, PA) connected to a standard laboratory wall vacuum system for 30 min at a pressure of ~110–120 kPa; (iii) exchange 100% ethanol with

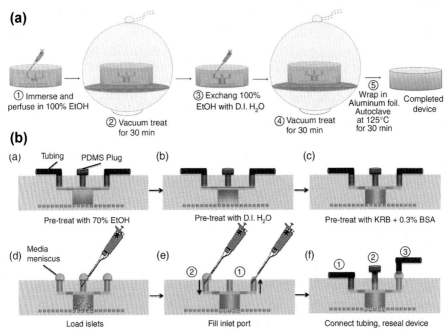

Figure 16.12 Preparation of microfluidic device (IPC device) for islet imaging. (a) Device debubbling and vacuum loading: five-step protocol of polydimethylsiloxane (PDMS) surface treatment and vacuum filling protocol for bubble formation prevention. (b) Device preconditioning and islet loading. (a) EtOH Pretreatment: Preconditioning begins by perifusing tubings and microfluidic devices with 70% ethanol (vol/vol) to apply a hydrophilic coating; (b) DI H$_2$O rinse; (c) BSA Rinse: 0.3% BSA in Krebs–Ringer Buffer (wt/vol) is then applied to prevent insulin and other organic species from being trapped in tubing and microfluidic device; (d) Islet Loading: Tubing is disconnected and inlet ports are filled and overflowed with perifusate to create a meniscus. Islets are then loaded with 20 μL pipette which is dialed down until empty; (e) Inlet Preparation: Medium from outlet (1) and inlet (2) is overflowed; (f) Final Connections: Inlet tubing is reconnected (1). Media at islet loading port and outlet port overflow. Loading port is sealed (2). Finally, outlet tubing is reconnected to outlet port (3) (Wang et al., 2013).
Reprinted with permission from Elsevier.

distilled (DI) water; (iv) vacuum treated for an additional 30 min; (v) Optional sterilization step: the device can now be wrapped in aluminum foil and autoclaved at 125°C for 30 min.
- 2| Connect a 10 mL syringe filled with 70% ethanol (vol/vol) to the inlet port with Tygon tubing. Flow the ethanol for 10 min through the device channels to sterilize and prevent the introduction of bubbles. Then, rinse with DI water for 5 min.
- **Critical step:** Pumping ethanol is important to minimize the introduction of bubbles. If bubbles cannot be completely removed, use a pipette to force DI water with repeated injection and withdrawal.

16.5.2.2 Islet cells preparation and loading (see Fig. 16.12)

- 3| Rinse tubing and device with KRB containing 0.3% BSA (wt/vol) for 5 min. Then, rinse with KRB containing 2 mM glucose for 5 min.
- **Critical step:** BSA coating prevents nonspecific absorption of released hormones to interior surfaces of tubing and microchannel walls, thus ensuring accuracy when later measuring bioanalyte or insulin secretion levels.
- **Critical step:** Whenever disconnecting or reconnecting tubing, care must be taken to minimize the introduction of bubbles into the microfluidic network. This can be accomplished by merging the fluid medial meniscus of the tubing with that of the inlet or outlet port prior to inserting the tubing.
- 4| Fluorescence labeling: Under the microscope, handpick 25 mouse islets and place in a Petri dish with 2 mL of KRB containing 2 mM glucose. In the Petri dish, use an ellipsoid swirling motion to aggregate a cluster for easier handling in subsequent steps. Add Fura-2 AM at a final concentration of 5 µM and Rh 123 at a final concentration of 2.5 µM.
- 5| Place the dish into the humidified incubator (37°C and 5% CO_2) for 30 min.
- 6| Islet loading: Disconnect the device from syringe pumps and place the device on a flat surface, making sure that a media meniscus bead of buffer overflows each unconnected port.
- 7| After 30 min incubation, pick up the islets using a 20 µL pipette inserted into the loading port and gently load the islets by dialing down the pipette.
- 8| Aspirate another 20 µL KRB from the outlet and inject it into the inlet port, dispensing the loaded islets into the bottom of the perifusion chamber.
- 9| Place the preconditioned device with the loaded islets on the 37°C heated microscope stage and connect the inlet to syringe pumps containing 2 and 25 mM glucose solutions via the Y-connector with the Tygon tubing. Connect the outlet of the microfluidic device to the fraction collector.
- **Critical step:** GSIS is sensitive to temperature changes, so maintain a temperature range of $37 \pm 3°C$ in the perifusion chamber and confirm with a temperature probe. To further avoid temperature change, place a hot plate set between 45°C and 60°C upstream of the device inlet to heat the incoming perifusing media.
- **Critical step:** In order to prevent sudden pressure changes and bubble formation in the perifusion chamber, islet loading is best done on a flat surface and when all the tubings are disconnected from the device. Rapid changes in pressure can cause islets to become dislodged and exit the perifusion chamber through the outlet.
- **Critical step:** Make sure the syringes, tubing, microfluidic device, and outlet are all on the same level surface or height. Different heights will cause different pressures and fluid flow which may eject islets. If perifusion is stopped, make sure to clamp outlet to prevent fluid flow which may eject islets.

16.5.2.3 Islet perifusion and fluorescence imaging

- 10| Start the syringe pump containing 2 mM glucose KRB solution to wash the excess dye from the perifusion chamber and islets at a speed of 250 µL min^{-1} for 10 min.
- **Critical step:** To maximize signal-to-noise ratio, make sure that there is enough time for hydrolysis and washing of excess fluorescent indicator dyes.

- 11| During the washing period, start searching the areas of interest (ROIs) using transmitted light illumination.
- **Critical step:** Start this step as soon as possible without waiting until the completion of the washing.
- 12| Open Simple PCI imaging software and LabVIEW.
- 13| Use the ROI tool of the imaging software to define the islets and islet regions to be imaged. Circle a nonislet area for later background subtraction.
- 14| Designate the excitation and emission filter sets for simultaneous imaging of Fura-2 for intracellular calcium changes and Rh 123 for mitochondrial potential changes. Fura-2 excitation occurs at 340 and 380 nm and detected at 510 nm ± 10. The Fura-2 excitation ratio (F380/F340) is obtained using Simple PCI. Rh 123 is excited at 490 nm and detected at 530 nm ± 10.
- 15| Initialize LabVIEW to create a defined linear glucose gradient (2−25 mM) and set the fraction collector at 1-min intervals.
- **Caution:** When programming LabVIEW, you can confirm the creation of the desired glucose gradient profile by sampling the perifusate and using a glucometer to measure glucose levels before experimentation.
- **Critical step:** Adjust fluorescence intensity gains at each wavelength to prevent artifacts.
- 16| Start acquiring a time series of Fura-2 and Rh 123 fluorescence at the ROIs at 15-second capture intervals.
- 17| Turn off the syringe pump containing 25 mM glucose after the completion of a glucose gradient. Let the low glucose pump continue to wash out the effect of the high glucose for 10 min.
- 18| Following the perifusion, export the data to excel for analysis. The amount of insulin secreted into the perifusate is determined by ELISA according to manufacturer protocol.
- 19| Flush out islets and cellular debris with 1 mL pipette and commence flushing the perifusion. Then, flush chambers with 70% ethanol (vol/vol) for 10 min and DI H_2O for 10 min. Cleaning is variable and dependent on media used.

16.5.3 Microencapsulation of islets on a chip
16.5.3.1 3D-printed coaxial flow device

- 1| Suspend rat islets in 3% alginate solution (ultrapure low-viscosity high-mannuronic acid (LVM) sodium alginate, NovaMatrix).
- 2| Connect two tubes with valves to the air vents on the top of the device. Set up the cell-suspending syringe with the syringe pump and connect the syringe to the alginate inlet with tubing.
- 3| Fix the device on a leveled support. Adjust the height of the device and let the distance between the bottom surface of the nozzle and top surface of the $CaCl_2$ collection bath to be 0.25 m.
- 4| Install a pressure regulator on a nitrogen tank. Connect the regulator to the air inlet located on the side of the device using a Tygon tubing. Open the tank and adjust the regulator knob until the reading reaches 5 psi.

- 5| Set up the syringe pump with a flow rate of 42 mL h^{-1}.
- 6| Collect the alginate beads in a 100 mM CaCl$_2$ bath where they were gelled during 15 min incubation. Following two washes with normal saline, incubate the microspheres in 0.1% (w/v) Poly-L-Ornithine for 10 min to provide them with permselectivity.

16.5.3.2 Internal gelation device

- 1| Prepare a solution of light mineral oil with 3% Span80 (v/v). The addition of Span80 to mineral oil prevents bead coalescence after generation at the flow-focusing junction.
- 2| Prepare a solution of 1.5% (w/v) alginate mixed with 100 mM Ca-EDTA at a 1:1 ratio while maintaining the concentration of alginate solution at 1.5% (w/v). Ca-EDTA complex mixed with the alginate at a 1:1 ratio is stable at pH 7.
- 3| To subject it to Aquapel treatment, withdraw about 0.1 mL of Aquapel with a 1 mL syringe. Use a 20-gauge syringe needle and a small polyethylene tube connected to the syringe needle to direct the fluid into one of the ports of the microfluidic device.
- **Critical step:** The tubing should be thread over the 20-gauge needle for a snug fit.
- 4| After all the solutions are drawn into 1 mL BD syringes, cap with 20-gauge needles. Fit a polyethylene tube over the needle. Place the solutions into the syringe pumps and manually prime until the fluid flows out of the tubing.
- 5| Start the slower flow rates first. This helps prime the channels with slower moving liquids (like alginate) and prevents the channels with faster moving liquids (mineral oil) from entering other channels and causing issues. It is very important that the solution from Inlet C does not backflow into Inlet B because it may result in premature alginate crosslinking that will clog the channel.
- 6| Usually within 2–3 min, the device will reach a steady state and run consistently for long periods of time until the syringes must be refilled.
- 7| A small cut end of a pipette tip (~5 mm long) can be snugly fit into the outlet port to direct the fluid into a dish, well, or other external collection item.
- 8| The beads-acid oil suspension streaming out of the channel is collected in a conical tube with a 1.1% (w/w) CaCl$_2$ solution. In the collection tube, acid oil will float to the top of the CaCl$_2$ solution due to its lower density, while beads will sediment at the bottom of the conical tube. Following the complete partitioning of beads to an aqueous phase, discard the oil and wash the beads twice with 1% Tween solution prior to a 20-min PLO (0.1%) coating for immunoisolation.

16.6 Conclusion and future trends

In summary, microfluidic techniques have been widely explored to help pancreatic islets and islet-like biologics study for human islets transplantation. Due to their strength on fluid control, microscale feature design, and easy integration of imaging, microfluidic technologies can be utilized to significantly improve the spatiotemporal resolution of traditional bioanalytical systems for islets and islet-like biologics. With several microfluidic devices described in this chapter, operation conducted in small dimensions offers the possibility of portable sample substances, multitasking, and parallel fluidic operations. Due to these advantages, microfluidic devices can be applied at the subcellular, single-cell, or cell-population levels in biomedical research to help better understanding of islets physiology and prediction of human islets transplantation outcomes.

In addition, microfluidic designs also provide opportunities of better control on biomanufacturing process of cell therapy product compared to conventional procedure. For human islets transplantation, the microfluidic platform offers a unique advantage in generating uniform-sized hydrogel microcapsules. Homogeneity can be seen in capsule size as well as cell distribution inside the capsule, leading to more sustained biomolecule penetration and islet graft survival for encapsulated islets.

Moving forward to the issue of limited islets resources, stem cells have been treated as a possible alternative resource of islet cells. Many research groups have put efforts to develop the stem cell derived islet cells, but not gotten much positive results. Benefit from the precise control of microenvironment, microfluidic dynamic cell culture showed potentials on better control on the fate of stem cells over the traditional static cell culture protocol. The combination of microfluidics and stem cell techniques may be the right path when facing the clinical challenges in human islets transplantation.

Acknowledgments

This study was supported by the Chicago Diabetes Project (CDP) and the National Institutes of Health (NIH) [R01 DK091526 (J.O)].

References

Adewola, A. F., Lee, D., Harvat, T., Mohammed, J., Eddington, D. T., Oberholzer, J., et al. (2010). Microfluidic perifusion and imaging device for multi-parametric islet function assessment. *Biomedical Microdevices, 12*(3), 409–417. https://doi.org/10.1007/s10544-010-9398-1.

Aguiari, P., Leo, S., Zavan, B., Vindigni, V., Rimessi, A., Bianchi, K., et al. (2008). High glucose induces adipogenic differentiation of muscle-derived stem cells. *Proceedings of the National Academy of Sciences, 105*(4), 1226–1231.

Alejandro, R., Barton, F. B., Hering, B. J., Wease, S., & Collaborative Islet Transplant Registry, I. (2008). 2008 update from the collaborative islet transplant Registry. *Transplantation, 86*(12), 1783–1788. https://doi.org/10.1097/TP.0b013e3181913f6a.

Armann, B., Hanson, M. S., Hatch, E., Steffen, A., & Fernandez, L. A. (2007). Quantification of basal and stimulated ROS levels as predictors of islet potency and function. *American Journal of Transplantation, 7*(1), 38–47. https://doi.org/10.1111/j.1600-6143.2006.01577.x.

Babenko, A. P., Aguilar-Bryan, L., & Bryan, J. (1998). A view of sur/KIR6.X, KATP channels. *Annual Review of Physiology, 60,* 667−687. https://doi.org/10.1146/annurev.physiol.60.1.667.

Bellin, M. D., Kandaswamy, R., Parkey, J., Zhang, H. J., Liu, B., Ihm, S. H., et al. (2008). Prolonged insulin independence after islet allotransplants in recipients with type 1 diabetes. *American Journal of Transplantation, 8*(11), 2463−2470. https://doi.org/10.1111/j.1600-6143.2008.02404.x.

Bertuzzi, F., & Ricordi, C. (2007). Prediction of clinical outcome in islet allotransplantation. *Diabetes Care, 30*(2), 410−417. https://doi.org/10.2337/dc06-1233.

Carvalho, C. P., Oliveira, R. B., Britan, A., Santos-Silva, J. C., Boschero, A. C., Meda, P., et al. (2012). Impaired beta-cell-beta-cell coupling mediated by Cx36 gap junctions in prediabetic mice. *American Journal of Physiology. Endocrinology and Metabolism, 303*(1), E144−E151. https://doi.org/10.1152/ajpendo.00489.2011.

Chen, D., Du, W., Liu, Y., Liu, W., Kuznetsov, A., Mendez, F. E., et al. (2008). The chemistrode: A droplet-based microfluidic device for stimulation and recording with high temporal, spatial, and chemical resolution. *Proceedings of the National Academy of Sciences of the United States of America, 105*(44), 16843−16848. https://doi.org/10.1073/pnas.0807916105.

Craighead, H. (2006). Future lab-on-a-chip technologies for interrogating individual molecules. *Nature, 442*(7101), 387−393. https://doi.org/10.1038/nature05061.

Dishinger, J. F., Reid, K. R., & Kennedy, R. T. (2009). Quantitative monitoring of insulin secretion from single islets of Langerhans in parallel on a microfluidic chip. *Analytical Chemistry, 81*(8), 3119−3127. https://doi.org/10.1021/ac900109t.

Duchen, M. R. (2000). Mitochondria and Ca(2+)in cell physiology and pathophysiology. *Cell Calcium, 28*(5−6), 339−348. https://doi.org/10.1054/ceca.2000.0170.

Easley, C. J., Rocheleau, J. V., Head, W. S., & Piston, D. W. (2009). Quantitative measurement of zinc secretion from pancreatic islets with high temporal resolution using droplet-based microfluidics. *Analytical Chemistry, 81*(21), 9086−9095. https://doi.org/10.1021/ac9017692.

El-Ali, J., Sorger, P. K., & Jensen, K. F. (2006). Cells on chips. *Nature, 442*(7101), 403−411. https://doi.org/10.1038/nature05063.

Gangemi, A., Salehi, P., Hatipoglu, B., Martellotto, J., Barbaro, B., Kuechle, J. B., et al. (2008). Islet transplantation for brittle type 1 diabetes: The UIC protocol. *American Journal of Transplantation, 8*(6), 1250−1261. https://doi.org/10.1111/j.1600-6143.2008.02234.x.

Gembal, M., Gilon, P., & Henquin, J. C. (1992). Evidence that glucose can control insulin release independently from its action on atp-sensitive K+ channels in mouse B-cells. *Journal of Clinical Investigation, 89*(4), 1288−1295. https://doi.org/10.1172/Jci115714.

Glieberman, A. L., Pope, B. D., Zimmerman, J. F., Liu, Q., Ferrier, J. P., Kenty, J. H. R., et al. (2019). Synchronized stimulation and continuous insulin sensing in a microfluidic human Islet on a Chip designed for scalable manufacturing. *Lab on a Chip, 19*(18), 2993−3010. https://doi.org/10.1039/c9lc00253g.

Gomez-Sjoberg, R., Leyrat, A. A., Pirone, D. M., Chen, C. S., & Quake, S. R. (2007). Versatile, fully automated, microfluidic cell culture system. *Analytical Chemistry, 79*(22), 8557−8563. https://doi.org/10.1021/ac071311w.

Goto, M., Holgersson, J., Kumagai-Braesch, M., & Korsgren, O. (2006). The ADP/ATP ratio: A novel predictive assay for quality assessment of isolated pancreatic islets. *American Journal of Transplantation, 6*(10), 2483−2487. https://doi.org/10.1111/j.1600-6143.2006.01474.x.

Headen, D. M., Aubry, G., Lu, H., & Garcia, A. J. (2014). Microfluidic-based generation of size-controlled, biofunctionalized synthetic polymer microgels for cell encapsulation. *Advanced Materials, 26*(19), 3003−3008. https://doi.org/10.1002/adma.201304880.

Henquin, J. C., Nenquin, M., Stiernet, P., & Ahren, B. (2006). In vivo and in vitro glucose-induced biphasic insulin secretion in the mouse: Pattern and role of cytoplasmic Ca^{2+} and amplification signals in beta-cells. *Diabetes, 55*(2), 441−451. https://doi.org/10.2337/diabetes.55.02.06.db05-1051.

Henquin, J. C., Schmeer, W., Nenquin, M., & Meissner, H. P. (1985). Effects of a calcium channel agonist on the electrical, ionic and secretory events in mouse pancreatic B-cells. *Biochemical and Biophysical Research Communications, 131*(2), 980−986. https://doi.org/10.1016/0006-291x(85)91336-1.

Hoshi, M., & Shreeve, W. W. (1973). Release and production of insulin by isolated, perifused rat pancreatic islets. Control by glucose. *Diabetes, 22*(1), 16−24. https://doi.org/10.2337/diab.22.1.16.

Ichii, H., Inverardi, L., Pileggi, A., Molano, R. D., Cabrera, O., Caicedo, A., et al. (2005). A novel method for the assessment of cellular composition and beta-cell viability in human islet preparations. *American Journal of Transplantation, 5*(7), 1635−1645. https://doi.org/10.1111/j.1600-6143.2005.00913.x.

Iglesias, I., Bentsi-Barnes, K., Umeadi, C., Brown, L., Kandeel, F., & Al-Abdullah, I. H. (2008). Comprehensive analysis of human pancreatic islets using flow and laser scanning cytometry. *Transplantation Proceedings, 40*(2), 351−354. https://doi.org/10.1016/j.transproceed.2008.01.037.

Ivanovic, Z. (2009). Hypoxia or in situ normoxia: The stem cell paradigm. *Journal of Cellular Physiology, 219*(2), 271−275. https://doi.org/10.1002/jcp.21690.

Jayaraman, S. (2008). A novel method for the detection of viable human pancreatic beta cells by flow cytometry using fluorophores that selectively detect labile zinc, mitochondrial membrane potential and protein thiols. *Cytometry, 73*(7), 615−625. https://doi.org/10.1002/cyto.a.20560.

Jun, Y., Kim, M. J., Hwang, Y. H., Jeon, E. A., Kang, A. R., Lee, S. H., et al. (2013). Microfluidics-generated pancreatic islet microfibers for enhanced immunoprotection. *Biomaterials, 34*(33), 8122−8130. https://doi.org/10.1016/j.biomaterials.2013.07.079.

Kang, A., Park, J., Ju, J., Jeong, G. S., & Lee, S. H. (2014). Cell encapsulation via microtechnologies. *Biomaterials, 35*(9), 2651−2663. https://doi.org/10.1016/j.biomaterials.2013.12.073.

Kennedy, E. D., Rizzuto, R., Theler, J. M., Pralong, W. F., Bastianutto, C., Pozzan, T., et al. (1996). Glucose-stimulated insulin secretion correlates with changes in mitochondrial and cytosolic Ca^{2+} in aequorin-expressing INS-1 cells. *Journal of Clinical Investigation, 98*(11), 2524−2538. https://doi.org/10.1172/JCI119071.

Kim, J. H., Park, S. G., Lee, H. N., Lee, Y. Y., Park, H. S., Kim, H. I., et al. (2009). ATP measurement predicts porcine islet transplantation outcome in nude mice. *Transplantation, 87*(2), 166−169. https://doi.org/10.1097/TP.0b013e318191e925.

Komjati, M., Bratusch-Marrain, P., & Waldhausl, W. (1986). Superior efficacy of pulsatile versus continuous hormone exposure on hepatic glucose production in vitro. *Endocrinology, 118*(1), 312−319. https://doi.org/10.1210/endo-118-1-312.

Lacy, L. R., Knudson, M. M., Williams, J. J., Richards, J. S., & Midgley, A. R., Jr. (1976). Progesterone metabolism by the ovary of the pregnant rat: Discrepancies in the catabolic regulation model. *Endocrinology, 99*(4), 929−934. https://doi.org/10.1210/endo-99-4-929.

Lacy, P. E., Walker, M. M., & Fink, C. J. (1972). Perifusion of isolated rat islets in vitro. Participation of the microtubular system in the biphasic release of insulin. *Diabetes, 21*(10), 987−998. https://doi.org/10.2337/diab.21.10.987.

Lee, D., Wang, Y., Mendoza-Elias, J. E., Adewola, A. F., Harvat, T. A., Kinzer, K., et al. (2012). Dual microfluidic perifusion networks for concurrent islet perifusion and optical imaging. *Biomedical Microdevices, 14*(1), 7−16. https://doi.org/10.1007/s10544-011-9580-0.

Liu, W. W., Goodhouse, J., Jeon, N. L., & Enquist, L. W. (2008). A microfluidic chamber for analysis of neuron-to-cell spread and axonal transport of an alpha-herpesvirus. *PloS One, 3*(6), e2382. https://doi.org/10.1371/journal.pone.0002382.

London, N. J., Thirdborough, S. M., Swift, S. M., Bell, P. R., & James, R. F. (1991). The diabetic "human reconstituted" severe combined immunodeficient (SCID-hu) mouse: A model for isogeneic, allogeneic, and xenogeneic human islet transplantation. *Transplantation Proceedings, 23*(1 Pt 1), 749. Retrieved from https://www.ncbi.nlm.nih.gov/pubmed/1990677.

Luciani, D. S., Misler, S., & Polonsky, K. S. (2006). Ca^{2+} controls slow NAD(P)H oscillations in glucose-stimulated mouse pancreatic islets. *Journal of Physiology, 572*(Pt 2), 379−392. https://doi.org/10.1113/jphysiol.2005.101766.

Maechler, P., Kennedy, E. D., Wang, H., & Wollheim, C. B. (1998). Desensitization of mitochondrial Ca^{2+} and insulin secretion responses in the beta cell. *Journal of Biological Chemistry, 273*(33), 20770−20778. https://doi.org/10.1074/jbc.273.33.20770.

McGuigan, A. P., Bruzewicz, D. A., Glavan, A., Butte, M., & Whitesides, G. M. (2008). Cell encapsulation in sub-mm sized gel modules using replica molding. *PloS One, 3*(5), e2258.

Mohammed, J. S., Wang, Y., Harvat, T. A., Oberholzer, J., & Eddington, D. T. (2009). Microfluidic device for multimodal characterization of pancreatic islets. *Lab on a Chip, 9*(1), 97−106. https://doi.org/10.1039/b809590f.

Morrison, S. J., & Spradling, A. C. (2008). Stem cells and niches: Mechanisms that promote stem cell maintenance throughout life. *Cell, 132*(4), 598−611.

Mosadegh, B., Huang, C., Park, J. W., Shin, H. S., Chung, B. G., Hwang, S. K., et al. (2007). Generation of stable complex gradients across two-dimensional surfaces and three-dimensional gels. *Langmuir, 23*(22), 10910−10912. https://doi.org/10.1021/la7026835.

Nair, G. G., Liu, J. S., Russ, H. A., Tran, S., Saxton, M. S., Chen, R., et al. (2019). Recapitulating endocrine cell clustering in culture promotes maturation of human stem-cell-derived beta cells. *Nature Cell Biology, 21*(2), 263−274. https://doi.org/10.1038/s41556-018-0271-4.

Nourmohammadzadeh, M., Xing, Y., Lee, J. W., Bochenek, M. A., Mendoza-Elias, J. E., McGarrigle, J. J., et al. (2016). A microfluidic array for real-time live-cell imaging of human and rodent pancreatic islets. *Lab on a Chip, 16*(8), 1466−1472. https://doi.org/10.1039/c5lc01173f.

Oppegard, S. C., Nam, K. H., Carr, J. R., Skaalure, S. C., & Eddington, D. T. (2009). Modulating temporal and spatial oxygenation over adherent cellular cultures. *PloS One, 4*(9), e6891. https://doi.org/10.1371/journal.pone.0006891.

Papas, K. K., Colton, C. K., Nelson, R. A., Rozak, P. R., Avgoustiniatos, E. S., Scott, W. E., et al. (2007a). Human islet oxygen consumption rate and DNA measurements predict diabetes reversal in nude mice. *American Journal of Transplantation, 7*(3), 707−713. https://doi.org/10.1111/j.1600-6143.2006.01655.x.

Papas, K. K., Pisania, A., Wu, H., Weir, G. C., & Colton, C. K. (2007b). A stirred microchamber for oxygen consumption rate measurements with pancreatic islets. *Biotechnology and Bioengineering, 98*(5), 1071−1082. https://doi.org/10.1002/bit.21486.

Papas, K. K., Suszynski, T. M., & Colton, C. K. (2009). Islet assessment for transplantation. *Current Opinion in Organ Transplantation, 14*(6), 674−682. https://doi.org/10.1097/MOT.0b013e328332a489.

Paredes Juarez, G. A., Spasojevic, M., Faas, M. M., & de Vos, P. (2014). Immunological and technical considerations in application of alginate-based microencapsulation systems. *Frontiers in Bioengineering and Biotechnology, 2*, 26. https://doi.org/10.3389/fbioe.2014.00026.

Penko, D., Mohanasundaram, D., Sen, S., Drogemuller, C., Mee, C., Bonder, C. S., et al. (2011). Incorporation of endothelial progenitor cells into mosaic pseudoislets. *Islets, 3*(3), 73−79. https://doi.org/10.4161/isl.3.3.15392.

Porksen, N., Hollingdal, M., Juhl, C., Butler, P., Veldhuis, J. D., & Schmitz, O. (2002). Pulsatile insulin secretion: Detection, regulation, and role in diabetes. *Diabetes, 51*(Suppl. 1), S245−S254. https://doi.org/10.2337/diabetes.51.2007.s245.

Qi, M., Kinzer, K., Danielson, K. K., Martellotto, J., Barbaro, B., Wang, Y., et al. (2014). Five-year follow-up of patients with type 1 diabetes transplanted with allogeneic islets: The UIC experience. *Acta Diabetologica, 51*(5), 833−843. https://doi.org/10.1007/s00592-014-0627-6.

Ricordi, C., Goldstein, J. S., Balamurugan, A. N., Szot, G. L., Kin, T., Liu, C., et al. (2016). National Institutes of health-sponsored clinical islet transplantation consortium phase 3 trial: Manufacture of a complex cellular product at eight processing facilities. *Diabetes, 65*(11), 3418−3428. https://doi.org/10.2337/db16-0234.

Ricordi, C., Lakey, J. R., & Hering, B. J. (2001). Challenges toward standardization of islet isolation technology. *Transplantation Proceedings, 33*(1−2), 1709. https://doi.org/10.1016/s0041-1345(00)02651-8.

Ricordi, C., Scharp, D. W., & Lacy, P. E. (1988). Reversal of diabetes in nude mice after transplantation of fresh and 7-day-cultured (24 degrees C) human pancreatic islets. *Transplantation, 45*(5), 994−996. https://doi.org/10.1097/00007890-198805000-00035.

Rocheleau, J. V., & Piston, D. W. (2008). Chapter 4: Combining microfluidics and quantitative fluorescence microscopy to examine pancreatic islet molecular physiology. *Methods in Cell Biology, 89*, 71−92. https://doi.org/10.1016/S0091-679X(08)00604-3.

Rocheleau, J. V., Walker, G. M., Head, W. S., McGuinness, O. P., & Piston, D. W. (2004). Microfluidic glucose stimulation reveals limited coordination of intracellular Ca^{2+} activity oscillations in pancreatic islets. *Proceedings of the National Academy of Sciences of the United States of America, 101*(35), 12899−12903. https://doi.org/10.1073/pnas.0405149101.

Roe, M. W., Worley, J. F., 3rd, Tokuyama, Y., Philipson, L. H., Sturis, J., Tang, J., et al. (1996). NIDDM is associated with loss of pancreatic beta-cell L-type Ca^{2+} channel activity. *American Journal of Physiology, 270*(1 Pt 1), E133−E140. https://doi.org/10.1152/ajpendo.1996.270.1.E133.

Ryan, E. A., Paty, B. W., Senior, P. A., Bigam, D., Alfadhli, E., Kneteman, N. M., et al. (2005). Five-year follow-up after clinical islet transplantation. *Diabetes, 54*(7), 2060−2069. https://doi.org/10.2337/diabetes.54.7.2060.

Schwarz, T. (2000). No eczema without keratinocyte death. *Journal of Clinical Investigation, 106*(1), 9−10.

Sharma, V., Hunckler, M., Ramasubramanian, M. K., Opara, E. C., & Katuri, K. C. (2017). Microfluidic approach to cell microencapsulation. *Methods in Molecular Biology, 1479*, 71−76. https://doi.org/10.1007/978-1-4939-6364-5_5.

Silva, P. N., Atto, Z., Regeenes, R., Tufa, U., Chen, Y. Y., Chan, W. C. W., et al. (2016). Highly efficient adenoviral transduction of pancreatic islets using a microfluidic device. *Lab on a Chip, 16*(15), 2921−2934. https://doi.org/10.1039/c6lc00345a.

Spigelman, A. F., Dai, X., & MacDonald, P. E. (2010). Voltage-dependent K(+) channels are positive regulators of alpha cell action potential generation and glucagon secretion in mice and humans. *Diabetologia, 53*(9), 1917−1926. https://doi.org/10.1007/s00125-010-1759-z.

Straub, S. G., & Sharp, G. W. (2002). Glucose-stimulated signaling pathways in biphasic insulin secretion. *Diabetes/Metabolism Research and Reviews, 18*(6), 451−463. https://doi.org/10.1002/dmrr.329.

Street, C. N., Lakey, J. R., Shapiro, A. M., Imes, S., Rajotte, R. V., Ryan, E. A., et al. (2004). Islet graft assessment in the Edmonton protocol: Implications for predicting long-term clinical outcome. *Diabetes, 53*(12), 3107−3114. https://doi.org/10.2337/diabetes.53.12.3107.

Sui, L., Danzl, N., Campbell, S. R., Viola, R., Williams, D., Xing, Y., et al. (2018). Beta-cell replacement in mice using human type 1 diabetes nuclear transfer embryonic stem cells. *Diabetes, 67*(1), 26−35. https://doi.org/10.2337/db17-0120.

Svensson, A. M., Sandler, S., & Jansson, L. (1994). Pancreatic islet blood flow in the rat after administration of islet amyloid polypeptide or calcitonin gene-related peptide. *Diabetes, 43*(3), 454−458. https://doi.org/10.2337/diab.43.3.454.

Sweet, I. R., & Gilbert, M. (2006). Contribution of calcium influx in mediating glucose-stimulated oxygen consumption in pancreatic islets. *Diabetes, 55*(12), 3509−3519. https://doi.org/10.2337/db06-0400.

Sweet, I. R., Gilbert, M., Scott, S., Todorov, I., Jensen, R., Nair, I., et al. (2008). Glucose-stimulated increment in oxygen consumption rate as a standardized test of human islet quality. *American Journal of Transplantation, 8*(1), 183−192. https://doi.org/10.1111/j.1600-6143.2007.02041.x.

Tan, W. H., & Takeuchi, S. (2008). Dynamic microarray system with gentle retrieval mechanism for cell-encapsulating hydrogel beads. *Lab on a Chip, 8*(2), 259−266. https://doi.org/10.1039/b714573j.

Taylor, A. M., Rhee, S. W., & Jeon, N. L. (2006). Microfluidic chambers for cell migration and neuroscience research. *Methods in Molecular Biology, 321*, 167−177. https://doi.org/10.1385/1-59259-997-4:167.

Tendulkar, S., Mirmalek-Sani, S. H., Childers, C., Saul, J., Opara, E. C., & Ramasubramanian, M. K. (2012). A three-dimensional microfluidic approach to scaling up microencapsulation of cells. *Biomedical Microdevices, 14*(3), 461−469. https://doi.org/10.1007/s10544-011-9623-6.

Wang, Y., Mendoza-Elias, J. E., Lo, J. F., Harvat, T. A., Feng, F., Li, Z., et al. (2013). Microfluidics for monitoring and imaging pancreatic islet and β-cells for human transplant. In X. Li, & Y. Zhou (Eds.), *Microfluidic devices for biomedical applications* (pp. 557−596e). Woodhead Publishing.

Wang, W., Upshaw, L., Strong, D. M., Robertson, R. P., & Reems, J. (2005). Increased oxygen consumption rates in response to high glucose detected by a novel oxygen biosensor system in non-human primate and human islets. *Journal of Endocrinology, 185*(3), 445−455. https://doi.org/10.1677/joe.1.06092.

Warnotte, C., Gilon, P., Nenquin, M., & Henquin, J. C. (1994). Mechanisms of the stimulation of insulin release by saturated fatty acids. A study of palmitate effects in mouse beta-cells. *Diabetes, 43*(5), 703−711. https://doi.org/10.2337/diab.43.5.703.

Weaver, D. C., McDaniel, M. L., Naber, S. P., Barry, C. D., & Lacy, P. E. (1978). Alloxan stimulation and inhibition of insulin release from isolated rat islets of Langerhans. *Diabetes, 27*(12), 1205−1214. https://doi.org/10.2337/diab.27.12.1205.

Weibel, D. B., Diluzio, W. R., & Whitesides, G. M. (2007). Microfabrication meets microbiology. *Nature Reviews Microbiology, 5*(3), 209−218. https://doi.org/10.1038/nrmicro1616.

Xing, Y., Nourmohammadzadeh, M., Elias, J. E., Chan, M., Chen, Z., McGarrigle, J. J., et al. (2016). A pumpless microfluidic device driven by surface tension for pancreatic islet analysis. *Biomedical Microdevices, 18*(5), 80. https://doi.org/10.1007/s10544-016-0109-4.

Zhang, Q., & Austin, R. H. (2012). Applications of microfluidics in stem cell biology. *Bionanoscience, 2*(4), 277−286. https://doi.org/10.1007/s12668-012-0051-8.

Zhang, X., & Roper, M. G. (2009). Microfluidic perfusion system for automated delivery of temporal gradients to islets of Langerhans. *Analytical Chemistry, 81*(3), 1162−1168. https://doi.org/10.1021/ac802579z.

3D printed microfluidic devices and applications

17

Sui Ching Phung, Qingfu Zhu, Kimberly Plevniak, Mei He
Department of Chemical and Petroleum Engineering, Department of Chemistry, University of Kansas, Lawrence, KS, United States

Guided-Reading Questions:

1. What are the 3D printing principles?
2. How can the 3D printing advance the microfluidic fabrication?
3. How do the 3D printed microfluidic devices aid biomedical research?

17.1 Introduction

In 1990, Manz et al., proposed a novel concept of "miniaturized total chemical analysis (µTAS)" for chemical sensing (Manz, Graber, & Widmer, 1990), which is well known as microfluidics nowadays. For making microfluidic devices and chips, the microfabrication process, called projection photolithography, was adapted from microelectromechanical system (MEMS) and is super tedious and costly (Manz et al., 1990; Xia & Whitesides, 1998). In this process, the entire geometric pattern of the photomask can be projected onto a thin film of photoresist that is photosensitive (Xia & Whitesides, 1998). As an alternative easier solution, Whitesides's Group introduced soft lithography using an elastomer known as poly(dimethylsiloxane) (PDMS) (Webster, Greenman, & Haswell, 2011; Xia & Whitesides, 1998) to cast microstructures from a photoresist-patterned silicon mold with featured sizes ranging from 30 nm to 100 µm. PDMS casting is more popular since then for rapid and low-cost fabricating microfluidic devices. The emerging of variable microfabrication approaches enabled researchers to push microfluidic applications to more broad biomedical research. However, creating silicon molds has to be done in a cleanroom and facility center using lengthy protocols and expensive equipment. Such limitations prevent powerful microfluidic technology from reaching researchers who are not familiar with design processes, even though the addition of microfluidics to such researchers' workflow could dramatically improve productivity and discovery. Thus, fabrication complications and extensive knowledge of design restrict the utility of microfluidics by biologists and clinicians.

In 1986, Charles W. Hull introduced the first three-dimensional (3D) printing (Hull, 1986; Murphy & Atala, 2014). He developed the "stereolithography" system that is capable of generating objects in 3D by using the ultraviolet (UV) light to cure layer-by-layer of a cross-sectional pattern (Hull, 1986; Murphy & Atala, 2014).

3D printing technology has evolved from additive manufacturing industry, food industry, to the biomedical field. Recently, the use of 3D printing has become a success in industries where quick prototyping, complex models for study, and variable biomedical applications (e.g., tissue scaffolding) are needed. 3D printing converts computer-assisted design (CAD) into a physical object in a single process, which is particularly attractive to the microfluidic field, owing to the low-cost, versatility, fast, and easy microscale fabrication capability. The application of 3D printing in microfluidic technology has shown tremendous potential in developing tissue engineering (Zhu, Hamilton, Vasquez, & He, 2019), sample preparation techniques (Ji & et al., 2018; Li, Smejkal, Macdonald, Guijt, & Breadmore, 2017; Pranzo, Larizza, Filippini, & Percoco, 2018), cell processing (Idaszek et al., 2019; Liu, Hwang, Wang, Whang, & Chen, 2016), and biochemical detection (Pranzo et al., 2018), which can facilitate a paradigm shift in methodology used in studying complex biological systems. For instance, researchers use microfluidic platforms to exploit living cells in a variety of ways to restore, maintain, or enhance tissues and organs (G.L.N, 2002).

The 3D printing technology can be classified into three main groups, including scalable additive technology that can be employed for both macro- and microscale, 3D direct writing technology, and the hybrid processes, as summarized in Fig. 17.1. Among these three groups, scalable addictive technology has been recognized as a promising approach for true 3D manufacturing that can be employed efficiently in fabricating complex 3D components, such as the selective laser sintering (SLS), inkjet printing processes, fused deposition modeling (FDM) laminated object manufacturing (LOM) and stereolithography (SLA) (Vaezi, Seitz, & Yang, 2013).

In SLS, a high temperature laser is used to sinter layers of fine powders selectively. Once each layer is produced, a roller is used to spread a fresh layer of the powder on the bed and repeats until the part is completed (Subramanian, 1993). However, drawbacks of this technology include needing a vacuum chamber to prevent smaller powder corrosion especially for printing finer details and thinner layers, due to the high reactivity against humidity and oxygen using smaller particle size (Petsch et al., 2004).

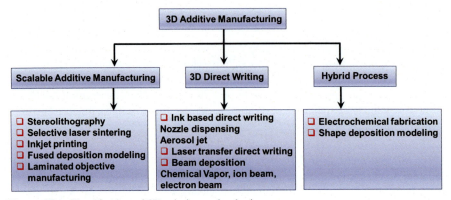

Figure 17.1 Classification of 3D printing technologies.

Additionally, the layers of the finer powders are very loose due to the interparticle forces, which require special collection approaches to prevent agglomerates. Thus, this technology requires high power consumption and has poor surface finished (Chua, Leong, & Lim, 2010).

The inkjet 3D printing technology was developed at Massachusetts Institute of Technology (MIT), which operates either in continuous or drop on demand (DoD) mode (Singh, Haverinen, Dhagat, & Jabbour, 2010; Waheed et al., 2016). The most common continuous mode is the use of light curable resin and a wax on paper printer (Waldbaur, Rapp, Länge, & Rapp, 2011). The wax is used to create a spatially constrained volume that is filled with the light curable resin. The fluids or ink materials are set, and this material turns into solid subsequently during the deposition process via cooling or solvent evaporation (Vaezi et al., 2013). The second layer is then applied directly on the top of the first layer and repeated until a complete building object is finished (Fig. 17.2(a)). In contrast, the droplets of binder materials for powder-based 3D printing are firstly deposited over the surface of a powder bed for sticking the powder particles together where the part will be shaped (Waldbaur et al., 2011). Afterward, lowering the powder bed using a piston allows fresh layer of the powder to be spread over the previous layer and repeat to complete (Fig. 17.2(b)). The advantages of this powder based droplets method include high speed for printing in seconds per layer, versatile, easy to operate, and no material waste. The powder materials, which are not printed during the cycle, can be reused. However, compared to SLS technology, this method has limited functional parts, and the building parts are much weaker. The materials have limited options and poor surface finishing which requires postprocessing protocols.

Scott Crump filed patents in 1989 for the FDM and cofounded the company Stratasys (USA) to commercialize the technology which is one of the most widely used additive manufacturing technology for rapid prototyping and production in the small

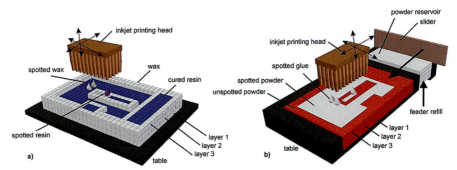

Figure 17.2 (a) Inkjet 3D printing—a movable array of nozzles is scanned across a table on which the part is manufactured. (b) Powder 3D printing—a movable nozzle array is used to spot droplets of glue into a bath of bulk material in powder form (Waldbaur et al., 2011). Permission of copyright from reference 19 was obtained from the Royal Society of Chemistry Rights Team.

scale. For FDM, a thermoplastic material is extruded through a high temperature nozzle to build a 3D model layer by layer (Pham & Gault, 1998). This nozzle is controlled by the computer, contains a temperature control unit that maintains the temperature of the thermoplastic material just above its melting point for melted thermoplastic material flowing through the nozzle and solidifying instantly in the desired area. Once a layer is built, the platform is lower and the extrusion nozzle deposits another layer for repeating until the desired object is formed.

SLA is the most essential 3D printing technology used for fabricating microfluidic devices, which is based on the UV-induced photopolymerization of light-sensitive polymers. The UV exposure is precisely controlled from a digital micromirors array or digital light projector (Derakhshanfar et al., 2018). Through selectively curing the photosensitive polymer resin in a layer-by-layer process, the polymerized and hardened resin layers additively build up to form 3D objects. No matter how complex the structure is, the entire pattern of the cross-sectional layer is projected. In turn, a precisely controlled microscale translational stage moves in the vertical direction to build up layers and form 3D objects, as illustrated in Fig. 17.3. One of the advantages of using SLA 3D printing technology in fabricating microfluidic devices is the high precision of 3D structures and surface finishing (Ho, Ng, Li, & Yoon, 2015; Horn & Harrysson, 2012; Gross, Erkal, Lockwood, Chen, & Spence, 2014), compared to other 3D printing technologies, such as the FDM and Polyjet 3D Printing. In addition to the acrylic photosensitive polymer, the SLA 3D printer can also print the light-sensitive hydrogels layer by layer rather than in straps or droplets (Salaris & Rosa, 2019). So far, the SLA 3D printing system can print layers with a thickness of 25 μm, and the minimum feature size as small as 25 μm. The typical printing time is less than an hour. Overall, the SLA resin materials are environment-friendly and can maintain high cell viability (>90%) (Carve & Wlodkowic, 2018).

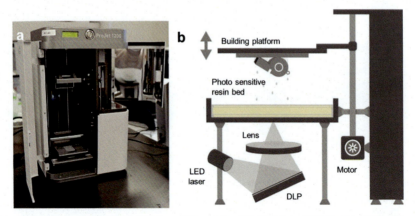

Figure 17.3 (a) A laptop-sized 3D stereolithography (SLA) printer (D3 ProJet 1200, 30-μm resolution); (b) The schematic illustration of SLA 3D printing mechanism.

It is important to note that 3D printed microfluidic devices could pose an issue related to the optical clarity from photohardenable resin material (Rusling, 2018; Urrios et al., 2016). Currently, there are no readily available printing materials that can replace the optical clarity and biocompatibility of PDMS. Although polyethylene glycol diacrylate-polyacrylic acid (PEGDA−PAA) hydrogels have been developed for 3D printing microfluidic devices, the printing resolution is over a few hundred microns and the optical clarity is still worse than PDMS material (Urrios et al., 2016). A printer with the ability to use PDMS, or the discovery of a suitable, printable material for making microfluidic devices is still under research and development (Macdonald et al., 2017). This chapter will focus on the 3D printing enabled microfabrication, including both monolithic, 3D-printed microfluidic device and 3D-printing of molds for casting PDMS microfluidic devices. The one-step 3D fabrication of molds does not require traditional soft photolithography and cleanroom usage, overcomes the lengthy and complicated protocols, and offers quick 3D microstructure prototyping. The 3D molding also allows the use of PDMS as the microfluidic material, which solves issues from using 3D resin with poor biocompatibility and optical clarity.

17.2 Direct 3D printing of microfluidic devices and applications

The direct 3D printing of monolithic microfluidic devices offers easy, cheap, and one-step fabrication for fast prototyping, which is particularly attractive for making microfluidic point-of-care biomedical devices. The benefit of utilizing 3D printing technology to prototype proof-of-concept (POC) devices is two-fold. Firstly, it allows manufacturers to increase design capability by increasing robustness and reducing fabrication cost and effort. Secondly, it allows rapid discovery of biological phenomena at the microfluidic level by making microfluidic technology readily and easily available to researchers unfamiliar with microfabrication, in turn, accelerating the scope of detection abilities in POC microfluidic devices. This chapter will discuss the key factors considered during direct 3D printing of microfluidic POC biomedical devices, including printing precision, microfluidic channel surface property, and 3D geometric influence on microfluidic profile. The application in anemia diagnosis is also demonstrated to show the capability of direct 3D printing of POC microfluidics.

17.2.1 Materials and methods

Three-dimensional design is always difficult within conventional microfabrication, due to complicated protocols for accurate alignment and multilayer bonding. Configured with smartphone solid modeling app (AutoCAD 360), a laptop-sized 3D printer (D3 ProJet 1200, 30-μm resolution) was used for fabrication of monolithic microfluidic chips. VisiJetFTX Clear resin consisting of triethylene glycol diacrylate, isobornyl methacrylate, and 2%−3% photoinitiator phenylbis (2,4,6-trimethylbenzoyl)-phosphine oxide was used to produce transparent 3D microfluidic chips per vendor's instruction. Printed 3D devices were cleaned using isopropyl alcohol and blown dry. The uncured resin within microchannel was flushed out by an air compressor. A field emission scanning electron microscope (SEM) characterized printed microstructures using a focus ion beam (FEI Versa) after gold sputtering coating in 20-nm thickness. Ethylene glycol chemistry was used to develop the hydrophilic surface of 3D printed devices: 1.82 M potassium hydroxide (KOH) was mixed into pure ethylene glycol solution (Sigma-Aldrich, anhydrous, 99.8%) and used to soak 3D devices at 55°C for 2 h. When needed, we also can bond the 3D printed objects with glass materials when 3% of photoinitiator 2-(2-bromoisobutyryloxy)ethyl methacrylate (BrMA, Sigma-Aldrich) was introduced into clear resin and mixed. The Silane-Prep glass slides pretreated with aminoalkylsilane (Sigma-Aldrich) were used to bond the 3D printed layer with open channels and microstructures. The clean 3D layer annealed very well with the glass slides. The two annealed layers were then exposed to 365-UV for 8 min. The bonding was irreversible via covalent chemical bond.

17.2.2 Precision of direct 3D printing approach

In this work, the desktop size D3 ProJet 1200 3D printer was used, which has a build area of 43 mm × 27 mm × 150 mm and provides a physical pixel size of 56 μm × 30 μm. A number of basic microstructures and three monolithic microfluidic mixing devices were directly 3D printed to evaluate printing capability and quality. The SEM imaging was used to characterize the precision of direct 3D printing microfabrication approach as shown in Fig. 17.4. Three monolithic microfluidic mixers were readily printed out in less than 10 min, as shown in Fig. 17.4(a–c). A smooth surface was observed in the microchannel and circular chamber. Other basic microstructures often used in microfluidic chips were also SEM imaged, including postarrays (Fig. 17.4(d) and (e)), microwells (Fig. 17.4(f)), and a D-shaped hollow microchannel. Close examination of SEM images revealed additional printing properties, and printing layers were observed due to the minimum pixel resolution (30 μm), such as the "stair"-looking of the D-shaped microchannel shown in Fig. 17.4(g) (diameter of 200 μm). Although a smaller channel could be printed, complete removal of uncured resin was difficult, due to high backpressure for cleaning. In order to avoid high backpressure for cleaning hollow channels, a bonding protocol was developed to attach a 3D printed open channel layer to a glass slide (Fig. 17.4(h)). An open channel with a diameter of 50 μm can be printed, resulting in a closed hollow microchannel. The bonding protocol follows the principle of saline chemistry by forming covalent chemical bonds between the glass surface and resin surface. As shown in Fig. 17.4(h), the ring-shaped channel in 50-μm deep and wide was bonded to a glass slide without leakage observed, which was proven by running through a red dye solution. This protocol could extend 3D printer capability for printing smaller hollow microchannels below 200 μm i.d.

17.2.3 Surface property of 3D-printed microfluidic devices

After 3D printing, the cured resin was slightly hydrophobic, as indicated by measuring contact angles (Fig. 17.2(a), $\Theta = 64$ degrees). A simple chemistry protocol can convert

3D printed microfluidic devices and applications

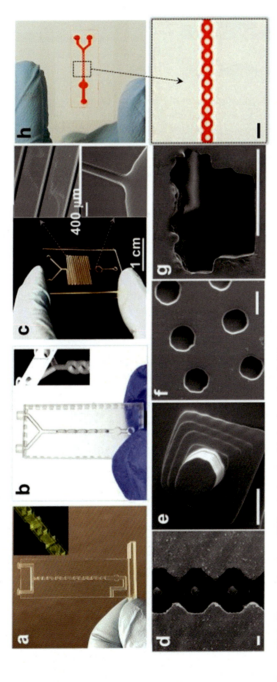

Figure 17.4 Characterization of 3D printing for fabricating microfluidic mixers: (a) Split and recombination (SAR) microfluidic mixer, (b) 3D ring-shaped micromixer, (c) and serpentine micromixer. Channel diameter is ∼500 μm. Scanning electron microscope (SEM) imaging was used to characterize variable 3D-printed microstructures: (d) posts in curved microfluidic channel, (e) pyramid postarrays, (f) microwells, and (g) a D-shaped hollow microchannel. Scale bar: 200 μm. (h) The bonded layer of a 3D-printed open channel with a glass slide. Permission of copyright from Plevniak, Campbell, Myers, Hodges, and He (2016) was obtained from the American Institute of Physics Publisher.

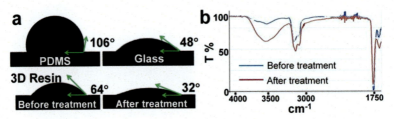

Figure 17.5 (a) Hydrophilic surface treatment of 3D-printed microfluidic chip for capillary-driven automixing; the contact angle (θ) of deionized (DI) water shows the hydrophilicity of polydimethylsiloxane (PDMS), glass, and printed resin before and after treatment. (b) Fourier transform infrared spectroscopy (FTIR) analysis of surface chemistry of 3D printed resin before and after surface treatment.
Permission of copyright from Plevniak et al. (2016) was obtained from the American Institute of Physics Publisher.

the 3D printed objects into hydrophilic property. The 3D printed micromixer chip was immersed into a pure ethylene glycol solution containing 1.82 M KOH and incubated at 55°C for 2 h. The contact angle of deionized (DI) water was measured to note the hydrophilicity of 3D printed microfluidic chip as compared to PDMS and glass materials. As shown in Fig. 17.5(a), hydrophilicity was significantly improved (θ = 32 degrees, RSD = 4.6%, n = 10), providing a stable capillary-driven force for inducing automixing. Hydrophilically treated 3D chip also can be stored in water solution for reuse for several days, thereby maintaining a stable surface chemistry. The surface chemistry was further characterized using Fourier Transform Infrared Spectroscopy (FTIR). Untreated surface spectra failed to show an OH stretch between 3000 and 3750 cm^{-1} (Fig. 17.5(b)) compared to treated 3D printing material which exhibits strong OH stretches, indicating a strong hydrophilic surface property.

17.2.4 3D geometric influence on microfluidic profile

Flow behaviors in several 3D-printed microfluidic channels and microstructures were studied in order to develop an effective capillary force driven automixing using 3D printed microfluidic mixer. The flow in microfluidic channels is characterized by low Reynold's numbers, which indicates the flow regime is laminar. The automixing flow rate is determined by a force balance between the capillary force and the frictional force. The capillary force can be represented based on the Young–Laplace equation:

$$\Delta P = \frac{4\sigma \cos \theta}{D} \qquad (17.1)$$

where ΔP is pressure drop, σ is surface tension, θ is the contact angle, and D is the channel diameter. The frictional drag force for laminar flow in a round channel can be represented by:

$$\Delta P = \frac{64}{Re} \times \frac{L}{D} \times \frac{\overline{V}^2}{2} \times \rho \qquad (17.2)$$

where Re is the Reynold's number ($\rho VD/\mu$), μ is the dynamic viscosity of the fluid, L is wetted length, V is flow velocity, and ρ is density. By equating frictional force to capillary force based on above two equations, we can determine the automixing velocity by the following relation:

$$\overline{V} = \frac{D\sigma \cos\theta}{8\,\mu L} \qquad (17.3)$$

Therefore, the capillary-force induced flow rate is governed by geometry, surface properties, and fluid profile properties. At a given fluid, geometry or characteristic dimension of microfluidic channel in given surface chemistry dominates the capillary-force induced flow rate. The velocity of capillary flow is fast at short wetted lengths while slow at long wetted lengths. On the other hand, at small diameters, the flow rate tends to be extremely slow due to the drag force overpowering the surface force. Hence, the theoretical analysis gives an applicable dimension regime of microchannels for a capillary force driven flow, ranging from ~100 μm to 2 mm in diameter with Reynold's numbers below 500. The typical capillary flow rate in a microchannel with 500 μm in diameter and 22 mm in wetted length is about 20 μL/s.

Based on above theoretical analysis, three microfluidic mixers with characteristic size of 500 μm in microchannel diameter were 3D printed: split and recombination (SAR) (Fig. 17.6(a)), serpentine channel (Fig. 17.6(b)), and ring channel (Fig. 17.6(c)). All three of these designs have Bo numbers less than 1, indicating capillary force is dominant, and have Reynold's numbers ranging from 11 to ~450. The computational fluid dynamics (CFD) modeling was used to evaluate the flow profile and automixing performance in these three 3D printed microfluidic mixer. If no 3D geometric influence as a straight flow-through channel, the two flows were unable to mix. By inclusion of SAR units in the straight flow-through channel, mixing can be completed after passing into view-window of SAR micromixer. Although ring channel directed flow to split and recombine, two flows were unable to crossover and continue to flow side-by-side. Thus, a novel design by rotating the ring structure 90° in the x-y plane with respect to the "Y" inlet was introduced (see Fig. 17.6(d), fourth figure), which led to the complete mixing due to the 3D geometric influence on flow split and causing interfaces to travel through the ring section. The food dyes in red and blue were used to experimentally demonstrate the automixing process, and the experimental results are consistent with simulation results (Fig. 17.6(e) and (f)).

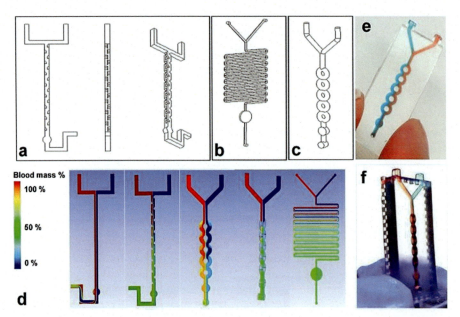

Figure 17.6 Design of three microfluidic mixers: (a) Split and recombination (SAR), (b) serpentine channel, and (c) ring-shaped channel. Channel diameter was ∼500 μm. (d) 3D computational fluid dynamics (CFD) simulation of blood mixing profile in three micromixers: red flow is blood mixed with aqueous solution (blue); green color indicates complete mixing. (e) Experimental image of 3D printed planner micromixer showing incomplete mixing under capillary force using colored dye solutions. (f) Experimental image of 3D printed, 3D-structured micromixer showing efficient mixing within 1s using colored dye solutions. Permission of copyright from Plevniak et al. (2016) was obtained from the American Institute of Physics Publisher.

17.2.5 Direct 3D printing of POC microfluidic device for anemia diagnosis

The automixing of reagents with blood via the capillary force can be very useful in point-of-care diagnosis using microfluidic devices, without requiring external pumps or power supply. A color-scale assay for rapid detection of blood hemoglobin level was developed using such POC microfluidic mixer, which was demonstrated for POC diagnosis and self-management of anemia. The current gold standard for anemia diagnosis is a complete blood count (CBC) using a hematology analyzer via venous blood, which requires a blood draw by a trained phlebotomist and needs electrical power to operate in centralized hospitals or clinics (Neufeld et al., 2019). Direct 3D printing enabled microfabrication allows the flexibility in making microfluidic POC devices in ultralow cost (∼$ 0.5 per test). Combined with smartphone camera and wireless function, this hemoglobin detection method represents a key step toward

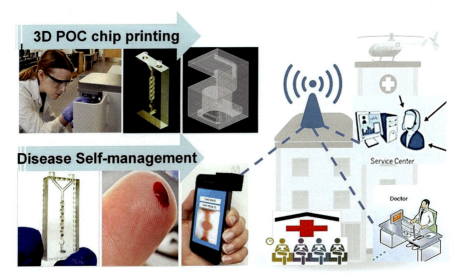

Figure 17.7 Low-cost, smartphone-based, 3D-printed proof-of-concept (POC) microfluidic chip for rapid diagnosis of anemia in 60 s.
Permission of copyright from Plevniak et al. (2016) was obtained from the American Institute of Physics Publisher.

advanced mobile health care for control of anemia (Fig. 17.7), which can eliminate substantial expenses related to clinic visits and facility resources, thereby providing dynamic access to high-quality health care.

The visual readout via smartphone camera from the micromixer reaction chamber was based on the 3,3′,5,5′-TMB (tetramethylbenzidine) oxidation—reduction reaction with blood Hgb as a catalyst (Levinson & Goldman, 1982). Depending on the ratio of charge transfer status of TMB, the resultant visual colors were blue, green, yellow, orange, or red (Fig. 17.8(a)) (Tyburski et al., 2014). The color images collected from an android phone with a micromixer housing system were consistently obtained in order to define region of interest (ROI) and quantitative red green blue (RGB) analysis. A rotated ring channel design was used to rapidly mix blood with oxidant reagents in 1s for observing color development. The standard hemoglobin protein spiked in diluted blood was used to establish calibration curve for correlating colorscales and validated by photospectrometer measurements for quantitative measurement of Hgb concentrations (Fig. 17.8(b)). Absorbance peaks of Hgb at 540 and 575 nm showed linear increase with increased Hgb concentrations. Combined with smartphone color-scale detection and analysis, point-of-care diagnosis of anemia from finger-prick blood was demonstrated using a training set of patient blood ($n_{anemia} = 16$, $n_{healthy} = 6$). The results showed consistent measurements of blood hemoglobin levels (a.u.c. = 0.97) and comparable diagnostic sensitivity and specificity, compared to standard clinical hematology analyzer (Fig. 17.8(c) and (d)).

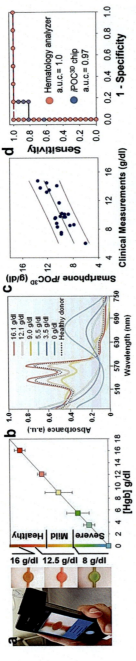

Figure 17.8 (a) Quantitative measurement of Hgb levels for color-scale anemia diagnosis using smartphone system via capillary-driven automixing of finger-prick blood. The calibration curve is established by measuring standard hemoglobin proteins spiked in diluted blood in 0, 5.5, 8.0, 9.0, 12.5, 16.0 g/dL, and correlated with color scale. (b) Spectrophotometric analysis of Hgb levels in blood reaction mixture for validating readout; Hgb peaks are at 540 and 575 nm, and tetramethylbenzidine (TMB) peak is at 630 nm. Blood from a healthy donor is indicated in the black dashed line. (c) Pilot study of anemia diagnosis ($n_{anemia} = 16$, $n_{healthy} = 6$) and the correlation of smartphone measurements with clinical standard hematology analyzer measurements using Durbin–Watson Statistic Normality Test with 95% confidence interval ($r = 0.8$, $P < .0001$). (d) Receiver operating characteristic (ROC) analysis of diagnostic accuracy using smartphone system, compared with standard clinical measurements using hematology analyzer. Permission of copyright from Plevniak et al. (2016) was obtained from the American Institute of Physics Publisher.

Capable of 3D fabrication flexibility and smartphone compatibility, this work presents a novel diagnostic strategy for advancing personalized anemia diagnosis and management, which could leverage global accessibility to high-quality health care.

17.3 3D-printing of molds for fabricating PDMS microfluidic devices and applications

Due to the limited 3D printing resolution, constructing complex 3D structures in microscale is still challenging. Thus, the 3D printing of molds for fabricating PDMS microfluidic devices is more attractive, which maintains the advantages of using PDMS materials, meanwhile, allows constructing complicated 3D microstructures for assembling into advanced microfluidic devices. This approach extended the capability and flexibility for 3D additive manufacturing by introducing geometrics-enabled structural functionality. For POC, the 3D fabrication and assembling of a micro 3D cell culture device with function of cell electrotransfection was demonstrated. The PDMS parts were molded from 3D-printed molds and assembled into a 3D-cell culture chamber, which connects arrays of perfusion channels and electrodes for cell transfection. Intracellular delivery of regulatory or therapeutic targets into the cell is crucial for pharmacology study as well as the tissue engineering and regenerative medicine (Chew, 2019). Among various delivery approaches such as using chemicals, ultrasound, and microneedle, electrotransfection has gained increasing popularity, due to its safe (chemical free) and effective transfection, and no restrictions on cell types (Suarez & McElwain, 2010; Xu & Jiang, 2011). To date, the investigation of electroporation on 3D cultured cells and tissues has not been explored in the microfluidic platform yet (Xu & Jiang, 2011). The benchtop method for electroporation study of 3D cells embedded in scaffolds showed very low transfection efficiency ($\sim 5\%$) (Suarez & McElwain, 2010). Therefore, a novel 3D microfluidic electrotransfection system will provide facile, fast, and automated control for electrotransfection of 3D cultured cells with high efficiency, which can be employed in tissue engineering and gene therapy.

17.3.1 Materials and methods

3D structures were designed and drawn by SOLIDWORKS 2017. The resin mold containing microstructures were printed by a laptop-sized 3D printer (D3 ProJet 1200, 30-μm resolution) using VisiJetFTX Clear resin (3D systems) for PDMS device production. The clear resin consists of triethylene glycol diacrylate, isobornyl methacrylate, and 2%−3% photoinitiator phenylbis (2,4,6-trimethylbenzoyl)-phosphine oxide as described in the product information. Freshly printed molds were cleaned using isopropyl alcohol in sonication and followed with 30-min postcure under UV light. A 20-nm thick palladium or gold coating was deposited onto the surface of the 3D-printed mold using a sputter coater (DENTON, DESK II). Prior to molding, the coated molds were conditioned with the surfactant solution (20% tween 20 in

80% isopropanol) for forming a dynamic micellar layer on the metal surface to facilitate the peel-off of polymer microstructures. PDMS was prepared using the standard 10:1 (base to curing agent) ratio. The PDMS mixture was degassed before pouring into the 3D-printed molds and then baked in 40°C for 12 h. The 3D printed molds are reusable after cleaning and conditioning. After the surface activation of molded PDMS pieces using a handheld corona discharge treater (Electro-Technic Product, Chicago), the PDMS blocks were then assembled and bound as the 3D μ-electrotransfection device (Fig. 17.9). The assembling was conducted on a flat stage under the microscope (here, we use the PDMS port creator stage, CorSolutions Inc.) which can guide the alignment easily. The assembled 3D μ-electrotransfection device was then bound to a glass slide to complete the fabrication.

17.3.2 3D-printing enabled microassembling of 3D μ-electrotransfection system

To build a 3D microfluidic electrotransfection system that is capable of uniform 3D electric field distribution as well as the effective 3D cell culture, the 3D-printing enabled microassembling approach was introduced as shown in Fig. 17.9. Conventional microfabrication approach is unable to construct such 3D microstructures, due to complicated protocols for accurate alignment and multilayer bonding. It is very challenging to 3D print monolithic microstructures, particularly microscale hollow channels. Thus, a 3D-printing assisted molding approach was introduced to cast PDMS parts as the LEGO blocks for assembling into a more complicated 3D device. As illustrated in Fig. 17.9(a), two designed parts were assembled as one transfer mold for PDMS molding. The assembled mold is detachable for easily releasing PDMS parts. The PDMS polymer was completely cured in the mold, and no microstructural defects were identified during the demolding process. Worth to mention that the high-temperature baking (e.g., > 40°C) should be avoided as the high temperature may cause physical structural distortion of 3D printed resin. The molded PDMS polymer replicates microstructures as a single assembling unit shown in Fig. 17.9(c) and (d). After four units assembling with permanent bonding using surface plasma treatment, the 3D microfluidic electrotransfection device can be formed with four main vertical microchannels (~350 μm) each connected with five horizontal microchannels (~200 μm) (Fig. 17.9(a)). To facilitate the precise production of microstructures, sputtering Ba or Au coating was deposited onto the mold surface in 20-nm thick as shown in Fig. 17.9(b) and (c). The final assembled device can be bound onto a glass slide after surface plasma treatment. The electrodes were fixed in a 3D printed holder (Fig. 17.9(e)), which fits the central culture chamber for electroporating 3D cultured cells (Fig. 17.9(f)). Four flat electrodes are mounted into the 3D culture chamber via a 3D-printed holder and controlled by a programmable power sequencer for multidirectional electric frequency scanning (3D μ-electro-transfection). This multidirectional scanning not only can create transient pores all over the cell membrane but also can generate local oscillation for enhancing mass transport and improving cell transfection efficiency.

3D printed microfluidic devices and applications 673

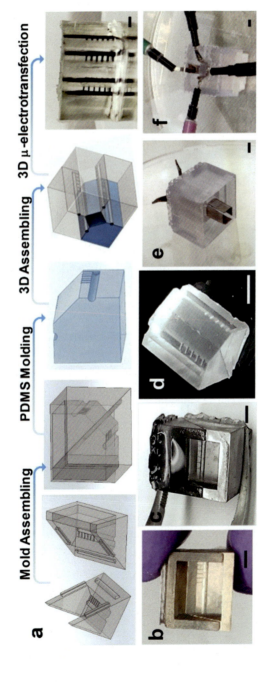

Figure 17.9 3D printing assisted assembling for building 3D μ-electroporation system. (a) The concept illustration of 3D printing, molding, and assembling. The last image shows the real four-piece assembled device bound to a glass slide with channels filled in black dye. The scale bar is 1 mm. (b) 3D printed mold (2 pieces assembled) with the surface deposited by 20-nm Au. The scale bar is 2 mm. (c) The mold (with 20-nm Ba coating) filled with polydimethylsiloxane (PDMS) and the molded PDMS part is shown in figure d. The scale bar is 2 mm. (e) Four electrodes mounted in a 3D printed holder. The scale bar is 2 mm. (f) The setup of four electrodes on top of cell culture chip for multidimensional electric frequency scanning. The electrodes are just fitting to the size of the culture chamber. The scale bar is 2 mm.
Permission of copyright from Zhu et al. (2019) was obtained from the Royal Society of Chemistry Rights Team.

17.3.3 3D μ-electrotransfection system for 3D cell culture and cellular engineering

Unlike the 3D cell culture in the well plate where the medium exchange only takes place from the top of well plates, the 3D-assembled μ-electrotransfection system allows multidirectional diffusion of the fresh medium from both the top of cell matrix and the side of microchannel arrays surrounded the culture chamber in vertical and horizontal directions (Fig. 17.10(a)). Such 3D perfusion microchannel network allows better nutrients support and waste exchange needed for the effective growth of 3D cells and tissues. The 3D perfusion microchannel network significantly improves the medium exchange, compared to the conventional 3D cell culture in the well plate. Due to high encapsulation stability, cell attachability, and biocompatibility, the peptide hydrogel was used as the scaffold for 3D cell growth in developed 3D μ-electrotransfection system shown in Fig. 17.10(a).

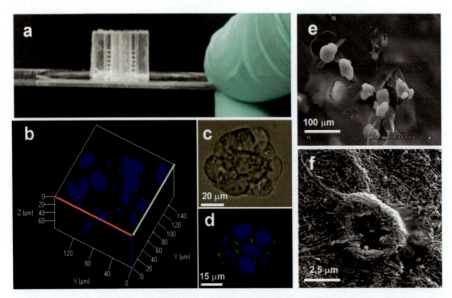

Figure 17.10 On-chip 3D cell culture and microscopy characterization. (a) Assembled polydimethylsiloxane (PDMS) chip bound to a glass slide for cell culture. (b) Distribution of 3D-cultured HeLa cell spheroids in peptide hydrogel under confocal microscope imaging. Nuclear DNA was stained by Hoechst. (c) The close look of a single 3D cell spheroid in bright field and in the fluorescence channels in d. The cell membrane was stained by fluorescein isothiocyanate (FITC) conjugated antibody-dye and the nuclear DNA was stained by Hoechst. (e) Scanning electron microscope (SEM) imaging the cell spheroid distribution and the single spheroid interacting with peptide fibers in (f).
Permission of copyright from Zhu et al. (2019) was obtained from the Royal Society of Chemistry Rights Team.

Upon crosslinking, the hydrogel forms a porous matrix with the pore size ranged from 200 to 400 nm, which gives a stable physical support for 3D cell growth as imaged in Fig. 17.10(e) and (f). The dense spheroid distribution in peptide hydrogel matrix in 3D as well as the morphology of a single spheroid has been characterized by confocal microscopy shown in Fig. 17.10(b−d). The side views demonstrated that cells are distributed along with the height of the cell chamber. The individual 3D spheroid with the size of ∼50 μm was observed after culturing for 4−5 days which composes of ∼10 cells as shown in Fig. 17.10(c) and (d). Such morphology characterization indicates that 3D μ-electrotransfection system provides suitable microenvironment for growing 3D cells and tissues, which is enabled by the implementation of 3D perfusion microchannels.

To assess the transfection efficiency and cell viability of 3D μ-electrotransfection system, a plasmid DNA (pAcGFP1-C1) encoding green fluorescence protein (GFP) was electroporated into 3D cultured HeLa cells. For conventional electrotransfection of 2D cell suspension, the critical electric field needs to reach a value in a range from 100 to 1000 V/cm (depending on cell size and electric field property) to disrupt cell membrane and ensure the reversible electroporation (Marrero & Heller, 2012; Wasungu, Escoffre, Valette, Teissie, & Rols, 2009). In contrast, delivery of plasmid directly to 3D cells embedded in the extracellular matrix has not been studied elsewhere, which is critical to mimic in vivo like tissue microenvironment. Thus, the key parameters that control the electroporation efficiency, including electric field strength, plasmid concentration, pulse duration, and duty cycles, were optimized as shown in Fig. 17.11(a−d). The electrotransfection experiments were carried out after the cells were seeded for 48 h. Fig. 17.11(h−e) show a typical image and flow cytometry analysis of 3D cultured cells after electrotransfection in the 3D-molded microfluidic electrotransfection system. The confocal microscopic imaging in Fig. 17.11(e−g) display a transfected 3D cell spheroid with a diameter around 60 μm. With a voltage of 300 V in multidirectional field scanning (equal to an electric field of 750 V/cm), 2.5% GFP expressed cells were identified from the total cell population with cell viability of ∼95% by flow cytometry analysis. The transfection efficiency was increasing while increasing the applied voltage from 300 to 600 V. However, the cell viability was decreased from ∼96% to ∼84%, due to more dead cells caused by the high voltage, which in turn decreases the transfection efficiency with a higher voltage of 600 V (1500 V/cm). Either increasing the pulse duration or adding more duty cycles can lead to an increase of transfection efficiency, but the dead cells were dramatically increased accordingly, due to the harsh electric interruption of cell membrane irreversibly. Applying four duty cycles lead to the 15.6% transfection efficiency but with 58.3% cell viability. To find the balance between the transfection efficiency and cell viability for the best transfection outcome, the optimized voltage is 500 V with ∼120 μg/mL plasmid concentration, which showed a more important role in the control of good cell viability compared to the electric duty cycle and pulse. Increasing the plasmid concentration will create more contact opportunities between cells and plasmids,

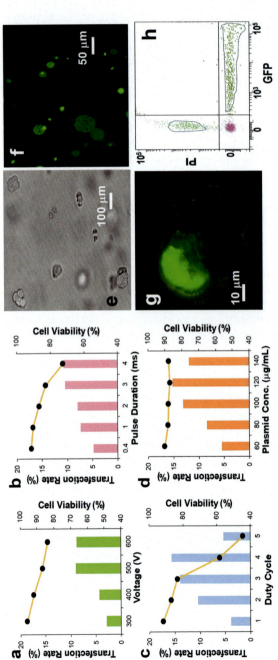

Figure 17.11 Electro delivery of GFP plasmid to 3D cultured HeLa cell spheroid within peptide hydrogel. (a) Investigation of the influence of transfection voltage on the transfection rate and cell viability. The plasmid concentration is 100 μg/mL, the pulse duration is 2 ms, and the duty cycle is 2. (b) Investigation of the influence of pulse duration on the transfection rate and cell viability. The plasmid concentration is 100 μg/mL, the transfection voltage is 500 V. (c) Investigation of the influence of duty cycle on the transfection rate and cell viability. The plasmid concentration is 100 μg/mL, the pulse duration is 3 ms, and the transfection voltage is 500 V. (d) Investigation of the influence of plasmid concentration on the transfection rate and cell viability. The pulse duration is 3 ms, the duty cycle is 3, and the transfection voltage is 500 V. The yellow dot lines in figure (a–d) indicate the cell viability. (e) Electroporated sample under the bright field and fluorescein isothiocyanate (FITC) channel in f. The transfection voltage was 500 V with a pulses duration of 3 ms for each direction, at the frequency of 1 Hz, and three duty cycles. (g) Confocal image of a transfected cell spheroid. (h) Representative flow cytometry graph to evaluate the green fluorescent protein (GFP) positive cell and propidium iodide (PI) labeling positive cell for estimating cell transfection efficiency and cell viability. The transfection voltage was 500 V with a pulses duration of 3 ms for each direction, at the frequency of 1 Hz, and three duty cycles. The cell transfection efficiency is 13.5% with 85% cell viability.

Permission of copyright from Zhu et al. (2019) was obtained from the Royal Society of Chemistry Rights Team.

reflecting an increasing number of transfected cells. The optimized conditions were chosen as 3 ms pulse duration, three duty cycles and transfection voltage of 500 V. Using the optimal plasmid concentration of ~120 μg/mL, 15.2% transfection efficiency with 87.1% cell viability can be achieved, which is 3-fold increase than currently reported benchtop 3D electrotransfection method with better cell viability (Murakami & Sunada, 2011). However, continuously increasing plasmid DNA concentration did not result in higher transfection efficiency. This observation agrees to the previous report that there is a maximum plasmid concentration for gene delivery. Compared to 2D cell transfection, the optimal plasmid concentration for 3D cell electroporation is much higher (110 vs. 40 μg/mL) (Murakami & Sunada, 2011). This is attributed to the porous peptide hydrogel matrix which limits the travel of plasmid to cells and requires more amount of plasmid to enhance contact opportunities with cells. In addition to the scaffold matrix effect, the 3D cell spheroid is much bigger than an individual cell and the plasmid needs to travel a long distance to reach the cells inside the cluster, which makes the gene delivery even difficult. Herein, the developed 3D electric field scanning strategy could improve mass transport to address this challenge.

17.4 Conclusions and future trends

3D printing has been increasingly applied in the fabrication of microfluidic devices. In this chapter, we discussed two microfabrication approaches for making microfluidic devices utilizing SLA 3D printing technology: (I) Direct SLA printing of channels and structures of a monolithic microfluidic POC device; (II) Indirect fabrication, utilizing SLA 3D printed molds for PDMS-based microfluidic device replication. Each microfabrication approach was demonstrated with applications in microfluidic POC diagnosis and cellular electrotransfection, respectively. The conventional microfabrication utilizes specialized techniques and infrastructure, making it difficult to access and time-consuming. 3D printing technology substantially simplify this microfabrication process with much lower cost.

Although the printing precision and material (3D resin) limitations are still not fully meeting the requirements from microfluidic technology, the new 3D printing technology is developing rapidly. Some specialized 3D printers for microfluidic device fabrication exclusively have been on market, such as Elveflow microfluidic 3D printer and Cellink LumenX 3D printer. However, current 3D printing precision is still above 50 μm and hard to print microscale hollow channels. For some 3D SLA printer with better printing resolution, the price is very high and not affordable for general users. Thus, 3D printing is still unable to completely replace complicated lithography process when submicron resolution is required. For future development, the high precision 3D printer with mass production capability will be on high demand, and represent the trend of novel microfabrication of microfluidic devices.

References

Carve, M., & Wlodkowic, D. (2018). 3D-Printed chips: Compatibility of additive manufacturing photopolymeric substrata with biological applications. *Micromachines, 9*.

Chew, S. Y. (2019). Sequential drug/gene delivery in tissue engineering & regenerative medicine. *Advanced Drug Delivery Reviews, 149–150*, 1.

Chua, C. K., Leong, K. F., & Lim, C. S. (2010). *Rapid prototyping: Principles and applications (with companion CD-ROM)*. World Scientific Publishing Company.

Derakhshanfar, S., et al. (2018). 3D bioprinting for biomedical devices and tissue engineering: A review of recent trends and advances. *Bioactive Materials, 3*, 144–156.

G.L.N, G. (2002). Tissue engineering- current challenges and expanding oppotunities. *Science, 295*, 1009.

Gross, B. C., Erkal, J. L., Lockwood, S. Y., Chen, C., & Spence, D. M. (2014). *Evaluation of 3D printing and its potential impact on biotechnology and the chemical sciences*. ACS Publications.

Ho, C. M., Ng, S. H., Li, K. H., & Yoon, Y. J. (2015). 3D printed microfluidics for biological applications. *Lab on a Chip, 15*, 3627–3637.

Horn, T. J., & Harrysson, O. L. (2012). Overview of current additive manufacturing technologies and selected applications. *Science Progress, 95*, 255–282.

Hull, C. W. (1986). *Apparatus for production of three-dimensional objects by stereolithography*. Google Patents.

Idaszek, J., et al. (2019). 3D bioprinting of hydrogel constructs with cell and material gradients for the regeneration of full-thickness chondral defect using a microfluidic printing head. *Biofabrication, 11*, 044101.

Ji, Q., et al. (2018). A modular microfluidic device via multimaterial 3D printing for emulsion generation. *Scientific Reports, 8*, 4791.

Levinson, S. S., & Goldman, J. (1982). Measuring hemoglobin in plasma by reaction with tetramethylbenzidine. *Clinical Chemistry, 28*, 471–474.

Li, F., Smejkal, P., Macdonald, N. P., Guijt, R. M., & Breadmore, M. C. (2017). One-step fabrication of a microfluidic device with an integrated membrane and embedded reagents by multimaterial 3D printing. *Analytical Chemistry, 89*, 4701–4707.

Liu, J., Hwang, H. H., Wang, P., Whang, G., & Chen, S. (2016). Direct 3D-printing of cell-laden constructs in microfluidic architectures. *Lab on a Chip, 16*, 1430–1438.

Macdonald, N. P., et al. (2017). Comparing microfluidic performance of three-dimensional (3D) printing platforms. *Analytical Chemistry, 89*, 3858–3866.

Manz, A., Graber, N., & Widmer, H. M. (1990). Miniaturized total chemical-analysis systems - a novel concept for chemical sensing. *Sensors and Actuators B: Chemical, 1*, 244–248.

Marrero, B., & Heller, R. (2012). The use of an in vitro 3D melanoma model to predict in vivo plasmid transfection using electroporation. *Biomaterials, 33*, 3036–3046.

Murakami, T., & Sunada, Y. (2011). Plasmid DNA gene therapy by electroporation: Principles and recent advances. *Current Gene Therapy, 11*, 447–456.

Murphy, S. V., & Atala, A. (2014). 3D bioprinting of tissues and organs. *Nature Biotechnology, 32*, 773–785.

Neufeld, L. M., et al. (2019). Hemoglobin concentration and anemia diagnosis in venous and capillary blood: Biological basis and policy implications. *Annals of the New York Academy of Sciences, 1450*, 172–189.

Petsch, T., et al. (2004). Industrial laser micro sintering. In *International congress on applications of lasers & electro-optics* (Vol. 2004)Laser Institute of America. M705.

Pham, D. T., & Gault, R. S. (1998). A comparison of rapid prototyping technologies. *International Journal of Machine Tools and Manufacture, 38*, 1257−1287.

Plevniak, K., Campbell, M., Myers, T., Hodges, A., & He, M. (2016). 3D printed auto-mixing chip enables rapid smartphone diagnosis of anemia. *Biomicrofluidics, 10*, 054113.

Pranzo, D., Larizza, P., Filippini, D., & Percoco, G. (2018). Extrusion-based 3D printing of microfluidic devices for chemical and biomedical applications: A topical review. *Micromachines, 9*.

Rusling, J. F. (2018). Developing microfluidic sensing devices using 3D printing. *ACS Sensors, 3*, 522−526.

Salaris, F., & Rosa, A. (2019). Construction of 3D in vitro models by bioprinting human pluripotent stem cells: Challenges and opportunities. *Brain Research, 1723*, 146393.

Singh, M., Haverinen, H. M., Dhagat, P., & Jabbour, G. E. (2010). Inkjet printing—process and its applications. *Advanced Materials, 22*, 673−685.

Suarez, C. E., & McElwain, T. F. (2010). Transfection systems for *Babesia bovis*: A review of methods for the transient and stable expression of exogenous genes. *Veterinary Parasitology, 167*, 205−215.

Subramanian, K. (1993). Selective laser sintering of A1203. In *1993 international solid freeform fabrication symposium*.

Tyburski, E. A., et al. (2014). Disposable platform provides visual and color-based point-of-care anemia self-testing. *Journal of Clinical Investigation, 124*, 4387−4394.

Urrios, A., et al. (2016). 3D-printing of transparent bio-microfluidic devices in PEG-DA. *Lab on a Chip, 16*, 2287−2294.

Vaezi, M., Seitz, H., & Yang, S. (2013). A review on 3D micro-additive manufacturing technologies. *International Journal of Advanced Manufacturing Technology, 67*, 1721−1754.

Waheed, S., et al. (2016). 3D printed microfluidic devices: Enablers and barriers. *Lab on a Chip, 16*, 1993−2013.

Waldbaur, A., Rapp, H., Länge, K., & Rapp, B. E. (2011). Let there be chip—towards rapid prototyping of microfluidic devices: One-step manufacturing processes. *Analytical Methods, 3*, 2681−2716.

Wasungu, L., Escoffre, J. M., Valette, A., Teissie, J., & Rols, M. P. (2009). A 3D in vitro spheroid model as a way to study the mechanisms of electroporation. *International Journal of Pharmaceutics, 379*, 278−284.

Webster, A., Greenman, J., & Haswell, S. J. (2011). Development of microfluidic devices for biomedical and clinical application. *Journal of Chemical Technology and Biotechnology, 86*, 10−17.

Xia, Y., & Whitesides, G. M. (1998). Soft lithography. *Angewandte Chemie International Edition in English, 37*, 550−575.

Xu, H., & Jiang, J. (2011). Application of microfluidics in cell transfection: A review. *Sheng Wu Gong Cheng Xue Bao, 27*, 1417−1427.

Zhu, Q., Hamilton, M., Vasquez, B., & He, M. (2019). 3D-printing enabled micro-assembly of a microfluidic electroporation system for 3D tissue engineering. *Lab on a Chip, 19*, 2362−2372.

Index

Note: 'Page numbers followed by "*f*" indicate figures and "*t*" indicate tables.'

A

Ablative methodologies, 238
Absorption, Distribution, Metabolism, Elimination, and Toxicology (ADMET), 284
Acetaminophen (ACT), 45
Acetic acid (CH$_3$COOH), 19
Acetylcholinesterase (AChE), 578
Acoustic(s), 126, 143—152
   basic principles of acoustic fluid and particle manipulation, 144—145
   bulk ultrasonic vibration, 145—147
   fluid, 144—145
   mechanisms, 357—360
      acoustic radiation force, 357—359
      acoustophoretic devices, 359—360
   surface acoustic waves, 147—152
Acoustofluidics. *See* Ultrasonic standing waves technology (USW technology)
Acoustophoresis, 144—145, 359—360
   devices, 359—360
Acoustophoretic cell synchronization (ACS), 370—371
Acrylic PSAs, 45—46
Activated cell sorting microdevices, 372
Active microfluidics, 174—175. *See also* Passive microfluidics
   control of individual droplets, 174—175
   control of multiple droplets, 174
Active pharmaceutical ingredients (APIs), 293—295
Actuation mechanisms for microfluidic biomedical devices
   acoustics, 143—152
   electrokinetics, 126—143
   limitations and future trends, 152—153

   mechanical and nonmechanical actuation mechanisms formicrofluidic actuation, 127t
Additive manufacturing process, 4
Adenosine triphosphate (ATP), 245
Adherent cell injection, 393
Adhesive, 45—46
   ligands (extracellular matrix) regulation, 451—453
Adsorption, 495
   adsorptive polymer coatings, 98—99
   PEMs, 99—101
   proteins, 96—98
   strategies, 96—102
   surfactants, 101—102
Adsorptive polymer coatings, 98—99
Adult stem cells, 437—438
Advanced microfluidic devices, 1—2
Affinity chromatography, 307
Aging, 238
Aldagen, 477—478
Alkenyl succinic acid anhydrate (ASA), 558—559
Alkyl ketene dimer (AKD), 556—557
Alternating current (AC), 137—138
   electrokinetics, 137—139
   electroosmosis, 139, 354
Aluminum oxide membrane (AOM), 526
Amalgamation of drug delivery, 247
Amine-reactive NHS ester, 495—497
(3-Aminopropyl)trimethoxysilane (APTMS), 84—85
Aminopropyltriethoxysilane (APTES), 83—84
Ammonium hydroxide (NH$_4$OH), 19
Amniotic fluid (AF), 475
Amniotic-fluid MSCs (AFMSCs), 475

Index

Amplification-free nucleic acid detection on microfluidics, 600
Analog plotter, 554–555
Anti-FluVax®-immunoglobulin G (AF-IgG), 245
Antibodies, 489–491
  antibody-free assay, 303
  detection, 499–503
Antiepileptic drugs (AEDs), 502
Antigens, 107
Antiresonant reflecting optical waveguide (ARROW), 600
Aquaporins, 331
Arraycount software, 277–280
Artificial cells, 187–188
Asymmetric pinched flow fractionation (AsPFF), 346
Automation, 392–393, 407
2, 2′-Azinobis {3-ethylbenzothiazoline-6-sulfonic acid}-diammonium salt (ABTS), 503

B

Bacillus cereus, 301–303
Bacteria-induced infectious diseases, 301–303
Baculovirus (BV), 600–603
Barcoded microchip for immunoassay, 603–606
BD Biosciences, 372
Becton Dickinson Soluvia (BD Soluvia), 248
Berkeley μCAE device, 532
β-Cyclodextrin (β-CD), 293–295
β-cells
  live-cell imaging of islets and, 628–629
  design and validation of microfluidic devices for β-cell perifusion and imaging, 633–635
Bilayer lipid membranes (BLMs), 264, 265f
Bio-microelectromechanical systems (Bio-MEMS systems), 329
Bioaffinity attachment, 495
Biofluid properties, 333–334
Biological
  cells, 331, 338
  fluids, 333
Biomanufacturing, 629–631
BioMark instrument, 459–460

Biomaterials, 176–181
  drug delivery, 179
  general perspective on droplet microfluidics and, 180–181
  materials, 177–179
  stem cells and tissue engineering, 179–180
Biomedical research, 659
Biomicrofluidics, 1–2
Biomimetics, 347–348
Biopolymers, 177
Bioreactors, 185–188
  artificial cells, 187–188
  drug screening, 185–187
  general perspective on droplet microfluidics and, 188
Biosensors, 244, 246
Biotin-avidin link, 495
Blood serum, lab-on-a-chip drug analysis of, 104–106
Boltzmann constant, 338–340
Bonding, 16–17
  of multilayer microfluidic device, 646
BOSCH-DIRE process, 244
Bovine serum albumin (BSA), 45, 96–97, 589
Brij-35, 101
Bubble extraction, 338
Bulk micromachining, 18–20
Bulk nanomachining, 214
Bulk ultrasonic vibration, 145–147
Buried channel technology, 214

C

C-reactive protein (CRP), 45, 86
Caenorhabditis elegans. See Roundworm (*Caenorhabditis elegans*)
Calcium, 628
Calibration factor, 242–243
Cancer cells manipulation in microfluidic systems, 368–372
  current challenges in sorting and detection, 372
  deformability and migration studies, 370
  microfluidic separation and sorting, 370–372
Cancer Genome Project, 511–512
Cancer stem cell (CSC), 477
Capillary array electrophoresis (CAE), 533–535

Index   683

Capillary electrophoresis (CE), 512
Capillary microdialysis, 240
Carbamazepine (CBZ), 502
Carbohydrate MN arrays, 228—229
Carbon nanotubes (CNTs), 88
Carboxylic acid, 87—88
Carcinoembryonic antigen (CEA), 45
Cardiac tissue engineering, 419
Cardiomyocytes, 414
Cardiopulmonary bypass procedures
    (CPB procedures), 448
Carry out LAMP (cLAMP), 598—600
Cartesian axis, 352
Cas13a, 606—607
Cavitational microstreaming, 146
Cell mechanics, 423—424
Cell seeding, 426
Cell wall integrity (CWI), 331
Cell(s), 391—392
    affinity—based stem cell isolation, 474
    analysis, 440—444
    cell-based assays, 97—98, 286
    cell-to-cell differences, 391—392
    cell/stem cell expansion and differentiation,
        420—421
    colonization of biomaterial scaffold,
        415—416
    cycle analysis, 459
    heterogeneity, 391—392
    holding devices, 396
    manipulation, 329
        cancer cells manipulation in microfluidic
            systems, 368—372
        key issues, 329—330
        manipulation technologies, 338—368
        microenvironment on cell integrity,
            330—332
        microscale fluid dynamics, 332—338
    microenvironment on cell integrity,
        330—332
    migration, 422—423
    structure and function, 331
    trapping techniques, 393—394
Cellular receptors, 268
Cellulose paper, 552—553
Central nervous system (CNS), 438—439
Centrifugal microfluidic platforms,
    270—271
Cetrimonium bromide (CTAB), 88

Charge-coupled device (CCD), 598—600
ChargeSwitch magnetic beads, 533—535
Chemical treatment, 24
Chemical vapor deposition method
    (CVD method), 85—86
Chemiluminescence (CL), 290, 497, 563
    detection, 497, 572
    signals, 499—500, 501f
Chip-based CE, 526—527
Christmas tree structure, 446—447
Chromatography paper, 552—553
Chronoamperometry, 570—571
Circular cross-section channels, 166
Circulating endothelial cells (CECs),
    306—307
Circulating tumor cells (CTCs), 306—307,
    370—371, 448, 522
Clausius—Mossotti factor, 141, 353
Clonidine (CLO), 295—296
Clustered regularly interspaced short
    palindromic repeats (CRISPR),
    606—607
Clusters of differentiation 4 (CD4),
    600—603
"Coat and poke" approach, 230—232
Coated microneedle arrays, 234
Coated MN arrays, 237
Codelink, 91
Colorimetric detection, 42—43, 563—570
Colorimetric substrate, 498
Colorimetry, 290
Combinatorial library in microarrays,
    277—280
Complementary metal-oxide semiconductor
    (CMOS), 400—401
Complete blood count (CBC), 668—669
Complex 3D microvascular networks,
    418—419
Complex microfluidic networks,
    336—338
Computational fluid dynamics (CFD), 336
Computer-aided simulation, 336
Computer-assisted design (CAD),
    659—660
Contactless DEP (cDEP), 357
Continuous flow microfluidic chip,
    290—291
Continuous flow microfluidic systems, 420
Continuous flow reactors, 273—274

Controlled drug delivery using microdevices
  future trends and challenges, 237—238
  micro/nanofluidics-based drug delivery systems, 234—235
  microreservoir-based drug delivery systems, 226—229
Convection-enhanced drug delivery (CED), 240
Conventional drug-delivery systems, 225—226
Cosmeceuticals
  MN-mediated skin appearance improvement and delivery of, 238—239
Cosmetic MN devices, 238—239
Cost reduction, 530—531
Cost-effective COP-based PCR chip, 107
Covalent attachment, 495—497
Covalent immobilization strategies
  glass devices, 92—95
  polymer devices, 81—92
    other polymer devices, 91—92
    PDMS devices, 81—86
    thermoplastic devices, 86—90
Covalent siloxane bonds (Si—O—Si), 103
Creatine kinase-MB (CK-MB), 300
CRISPR RNAs (crRNAs), 606—607
CRISPR-Cas13a-based virus detection on microchip, 606—607
Current good manufacturing practices (cGMPs), 620
Curved channels, 344—345
Cutting, 2
  plotter, 46
  tools, 46
Cyclic olefin copolymers (COC), 5—6, 39—41, 88—90, 514
Cyclic olefin polymer (COP), 39—41, 88—90
Cyclicvoltammogram (CV), 45
Cytokine(s), 489—491
  assay using single antibody, 504f
  detection, 503—505

D

2000-Da diaminopolyethyleneglycol (DAPEG), 499—500
Danio rerio. See Zebrafish (*Danio rerio*)
Debye double layer, 126
Debye—Hückel approximation, 131
Deep reactive-ion etching (DRIE), 13
Deformability, 370
Deionized water (DI water), 664—666
Deoxyribonucleic acid (DNA), 519—520, 595
  analysis, 106
  sequencing, 518
Derivatized silanes, 84—85
Detection, 628—629
Detection methods, 497—499
Deterministic lateral displacement (DLD), 340—343
Device designs, 398—399
Device fabrication process, 394
Diagnostics, 588—589
Diamond blades, 13—15
Diamond coating, 246—247
Diclofenac (DCF), 45, 232—234
Dielectrophoresis (DEP), 140—143, 351—353, 393—394
Dielectrophoretic assisted cell sorting (DACS), 474—475
Dielectrophoretic field flow fractionation (DEP-FFF), 355—356
Differential environmental spatial patterning (dESP), 453
Differential interference contrast microscopy (DIC microscopy), 393
Differential pulse voltammetry (DPV), 42—43
Differential strategies for fluid extraction, 242—243
Differentiation, 420—421
Diffusion-based gradient generator, 46
Digital LAMP, 184
Digital microfluidics (DMF), 282—283, 519—520
Digital PCR (dPCR), 530
Dimensionless numbers, 165—166, 332—333
Direct 3D printing of microfluidic devices and applications, 663—671
  3D geometric influence on microfluidic profile, 666—667
  direct 3D printing of POC microfluidic device for anemia diagnosis, 668—671
  materials and methods, 663—664
  precision of direct 3D printing approach, 664

surface property of 3D-printed microfluidic devices, 664–666
Direct current (DC), 137–138
Direct reprogramming approaches, 415
Dissolving microneedle arrays, 234–235, 238
Dithiothreitol (DTT), 567–568
DNA extraction and amplification (DEA), 533–535
Docetaxel (DTX), 232–234
Dosing indicator, 248
Downstream signal transduction pathways, 268
Dried blood spot (DBS), 301
"Drop-Seq" technique, 525
Droplet interface bilayer techniques (DIB techniques), 266
Droplet microfluidics, 164–175, 275
　active microfluidics, 174–175
　advantages of, 170
　biomedical applications, 175–188
　　biomaterials, 176–181
　　bioreactors, 185–188
　　isolated element screening, 181–185
　comparison and contrast of single-phase and droplet microfluidics, 168–171
　disadvantages of, 170–171
　droplet flow in microchannels, 165–168
　droplet in wider context of microfluidics, 163–165
　passive microfluidics, 171–174
Droplet mode, 282
Droplet-based single-exosome-counting enzyme-linked immunoassay (droplet digital ExoELISA) approach, 308–309
Drosophila larvae
　microfabricated device for immobilization and mechanical stimulation of, 401–405
　　Drosophila larva immobilization device, 405f
　　experimental validation of worm body expansion, 404f
　　fluorescent images of *Drosophila larva*, 406f
　　image frame sequence of injection area, 403f
　　inlet/valve operation states, 402t

Drosophila melanogaster. See Fruit fly (*Drosophila melanogaster*)
Drug candidates, 398
Drug delivery, 179, 225
　coated microneedle arrays, 234
　dissolving microneedle arrays, 234–235
　hollow microneedle arrays, 235–236
　hydrogel-forming microneedle arrays, 236–237
　solid microneedle arrays, 232–234
　strategies using MN arrays, 230–237
Drug discovery
　hit identification and lead optimization, 271–284
　　high throughput screening, 276–284
　　preclinical evaluation, 284–288
　　synthesis of drug libraries, 273–276
　identification of druggable targets, 263–271
　microfluidics for, 263–288
Drug libraries, synthesis of, 273–276
Drug screening, 185–187
　application, 280–282
Drug targets, 263–264
Druggable targets identification, 263–271
Dry etching of silicon, 19–20
Dynamic seeding methodologies, 416–417

E
Eckart streaming, 145
Edmonton Protocol, 617–618
Effective cell seeding and scaffold colonization, 415–417
Effective drug delivery, 225
Electric double layer, 126–132
Electrical FFF (EIFFF), 340
Electrochemical detection (ECD), 244, 498–499, 552–553, 570–572
Electrochemical impedance spectroscopy (EIS), 42–43, 300, 571–572
Electrochemical method (EC method), 42–43
Electrochemiluminescence (ECL), 42–43, 563
　detections, 572
Electrokinetics (EK), 126–143, 291–292
　AC, 137–139
　actuator, 239–240
　devices, 354–357

Electrokinetics (EK) (*Continued*)
  dielectrophoresis, 140–143
  electric double layer, 126–132
  electroosmosis, 132–135
  electrophoresis, 135–137
  mechanisms, 351–357
    AC electroosmosis, 354
    dielectrophoresis, 352–353
    electrokinetic devices, 354–357
Electrolyte, 266
Electron transport chain (ETC), 618–619
Electroosmosis, 132–135
  electroosmotic mixing, 134–135
  electroosmotic pumping, 133–134
  electroosmotic slip, 132
Electroosmotic flow (EOF), 83–84
Electroosmotic mixing, 134–135
Electroosmotic pumping, 133–134
Electroosmotic slip, 132
Electrophoresis, 135–137
Electrophoretic separations, 79
Electroplating, 228
Electrospun nanofibrous membranes, 593–594, 593f
Electrothermal induction, 229
Electrotransfection, 671
Electrowetting-on-dielectric (EWOD), 275–276
Embryoid bodies (EBs), 444–445
Embryonic stem cells (ESCs), 437–438
Emulsification, 623, 624f
Endothelial cell function, 424
Endothelial cell function, shear stress impacts on, 423–424
Endothelial progenitor cells (EPCs), 371–372, 474
Energy-transfer (ET), 518
Environmental monitoring, 573
Environmental testing, 578–579
Enzyme-linked immunosorbent assay (ELISA), 83–84, 107, 303–304, 489–491, 503, 571–572, 587–589, 589f, 628
Enzyme(s), 268, 331
  immobilisation, 244, 299
ePADs, 571
Ephedrine (EPH), 295–296
Epidermal growth factor (EGF), 451

Epithelial cell adhesion molecules (EpCAM), 370–371
Escherichia coli, 282, 301–303, 497, 498f, 501
Etching techniques, 2–3
1-Ethyl-3-(3-dimethylaminopropyl) carbodiimide (EDC), 495–497
Ethylene diamine pyrocatechol (EDP), 19
Ex vivo evaluation, 287–288
Exosomes, 308–309
External stresses on cells, 331–332
Extracellular matrix (ECM), 331, 413, 439
Extrusion, 623, 624f

F
Fabrication, 8
  glass, 9
  of microfluidic devices
    using parylene, 27
    using PDMS, 21–23
    using PMMA, 35
  silicon, 18
Fast Lithographic Activation of Sheets (FLASH), 553–554, 554f
Ferromagnets, 365–366
Fibroblast growth factor 2 (FGF2), 451
Fibroblasts, 370–371
Field flow fractionation (FFF), 338–340
Field-amplified sample injection (FASI), 291–292
Field-amplified sample stacking (FASS), 291–292
Field-enhanced sample injection (FESI), 291–292
Flexographic printing, 556–557, 556f
Flinders Technology Associates (FTA), 530–531, 598–600
Flow cytometry, 600–603
Flow dynamics in microchannels, 334–336
Flow FFF (FlFFF), 340
Flow patterns, 166–167
Fluid control, 627–628
Fluid extraction, differential strategies for, 242–243
Fluid flow, 240–242
Fluidigm C1, 311
Fluidigm Dynamic Array, 270–271
Fluorescein isothiocyanate dye (FITC dye), 401

Index 687

Fluorescence in-situ hybridization (FISH), 522
Fluorescence Ubiquitination Cell Cycle Indicator system (FUCCI system), 459
Fluorescence-activated cell sorter (FACS), 361−363, 448, 620
Fluorescence-activated stem cell sorting, 471
FluoZin-3, 620
FOTURAN glass, 16
Fourier transform infrared spectroscopy (FTIR), 664−666
Fruit fly (*Drosophila melanogaster*), 392
Fused deposition modeling (FDM), 660
Fused silica, 9

G
Gabapentin (GPN), 293−295
Gadolinium diethylenetriamine pentaacetic acid (Gd-DTPA), 372
Gas bubble formation, 338
Gas chromatography (GC), 17−18
    gas chromatography−mass spectrometry, 298−299
Gene expression, 106
    analysis, 521
    profiling, 459−461
Generic materials, 398
Genetic analysis, 511−512
Geometrically enhanced differential immunocapture (GEDI), 307−308
Glass, 9−17, 514
    applications and future trends, 17
    bonding, 16−17
    devices, 92−95
        other strategies, 95
        silanization, 93−95
    fabrication, 9
    other methods, 13−16
    plasma etching, 13
    wet chemical etching, 9−13
Glass microfluidic device, 393−396. *See also* Paper-based microfluidic devices (μPADs)
    immobilization on 5 x 5 array of mouse zygotes, 396f
    microfabrication process, 395f
    microfluidic device for high-speed microinjection of *C. elegans*, 400f

mouse zygote penetrated by micropipette before material deposition, 397f
robotic system for automated mouse zygote microinjection, 397f
system setup for automated *C. elegans* injection, 400f
Glass transition temperature (Tg), 45−46
GlaxoSmithKline (GSK), 273
Glucose-induced insulin secretion, 618−619
Glucose-stimulated insulin secretion (GSIS), 618−619
Glutaraldehyde (GA), 495−497
Gold microelectrodes, 244
Gold nanoparticles (AuNPs), 578, 603−606
Gravitational FFF (GrFFF), 340
Green fluorescent protein (GFP), 404−405, 448

H
Haemopoieticstem cells (HSCs), 371−372
Hagen−Poiseuille flow, 335
Handheld advanced nucleic acid analyser (HANAA), 526
Healthcare professional (HCP), 234−235
Hele-Shaw flow, 335
Helicase-dependent amplification (HDA), 530−531
Hematopoietic stem cells (HSCs), 437−438
Hepatitis delta virus (HDV), 270−271
Hepatotoxicity, 285
Heterogeneous immunoassay, 494
High performance liquid chromatography (HPLC), 290
High resolution fabrication techniques, 17
High resolution melt (HRM), 530
High throughput microfluidic devices, 263
High throughput screening, 276−284
High-gradient magnetic field concentrator (HGMC), 448
High-throughput microfluidic flow cytometry devices, 372
Hit identification (HI), 271−284
Hollow microneedle arrays, 235−236
Homocysteine (Hcy), 567−568
Hormones, 225−226, 331
Horseradish peroxidase (HRP), 497, 593−594
Hot embossing, 5−6
Hue-saturation-value (HSV), 566−567

Human bone marrow—derived
   mesenchymal stromal
   cell (hMSC), 423
Human embryonic stem cells (hESCs), 414,
   451—452
Human genome project (HGP), 511—512
Human immunodeficiency virus (HIV), 84,
   587—588
Human liver cancer cells (HepG2),
   370—371
Human mesenchymal stem cells (hMSCs),
   349—350
Human NSPCs (hNSPC), 451
Human papillomavirus (HPV), 596—597
Human pluripotent stem cell (hPSC),
   414, 631
Human primary mesenchymal stem cells
   (hMSCs), 631—632
Human umbilical vein endothelial cells
   (HUVEC), 306—307, 426, 467—469
Hydraulic-electric circuit analogy concept,
   336—337
Hydrodynamic devices, 349—351
Hydrodynamic filtration (HDF), 337—338
   and microfluidic networks, 345—346
Hydrodynamic mechanisms,
   340—351, 372. *See also*
   Electrokinetic mechanisms
   biomimetics, 347—348
   curved channels, 344—345
   DLD, 340—343
   hydrodynamic devices, 349—351
   hydrodynamic filtering and microfluidic
      networks, 345—346
   hydrophoresis and microstructure
      inclusions, 348—349
   inertial migration, 343—344
   traps, 393—394
Hydrofluoric acid (HF), 394
   wet etching, 2—3
Hydrogel, 446, 600
   hydrogel-forming microneedle arrays,
      236—237
   hydrogel-forming MN arrays, 240,
      248—249
Hydrophobic nitrocellulose membranes, 553
Hydrophoresis, 348—349
Hydrostatic pressure approach, 299—300
Hydroxyflutamide (HF), 296—298

I

i-STAT system device, 310—311
Ibuprofen, 232—234
Immiscible fluid, 163
Immobilization, 395
   chemistry, 494—497
   comparison of immobilization
      techniques, 496t
Immunoassays, 489—491
   applications, 499—505
   comparison of different commercial
      bioarray methods, 490t—491t
   detection methods, 497—499
   immobilization chemistry, 494—497
   technologies, 491—494
Immunochromatographic strips (ICS), 551
Immunoglobulin G (IgG), 92, 501, 590—591
Immunogold silver staining (IGSS), 498,
   499f, 501f
Immunological detection, 588—589
Immunosensor, 92
   to detect pathogenic bacteria, 107—108
In vitro evaluation, 285—287
In vitro toxicological testing, 284—285
In vivo evaluation, 288
In vivo tissue regeneration, 413
In vivo tissue repair, 413
In-plane MNs, 226
In-plane silicon hollow MN, 244
Indium tin oxide (ITO), 514—515
Individual droplets control, 174—175
Induced pluripotent stem cells (iPSCs), 414,
   437—438
Inertial migration, 343—344
Infrared (IR), 361, 514—515
Injection molding, 6—7
Inkjet 3D printing technology, 661
Inkjet etching process, 555—556
Inkjet printing technology, 283—284,
   493, 560
Institute of Cancer Research (ICR), 396
Insulator-based dielectrophoresis (iDEP),
   357
Insulin, 225—226
   secretory pathway, 618—620, 619f
Integrated "everything-on-a-chip" systems,
   311
Integrated bubble traps (IBT), 338
Integrated designs, 243—247

Integrated fluidic circuit (IFC), 270—271, 519—520
Integrated microfluidic systems, 513
  future trends, 535—536
  genetic analysis
    applications of fully integrated systems in, 518—535
    integrated microdevices development, 513—517
    integrated microsystem for preparing DNA libraries, 520f
Interdigital transducer (IDT), 143—144
Interdigitated transducers (IDTs), 360
Interfacial tension, 167
Interleukins (IL), 503
Internal gelation device, 651
Intersection bioarray approach, 504—505
Interstitial fluid (ISF), 230—232
Intracytoplasmic sperm injection (ICSI), 391—392
Intramuscular route (IM route), 237
Ion channels, 331
Islet
  cells preparation and loading, 649
  design and validation of microfluidic devices
    for islet microencapsulation, 635—639
    for islet perifusion and imaging, 633—635
  immobilization, 625—627
  methods for islet encapsulation, 623
  microencapsulation, 629—631
  obstacles toward clinical use of islet products, 620—621
  perifusion and fluorescence imaging, 649—650
  standard assays used to determine islet potency, 622—623
  study and transplantation, design and validation of microfluidic devices for, 632—639
  transplantation, 618
    emergence of microfluidics applied to, 623—632
Islet Equivalent (IEq), 622
Islet on-chip microencapsulation, 642—643
  equipment and materials, 643
  reagents, 642—643
Islet perifusion array (IPA), 634

Islet perifusion chamber (IPC), 633—634
Isolated element analysis, 185
Isolated element screening, 181—185
  general perspective on droplet microfluidics and isolated element analysis, 185
  on-chip analysis tools, 183—185
  single-cell encapsulation, 182—183
Isothermal amplification technologies, 595

K
Ketone, 45
Ketoprofen, 232—234
KOH wet etching. *See* Potassiumhydroxide wet etching (KOH wet etching)
KSOM. *See* Potassium-supplemented simplex optimized medium (KSOM)

L
Lab-on-a-chip
  devices, 1—2, 439—440, 513, 551
  drug analysis of blood serum, 104—106
  systems, 367—368
Label-free approach, 474—475
  electrophysiological properties, 474—475
  size differences, 475
Laboratories-on-a-chip (LOC), 329
Laser
  cutters, 7—8, 46
  cutting, 228
  micromachining technique, 16
  printing and treatment, 561
Laser-based fabrication method, 229
Lateral droplet motion (LOET), 361—363
Lateral flow assay (LFA), 305—306
Lead identification (LI), 271
Lead optimization, 271—284
Leveraging techniques, 392—393
Ligand type, 421—423
Limit of detection (LOD), 308—309, 567—568
Limit of quantitation (LOQ), 295—296
Lipid bilayer, 331
Lithium aluminum hydride (LAH), 87
Lithographie, Galvanoformung, Abformung process (LIGA process), 3
Live cell imaging, design considerations and strategies for, 625—627
Live-cell imaging of islets and β-cells, 628—629

Live/Dead assay, 283−284
Loop-mediated isothermal amplification (LAMP), 530−531, 595, 597−598
Low-cost assays
  paper-based microfluidic devices
    application, 573−579
    current limitations and future perspectives in, 579−580
    detection and read-out technologies, 563−572
    fabrication techniques for, 552−563

M

M-H hysteresis loops, 365−366
Macro-to-micro interface, 517
Magnet-activated cell sorting (MACS), 366−367
Magnetic force, 365−366
Magnetic mechanisms, 364−368
  magnetic force, 365−366
  magnetophoretic devices, 366−368
Magnetic susceptibilities (MACS), 372
Magnetic trapping, 393−394
Magnetic-activated cell sorters (MACS), 448
Magnetic-activated stem cell sorting, 471−474
Magnetophoretic devices, 366−368
Magnetotactic bacteria (MTB), 366−367
Male master mold, 228−229
Mammalian cells, 331−332
Manipulation technologies, 338−368
  acoustic mechanisms, 357−360
  electrokinetic mechanisms, 351−357
  FFF, 338−340
  hydrodynamic mechanisms, 340−351
  magnetic mechanisms, 364−368
  optical mechanisms, 360−363
Marker-dependent approach, 471−474
  cell affinity−based stem cell isolation, 474
  fluorescence-activated stem cell sorting, 471
  magnetic-activated stem cell sorting, 471−474
Massachusetts Institute of Technology (MIT), 661
Matrix metalloproteinase-8 (MMP-8), 303
Matrix-assisted laser/desorptionionization−mass spectrometry (MALDI-MS), 288

Mechanical actuation mechanisms for microfluidic actuation, 126, 127t
Mechanical microspotting, 492
Mechanosensitive ion channel (MscL), 268
Merging, 172−173
Mesenchymal stem cells (MSCs), 415, 437−438
"Metabolomics-on-a-chip" approach, 296−298
Metal sputtering methods, 103−104
Metallic hollow MN arrays, 240
Metal−oxide−semiconductor field-effect transistor (MOSFET), 607
Metals, 228
Methylene blue (MB), 301−303
Micellar electrokinetic chromatography technique (MEKC technique), 291−292
Micelle-to-solvent stacking (MSS), 291−292
Micro total analysis systems (μTAS), 163, 289−290, 439−440
Microarray methods, 493−494, 494t
Microbioreactor arrays, 420
Microchannels
  droplet flow in, 165−168
    dimensionless numbers, 165−166
    flow patterns, 166−167
    independent variables for experiments, 167
    interfacial tension and surfactants, 167
    surface wetting conditions, 168
  layers, 399−400
Microchannels, flow dynamics in, 334−336
Microchip electrophoresis (MCE), 291−292
Microchip technology, 525−526
Microcirculatory networks creation, microdevices for, 425−427
Microdevices for label-free and noninvasive monitoring of stem cell differentiation, 461−467, 464f
  DEP-well system used to measure cellular dielectric properties, 465f
  dielectric characterization of complete mononuclear and polymorphonuclear blood-cell subpopulations, 465f
  microfluidic impedance cytometry, 466f
Microdilutor network (μDN), 590−591

Index

Microelectromechanical systems (MEMS), 1–2, 226, 276–277, 392–393, 659
Microemulsions, 525
Microencapsulation of islets on chip, 650–651
Microenvironment on cell integrity, 330–332
  cell structure and function, 331
  external stresses on cells, 331–332
Microfabricated capillary array electrophoresis (μCAE), 532
Microfabricated device, 401–405
Microfabricated FACS (ìFACS), 448
Microfabrication methods, 2–8, 261–262, 419, 455, 513, 659
  materials, 8–46
    glass, 9–17
    paper, 41–43
    polymers, 21–41
    PSA, 45–46
    silicon, 17–21
    thread, 43–45
  photolithography-based microfabrication, 2–4
  replication-based methods, 4–7
  xurography-based microfabrication, 7–8
Microfiber, 629–631
Microfluidic device, 79–81, 270, 393
  for automated, high-speed microinjection of *C. elegans*, 397–401
  fabrication, 639–640
    equipment, 640
    reagents and tools, 639
  glass microfluidic device, 393–396
  microfabricated device for immobilization and mechanical stimulation of *Drosophila larvae*, 401–405
  platforms for tissue scaffolds, 419–427
Microfluidic drug delivery with inorganic light-emitting diode arrays (m-ILED arrays), 240
Microfluidic electrochemical device (μFED), 498–499, 500f
Microfluidic flow cytometer, 600–603
  for monitoring HIV infection, 607–608
Microfluidic immunoassay, 588–594, 590f
  for detecting HIV infection, 591f
Microfluidic loop-mediated isothermal amplification (μLAMP), 597–598, 599f
Microfluidic network (μFN), 589
  hydrodynamic filtering and, 345–346
Microfluidic nucleic acid
  amplification, 595–600
  detection, 595–600
Microfluidic paper analyticaldevices (μPAD), 304–305
Microfluidic paper-based electrochemical device (μPED), 570–571
Microfluidic PCR, single cell transcriptome analysis with, 106–107
Microfluidic Western blot (μWB), 594
Microfluidic(s), 262, 439–440
  3D cell culture platforms, 285
  biosensors, 299
  diagnostic
    applications, 298–310
    system, 592, 592f
  for drug discovery, 263–288
  examples of commercial microfluidic devices, 310–311
  future trends, 311–312
  microfluidics-based drug delivery systems, 234–235
    applications, 237–239
    fabrication of microfluidic drug delivery systems, 236–237
    working principle, 235–236
  microwell arrays, 276–277
  for pharmaceutical analysis, 289–298
  protocol on materials, 639–643
  protocol on procedures, 643–651
    bonding of multilayer microfluidic device, 646
    device preconditioning, 647–648
    islet cells preparation and loading, 649
    islet perifusion and fluorescence imaging, 649–650
  separation and sorting, 370–372
  stem cell separation technology, 467–475
    DEP-based microfluidics cell sorter, 470f
    label-free approach, 474–475
    layout of microfluidic based cell sorting system, 469f
    marker-dependent approach, 471–474
    microfluidic cell sorting, 468f

Microfluidic(s) (*Continued*)
microfluidic device for separation of AFMSCs, 471f
microfluidics devices for stem cell isolation/separation, 472t—473t
micromagnetic separators for stem cell sorting, 470f
systems, 329
cancer cells manipulation in, 368—372
technologies, 623—632
viral detection, 588—603
Microinjection
Glass microfluidic device for, 393—396
Microinjection, 398
Micron-sized BLMs, 264
Microneedle (MN), 225
array applications
MN-mediated skin appearance improvement and delivery of cosmeceuticals, 238—239
MN-mediated vaccine delivery, 237—238
clinical translation and commercialisation of MN products, 247—250
design parameters and structure, 226—229
geometry, 226—227
materials, 227—229
drug delivery strategies using MN arrays, 230—237
microneedle-mediated patient monitoring and diagnosis, 239—247
differential strategies for fluid extraction, 242—243
fluid flow, 240—242
integrated designs, 243—247
shapes, 227f
Microneedle-mediated vaccine delivery, 237—238
Microreservoir-based drug delivery systems, 226—229
microreservoir fabrication, 227—229
polymer-based device, 234
silicon-based devices, 232—234
working principle, 226—227
Microscale cell culture analog (µCCA), 286
Microscale fluid dynamics, 332—338
dimensionless numbers, 332—333
flow dynamics in microchannels, 334—336
properties of biofluids, 333—334
system design and operation, 336—338
bubble extraction, 338
complex microfluidic networks, 336—338
Microscale technologies, 420
Microspheres for cytokine capture, 503—504, 505f
Microspot array, 491—493, 492f
Microstructure inclusions, 348—349
Microtechnologies, 420
Micrototal analysis systems (µTAS), 513
Microvalves, 515—516
for fluidic control on integrated devices, 516t
Middle East respiratory syndrome (MERS), 600
Migration studies, 370
Miniaturised conventional technologies for cell analysis, 447—448
Miniaturised devices for cell culture, 440—447
biochemical regulation, 446—447
biophysical regulation, 444—445
cell surface marker targeting cell sorter, 443f
cell—cell interaction, 446
dielectrophoresis (DEP) based cell sorter, 443f
emerging microfluidic platforms for advancing cell analysis, 441f
fluorescence-activated sorting, 442f
microfluidics concentration gradient generators, 441f
microfluidics-based polymerase chain reaction, 442f
microfluidics-based stem cell culture platform, 450—458
Miniaturised system, 246—247
Miniaturized total chemical analysis (µTAS), 659
Minimally invasive monitoring methods, 240
Mixing process, 173
Monomers, 1—2
Mosaic arrays, 493—494, 493f
Mouse ESCs (mESC), 452—453
Mouse islet isolation and culture, 640
cell culture media, 640
equipment and materials, 640
reagents, 640

Index

Mouse pancreatic islet isolation, 646–647
Multidrug resistant (MDR), 286–287
Multilayer soft lithography, 311, 336
Multiple displacement amplification (MDA), 521
Multiple droplets control, 174
Multiple pneumatic microvalves, 399–400
Multiple pulse amperometry (MPA), 45
Multiplexed screening platforms, 282
Multistage-multiorifice flow fractionation (MS-MOFF), 351
Multitarget cells (MT-DACS), 372
Murine embryonic fibroblasts (MEFs), 455
Myocardial infarction, 414

N

N-hydroxysuccinimide (NHS), 495–497
Nano-HPLC integrated to tandem massspectrometry (nano-HPLC-Chip-MS/MS), 295–296
Nanobioarray chip method (NBA chip method), 502–503, 502f
Nanodrugs, 239
Nanoelectrospray ionization mass spectrometry (nESI-MS), 301
Nanofluidics-based drug delivery systems, 234–235. *See also* Microfluidics-based drug delivery systems; Microreservoir-based drug delivery systems
Nanoimprinted lithography (NIL), 237
Nanoimprinting, 5–6
Nanoparticles (NPs), 567–568
Nanoprinting lithography, 238
National Health Service (NHS), 239–240
National Institute of Health (NIH), 518
Natural rubber, 45–46
Navier–Stokes equation, 334
Near-infrared radiation (NIR radiation), 234–235
Negative DEP (nDEP), 353
Neural stem cells (NSCs), 437–438
Neural stem/progenitor cells (NSPCs), 451
Newport Green (NP Green), 620
Newton's law of viscosity, 333
Newton's second law, 334
Next-generation sequencing (NGS), 518
Nicking enzyme amplificationreaction (NEAR), 595

Nitric acid (HNO$_3$), 19
Nitrite, 45
Nitrocellulose (NC), 553
Non-steroidal anti-inflammatories (NSAIDs), 232–234
Noncommunicable diseases (NCDs), 305–306
Nonimmunoassays, 300
Nonmechanical actuation mechanisms for microfluidic actuation, 126, 127t
Nucleic acid sequence-based amplification (NASBA), 530–531, 595–597

O

o-nitrophenol (ONP), 575–578
On-chip analysis tools, 183–185
Optical devices, 361–363
Optical mechanisms, 360–363
  optical devices, 361–363
Optical traps. *See* Optical tweezers
Optical tweezers, 361, 393–394
Optically induced DEP (ODEP), 361–363
Optofluidic neural probe, 240
Organ-on-a-chip devices, 285–286
"Osmotic shock", 332
Out-of-plane MNs, 226
Oxygen consumption rate (OCR), 622–623
Oxygen plasma treatment, 103

P

p-aminophenol (PAP), 575–578
p-nitrophenol (PNP), 575–578
Pancreatic islet, 618–619
Paper, 41–43, 551
  cutting and taping, 561–563
  substrates, 552–553
Paper-based microfluidic devices (μPADs), 551. *See also* Glass microfluidic device
  application, 573–579
    on-demand, 574
    ready-to-use, 574–579
  current limitations and future perspectives in, 579–580
  detection and read-out technologies, 563–572
    chemiluminescent and electrochemiluminescent detections, 572

Paper-based microfluidic devices
(μPADs) (*Continued*)
  colorimetric detection, 563–570
  ECD, 570–572
  fabrication techniques for, 552–563
    chemical modification of paper surface, 558–560
    chromatography paper with patterned channels, reservoirs and folding frame, 565f
    other techniques, 561–563
    paper substrates, 552–553
    physical filling of pores with hydrophobic polymer, 553–555
    preparation and demonstration of 3D PAD, 562f–563f
    soaking of paper with hydrophobic chemical, 555–558
Paracetamol, 232–234
Paracrine and autocrine signaling control, 453–455
Particle manipulation, 144–145
Parylene, 27–31
  applications and future trends, 29–31
  fabrication of microfluidic devices using, 27
  interconnection and bonding, 27–29
Passive microfluidics, 171–174. *See also* Active microfluidics
  generation, 171–172
  incubation, 173
  merging, 172–173
  mixing, 173
  sorting, 173–174
  splitting, 172
Pathogen
  detection, 525–526
  pathogen/infectious disease detection, 525
Pathogenic bacteria, immunosensor to detect, 107–108
Patient safety, 248–249
Patterning threads, 44
Péclet number (Pe), 340–343
Perfusion flow mode of drug screening, 280–282
Permanent magnets. *See* Ferromagnets
Pharmacokinetics (PK), 286
Phenytoin (PHT), 502
Phosphosilicate glass (PSG), 23–24
Photochemical etching, 228

Photodefinable polymers, 3
Photolithographic microfabrication, 2
Photolithography, 18–19, 226–227, 492, 553–554
  photolithography-based microfabrication, 2–4
Photomask for SU-8 negative master, 643
Photomultiplier tube (PMT), 600–603
Photosensitive material, 2
Physical filling of pores with hydrophobic polymer, 553–555
  photolithography, 553–554
  plotting with analog plotter, 554–555
Physiologically based pharmacokinetic modeling (PBPK), 286
Pinch flow fractionation (PFF), 346
Plaque-forming units (PFUs), 600–603
Plasma etching method, 13
Plasma oxidation etching method, 560
Plasma treatment, 23–24, 29
Plasma-enhanced chemical vapor deposition (PECVD), 226
Platelet-derived growth factor (PDGF), 451
Pneumatic valve–regulated microfluidic device, 399
Point-of-care (POC), 587–588
  diagnostic devices, 304–305
  testing, 551
Poiseuilleprofile flow, 334
"Poke and release" approach, 230–232
Poly methyl vinyl ether and maleic anhydride (PMVE/MAH), 236–237
Poly-lysine (PLL), 504–505
Poly(methyl methacrylate) (PMMA), 5–6, 35–37, 86–88, 226–227, 264–266, 514
  fabrication of microfluidic devices using, 35
  interconnection and bonding, 35–37
Poly(*N*, *N*-dimethylacrylamide) (pDMA), 518
Poly(*N*-hydroxyethylacrylamide) (pHEA), 518
Poly(o-phenylenediamine) (PPD), 245
Poly(styrene), 555–556
Polycarbonate (PC), 5–6, 37–39, 91–92, 514, 590–591
  MN arrays, 243

Index

Polydimethylsiloxane (PDMS), 5, 21, 81–82, 168, 228–229, 337–338, 418–419, 444–445, 493, 514, 554–555, 590–591, 623, 659
  casting, 645–646
  device fabrication, 643–647
    photomask for SU-8 negative master, 643
    SU-8 negative master fabrication, 643–645
  devices, 81–86, 633
    other immobilization schemes on PDMS, 85–86
    silanization strategies, 82–85
  fabrication of microfluidic devices using, 21–23
Polyelectrolyte multilayers (PEMs), 99–101
Polyester, 5
Polyethylene glycol (PEG), 83–84, 179, 236–237, 444–445
Polyethylene terephthalate (PET), 8, 514
Polyethylene terephthalate glycol (PETG), 23–24
Polyimide (PI), 4
Polylactic-co-glycolic acid (PLGA), 179, 230–232
Polymer(s), 1–2, 21–41
  devices, 81–92
    PDMS devices, 81–86
    polycarbonate, 91–92
    polystyrene, 92
    thermoplastic devices, 86–90
  films, 2
  MN arrays, 228–229
  polymer-based device, 234
  polymer-based devices, 226–227
  siloxane elastomers, 21–24
  thermoplastic polymers, 34–41
  thermosetting polymers, 24–34
Polymerase chain reaction (PCR), 17, 301–303, 512, 587–588
Polymeric microfluidic devices, 264–266
Polymethacrylate (PMMA), 242
Polystyrene (PS), 23–24, 92, 504–505, 514
Polyurethane (PU), 5, 33–34
Polyvinyl chloride (PVC), 8
Polyvinylidenefluoride (PVDF), 594
Pore geometry, 421–423
Potassium-supplemented simplex optimized medium (KSOM), 396
Potassiumhydroxide wet etching (KOH wet etching), 2–3
Powder machining technique, 15
Precision of direct 3D printing approach, 664
Preclinical evaluation, 284–288
  ex vivo evaluation, 287–288
  in vitro evaluation, 285–287
  in vivo evaluation, 288
Pregabalin (PGN), 293–295
Preimplantation genetic screening (PGS), 391–392
Prepolymer, 226–227
Pressure sensitive adhesives (PSA), 2, 45–46
Pressure-driven laminar flow, 336–337
Print-to-screen platform (P2S platform), 277–280
Printed circuit board (PCB), 600–603
Projection photolithography, 659
Proof-of-concept experiment (POC experiment), 399, 663
Prostate-specific antigen (PSA), 300
Proteins, 96–98
  microarray fabrication surfaces and properties, 495–497, 496t
  protein–ligand binding assay, 270–271
Turtle, 401–403
Pseudorabies virus (PRV), 597–598
Pulsed laser beam, 229
Pumpless islet perifusion array (p-IPA), 635
Pyrex Corning 7740, 9

Q

Quantitative polymerase chain reaction (qPCR), 521
Quantum dots (QDs), 568–570

R

Radioactivity, 499
Radioimmunoassay (RIA), 628
Raman spectroscopy (RACS), 372
Rapid DNA sequencing, 79
Reactive oxygen species (ROS), 622–623
Reactive-ion etching (RIE), 2–3
Recombinase polymerase amplification (RPA), 530–531
Red blood cells (RBC), 332
Replica molding, 226–227

Replication-based methods, 2, 4—7
  hot embossing, 5—6
  injection molding, 6—7
  soft lithography, 5
Retention equation, 338—340
Reverse iontophoresis, 240
Reverse transcriptase polymerase chain reaction amplification (RT-PCR), 106, 523, 526
Reynolds numbers (Re), 125, 332—333
Ribonucleic acid (RNA), 595—596
Robotic micromanipulation systems, 392—393
Rolling circle amplification (RCA), 600
Rotate & react SlipChip (RnR-SlipChip), 301—303
Roundworm (*Caenorhabditis elegans*), 392
  microfluidic device for automated, high-speed microinjection of, 397—401

S
Salmonella enterica, 301—303
Sample preparation modules (SPMs), 533—535
Sanger sequencing, 518—519
Scaffold architecture on cell migration, 421—423
Scaffold colonization, 415—417, 421—423
Scanning electron microscope (SEM), 663—664
Screen printing, 558
Screen-printed electrodes (SPEs), 300
Sedimentation FFF (SdFFF), 340
Sedimentation potential, 131
Seeding methodologies, 416—417
Selective laser sintering (SLS), 660
Selective laser-induced etching process (SLE process), 16
Self-assembled monolayers (SAMs), 103—104
Sequential operation droplet array (SODA), 277—280
SERS biotags (SBTs), 307—308
Short synthetic oligonucleotides, 275
Short tandem repeat (STR analysis), 513, 531
Signal transduction, 268
Silanization, 29, 82—85, 93—95
Silica (SiO_2), 17—18
Silicon, 17—21
  applications and future trends, 20—21
  bulk micromachining, 18—20
  elastomer, 228—229
  fabrication, 18
  MN arrays, 227—228
  PSAs, 45—46
  silicon-based devices, 232—234
  silicone laser-engineered MN array molds, 229
  surface micromachining, 20
Siloxane elastomers, 21—24
  applications and future trends, 24
  fabrication of microfluidic devices using PDMS, 21—23
  interconnection and bonding, 23—24
  PDMS, 21
Simian virus 40 (SV40), 270—271
Simultaneous islet perifusion and fluorescence imaging, 641—642, 647—650
  cell culture media, 641
  device preconditioning, 647—648
  equipment and experimental setup, 642
  equipment and materials, 641—642
  reagents, 641
Single cell
  analysis, 268—270, 391—392
  culture platform, 458
  encapsulation, 182—183
  genome sequencing, 521
  immobilization, 393
    glass microfluidic device for rapid, 393—396
  microsurgery, 391—392
  transcriptome analysis with microfluidic PCR, 106—107
Single nucleotide polymorphisms (SNPs), 598—600
Single stem cell analysis, 458—461
  cell cycle analysis, 459
  cell cycle analysis of single stem cells with microfluidics, 460f
  gene expression profiling, 459—461
  high-throughput analysis of single HSC proliferation in microfluidic, 459f
  single-cell culture platform, 458
  single-cell gene expression analysis, 461f

Index   697

Single stranded deoxyribonucleic acid (ssDNA), 596–597
Single-phase microfluidics, 168–171
  disadvantages of, 169
  general advantages of, 169
Size-based chromatography method, 309–310
Skin trauma, 225–226
Small organisms, 392
"Smeared-out" approach, 353
Smoluchowski slip velocity, 132
Smooth muscle cell function, shear stress impacts on, 423–424
Soaking of paper with hydrophobic chemical, 555–558
  flexographic printing, 556–557
  inkjet etching, 555–556
  screen printing, 558
  wax dipping, 558, 559f
  wax printing, 557
Soda lime glass, 17
Sodium dodecyl sulfate polyacrylamide gel electrophoresis (SDS-PAGE), 594
Sodium hydroxide (NaOH), 19
Soft lithography, 5, 336
Sol–gel translation, 398–399
Solid microneedle arrays, 232–234
Solid MN arrays, 230–232
Solvent free method, 266
Solvent molding techniques, 33–34
Sorting, 173–174
Spatially distinct biochemical profile exposure, 451
Spatially distributed gradient generation, 451
Specific membrane capacitance (Cspec), 461–463
Specific membrane conductance (Gspec), 461–463
Spinal cord injury (SCI), 438–439
Split and recombination (SAR), 667
Splitting, 172
Stainless steel, 228
Standing surface acoustic waves (SSAWs), 360
Staphylococcal Enterotoxin B (SEB), 88
Staphylococcus aureus, 501
Stem cells, 179–180, 414–415, 437–439, 631–632
  biochemical regulation, 450–453

adhesive ligands (extracellular matrix) regulation, 451–453
microfluidics-based biochemical regulation, 452f
spatially distinct biochemical profile exposure, 451
spatially distributed gradient generation, 451
biophysical regulation, 455–458
  control of biophysical factors at microscale, 456f
  controlling environmental mechanical influence, 456–457
  controlling external shear stress, 457–458
  microfluidics-based single stem cell analysis, 457f
cell–cell interaction, 453–455
  controlling cell shape, 455
  microfluidics-based cell–cell interaction study, 454f
  paracrine and autocrine signaling control, 453–455
culture and analysis, 439
current status of stem cells, 437–439
derivation and differentiation of human stem cells, 438f
emerging technologies for cell research, 439–440
microdevices for label-free and noninvasive monitoring of stem cell differentiation, 461–467, 464f
  DEP-well system used to measure cellular dielectric properties, 465f
  dielectric characterization of complete mononuclear and polymorphonuclear blood-cell subpopulations, 465f
  microfluidic impedance cytometry, 466f
microfluidics stem cell separation technology, 467–475
  DEP-based microfluidics cell sorter, 470f
  label-free approach, 474–475
  layout of microfluidic based cell sorting system, 469f
  marker-dependent approach, 471–474
  microfluidic cell sorting devices based on marker-dependent or label-free approaches, 468f

Stem cells (*Continued*)
  microfluidic device for separation of AFMSCs utilising louver-array structures, 471f
  microfluidics devices for stem cell isolation/separation, 472t–473t
  micromagnetic separators for stem cell sorting, 470f
  miniaturised devices for cell culture, 440–447
    biochemical regulation, 446–447
    biophysical regulation, 444–445
    cell surface marker targeting cell sorter, 443f
    cell–cell interaction, 446
    dielectrophoresis (DEP) based cell sorter, 443f
    emerging microfluidic platforms for advancing cell analysis, 441f
    fluorescence-activated sorting, 442f
    microfluidics concentration gradient generators, 441f
    microfluidics-based polymerase chain reaction, 442f
    microfluidics-based stem cell culture platform, 450–458
  single stem cell analysis, 458–461
    cell cycle analysis, 459
    cell cycle analysis of single stem cells with microfluidics, 460f
    gene expression profiling, 459–461
    high-throughput analysis of single HSC proliferation in microfluidic, 459f
    single-cell culture platform, 458
    single-cell gene expression analysis, 461f
  technologies used, 440–450
    emerging microfluidics technologies, 449–450
    miniaturised conventional technologies for cell analysis, 447–448
Stereolithography, 4, 659–660, 662
Steric FFF mode, 340
Stratum corneum (SC), 225
Streaming potential, 131
Streptavidin, 97
SU-8, 226–227
  negative master fabrication, 643–645
Substrate, 421–423
Subtractive manufacturing process, 4

Surface acoustic waves (SAW), 143–144, 147–152, 357
  fluid actuation and manipulation, 148–152
  particle manipulation, 148
Surface assembled monolayer (SAM), 571–572
Surface chemistry, 108
Surface chemistry, 393–394
Surface coatings for microfluidic biomedical devices
  adsorption strategies, 96–102
  covalent immobilization strategies, 81–92
  examples of applications, 104–108
    immunosensor to detect pathogenic bacteria, 107–108
    lab-on-a-chip drug analysis of blood serum, 104–106
    single cell transcriptome analysis with microfluidic PCR, 106–107
  other strategies utilizing surface treatments, 102–104
Surface machining, 226–227
Surface micromachining, 20
Surface modification techniques, 1–2
Surface property of 3D-printed microfluidic devices, 664–666
Surface receptors, 331
Surface roughness of glass, 17
Surface wetting conditions, 168
Surface-enhanced Raman spectroscopy (SERS), 290
Surfactants, 101–102, 167
Suspended cell injection, 393
Swift analysisis, 79
Synthetic polymers, 234–235

T
"Taylor dispersion", 166
TCA cycle. *See* Tricarboxylic acid cycle (TCA cycle)
3, 3′, 5, 5′-Tetramethylbenzidine, 498
Therapeutic patient monitoring, 239–240
Thermomechanical method, 29
Thermoplastic devices, 86–90
  cyclic olefin polymers and copolymers, 88–90
  PMMA, 86–88

Thermoplastic polymers, 34–41
  COC/COP, 39–41
  PMMA, 35–37
  polycarbonate, 37–39
Thermosetting polymers, 4, 24–34
  parylene, 27–31
  polyurethane, 33–34
Thread, 43–45
  applications, 45
  patterning, 44
Three dimension (3D)
  3D μ-electrotransfection system for 3D cell culture and cellular engineering, 674–677
  3D-printed coaxial flow device, 650–651
  3D-printing enabled microassembling of 3D μ-electrotransfection system, 672
  cell culture, 285
  dynamic microenvironment, 439
  microenvironment, 413
  printing, 659–660
    direct 3D printing of microfluidic devices and applications, 663–671
    future trends, 677
    materials and methods, 671–672
    of molds for fabricating PDMS microfluidic devices and applications, 671–677
    technologies, 660f
Three-degree-of-freedom micromanipulator (3-DOF micromanipulator), 400–401
Tissue development, 421–423
Tissue engineering, 179–180, 413
Tissue scaffolds, microfluidic devices for
  microfluidic device platforms, 419–427
    microdevices for microcirculatory networks creation, 425–427
    optimization of microenvironments for cell/stem cell expansion and differentiation, 420–421
    studying cell mechanics and impacts of shear stress, 423–424
    studying effects of substrate and ligand type, pore geometry, and scaffold architecture, 421–423
  technical challenges for successful tissue engineering, 414–419
    clinically relevant cell numbers, 414–415
    effective cell seeding and scaffold colonization, 415–417
    vascularization, 417–419
Titanium, 228
Transdermal delivery market, 247
Transdifferentiation, 415
Transfer adhesives, 46
Traveling wave DEP (twDEP), 353
Treponema pallidum (TP), 603–606
Tricarboxylic acid cycle (TCA cycle), 618–619
Triggered system, 226
  NIR-triggered device, 234–235
  thermal-triggered microfluidic drug delivery, 240
Triphasic PMMA-based BLMs, 266
Turtle (cell-surface protein), 401–403
Two-dimensional adhesion cultures (2D adhesion cultures), 439
Type I diabetes mellitus (T1DM), 617–618
Tyrosine kinase, 268

U

U. S. Food and Drug Administration (FDA), 620
Ultrasonic standing waves technology (USW technology), 357
Ultrasound-induced bubble oscillation, 146
Ultraviolet (UV), 5, 81–82
  exposure, 102–103
  light, 659–660
  UV/ozone exposure, 102–103
Undoped silicate glass (USG), 23–24
Unique molecular identifier (UMI), 525
United States Food and Drug Administration (USFDA), 234–235, 263

V

Vaccines, 237
  microneedle-mediated vaccine delivery, 237–238
Vacuum-based confinements, 393–394
Valproic acid (VPA), 502
Vascular endothelial growth factor (VEGF), 416–417
Vascularization, 416–419

Vibrio parahaemolyticus, 301–303
Vibriofluvialis, 301–303
Viral detection
  examples of applications, 603–608
  future trends, 609–610
  microfluidic devices, 588–603
  microfluidic flow cytometry, 600–603
  microfluidic nucleic acid detection, 595–600
Viral infection, 593–594
Voltage-dependent calcium channels (VDCCs), 618–619
Volumetric flow rate, 335

W
Wafer bonding, 16–17
Water-assisted femtosecond laser drilling (WAFLD), 16
Water-in-oil-in-water emulsion (W/O/W emulsion), 275
Wax
  dipping, 558, 559f
  printing, 557
West Nile Virus (WNV), 571–572
Wet chemical etching process, 9–13
Whatman filters, 552–553
Whole genome amplification (WGA), 521
World-to-chip interface, 517
Worm immobilization method, 398–399
Worm-based drug testing, 398
Wound healing assay, 422

X
Xurography, 46
Xurography-based microfabrication, 2, 7–8

Y
Young–Laplace equation, 666–667

Z
Zebrafish (*Danio rerio*), 392
Zeta potential, 131
Zinc, 628
Zygote, 396
    immobilization process, 395

Printed in the United States
by Baker & Taylor Publisher Services